CLINICAL LEARNING GUIDES

CASE-BASED ANESTHESIA

CLINICAL LEARNING GUIDES
CASE-BASED ANESTHESIA

GEORGE SHORTEN

Professor of Anaesthesia and Intensive Care Medicine
Department of Anaesthesia
University College of Cork
Consultant Anaesthetist
Department of Anaesthesia
Cork University Hospital
Cork, Ireland

STEPHEN F. DIERDORF, MD

Professor and Vice Chairman
Department of Anesthesia
Indiana University School of Medicine
Indianapolis, Indiana

GABRIELLA IOHOM, MD, PhD

Consultant Anaesthetist/Senior Lecturer
Cork University Hospital
University College Cork
Cork, Ireland

CHRISTOPHER J. O'CONNOR, MD

Professor of Anesthesiology
Rush University Medical Center
Chicago, Illinois

CHARLES W. HOGUE, JR., MD

Associate Professor
Department of Anesthesiology and Critical Care Medicine
The Johns Hopkins Medical Institutions and The Johns Hopkins Hospital
Baltimore, Maryland

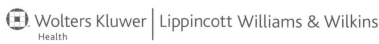

Wolters Kluwer | Lippincott Williams & Wilkins
Health

Philadelphia · Baltimore · New York · London
Buenos Aires · Hong Kong · Sydney · Tokyo

Acquisitions Editor: Frances DeStefano
Product Manager: Nicole Dernoski
Marketing Manager: Angela Panetta
Production Editor: Julie Montalbano
Design Coordinator: Terry Mallon
Compositor: Maryland Composition/ASI

Copyright © 2009 Lippincott Williams & Wilkins, a Wolters Kluwer business.

351 West Camden Street
Baltimore, MD 21201

530 Walnut Street
Philadelphia, PA 19106

Printed in China.

9 8 7 6 5 4 3 2 1

Library of Congress Cataloging-in-Publication Data

Case-based anesthesia : clinical learning guides / [edited by] George Shorten.
    p. ; cm.
  Includes bibliographical references and index.
  ISBN 978-0-7817-8955-4
 1. Anesthesia—Case studies. I. Shorten, George.
  [DNLM: 1. Anesthesia—Case Reports. 2. Anesthesia—Problems and Exercises. 3. Anesthesiology—methods—Case Reports. 4. Anesthesiology—methods—Problems and Exercises. 5. Anesthetics—Case Reports. 6. Anesthetics—Problems and Exercises. 7. Perioperative Care—methods—Case Reports. 8. Perioperative Care—methods—Problems and Exercises.
  WO 218.2 C337 2009]
  RD82.45.C37 2009
  617.9'6—dc22
                      2008052575

DISCLAIMER

Care has been taken to confirm the accuracy of the information present and to describe generally accepted practices. However, the authors, editors, and publisher are not responsible for errors or omissions or for any consequences from application of the information in this book and make no warranty, expressed or implied, with respect to the currency, completeness, or accuracy of the contents of the publication. Application of this information in a particular situation remains the professional responsibility of the practitioner; the clinical treatments described and recommended may not be considered absolute and universal recommendations.

The authors, editors, and publisher have exerted every effort to ensure that drug selection and dosage set forth in this text are in accordance with the current recommendations and practice at the time of publication. However, in view of ongoing research, changes in government regulations, and the constant flow of information relating to drug therapy and drug reactions, the reader is urged to check the package insert for each drug for any change in indications and dosage and for added warnings and precautions. This is particularly important when the recommended agent is a new or infrequently employed drug.

Some drugs and medical devices presented in this publication have Food and Drug Administration (FDA) clearance for limited use in restricted research settings. It is the responsibility of the health care provider to ascertain the FDA status of each drug or device planned for use in their clinical practice.

To purchase additional copies of this book, call our customer service department at **(800) 638-3030** or fax orders to **(301) 223-2320**. International customers should call **(301) 223-2300**.

Visit Lippincott Williams & Wilkins on the Internet: http://www.lww.com. Lippincott Williams & Wilkins customer service representatives are available from 8:30 am to 6:00 pm, EST.

Dedicated to the memory of Gerard McDonnell.

Dr. Shorten wishes to thank Ms. Renee Mooney for her incomparable efficiency and hard work.

FOREWORD

The discovery and application of anesthesia is the most important contribution of American medicine to mankind. Its impact exceeds even the elucidation of the human genome. Without visionary discoveries by pioneers in anesthesiology, the explosive growth in type, complexity, and safety of surgical procedures would not have occurred. More importantly, anesthesiology is considered to be the lead specialty in patient safety.

The core principle that drives these advances is training and continuing education. It is interesting to note that, in the 19th century, anesthesiology was considered a "technique" with little scientific merit. It was not until 100 years later that the specialty developed a rigorous scientific foundation with postgraduate training programs. Even more astounding is the fact that, into the late 20th century, there was a paucity of books authored by North Americans. Textbooks supporting resident education, preparation for board examinations, and reference for clinical care were predominantly British in origin.

In the 1980s the educational scene changed dramatically. Residents and fellows were recruited from the upper tier of medical school graduates. In addition to publication of core and specialty textbooks and journals, application of electronic media, such as the Internet, has revolutionized the specialty of anesthesiology. The American Board of Anesthesiology has stated, "The ability to independently acquire and process information in a timely manner is central to assure individual responsibility for all aspects of patient care." Although use of the Internet and other electronic media assist in rapidly answering questions related to patient care, most residents, fellows, and experienced clinicians still use the printed word to comprehensively learn about a new topic, prepare for board examination and recertification, and even organize a clinical management plan for the patient with a complex array of coexisting diseases.

So in this setting, where does *Case-Based Anesthesia: Clinical Learning Guides* edited by Drs. Shorten, Dierdorf, O'Connor, Iohom, and Hogue fit in? In other words, do we need yet another anesthesiology text? The answer, in this case, is a resounding yes! Why? First starting with the title, *Clinical Learning Guides*, the editors have chosen to emphasize learning in the broader sense, not just Board exam preparation and re-certification, but acquisition of knowledge as part of the process of responsibility and accountability for one's education and lifelong learning. By viewing education through this lens, the practitioner can apply information gained from this text into a variety of clinical and examination settings. The Editors accomplish their goal through the innovative approach of using two formats for case-based learning: "Step-by Step" or "Reflection." This is a unique approach for a textbook. Importantly, it recognizes different learning styles to help reinforce important clinical concepts. This is the first time such diverse information has been organized on these educationally sound principles in a clinical textbook. The editors have coupled this with the use of "hot topics" where new evidence can be applied to clinical conundrums as well as to responses to examination questions. This is accomplished by a list of all-star contributors, each an authority in his/her own area of expertise. It is as if the reader is being taken through a clinically challenge case with an expert at their side.

As Thomas L. Friedman implies in his best-selling book *The World is Flat* (Picador 2007), anesthesiologists worldwide are truly interconnected, as globalization brings us into wide-reaching contact with our peers and new opportunities arise. Thus, *Case-Based Anesthesia: Clinical Learning Guides* is targeted at an international array of inquisitive trainees and clinicians whose basic goal is safe and unsurpassed clinical care of our patients.

Paul G. Barash, MD
Professor, Department of Anesthesiology
Yale University School of Medicine
Attending Anesthesiologist
Yale-New Haven Hospital
New Haven, Connecticut

CONTRIBUTORS

Hassan M. Ahmad, MD
The Johns Hopkins School of Medicine
The Johns Hopkins Hospital
Baltimore, Maryland

Ioanna Apostolidou, MD
Associate Professor of Anesthesiology
School of Medicine
University of Minnesota
Minneapolis, Minnesota

Ashit Bardhan, MBBS, FCARCSI
Specialist Registrar
Cork University Hospital
Cork, Ireland

Dorothy Breen, FCARCSI, FJFICM
Specialist Registrar in Anaesthesia
Cork University Hospital
Cork, Ireland

Siun Burke, FCARCSI
Research Fellow
Cork University Hospital
Cork, Ireland

Asokumar Buvanendran, MD
Associate Professor of Anesthesiology
Rush University Medical Center
Chicago, Illinois

Charles D. Collard
Professor and Vice-Chairman
Department of Anesthesiology
Baylor College of Medicine
Houston, Texas

W. Christopher Croley, MD, FCCP
Assistant Professor of Anesthesiology and Critical Care Medicine
Rush University Medical Center
Chicago, Illinois

Stephen F. Dierdorf, MD
Professor and Vice Chairman
Department of Anesthesia
Indiana University School of Medicine
Indianapolis, Indiana

John Dowling, BDS, MB, BCh, BAO(Hons), BMedSc(NUI)
Specialist Registrar in Anaesthesia
Cork University Hospital
Cork, Ireland

Craig Dunlop, MBBS, FCARCSI
Specialist Registrar in Anaesthesia
Cork University Hospital
Cork, Ireland

Amanda A. Fox
Staff Anesthesiologist
Brigham & Women's Hospital
Harvard Medical School
Boston, Massachusetts

Kelly Grogan, MD
Assistant Professor of Anesthesiology and Critical Care Medicine
The Johns Hopkins School of Medicine
The Johns Hopkins Hospital
Baltimore, Maryland

Anthony Hennessy, FCARCSI
Specialist Registrar in Anaesthesia
Cork University Hospital
Cork, Ireland

Charles W. Hogue, Jr., MD
Associate Professor
Department of Anesthesiology and Critical Care Medicine
The Johns Hopkins Medical Institutions and The Johns Hopkins Hospital
Baltimore, Maryland

Michelle Isac, MD
Assistant Clinical Professor of Anesthesia
McMaster University
Hamilton, Ontario, Canada

Jason S. Johnson, MD
Associate Professor of Anesthesiology
School of Medicine
University of Minnesota
Minneapolis, Minnesota

Roy Kan, MBBS(Singapore), MMed (Anesth)
Department of Anesthesiology and Critical Care Medicine
The Johns Hopkins School of Medicine
The Johns Hopkins Hospital
Baltimore, Maryland

Justin Lane, FCARCSI
Specialist Registrar in Anaesthesia
Cork University Hospital
Cork, Ireland

Peter John Lee, MB, BCh, BAO, FCARCSI
Specialist Registrar in Anaesthesia
Cork University Hospital
Cork, Ireland

Audrey R. Leverich, MD
Fellow in Cardiothoracic Anesthesiology
Department of Anesthesiology
Weill Cornell Medical College
New York-Presbyterian Hospital
New York, New York

Jay K. Levin, MD
Department of Anesthesiology and Critical Care Medicine
The Johns Hopkins School of Medicine
The Johns Hopkins Hospital
Baltimore, Maryland

Bryan V. May, MD
Southeast Anesthesiology Consultants
Charlotte, North Carolina

Nanhi Mitter, MD
Assistant Professor
Department of Anesthesiology
Rush University Medical Center
Chicago, Illinois

Laurel E. Moore, M.D.
Department of Anesthesiology
The University of Michigan
Ann Arbor, Michigan

Mohan Mugawar, FCARCSI
Specialist Registrar in Anaesthesia
Department of Anaesthesia
Cork University Hospital
Cork, Ireland

Christopher J. O'Connor, MD
Professor of Anesthesiology
Rush University Medical Center
Chicago, Illinois

Brian D. O'Donnell, MB, FCARCSI, MSc
Clinical Lecturer in Anaesthesia
Cork University Hospital
Cork, Ireland

James O'Driscoll, FCARCSI
Specialist Registrar in Anaesthesia
Cork University Hospital
Cork, Ireland

Owen O'Sullivan, MB, BCh, BAO
Specialist Registrar in Anaesthesia
Cork University Hospital
Cork, Ireland

Richard J. Pollard, MD
Southeast Anesthesia Consultants
Charlotte, North Carolina

David M. Rothenberg, MD, FCCM
The Max S. Sadove, MD Professor of Anesthesiology
Associate Dean, Academic Affiliations
Rush University Medical Center
Chicago, Illinois

Leon Serfontein, MBChB, FANZCA
Consultant Anaesthetist
Cork University Hospital
Cork, Ireland

Mansoor A. Siddiqui, MBBS, FCPS, FCARCSI
Specialist Registrar in Anaesthesia
Cork University Hospital
Cork, Ireland

Nikolaos J. Skubas, MD
Associate Professor of Anesthesiology
Weill Cornell Medical College
Department of Anesthesiology
New York, New York

Joshua D. Stearns, MD
Assistant Professor of Anesthesiology and Critical Care Medicine
The Johns Hopkins School of Medicine
The Johns Hopkins Hospital
Baltimore, Maryland

Jason Van der Velde, BAA, MBChB, EMDM-A
Trauma Research Registrar
Cork University Hospital
Cork, Ireland

John Vullo, MD
Southeast Anesthesiology Consultants
Charlotte, North Carolina

Adrienne Wells, MD
Assistant Professor of Anesthesiology
Rush University Medical Center
Chicago, Illinois

CONTENTS

CHAPTER 1

Statins and Perioperative Risk

Amanda A. Fox and Charles D. Collard

CASE FORMAT: REFLECTION

A 75-year-old, 50-kg, Caucasian female presented for left heart cardiac catheterization after having a positive finding on a dobutamine stress echocardiogram. She had a history of exertional chest pain, hypertension, dyslipidemia, and a 45 pack-year history of cigarette smoking. The patient's history was also significant for peripheral vascular disease, with bilateral lower extremity claudication. A right carotid endarterectomy (CEA) was performed in 2002. The patient's serum creatinine level was 1.3 mg/dL, with an estimated creatinine clearance of 30 mL/min. She was receiving the following medications: intravenous nitroglycerin and heparin infusions, atenolol 25 mg orally once per day, and aspirin 81 mg orally once per day.

Cardiac catheterization revealed significant three-vessel coronary artery disease (90% proximal left main coronary artery, 90% proximal right coronary artery, 60% first obtuse marginal) and a left ventricular ejection fraction of 60%. Carotid ultrasound showed no significant stenosis of the right carotid artery, but there was 85% to 90% stenosis of the left proximal internal carotid artery. Thus, the patient was scheduled for combined left CEA and coronary artery bypass graft (CABG) surgery.

On the day of surgery, a right radial arterial line was placed preinduction with midazolam sedation and local anesthesia. The patient then underwent intravenous induction of anesthesia with 8 mg of midazolam, 100 mg of thiopental, 200 μg of fentanyl, and 10 mg of pancuronium. Anesthesia was maintained with 0.6% to 0.8% end-tidal isoflurane. A right internal jugular central line was placed. Electroencephalogram monitoring was conducted throughout the CEA without evidence of complications. Three-vessel CABG surgery was performed (left internal mammary arterial conduit to the left main artery and saphenous vein grafts to the right coronary artery and first obtuse marginal artery), and the patient was separated uneventfully from cardiopulmonary bypass. After heparin reversal with protamine and chest closure, the surgeons closed the left CEA neck incision. The patient was extubated 3 hours after surgery and had an uneventful postoperative course. She was monitored for 24 hours in the intensive care unit and was then transferred to the hospital ward. The patient's postoperative serum creatinine peaked at 1.6 mg/dL and returned to her preoperative value of 1.3 mg/dL before discharge. The patient was discharged to home on postoperative day 7, at which time in addition to her previous preoperative medications, she was started on rosuvastatin 5 mg orally per day.

CASE DISCUSSION

Pharmacologic Mechanisms of Statins

3-hydroxy-3-methylglutaryl coenzyme A reductase inhibitors, commonly known as *statins*, are frequently prescribed cholesterol-lowering medications that decrease circulating plasma low-density lipoprotein (LDL) cholesterol. Statins are not only associated with reduced atherosclerotic plaque formation, but there is mounting evidence that statins may help prevent atherosclerotic plaque rupture.[1] Atherosclerotic plaques that are vulnerable to rupture have a prothrombotic, lipid-rich core that is infiltrated with active macrophages and is covered by a thin fibrous cap. Surgical insults such as trauma to tissues, vascular cross clamping, extracorporeal circulation, or blood transfusion can trigger profound systemic proinflammatory responses that may prompt vulnerable plaque rupture resulting in arterial occlusion and end-organ ischemia (e.g., myocardial infarction [MI], stroke, renal and gastrointestinal infarction). Potential mechanisms by which statins may stabilize vulnerable plaques, as well as reduce the impact of plaque rupture include:

1. Increasing the collagen content of the lipid-rich plaque core.[2]
2. Decreasing plaque macrophage content[2] and T-cell activity.[2,3]
3. Inhibition of cellular matrix metalloproteinases involved with erosion of the fibrous plaque cap.[2,4]
4. Inhibition of cellular transcription factors that modify G proteins involved in regulating endothelial, leukocyte, and platelet function.[4]
5. Decreasing inflammatory mediators such as interleukin-6, C-reactive protein, tumor necrosis factor-α, and serum amyloid A.[3,5]

Thus, the benefits of statin therapy are not limited to cholesterol alone, and statin therapy in the perioperative setting may be particularly beneficial because of antiatherosclerotic, anti-inflammatory, and antithrombotic properties. However, the precise underlying mechanisms by which statins prevent or reduce adverse postoperative outcomes, such as mortality or postoperative atrial fibrillation, are not yet clearly defined.[6]

Perioperative Statins: The Evidence in Cardiac and Vascular Surgery

A recent meta-analysis of 223,010 patients undergoing cardiovascular surgery found that preoperative statin therapy was associated with 38% and 59% reductions in the risk of 30-day

1

mortality after cardiac (1.9% vs. 3.1%; $p = 0.0001$) and vascular (1.7% vs. 6.1%; $p = 0.0001$) surgery, respectively.[7] Additionally, a retrospective, case-control study of more than 2600 primary, elective CABG surgery patients found that preoperative statin therapy was independently associated with a reduced risk of in-hospital cardiovascular death (adjusted odds ratio [OR], 0.25; 95% confidence interval [CI], 0.07–0.87) but not nonfatal postoperative MI.[8] Thus, perioperative statin therapy has been shown to be associated with a reduced incidence of acute, in-hospital adverse outcomes.

However, the benefits of perioperative statin therapy extend beyond the acute perioperative period. For example, a study of post-CABG surgery patients with moderately elevated LDL cholesterol levels who were placed on aggressive, long-term lovastatin therapy (goal LDL concentration <100 mg/dL) showed that during the 4-year follow-up period after starting statin therapy, patients on aggressive therapy experienced significantly reduced saphenous vein graft occlusion and need for revascularization as compared with patients on lower-dose statin therapy.[9] This clinical observation is also supported by in vitro evidence that statins prolong arterial bypass graft patency.[10] Finally, at least one retrospective study suggests that statin therapy may slow the progression of bioprosthetic aortic valve degeneration after surgical implantation.[11]

Cardiovascular morbidity and mortality after vascular surgery is also relatively frequent, with mortality and nonfatal MI occurring in up to 5% to 6% and 30% of patients, respectively.[1] Retrospective studies of preoperative statin therapy in patients undergoing major vascular surgery have shown that statins are associated with a reduced risk in both in-hospital and long-term, all-cause cardiovascular mortality.[12,13] Additionally, a recent prospective randomized study of vascular surgery patients found that preoperative atorvastatin therapy significantly reduced adverse cardiovascular events up to 6 months after surgery.[14] Based on these data, it seems reasonable that the patient who underwent combined major cardiac and vascular surgery in the case presentation might have benefited from statin therapy initiated preoperatively.

Perioperative Statins: The Evidence in Noncardiovascular Surgery

Although the present case involves both major cardiac and vascular surgery, cardiovascular complications after noncardiac surgery are also an important cause of morbidity and mortality. A recent retrospective cohort study investigated the association between perioperative statin therapy and in-hospital postoperative mortality in 780,591 patients undergoing major noncardiac surgery at 329 hospitals in the United States. Moreover, this study only assessed patients whose preoperative statin therapy was reinitiated within 2 days after surgery, and it found that perioperative statin therapy was associated with a significant reduction in all-cause mortality (adjusted OR, 0.62; 95% CI, 0.58–0.67).[15] Not only do these data further suggest the usefulness of preoperative statin therapy, but they also suggest the importance of continuing statins throughout the postoperative period.

Effect of Statin Withdrawal

In a study of ambulatory patients, statin therapy initiated before the occurrence of acute MI was associated with a signifi-

cantly decreased incidence of adverse cardiovascular events.[16] If statin therapy was discontinued after the MI occurred, however, the incidence of 30-day death and nonfatal MI was significantly increased compared with patients receiving continuous statin therapy (OR, 2.93; 95% CI, 1.64–6.27).[16] This finding may explain in part why studies of the benefits of preoperative statin therapy have reported mixed results regarding postoperative nonfatal MI outcomes, as many of these surgical studies did not assess whether statins were continued in the postoperative period. Supporting this hypothesis is a recent multicenter study of 2666 CABG surgical patients in which preoperative statin therapy was independently associated with a significant reduction (adjusted OR, 0.25; 95% CI, 0.07–0.87) in the risk of cardiac death within the first 3 days following primary, elective CABG surgery (0.3 vs. 1.4%; p <0.03) but was not associated with a reduced risk of postoperative nonfatal, in-hospital MI (7.9% vs. 6.2%; p = NS). In this same study, however, discontinuation of statin therapy after surgery was independently associated with a significant increase in late (postoperative day 4 though hospital discharge) all-cause mortality (adjusted OR, 2.64; 95% CI, 1.32–5.26) as compared with patients in whom statin therapy was continued (2.64 vs. 0.60%; p <0.01). This was true even after controlling for the postoperative discontinuation of aspirin, β-blockers, or angiotensin-converting enzyme inhibitor therapy. Discontinuation of statin therapy after surgery was also independently associated with a significant increase in late, in-hospital cardiac mortality (adjusted OR, 2.95; 95% CI, 1.31–6.66) compared with patients in whom statin therapy was continued (1.91% vs. 0.45%; p <0.01).[8]

Despite guidelines by the American College of Cardiology and American Heart Association recommending statin therapy for CABG patients with LDL concentrations >100 mg/dL,[17] two thirds of such patients may not be receiving statin therapy when discharged from the hospital after their CABG surgeries.[18] Reasons for not initiating or reinitiating statin therapy after CABG surgery may include patients' decreased tolerance of oral medications secondary to postoperative nausea and vomiting, transient renal dysfunction, concerns pertaining to hepatic toxicity or myositis, or failure of the responsible physician to reimplement preoperative medications. Thus, it may be warranted to educate physicians about the potential benefits of perioperative statin therapy that continue in the postoperative period. In the present case, although the patient was discharged on rosuvastatin, not only was she not receiving preoperative statin therapy, but there was also failure to initiate a statin in the immediate preoperative period. Both are measures that might have decreased her risk for both in-hospital and long-term adverse cardiovascular outcomes.

2007 American College of Cardiology and American Heart Association Guidelines on Perioperative Cardiovascular Evaluation and Care for Noncardiac Surgery

In light of the previously mentioned evidence, the American College of Cardiology and the American Heart Association recently published perioperative guidelines that for the first time specifically address the role of perioperative statin therapy.[19] Specifically, these new guidelines state that:

1. For patients currently taking statins and scheduled for noncardiac surgery, statins should be continued.[19]
2. For patients undergoing vascular surgery with or without clinical risk factors, statin use is reasonable.[19]
3. For patients with at least one clinical risk factor who are undergoing intermediate-risk procedures, statins may be considered.[19]

Thus, based on these guidelines, it would have been reasonable to initiate and maintain statin therapy throughout the perioperative period for the patient in the case presentation.

Safety of Statin Therapy

Severe hepatotoxicity or myopathy associated with statin use has been reported but is rare.[20] This is true for all available statins, although the risk profile for atorvastatin might be the most favorable.[20] Although mild, dose-related elevations in serum aspartate aminotransferase and alanine aminotransferase occur in about 1% of patients on statins, and acute liver injury has been isolated to a few cases.[21] Although statins are considered contraindicated in patients with chronic liver disease, a recent multicenter, randomized, double-blind, placebo-controlled trial of pravastatin therapy in hyperlipidemic patients with chronic, compensated liver disease showed no increase in statin-associated hepatotoxicity in these patients.[21] Caution should be exercised in initiating statin therapy in patients with chronic liver disease, however, and should probably only be done in conference with such patients' gastroenterologists.

The most serious potential statin side effect is rhabdomyolysis. Across a spectrum of ambulatory trials, rhabdomyolysis was reported to occur in $\leq 0.7\%$ of patients receiving a broad range of statins and doses.[22] Cerivastatin, which is no longer on the market, is known to have the greatest associated rhabdomyolysis risk (3.16 per million prescriptions).[20] In contrast, the risk of statin-related rhabdomyolysis is only in the range of 0 to 0.19 per million prescriptions for other commonly used statins.[20] The risk for rhabdomyolysis is associated with factors that increase serum statin concentrations, such as small body size, advanced age, renal or hepatic dysfunction, diabetes, hypothyroidism, and drugs that interfere with statin metabolism, such as cyclosporin, antifungal agents, calcium-channel blockers, and amiodarone.[20] Because these characteristics are prevalent in surgical populations, it is advisable to monitor for statin side effects in patients on perioperative statin therapy, particularly in those with muscle disease, or hepatic or renal dysfunction. The present case involving a small, elderly patient with renal insufficiency should have been closely monitored in the acute perioperative period for evidence of acidosis, muscle pain or weakness, or a rise in creatinine kinase level.

Although statin-related rhabdomyolysis is extremely rare, early recognition and treatment are important to avoid serious morbidity. In a recent study by Schouten et al., perioperative statin use was not associated with an increased risk of perioperative myopathy or increased postoperative creatine phosphokinase concentrations in a large group of major vascular surgical patients.[23] After correcting for cardiac risk factors and clinical risk factors for myopathy, length of surgery remained the only independent predictor for myopathy.[23] No case of rhabdomyolysis was observed, and there was no difference in creatine phosphokinase levels between patients on long-term preoperative statin therapy and patients who started statin therapy shortly before surgery.[23]

Need for Future Studies

Presently available data and guidelines suggest that perioperative statin therapy is both appropriate and beneficial, but further studies are needed to determine optimal statin duration and dosage. For example, although a recent meta-analysis of more than 300,000 patients with an acute MI suggests that initiating statin therapy within 24 hours of MI onset reduces mortality, it is not clear if this holds true for cardiovascular surgical patients with acute coronary syndromes, if they require longer periods of statin administration.[24] There thus remains a need for further randomized controlled trials conducted in specific cardiac and noncardiac surgical populations to identify patients who will benefit most from perioperative statin therapy and to determine the optimal duration of perioperative statin therapy.

KEY MESSAGES

1. Statin administration is associated with decreased atherosclerotic plaque formation and may contribute to prevention of atherosclerotic plaque rupture.

2. A recent meta-analysis demonstrated that preoperative statin therapy was associated with a 38% and 59% reduction in the risk of 30-day mortality after cardiac (1.9% vs. 3.1%; $p = 0.0001$) and vascular (1.7% vs. 6.1%; $p = 0.0001$) surgery, respectively.

3. Perioperative statin therapy is associated with a reduced incidence of acute, in-hospital adverse outcomes.

4. Preoperative atorvastatin therapy significantly reduces adverse cardiovascular events up to 6 months after vascular surgery.

5. Following noncardiac surgery, perioperative statin therapy is associated with a significant reduction in all-cause mortality.

6. American College of Cardiology/American Heart Association guidelines state:

   a. For patients currently taking statins and scheduled for noncardiac surgery, statins should be continued.

   b. For patients undergoing vascular surgery with or without clinical risk factors, statin use is reasonable.

   c. For patients with at least one clinical risk factor who are undergoing intermediate-risk procedures, statins may be considered.

QUESTIONS

1. **What is the mechanism by which statins lower circulating LDL cholesterol?**

   Answer: They act as inhibitors of 3-hydroxy-3-methylglutaryl coenzyme A reductase.

2. **How do statins stabilize atheromatous plaques or limit the adverse effects of rupture?**

   Answer: Suggested mechanisms include:
   Increasing the collagen content of the lipid-rich plaque core.
   Decreasing plaque macrophage content[2] and T-cell activity.
   Inhibition of cellular matrix metalloproteinases involved with erosion of the fibrous plaque cap.
   Inhibition of cellular transcription factors that modify G proteins involved in regulating endothelial, leukocyte, and platelet function.
   Decreasing inflammatory mediators such as interleukin-6, C-reactive protein, tumor necrosis factor-α, and serum amyloid A.

3. **What adverse effects are associated with statin administration?**

   Answer: The most serious potential statin side effect is rhabdomyolysis. Mild, dose-related elevations in serum aspartate aminotransferase and alanine aminotransferase occur in about 1% of patients on statins; acute liver injury has been observed in a few cases. Severe hepatotoxicity or myopathy is rare.

References

1. Hindler K, Eltzschig HK, Fox AA, et al. Influence of statins on perioperative outcomes. J Cardiothorac Vasc Anesth 2006;20:251–258.
2. Crisby M, Nordin-Fredriksson G, Shah PK, et al. Pravastatin treatment increases collagen content and decreases lipid content, inflammation, metalloproteinases, and cell death in human carotid plaques: implications for plaque stabilization. Circulation 2001;103:926–933.
3. Crisby M. Modulation of the inflammatory process by statins. Drugs Today (Barc) 2003;39:137–143.
4. Kinlay S, Ganz P. Early statin therapy in acute coronary syndromes. Semin Vasc Med 2003;3:419–424.
5. Kinlay S, Schwartz GG, Olsson AG, et al. High-dose atorvastatin enhances the decline in inflammatory markers in patients with acute coronary syndromes in the MIRACL study. Circulation 2003;108:1560–1566.
6. Blanchard L, Collard CD. Non-antiarrhythmic agents for prevention of postoperative atrial fibrillation: role of statins. Curr Opin Anaesthesiol 2007;20:53–56.
7. Hindler K, Shaw AD, Samuels J, et al. Improved postoperative outcomes associated with preoperative statin therapy. Anesthesiology 2006;105:1260–1272.
8. Collard CD, Body SC, Shernan SK, et al. Preoperative statin therapy is associated with reduced cardiac mortality after coronary artery bypass graft surgery. J Thorac Cardiovasc Surg 2006;132:392–400.
9. The Post Coronary Artery Bypass Graft Trial Investigators. The effect of aggressive lowering of low-density lipoprotein cholesterol levels and low-dose anticoagulation on obstructive changes in saphenous-vein coronary-artery bypass grafts. N Engl J Med 1997;336:153–162.
10. Nakamura K, Al-Ruzzeh S, Chester AH, et al. Effects of cerivastatin on vascular function of human radial and left internal thoracic arteries. Ann Thorac Surg 2002;73:1860–1865; discussion 5.
11. Antonini-Canterin F, Zuppiroli A, Popescu BA, et al. Effect of statins on the progression of bioprosthetic aortic valve degeneration. Am J Cardiol 2003;92:1479–1482.
12. Poldermans D, Bax JJ, Kertai MD, et al. Statins are associated with a reduced incidence of perioperative mortality in patients undergoing major noncardiac vascular surgery. Circulation 2003;107:1848–1851.
13. Kertai MD, Boersma E, Westerhout CM, et al. Association between long-term statin use and mortality after successful abdominal aortic aneurysm surgery. Am J Med 2004;116:96–103.
14. Durazzo AE, Machado FS, Ikeoka DT, et al. Reduction in cardiovascular events after vascular surgery with atorvastatin: a randomized trial. J Vasc Surg 2004;39:967–975; discussion 75–76.
15. Lindenauer PK, Pekow P, Wang K, et al. Lipid-lowering therapy and in-hospital mortality following major noncardiac surgery. JAMA 2004;291:2092–2099.
16. Heeschen C, Hamm CW, Laufs U, et al. Withdrawal of statins increases event rates in patients with acute coronary syndromes. Circulation 2002;105:1446–1452.
17. Eagle KA, Guyton RA, Davidoff R, et al. ACC/AHA Guidelines for Coronary Artery Bypass Graft Surgery: a Report of the American College of Cardiology/American Heart Association Task Force on Practice Guidelines (Committee to Revise the 1991 Guidelines for Coronary Artery Bypass Graft Surgery). American College of Cardiology/American Heart Association. J Am Coll Cardiol 1999;34:1262–1347.
18. Khanderia U, Faulkner TV, Townsend KA, Streetman DS. Lipid-lowering therapy at hospital discharge after coronary artery bypass grafting. Am J Health Syst Pharm 2002;59:548–551.
19. Fleisher LA, Beckman JA, Brown KA, et al. ACC/AHA 2007 guidelines on perioperative cardiovascular evaluation and care for noncardiac surgery: a report of the American College of Cardiology/American Heart Association Task Force on Practice Guidelines (Writing Committee to Revise the 2002 Guidelines on Perioperative Cardiovascular Evaluation for Noncardiac Surgery) developed in collaboration with the American Society of Echocardiography, American Society of Nuclear Cardiology, Heart Rhythm Society, Society of Cardiovascular Anesthesiologists, Society for Cardiovascular Angiography and Interventions, Society for Vascular Medicine and Biology, and Society for Vascular Surgery. J Am Coll Cardiol 2007;50:e159–241.
20. Lazar HL. Should all patients receive statins before cardiac surgery: are more data necessary? J Thorac Cardiovasc Surg 2006;131:520–522.
21. Lewis JH, Mortensen ME, Zweig S, et al. Efficacy and safety of high-dose pravastatin in hypercholesterolemic patients with well-compensated chronic liver disease: results of a prospective, randomized, double-blind, placebo-controlled, multicenter trial. Hepatology 2007;46:1453–1463.
22. Davidson MH, Robinson JG. Safety of aggressive lipid management. J Am Coll Cardiol 2007;49:1753–1762.
23. Schouten O, Poldermans D, Visser L, et al. Fluvastatin and bisoprolol for the reduction of perioperative cardiac mortality and morbidity in high-risk patients undergoing non-cardiac surgery: rationale and design of the DECREASE-IV study. Am Heart J 2004;148:1047–1052.
24. Fonarow GC, Wright RS, Spencer FA, et al. Effect of statin use within the first 24 hours of admission for acute myocardial infarction on early morbidity and mortality. Am J Cardiol 2005;96:611–616.

CHAPTER 2

Perioperative β-Blockade

Stephen F. Dierdorf

CASE FORMAT: STEP BY STEP

A 67-year-old male was scheduled for an exploratory laparotomy and probable colectomy for colon cancer. The patient had first noticed blood in his stool 4 months before the scheduled surgery, but he had only sought medical attention 2 weeks prior to surgery. Colonoscopy performed at that time revealed a mass in the descending colon, and a biopsy result was positive for adenocarcinoma. He was scheduled for surgery at the first available date. The patient had a 24-year history of hypertension treated with lisinopril and a 12-year history of non–insulin-dependent diabetes treated with diet and an oral hypoglycemic agent. He denied chest pain or exertional dyspnea. The patient, a retired accountant with a sedentary lifestyle, underwent a lumbar laminectomy and spinal fusion at age 53.

The patient's vital signs were as follows: heart rate, 86 beats per minute; blood pressure, 152/95 mm Hg; and respiratory rate, 16 breaths per minute. His height was 70 inches (1.8 meters), and his weight was 225 pounds (102 kg). Laboratory studies indicated that his resting electrocardiogram reading was normal; hematocrit level, 41%; sodium, 137 mmol/L; potassium, 4.1 mmol/L; creatinine, 1.2 mg/dL; blood urea nitrogen, 13 mg/dL; and glucose, 130 mg/dL.

The patient's internist recommended perioperative metoprolol. Would this reduce the patient's perioperative risk of an adverse cardiac event?

Ischemic heart disease is the major cause of morbidity and mortality in developed countries throughout the world. Approximately 100 million adults undergo noncardiac surgery per year, and 500,000 to 1 million will suffer a perioperative cardiac complication. The efficacy of β-blockers for the treatment of ischemic heart disease is well documented, and it is only logical that β-blocker therapy should be applied to patients with coronary artery disease undergoing noncardiac surgery.

Surgery produces an increase in stress hormones and catecholamine levels and a hypercoagulable state. Effects of these increases include tachycardia, hypertension, enhanced myocardial contractility, and increased myocardial oxygen demand. In susceptible patients, adverse cardiac events such as myocardial ischemia and dysrhythmias can occur. β-Adrenergic blockers reduce myocardial oxygen demand by reducing heart rate, cardiac contractility, and blood pressure. Slowing of the heart rate increases diastole

and allows more time for coronary artery filling. β-Blockers also act at the cellular level to improve the balance between oxygen supply and demand by protecting myocardial mitochondria by means of antioxidation. All of these effects can reduce the incidence of perioperative myocardial ischemia and cardiac dysrhythmias.

Although the initial report of the efficacy of β-blockers to reduce perioperative cardiac events was published in 1987, two studies from the 1990s sparked widespread interest in perioperative β-blockers.[1–3] By 2002, the indications for the administration of perioperative β-blockers had been expanded.[4,5]

The patient's internist recommended the oral administration of long-acting metoprolol for 72 hours before surgery. Intravenous metoprolol was to be administered if the patient's heart rate was greater than 65 beats per minute immediately before surgery. In the preoperative holding area, the patient's heart rate was 76 beats per minute, and his blood pressure was 138/80 mm Hg. After intravenous metoprolol (5 mg), his heart rate was 63 beats per minute, and his blood pressure was 124/68 mm Hg.

Are there differences in the pharmacologic effects of different β-blockers?

Although differences in the effects of different β-blockers have been demonstrated in basic research and animal studies, there have been no compelling reports of clinically significant differences. β-1 and β-2 receptors are found in cardiac muscle; however, β-1 receptors are dominant. β-2 Receptors are the primary β-receptors in bronchi.

Propranolol, a first-generation β-blocker, is a nonselective antagonist with equal antagonistic effects on β-1 and β-2 receptors. Second-generation β-blockers such as atenolol, metoprolol, and bisoprolol have much greater selectivity for blockade of β-1 receptors. Third-generation β-blockers such as labetalol, carvedilol, and nebivolol have varying β- adrenergic blocking effects (β-1 and β-2) and vasodilating capabilities. Labetalol is a nonselective β-blocker with strong β-1 receptor blocking effects thereby causing vasodilation. Carvedilol blocks β-1 and β-2 receptors. Nebivolol is a highly selective antagonist of β-1 receptors and causes vasodilation by activation of L-arginine and nitric oxide (Table 2.1). For diabetic patients, carvedilol increases insulin sensitivity, whereas atenolol and metoprolol decrease insulin sensitivity.[6] The lack of β-selectivity of propranolol and labetalol explains the increased incidence of bronchoconstriction with both drugs.

TABLE 2.1 β-Adrenergic Antagonists

First-generation β-blockers

Propranolol

Second-generation β-blockers

Metoprolol

Atenolol

Bisoprolol

Third-generation β-blockers

Labetalol

Bucindolol

Carvedilol

Nebivolol

Bisoprolol, metoprolol, and carvedilol have been shown to significantly reduce mortality in patients with heart failure. No clinical studies have been performed that demonstrate the superiority of one β-blocker over the others with respect to reducing perioperative risk. Limited evidence suggests that β-blockers with vasodilating properties may be better for patients after myocardial infarction and for patients with chronic ischemic heart disease.

Induction of anesthesia was performed with propofol (1.5 mg/kg), and rocuronium (0.6 mg/kg) was administered to facilitate tracheal intubation. Oxygen in sevoflurane was administered by face mask until adequate muscle relaxation was achieved for tracheal intubation. Direct laryngoscopy and tracheal intubation were performed without difficulty. The patient's vital signs immediately after tracheal intubation were: heart rate 68 beats per minute and blood pressure 80/45 mm Hg. Two 5-mg doses of ephedrine did not significantly affect the heart rate or blood pressure. Phenylephrine (100 μg) increased the blood pressure to 100/60 mm Hg and decreased the heart rate to 58 beats per minute. Maintenance of anesthesia was done with desflurane in an air-oxygen mixture. The operative course was marked by blood pressure lability that required a phenylephrine infusion and repeated boluses of intravenous fluids to maintain a satisfactory blood pressure. Emergence was slower than expected, but the patient was extubated in the operating room without difficulty. He was confused for the first 48 hours after surgery. At the time of discharge from the hospital, his wife felt that he had returned to his normal mental status.

Are there risks to perioperative β-adrenergic blockade?

Aggressive β-blockade can cause bradycardia as well as hypotension and may increase the risk of stroke and death. The enthusiasm for widespread perioperative β-blocker administration has been dampened by reports concerning the lack of effect of β-blockers in some studies and an increased risk of adverse effects reported in others.[7–9] Studies such as these that report conflicting results present a dilemma for the clinical anesthesiologist. Advisory and regulatory groups have been quick to advocate routine β-blocker therapy for a large number of patients. Unfortunately, data have been accumulating faster than these groups can revise guidelines.

Can the differences in outcome from these studies be resolved to formulate a logical plan for perioperative β-blocker therapy that has the highest benefit potential?

Resolving three questions concerning perioperative β-blockade would provide much-needed information.

1. Do current β-blocker regimens provide maximal cardio-protection?

   Administration of β-blockers for 7 to 10 days before surgery may be required for optimal effect at the cellular level. This period of time may also be important for patients with hypertension to normalize cerebral autoregulation. Cooperative efforts among internists, surgeons, and anesthesiologists would be required to achieve this goal.

2. Is more precise perioperative hemodynamic control required?

   There is evidence that β-blockade and tight heart rate control are associated with a lower incidence of myocardial ischemia and better long-term outcome.[10]

3. Are there differences in individual patients that explain the inconsistencies in the results from published studies?

   Polymorphism in adrenergic receptors may affect a patient's response to β-blockers and have a significant effect on ultimate outcome. It is known that patients with hypertension have a variable response to β-blockers based on genetic variations in adrenergic receptors. Ser49Gly and Arg389Gly are two single nucleotide polymorphisms of β1-adrenergic receptor genes. Patients with hypertension and Arg389Arg receptors have a greater decrease in systolic and diastolic blood pressure when treated with metoprolol.[11] A study of patients undergoing surgery with spinal anesthesia found that the polymorphism of the β-adrenergic receptor was more predictive of outcome than the influence of β-blockers.[12] Because no previous perioperative studies evaluated genetic variations, differences in genetic patterns might explain variable responses to β-blockers. Further study of the relationship between perioperative outcome and genetic variations in adrenergic receptors is clearly warranted.

This patient had no adverse perioperative cardiac events but did have significant blood pressure lability and possible central nervous system morbidity (delayed emergence and postoperative confusion). Was he, in fact, a suitable candidate for perioperative β-blockers?

Recommendations for treatment can be divided into three classes based on risk-to-benefit ratio and degree of evidence.

Class I: benefit >>> risk. Treatment should be administered.
Class IIa: benefit >> risk. It is reasonable to administer treatment.
Class IIb: benefit ≥ risk. Treatment may be considered.
Class III: risk ≥ benefit. Treatment should not be administered.

TABLE 2.2 Risk for Noncardiac Surgery

Low-risk surgery

Ambulatory surgery

Breast surgery

Cataract surgery

Endoscopy (gastrointestinal and gastric ulcers)

Intermediate risk surgery

Intraperitoneal surgery

Intrathoracic surgery

Carotid endarterectomy

Head and neck surgery

Orthopedic surgery

High-risk surgery

Aortic surgery

Peripheral vascular surgery

Patients require stratification regarding preoperative medical condition and degree of risk of the surgery (Table 2.1). Patients receiving preoperative β-blockers for cardiac disease should have β-blockers continued regardless of the risk of surgery (class I). High-risk patients undergoing vascular surgery should also receive perioperative β-blockers (class I).[13] There are several risk factors for adverse perioperative outcomes (Table 2.2). Patients with active cardiac diseases such as unstable angina, recent myocardial infarction, heart failure, significant dysrhythmias (high-grade atrioventricular block), and severe valvular disease require evaluation and treatment prior to noncardiac surgery. Provocative testing for myocardial ischemia need only be performed if testing will alter management (e.g., revascularization). Patients with only one or two risk factors undergoing intermediate risk surgery do not require stress testing but may benefit from perioperative β-blockers.

The patient had two preoperative risk factors: hypertension and diabetes mellitus and was undergoing intermediate-risk surgery. The indication for perioperative β-blockers was weak and intraoperative hemodynamic instability did develop.

Patients with risk factors for cardiac disease present many challenges for perioperative management. Recommendations

TABLE 2.3 Cardiac Risk Factors

Ischemic heart disease

Compensated heart failure

Cerebrovascular disease

Diabetes mellitus

Renal insufficiency

for evaluation and management of the patient with some risk factors but no overt evidence of cardiac disease have not been sufficiently elucidated to provide the anesthesiologist with clear and unambiguous guidelines. It is difficult for advisory and regulatory groups to revise recommendations as rapidly as new information accumulates. Although β-blockers can certainly reduce the incidence of perioperative cardiac events, there are potential risks, and accurate patient stratification is necessary to obtain maximum benefit with the least risk.[14] The effect of the perioperative use of statins and α-2 adrenergic agonists on outcome needs to be more thoroughly evaluated. The judicious use of these drugs in combination with β-blockers may achieve an even greater perioperative risk reduction (Table 2.3).[15]

KEY MESSAGES

1. β-Adrenergic blockers produce pharmacologic effects that can reduce the incidence of perioperative myocardial ischemia and cardiac dysrhythmias. These effects include decreasing myocardial oxygen demand by reducing heart rate, cardiac contractility, and blood pressure; slowing of the heart rate to prolong diastole during which coronary artery flow occurs; and protection of myocardial mitochondria by means of antioxidation.

2. No clinical studies have been performed that demonstrate the superiority of one β-blocker over the others with respect to reducing perioperative risk.

3. Administration of β-blockers for 7 to 10 days before surgery may be required for optimal effect at the cellular level.

QUESTIONS

1. By what mechanism do β-adrenergic blockers reduce the risk of myocardial ischemia?

   Answer: β-blockers reduce myocardial oxygen consumption by reducing heart reate, myocardial contractility, blood pressure, and protecting mitochondria by antioxidation. The reduction in heart rate increases diastole and provides more time for coronary perfusion.

2. What does class IIB recommendation imply?

   Answer: Treatment recommendations are based on strength of evidence supporting a treatment. A class IIB recommendation suggests that enough evidence exists that a treatment should be considered.

3. What are the risks of perioperative β-adrenergic blockade?

   Answer: Although perioperative β-adrenergic blockade can reduce the incidence of myocardial ischemia, the risk of intraoperative hypotension, stroke, and death are increased.

References

1. Pasternack PF, Imperato AM, Baumann FG, et al. The hemodynamics of beta-blockade in patients undergoing abdominal aortic aneurysm repair. Circulation 1987;76:III 1–7.

2. Mangano DT, Layug EL, Wallace A, Tateo I. Effect of atenolol on mortality and cardiovascular morbidity after noncardiac surgery. N Engl J Med 1996;335:1713–1720.

3. Poldermans D, Boersma E, Bax JJ, et al. The effect of bisoprolol on perioperative mortality and myocardial infarction in high-risk patients undergoing vascular surgery. N Engl J Med 1999;341: 1789–1794.

4. Auerbach AD, Goldman L. β-blockers and reduction of cardiac events in noncardiac surgery. JAMA 2002;287:1445–1447.

5. Fleisher LA, Eagle KA. Lowering cardiac risk in noncardiac surgery. N Engl J Med 2001;345:1677–1682.

6. Weber MA. The role of new β-blockers in treating cardiovascular disease. Am J Hypertens 2005;18:169S–176S.

7. POBBLE Trial Investigators. Perioperative β-blockade (POB-BLE) for patients undergoing infrarenal vascular surgery: results of a randomized double-blind controlled trial. J Vasc Surg 2005; 41:602–609.

8. Yang H, Raymer K, Butler R, et al. The effects of perioperative β-blockade: results of the metoprolol after vascular surgery (MaVS) study, a randomized controlled trial. Am Heart J 2006; 152:983–990.

9. POISE Study Group. Effects of extended-release metoprolol succinate in patients undergoing non-cardiac surgery (POISE trial): a randomized controlled trial. Lancet 2008;371: 1839–1847.

10. Feringa HHH, Bax JJ, Boersma E, et al. High dose β-blockers and tight heart rate control reduce myocardial ischemia and troponin T release in vascular surgery patients. Circulation 2006;114 (Suppl I):I-344-I-49.

11. Shin J, Johnson JA. Pharmacogenetics of β-blockers. Pharmacotherapy 2007;27:874–887.

12. Zaugg M, Bestmann L, Wacker J, et al. Adrenergic receptor genotype but not perioperative bisoprolol therapy may determine cardiovascular outcome in at-risk patients undergoing surgery with spinal block. Anesthesiology 2007;107:33–44.

13. Fleisher LA, Beckman JA, Brown KA, et al. ACC/AHA 2007 guidelines on perioperative cardiovascular evaluation and care for noncardiac surgery: executive summary. Anesth Analg 2007; 106:685–712.

14. Fleisher LA, Poldermans D. Perioperative β blockade: where do we go from here? Lancet 2008;371:1813–1814.

15. London MJ. Beta blockers and alpha-2 agonists for cardioprotection. Best Pract Res Clin Anaesth 2008;22:95–110.

Perioperative Glycemic Control

Kelly Grogan

FORMAT: REFLECTION

A 72-year-old male with a history of type 2 diabetes mellitus, hypertension, and remote tobacco use presented for coronary artery bypass graft surgery. His medications included aspirin daily, metoprolol 50 mg daily, metformin 500 mg twice daily, omeprazole 20 mg daily, and atorvastatin 10 mg daily. He had no known drug allergies. Preoperatively, an echocardiogram showed mild mitral regurgitation, nonsignificant aortic sclerosis, and a left ventricular ejection fraction of 40% with mild inferior hypokinesis. Laboratory test results included a fasting serum glucose level of 165 mg/dL; HgbA1C, 7.6%; hematocrit, 36%; and creatinine, 1.3 mg/dL. On the morning of surgery, the patient's serum glucose level was 134 mg/dL. He had received metoprolol the morning of surgery, and was fasting since 10:00 PM on the previous evening.

After induction of general anesthesia and tracheal intubation, central venous access was obtained, and a transesophageal echocardiography probe was placed. The patient's initial serum glucose level was 155 mg/dL. An intravenous insulin infusion was started at 2 units per hour. Serum glucose testing was repeated every hour during the procedure, and the insulin dosage was adjusted based on the institutional intraoperative insulin protocol (Table 3.1).

What is the epidemiology of diabetes mellitus?

From 1980 through 2004, the number of Americans with diabetes mellitus increased from 5.8 to 14.7 million. Diabetes now affects nearly 21 million Americans, or 7% of the U.S. population; more than 6 million of the affected do not know they have diabetes. Compelling evidence continues to accumulate suggesting that poorly controlled glucose levels are associated with increased morbidity and mortality rates, as well as higher health care costs. Further, long-term strict glycemic control reduces the frequency of diabetes complications, particularly microvascular complications and renal dysfunction. The United States spends approximately $132 billion each year on diabetes—$92 billion in direct medical costs and another $40 billion in indirect costs because of missed workdays or other losses in productivity.[1]

What is (are) the relationship(s) between the mechanisms underlying hyperglycemia and poor patient outcome?

The mechanisms of harm from hyperglycemia center on the immune system, mediators of inflammation, vascular perturbations, altered hemodynamics, and enhanced neuronal damage following brain ischemia. The association of hyperglycemia and infection appears to primarily result from phagocyte dysfunction involving impaired neutrophil and monocyte adherence, chemotaxis, phagocytosis, and bacterial killing.[2] Classic microvascular complications of diabetes are caused by alterations in the aldose reductase pathway, advanced glycation end-product pathway, enhanced reactive oxygen species production, and the protein kinase C pathway. Several of these pathways may contribute to immune dysfunction.[3]

Acute hyperglycemia also has numerous effects on the cardiovascular system. Hyperglycemia impairs myocardial ischemic preconditioning that might contribute to larger myocardial infarct size in diabetics compared with nondiabetics.[4] Hyperglycemia is associated with reduced coronary collateral blood flow[5] and increased cardiac myocyte death through apoptosis[6] or by exaggerating ischemia-reperfusion cellular injury.[7] Multiple studies have identified a variety of hyperglycemia-related abnormalities in hemostasis that favor thrombosis.[8,9]

Acute hyperglycemia is associated with enhanced neuronal damage following induced brain ischemia.[2] This enhanced injury is mostly in the ischemic penumbra thus contributing to stroke expansion.[10–13] Elevated glucose concentrations have been associated with enhanced cerebral ischemic damage secondary to increased tissue acidosis and lactate levels. Lactate has been associated with damage to neurons, astrocytes, and endothelial cells.[14]

Other than glycemic regulation, how does insulin influence metabolic regulation?

There may be beneficial effects of insulin therapy that are separate from mere glycemic control. First, insulin inhibits lipolysis, reducing free fatty acid levels that are believed to contribute to cardiac arrhythmias. Next, insulin stimulates endothelial nitric oxide synthase enhancing nitric oxide secretion, resulting in arterial vasodilation in addition to a variety of other beneficial effects on oxidation and inflammation. Finally, insulin, in the environment of euglycemia or near-euglycemia,

TABLE 3.1A Insulin Loading Dose and Initial Infusion Rate

Glucose (mg/dL)	Recommended Action	
	Intravenous Loading Bolus	**Infusion Rate**
>300	12 units	8–10 U/h
261–300	9 units	7–8 U/h
231–260	7 units	6–7 U/h
201–230	3 units	5–6 U/h
171–200	2 units	3–5 U/h
141–170	0 units	2–3 U/h
120–140	0 units	1–2 U/h
100–119	0 units	0.5 U/h

appears to inhibit proinflammatory cytokines, adhesion molecules, and chemokines, in addition to acute-phase proteins.[15]

Is in-hospital hyperglycemia associated with adverse patient outcomes?

Data from observational studies have linked hyperglycemia with poor outcome in acutely ill patients. In cardiac surgical patients, hyperglycemia is associated with a greater risk for sternal wound infections.[16,17] More aggressive treatment of hyperglycemia with intravenous insulin targeting serum glucose levels of 100 to 150 mg/dL reduced the risk of deep sternal wound infections by 57% compared with historical controls in which the goal was to maintain glucose levels between 150 to 200 mg/dL.[18,19] In those analyses, there was a

significant correlation between average postoperative glucose level and mortality with the lowest mortality rates found in patients with postoperative glucose levels <150 mg/dL. In patients undergoing general surgery, a single blood glucose level >220 mg/dL is associated with a nearly threefold greater risk for infection compared with blood glucose levels <220 mg/dL.[20] Multiple other retrospective studies have linked hyperglycemia with worse outcomes in patients with acute myocardial infarction.[21,22] Hyperglycemia is further associated with more severe brain damage and mortality after ischemic but not hemorrhagic stroke.[23,24]

Until recently, data linking hyperglycemia with poor outcomes in hospitalized patients were retrospective. In a landmark series of prospectively randomized, double-blinded studies, Van den Berghe et al.[25] reported that criti-

TABLE 3.1B Insulin Dose for Infusion Titration Based on Hourly Glucose Checks

Glucose (mg/dL)	Rising Glucose		Falling Glucose	
	Re-Bolus	**Increase Rate**	**Hold Infusion**	**Decrease Rate**
>350	12 units	5–6 U/h	—	0%
301–350	9 units	4–5 U/h	—	0%
251–300	7 units	3–4 U/h	—	0%
201–250	5 units	2–3 U/h	—	0%–10%
161–200	3 units	1–2 U/h	—	0%–10%
121–160	0 units	No change	0–30 min	0%–25%
81–120	0 units	No change	0–60 min	0%–50%
61–80	0 units	No change	0–60 min	25%–75%
40–60		Stop infusion; ensure adequate glucose administration	30–60 min	Do not restart infusion until glucose is >120 mg/dL
<40		Stop infusion; administer one-half amp D50 and check glucose in 30–60 min	Until adequate rebound in glucose is ensured	Do not restart infusion until glucose is >120 mg/dL

cally ill patients in a mixed medical surgical intensive care unit (ICU) had improved outcomes with intensive insulin therapy targeted to serum glucose levels of 80 to 110 mg/dL compared with standard treatment. Patients in the intensive insulin treatment group had a 34% reduction in mortality, a 46% lower incidence of sepsis, a 41% reduction in the rate of renal failure requiring dialysis, a 50% reduction in the frequency of blood transfusion, and a 44% reduction in the rate of critical illness polyneuropathy compared with the control group. These benefits, however, were restricted to patients hospitalized in the ICU for 3 to 5 days. When the data were limited to medical ICU patients, intensive insulin treatment was associated with worse outcomes, in fact, for patients with a shorter duration of ICU admission. A meta-analysis of 35 clinical trials evaluating the effect of insulin therapy on mortality rates in hospitalized patients with critical illness found that insulin therapy decreased short-term mortality by 15% in a variety of clinical settings.[26] These studies, however, did not investigate the risk versus benefits of intraoperative intensive insulin management. In fact, Gandhi et al.[27] found a higher mortality rate for patients randomized to receiving intensive insulin therapy (targeted glucose levels of 80 to 110 mg/dL) during cardiac surgery compared with controls.

What glucose level should be targeted?

Based on the available data, recommendations have been advanced as to what serum glucose level to target with insulin therapy for patients in critical care settings. The targets for non–intensive care patients including those during surgery are less well defined and are somewhat controversial. Regardless, guidelines from the American Diabetes Association and the American College of Endocrinology recommend intensive insulin management for both ICU and non-ICU patients (Table 3.2).[15,28] Guidelines for the management of patients with acute stroke from the American Heart Association, however, acknowledge that the exact glucose level that should be targeted with insulin therapy for patients with stroke are not known and are probably <140 mg/dL.[29]

TABLE 3.2 Recommended Targets for Serum Glucose Levels in Hospitalized Patients from the ADA and the ACE

	ADA (28)	ACE (15)
Intensive care unit	As close to 110 mg/dL as possible	<110 mg/dL
Non–critical care units	As close to 90–130 mg/dL as possible; maximal <180 mg/dL	<110 mg/dL preprandial; maximal <180 mg/dL

To convert mg/dL of glucose to mmol/L, divide by 18 or multiply by 0.055.
ACE, American College of Endocrinology; ADA, American Diabetes Association.

What are the principles of perioperative management of the diabetic patient?

Insulin resistance and insulin secretory capacity in hospitalized patients is influenced by numerous factors, including severity of illness, medications (e.g., glucocorticoids and catecholamines), procedures, and diet that is often interrupted. The ability to control glucose in diabetic patients will, in part, depend on the quality of their control before admission. This can be assessed by measuring hemoglobin A1C value (a value >6% indicates poor control).

Hospitalized patients are usually not managed with oral hypoglycemic agents because of their long half-life, potential for side effects caused by an acute illness, and the inability to rapidly titrate the dose. Nonetheless, continuing oral hypoglycemic agents taken before hospitalization is considered for non–critically ill patients who had good pre-hospital glucose control and who are expected to eat a normal diet. Important considerations for the use of oral hypoglycemic agents in hospitalized patients include:

- Sulfonylureas have a long duration of action (that varies from patient to patient) predisposing to hypoglycemia especially in patients who are not eating (nothing by mouth [NPO]). These agents do not allow rapid dose adjustment to meet the changing needs of acutely ill patients. Further, sulfonylureas block ATP-sensitive potassium channels that mediate in part myocardial ischemic preconditioning. Patients at risk for myocardial ischemia, thus, might experience greater myocardial damage if given sulfonylureas (e.g., during cardiac surgery or when a perioperative myocardial infarction occurs).
- Metformin may lead to potentially fatal lactic acidosis particularly during the stress associated with surgery or acute illness. Risk factors for this side effect include cardiac disease, heart failure, hypoperfusion, renal insufficiency, old age, and chronic pulmonary disease. Nonetheless, predicting individual susceptibility is limited, and most data regarding this condition are from case series in which other factors might have confounded the findings. Regardless, metformin is typically stopped the morning of surgery or at least 8 hours before surgery.
- Thiazolidinediones have few side effects, but these drugs do increase intravascular volume that might predispose to congestive heart failure. Their use is associated with abnormal liver function tests, and they should not be given to patients with liver dysfunction.

Previously diagnosed and newly diagnosed diabetics will likely require insulin management perioperatively or during an acute illness. The commonly used "sliding scale insulin therapy" with regular insulin is generally inappropriate as a sole insulin management strategy. A key component to providing effective insulin therapy is determining whether a patient has the ability to produce endogenous insulin. Patients with type 1 diabetes are by definition insulin deficient. Patients with prior pancreatectomy or with pancreatic dysfunction, those who have received insulin for greater than 5 years, and patients with wide fluctuations in serum glucose levels may all have a significant degree of insulin deficiency. Patients determined to be insulin deficient require basal insulin replacement at all times to prevent iatrogenic diabetic ketoacidosis. A subcutaneous insulin regimen consists of three elements:

- Basal insulin requirement provided in the form of intermediate or long-acting analogs such as lente insulin. Some non–insulin-deficient patients may not require basal insulin if they are to take nothing by mouth. However, withholding basal insulin in insulin-deficient patients may result in ketoacidosis.
- Prandial insulin is given before meals. The rapid-acting insulin analogs, insulin lispro and aspart, are excellent prandial insulins. Some patients do receive their prandial coverage immediately after eating, and the dose is based on carbohydrate counting.
- Correction-dose or supplemental insulin is given to treat hyperglycemia. This should not be confused with "sliding scale insulin," which usually refers to a set amount of insulin administered for hyperglycemia without regard to the timing of food, the presence or absence of pre-existing insulin administration, or individualization of the patient's sensitivity to insulin. Correctional-dose insulin can be used to accommodate the increased insulin requirements that accompany acute illness and insulin resistance secondary to counterregulatory responses to stress and/or illness.

By far, intravenous insulin is the most reliable means for achieving glycemic control particularly in critically ill patients who may have severe or rapidly changing insulin requirements, generalized edema, impaired perfusion of subcutaneous sites and extremities, and those who are receiving total parenteral nutrition and/or sympathomimetic drugs. Most institutions now have standardized algorithms. The most effective are those that use dynamic scales, incorporating the rate of change in glucose into dose adjustments. Frequent glucose level monitoring is imperative to ensure good control and minimize hypoglycemic events. As a patient's clinical status improves, he or she can be transitioned to subcutaneous insulin. This step requires using the most recent infusion rate to approximate the overall daily requirement, dividing this into basal and prandial components. It is often necessary to overlap the intravenous and subcutaneous insulin to ensure a proper conversion.

PREVENTION AND MANAGEMENT OF HYPOGLYCEMIA

Hypoglycemia, if unrecognized and prolonged, can have severe and permanent negative outcomes. Hospitalized patients are at an increased risk of developing hypoglycemia because of altered nutritional state, liver and kidney dysfunction, infection, malignancy, and sepsis. Changes in medications (particularly steroids and catecholamines), decreased oral intake, vomiting, procedures that require the patient to take nothing by mouth, unexpected interruptions of enteral feedings or parenteral nutrition, and patients' mental status all contribute to the complexity of glucose management. Patients that are sedated or under general anesthesia, having delirium, or are hospitalized for neurologic events will be unable to communicate the typical signs and symptoms of hypoglycemia. Decreased levels of consciousness, confusion, or diaphoresis may be the only signs. Acute hypoglycemia is treated by administering 25 to 50 g of glucose intravenously.

KEY MESSAGES

1. Diabetes now affects nearly 21 million Americans, or 7% of the U.S. population.

2. The mechanisms of harm from hyperglycemia center on the immune system, mediators of inflammation, vascular perturbations, altered hemodynamics, and enhanced neuronal damage following brain ischemia.

3. Van den Berghe et al. reported that critically ill patients in a mixed medical surgical ICU had improved outcomes with intensive insulin therapy targeted to serum glucose levels of 80 to 110 mg/dL compared with standard treatment.

4. Intravenous insulin is the most reliable means for achieving glycemic control, particularly in critically ill patients.

QUESTIONS

1. By what mechanism(s) does diabetes mellitus result in microvascular complications?

   Answer: These mechanisms are alterations in the aldose reductase pathway, advanced glycation end-product pathway, enhanced reactive oxygen species production, and the protein kinase C pathway.

2. What is the most important adverse effect associated with metformin administration?

   Answer: Metformin may lead to potentially fatal lactic acidosis, particularly during the stress associated with surgery or acute illness.

3. What factors may contribute to hypoglycemia in acutely ill patients?

   Answer: Decreased nutritional intake (decreased oral intake, vomiting, procedures that require the patient to take nothing by mouth, unexpected interruptions of enteral feedings or parenteral nutrition, altered level of consciousness), liver and kidney dysfunction, infection, malignancy, and sepsis may be contributing factors.

References

1. Centers for Disease Control and Prevention. National diabetes surveillance system: prevalence of diabetes number (in millions) of persons with diagnosed diabetes, United States, 1980–2004. Available at: http://www.sds.gov/diabetes/statistics/prev/national/figpersons.htm. Accessed March 3, 2009.
2. Clement S, Braithwaite SS, Magee MF, et al. Management of diabetes and hyperglycemia in hospitals. Diabetes Care 2004; 27:553–591.
3. Sheetz M, King G. Molecular understanding of hyperglycemia's adverse effects for diabetic complications. JAMA 2002;288:2579–2588.
4. Kersten J, Schmeling T, Orth K, et al. Acute hyperglycemia abolishes ischemic preconditioning in vivo. Am J Physiol 1998; 275:H721–725.

5. Kersten J, Toller W, Tessmer J, et al. Hyperglycemia reduces coronary collateral blood flow through a nitric oxide-mediated mechanism. Am J Physiol 2001;281:H2097–2104.

6. Ceriello A, Quagliaro L, D'Amico M, et al. Acute hyperglycemia induces nitrotyrosine formation and apoptosis in perfused heart from rat. Diabetes 2002;51:1076–1082.

7. Verma S, Mailand A, Weisel R, et al. Hyperglycemia exaggerates ischemia-reperfusion-induces cardiomyocyte injury: reversal with endothelin antagonism. J Thorac Cardiovasc Surg 2002;123:1120–1124.

8. Davi G, Catalano I, Averna M, et al. Thromboxane biosynthesis and platelet function in type II diabetes mellitus. N Engl J Med 1990;322:1769–1774.

9. Knobler H, Sanion N, Shenkman B, et al. Shear-induced platelet adhesion and aggregation on subendothelium are increased in diabetic patients. Throm Res 1998;80:181–190.

10. Prado R, Ginsberg MD, Dietrich WD, et al. Hyperglycemia increases infarct size in collaterally perfused but not end-arterial vascular territories. J Cereb Blood Flow Metab 1988;8:186–192.

11. Ginsberg MD, Prado R, Dietrich WD, et al. Hyperglycemia reduces the extent of cerebral infarction in rats. Stroke 1987;18:570–574.

12. Venables GS, Miller SA, Gibson G, et al. The effects of hyperglycemia on changes during reperfusion following focal cerebral ischemia in the cat. J Neurol Neurosurg Psychiatry 1985;48:663–669.

13. Anderson RE, Tan WK, Martin HS, Meyer FB. Effects of glucose and PaO$_2$ modulation on cortical intracellular acidosis, NADH redox state, and infarction in the ischemic penumbra. Stroke 1999;30:160–170.

14. Petito CK, Kraig RP, Pulsinelli WA. Light and electron microscopic evaluation of hydrogen ion-induced brain necrosis. J Cereb Blood Flow Metab 1987;7:625–632.

15. Garber AJ, Moghissi ES, Bransome ED, et al. American college of endocrinology position statement on inpatient diabetes and metabolic control. Endocr Pract 2004:10:77–82.

16. Golden S, Peart-Vigilence C, Kao W, Brancati F. Perioperative glycemic control and the risk of infectious complications in a cohort of adults with diabetes. Diabetes Care 1999;22:1408–1414.

17. Latham R, Lancaster AD, Covington JF, et al. The association of diabetes and glucose control with surgical site infection among cardiothoracic surgery patients. Infec Control Hosp Epidemiol 2001;22:607–612.

18. Furnary AP, Zerr K, Grunkemeier G, Starr A. Continuous intravenous insulin infusion reduces the incidence of deep sternal would infection in diabetic patients after cardiac surgical procedures. Ann Thorac Surg 1999;67:352–362.

19. Furnary AP, Gao G, Grunkemeier GL, et al. Continuous insulin infusion reduces mortality in patients with diabetes undergoing coronary artery bypass grafting. J Thorac Cardiovasc Surg 2003;125:1007–1021.

20. Pomposelli J, Baxter J, Babineau T, et al. Early postoperative glucose control predicts nosocomial infection rate in diabetic patients. J Parenter Enter Nutr 1998;22:77–81.

21. Kasiobrod M, Rathore SS, Inzucchi S, et al. Admission glucose and mortality in elderly patients hospitalized with acute myocardial infarction: implications for patients with and without recognized diabetes. Circulation 2005;111:3078.

22. Capes SE, Hunt D, Malmberg K, Gerstein HC. Stress hyperglycemia and increased risk of death after myocardial infarction in patients with and without diabetes: a systematic overview. Lancet 2000;355:773–778.

23. Capes S, Hunt D, Malmberg K, et al. Stress hyperglycemia and prognosis of stroke in nondiabetic and diabetic patients: a systematic overview. Stroke 2001;32:2426–2432.

24. Kiers I, Davis SM, Larkins R, et al. Stroke topography and outcome in relation to hyperglycemia and diabetes. J Neurol Neurosurg Psychiatry 1992;55:263–270.

25. Van den Berghe G, Wouters P, Weekers F, et al. Intensive insulin therapy in critically ill patients. N Engl J Med 2001;345:1359–1367.

26. Pittas AG, Siegel RD, Lau J. Insulin therapy for critically ill hospitalized patients: a meta-analysis of randomized, control trial. Arch Inter Med 2004;164:2005–2011.

27. Gandhi GY, Nuttall GA, Adel MD, et al. Intensive intraoperative insulin therapy versus conventional glucose management during cardiac surgery. Ann Intern Med 2007;146:233–243.

28. American Diabetes Association. Standards of medical care in diabetes. Diabetes Care 2005;28:S4–36.

29. Adams HP, del Zoppo G, Alberts MJ, et al. Guidelines for the early management of adults with ischemic stroke. A guideline from the American Heart Association/American Stroke Association Stroke Council, Clinical Cardiology Council, Cardiovascular Radiology and Intervention Council, and the Atherosclerotic Peripheral Vascular Disease and Quality of Care Outcomes in Research Interdisciplinary Working Groups. Stroke 2007;38:1655–1711.

CHAPTER 4

Neuraxial Analgesic Techniques for Cardiac Anesthesia

Hassan M. Ahmad

CASE FORMAT: STEP BY STEP

A 62-year-old, 85-kg man with a history of cigarette smoking, hypertension, and hyperlipidemia was referred by his primary care physician for a routine exercise stress test. Electrocardiogram changes occurred in the anterior leads when his heart rate was 50% of the maximal predicted rate, although the patient remained asymptomatic. He was then referred for diagnostic and possible interventional cardiac catheterization. Angiography confirmed the presence of a 90% distal stenosis of the left anterior descending coronary artery and a 75% stenosis of the circumflex coronary artery. Because the former lesion was not amenable to percutaneous intervention, he was referred for coronary artery bypass graft surgery (CABG).

During the preoperative interview, the cardiac anesthesiologist learned that the patient had an active lifestyle with frequent exercise and a past medical history of hypertension. His current medications were hydrochlorothiazide, atorvastatin, and aspirin. He had no known allergies and had undergone an appendectomy 20 years previously. The patient had been smoking one pack of cigarettes per day for approximately 40 years, and his family history was positive for coronary artery disease (both parents having suffered "heart attacks" in their late 50s). Physical examination revealed faint wheezing in both lung fields. Blood pressure was 142/67 mm Hg; heart rate, 72 beats per minute; room air oxygen saturation, 96%; and temperature, 36.7°C. All baseline investigations (hematology, chemistries, and coagulation studies) were normal.

The surgical plan was perform a median sternotomy and "off-pump" CABG surgery with the left internal mammary artery to the left anterior descending artery and saphenous vein graft to the circumflex coronary artery. After a discussion with the patient, the anesthetic plan was combined general and thoracic epidural anesthesia.

Are there benefits to epidural anesthesia and analgesia for cardiac surgery?

Several studies have compared general with combined general/epidural anesthesia for cardiac surgery. There is some evidence to indicate that the use of epidural analgesia facilitates early tracheal extubation postoperatively. Other outcomes, including duration of hospital stay and overall cost are similar when the two techniques are compared.[6,7]

The more theoretical benefits of epidural anesthesia/analgesia for cardiac surgery are related to sympathetic blockade. Decreased heart rate and coronary vasodilation result in improved subendocardial blood flow, which might be beneficial for patients undergoing CABG surgery. Attenuation of stress reactions and attenuation of postoperative pain are other proposed benefits. Several (although not all) investigations have suggested that postoperative sympathetic blockade decreases the incidence of atrial fibrillation typically on postoperative day 2 or 3 in greater than one third of patients. Overall, potential theoretical benefits of thoracic epidural anesthesia/analgesia for CABG surgery have not been shown to lead to clinically important patient benefit.[8,9,10]

On the morning of surgery, the patient was transported to the preoperative area, where the anesthesiologist inserted a thoracic epidural at the T5-6 level. A 17-gauge Tuohy needle was used to the access the epidural space, utilizing a loss-of-resistance technique. An epidural catheter was inserted 4 cm into the epidural space, and a 3-mL test dose of 1.5% lidocaine with 1:200,000 epinephrine was administered with no evidence of intravascular or intrathecal injection.

What are the potential risks and complications of using epidurals in cardiac surgery?

Placing an epidural before surgery requiring subsequent anticoagulation has been shown to be quite safe in several different settings. In general, the possibility of infection, bleeding, and nerve injury should be clearly disclosed to patients before placing an epidural catheter.[2]

The greatest concern in inserting an epidural prior to cardiac surgery is the potential risk of epidural hematoma secondary to anticoagulation. Large series indicate that epidural catheter placement before anticoagulation with unfractionated or low-molecular-weight heparin can be performed with a minimal risk for epidural hematoma if certain precautions are taken.

Other complications from epidural anesthesia include hypotension resulting from sympathectomy and systemic toxic effects of opioids and local anesthetics.

What are the guidelines for the use of epidurals in the setting of anticoagulation with heparin?

It is not uncommon for patients undergoing cardiac surgery to have been on a heparin infusion before surgery. The American Society of Regional Anesthesia has issued guidelines that may reduce the risk of epidural hematoma related to epidurals in anticoagulated patients. Typically, heparin infusion should be discontinued 4 hours before epidural placement, and the interval between epidural placement and complete anti-coagulation for bypass should exceed 60 minutes. Also, epidural catheters should be removed only when normal coagulation has been restored; if a heparin infusion is required in the postoperative period, the infusion should be discontinued 2 to 4 hours prior to catheter removal. In general, epidurals should be avoided in patients with known coagulopathy. It is unclear whether a traumatic epidural placement necessitates canceling cardiac surgery, but the consensus is to delay the operation for at least 24 hours, should a "bloody tap" occur.[5]

Can intrathecal opioids be used for cardiac surgery?

It has been shown that inadequate analgesia in the postoperative period leads to increased likelihood of myocardial ischemia associated with the stress response to pain. Adverse changes in hemodynamics, metabolic activity, immune function, and hemostasis can be attenuated with better pain control.

Several studies have evaluated the potential benefit of intrathecal opioids as a method of providing postoperative analgesia. Most investigations have studied the use of intrathecal morphine and its effect on time to tracheal extubation, use of additional intravenous opioids, and duration of hospital stay. Generally, the long-acting effect of intrathecal morphine provided better analgesia compared to placebo. No clear benefit has been demonstrated regarding tracheal extubation and overall outcomes, however, in part because of the adverse respiratory effects. The combined use of intrathecal morphine and intrathecal clonidine provides better postoperative analgesia and facilitates earlier tracheal extubation.[1]

What dosing regimen should be used?

The goals for an epidural technique in cardiac surgery are establishing surgical anesthesia, thereby minimizing systemic opioid use and to create a significant sympathectomy. This means a block level as high as T1.

The dosing should begin with a test dose of 1.5% lidocaine with epinephrine 1:200,000 to detect an unwanted intrathecal or intravascular catheter. Then, a loading dose of preservative-free morphine 20 μg/kg is given, followed by 0.5% bupivacaine given in 5-mg increments to a total of 25 to 35 mg. A continuous infusion of 0.5% bupivacaine with morphine 25 μg/mL is started at 4 mL per hour and adjusted to achieve adequate analgesia.

Is the use of a total spinal technique justified?

Much of the proposed benefit of regional anesthesia in cardiac surgical patients is based on the sympathetic blockade, which cannot be reliably achieved with intrathecal opioids alone. Administration of large doses of intrathecal local anesthetics to achieve this goal has been studied. Typically, the Trendelenburg position is used to achieve an adequate cephalad spread to above T1, resulting in a "total spinal." Although the subsequent sympathectomy is observed by serum markers and hemodynamics, no significant clinical benefit results. Moreover, the resultant hypotension and bradycardia may make this technique inappropriate for cardiac surgical patients.[4]

Are there any other regional techniques that can favorably influence the postoperative course?

Parasternal block entails the surgeon injecting local anesthetic along the sternal border to anesthetize the intercostal nerves and their branches. Using this technique has been shown to significantly decrease the dose of morphine required in the immediate postoperative period and was associated with better oxygenation at the time of tracheal extubation (although not an earlier time of extubation). Nonetheless, it is a relatively safe and easy procedure that can provide excellent analgesia.[3]

KEY MESSAGES

1. Epidural analgesia and anesthesia is an option in cardiac surgery and has the potential for earlier extubation and improved pain control in the immediate postoperative period.

2. The complete systemic anticoagulation associated with cardiopulmonary bypass is a concern with placement of epidural catheters, particularly the risk of developing an epidural hematoma.

3. A combination of local anesthetics and opioids can be administered via epidural, and there are several potential effects related to the attenuated stress response that may be beneficial to cardiac surgical patients.

QUESTIONS

1. What spinal levels are associated with sympathetic nervous supply to the heart?

   Answer: T1-T5.

2. What are the early clinical signs of epidural hematoma?

   Answer: Back pain, lower extremity weakness and diminished sensation, and loss of bowel and bladder control.

3. What long-acting local anesthetic has been shown to have less cardiovascular toxicity than bupivacaine?

   Answer: Ropivacaine

References

1. Chaney MA. Intrathecal and epidural anesthesia and analgesia for cardiac surgery. Anesth Analg 2006;102:45–64.
2. Chaney MA, Labovsky JK. Thoracic epidural anesthesia and cardiac surgery: balancing postoperative risks associated with hematoma formation and thromboembolic phenomenon. J Cardiothorac Vasc Anesth 2005;19:768–771.
3. McDonald SB, Jacobsohn E, Kopacz DJ, et al. Parasternal block and local anesthetic infiltration with levobupivacaine after cardiac surgery with desflurane: the effect on postoperative pain, pulmonary function, and tracheal extubation times. Anesth Analg 2005;100:25–32.

4. Lee TW, Grocott HP, Schwinn D, et al. Winnipeg High-Spinal Anesthesia Group. High spinal anesthesia for cardiac surgery: effects on beta-adrenergic receptor function, stress response, and hemodynamics. Anesthesiology 2003;98:499–510.

5. Horlocker TT, Wedel DJ, Benzon H, et al. Regional Anesthesia in the Anticoagulated Patient: Defining the Risks (The Second ASRA Consensus Conference on Neuraxial Anesthesia and Anticoagulation) Regional Anesthesia and Pain Medicine, Vol 28, No. 3 (May–June), 2003: 172–197.

6. Karagoz HY, Kurtoglu M, Bakkaloglu B, et al. Coronary artery bypass grafting in the awake patient: three years' experience in 137 patients. J Thorac Cardiovasc Surg 2003;125:1401–1404.

7. Priestley MC, Cope L, Halliwell R, et al. Thoracic epidural anesthesia for cardiac surgery: the effects on tracheal intubation time and length of hospital stay. Anesth Analg 2002;94:275–282, table of contents.

8. Fillinger MP, Yeager MP, Dodds TM, et al. Epidural anesthesia and analgesia: effects on recovery from cardiac surgery. J Cardiothorac Vasc Anesth 2002;16:15–20.

9. Hansdottir V, Philip J, Olsen MF, et al. Thoracic epidural versus intravenous patient-controlled analgesia after cardiac surgery: a randomized controlled trial on length of hospital stay and patient-perceived quality of recovery. Anesthesiology 2006;104: 142–151.

10. Barrington MJ, Kluger R, Watson R, et al. Epidural anesthesia for coronary artery bypass surgery compared with general anesthesia alone does not reduce biochemical markers of myocardial damage. Anesth Analg 2005;100:921–928.

CHAPTER 5

Off-Pump Coronary Artery Surgery

Audrey R. Leverich and Nikolaos J. Skubas

CASE FORMAT: STEP BY STEP

A 62-year-old man with triple-vessel coronary artery disease presented for off-pump coronary artery bypass graft surgery (OPCAB). His past medical history included hypertension and hyperlipidemia. A coronary angiogram revealed a 95% obstruction of the left anterior descending artery (LAD), 60% stenosis of the circumflex artery (CX), and 70% narrowing of the right coronary artery (RCA). Left ventricular (LV) ejection fraction was preserved (>50%); there was mild mitral regurgitation, and LV pressures were 135/12 mm Hg. Carotid ultrasound revealed 80% obstruction of the right carotid artery. Physical examination, vital signs, and laboratory work were within normal limits, except for a bruit audible over the right side of the patient's neck. His medication list included an antihypertensive, a β-blocker, aspirin, and a statin.

How does OPCAB differ from CABG?

Standard coronary revascularization procedures in the past relied on the use of extracorporeal circulation (cardiopulmonary bypass [CPB]). The use of CPB during CABG surgery, however, is associated with undesirable effects including coagulation abnormalities, activation of the inflammatory response, and the potential for multiple organ system dysfunction. OPCAB involves performing coronary revascularization on a beating heart.[1] High-risk patients such as those who have cerebral, renal, or pulmonary dysfunction as well as the elderly (>80 years), might likely benefit the most from OPCAB by avoiding the deleterious consequences of CPB. Patients with severe atherosclerosis of the ascending aortas might further benefit from OPCAB because aortic cross clamping is not necessary. Contraindications to OPCAB are mostly limited to technical considerations such as an intramyocardial coronary artery that is difficult to dissect, intracavitary thrombus that can be dislodged during heart manipulation, and combined surgical procedures that include open-chamber valve replacement surgery. Patients with a history of malignant ventricular arrhythmias, as well as patients who would not tolerate periods of myocardial ischemia, are not optimal candidates for OPCAB procedures (Table 5.1).

What are the surgical approaches to OPCAB?

There are two surgical approaches to OPCAB: (a) the minimally invasive direct access coronary artery bypass graft (MID-CAB) procedure, which involves a small left thoracotomy incision, through which the left internal mammary artery (LIMA) is anastomosed to the target vessel (usually the LAD); and (b) the typical OPCAB in which multiple coronary artery bypass grafts are constructed via a median sternotomy incision. Exposure of the target coronary vessels is achieved with displacement of the heart.[2] The LAD, diagonal branches, and proximal RCA can be adequately exposed with a suction stabilizer device and sponges in the pericardial sac (Fig. 5.1), and the displacement is minimal. Targets in the posterior (distal RCA) and lateral (CX) surface of the heart, however, require rotating the heart out of the thoracic cavity with anterior displacement ("verticalization"). This is typically achieved with an aspirating device placed on the cardiac apex. In either case, stabilizing the epicardium is necessary to carry out coronary arteriotomy and graft anastomosis. Stabilizer devices use a combination of pressure and suction to immobilize the planned anastomotic site (Fig. 5.2). Transient interruption of coronary flow is achieved with elasticized sutures placed around the proximal and distal target vessel. Anastomoses are then performed on a relatively bloodless, motionless field.

Does the patient's history affect the anesthesia plan?

This patient has extensive coronary artery disease, but his LV function is preserved, and there are no significant valvular lesions. The presence and degree of collateral coronary blood supply should dictate the sequence of distal anastomoses. The presence of a carotid bruit at the site of a documented carotid stenosis raises concerns regarding preservation of cerebral blood flow to the brain perioperatively. For these reasons, hypotension may not be tolerated in this patient. This patient might further have atherosclerosis of the ascending aorta or of other arteries such as the renal and splanchnic arteries (Fig. 5.3). Blood flow to the latter might be sensitive to reduce blood pressure during cardiac manipulations while OPCAB is being performed .

Which monitors should be used during the intraoperative period?

Conventional five-lead electrocardiogram (ECG), pulse oximetry, and intra-arterial blood pressure monitoring should be performed in all patients undergoing an OPCAB procedure. In addition, a pulmonary artery catheter can be considered depending on ventricular function, pulmonary arterial hypertension, or other complicating factors. External defibrillator/pacing pads should be placed particularly for MIDCAB where

TABLE 5.1 Differences Between Traditional CABG and OPCAB

	CABG	OPCAB
Incision	Sternotomy	Sternotomy or Thoracotomy
Heparinization	Full: ACT >480 s	Partial: ACT ~250–300 s
Cannulation	Aortic, venous	Neither
Aortic cross clamp	Yes	No
Cardioplegia	Yes	No
Partial aortic cross clamp for construction of proximal anastomosis	Yes	Yes, if > two vessels No, if all arterial grafts on a "Y" or "T" anastomosis to LITA

ACT, activated clotting time; CABG, coronary artery bypass graft; LIMA, left internal mammary artery; OPCAB, off-pump coronary artery bypass graft surgery.

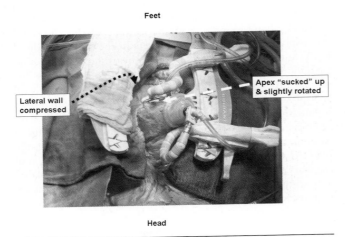

Feet

Lateral wall compressed

Apex "sucked" up & slightly rotated

Head

Figure 5.1 • A Stabilizer Device Used for Off-Pump Coronary Revascularization. A combination of suction (applied to the cardiac apex) and stabilization (applied at the anastomotic site; here at the lateral wall of the heart) provides an immobile and bloodless field.

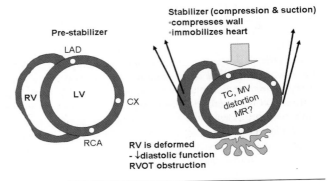

Pre-stabilizer

LAD

RV   LV   CX

RCA

Stabilizer (compression & suction)
•compresses wall
•immobilizes heart

TC, MV distortion MR?

RV is deformed
- ↓diastolic function
RVOT obstruction

Figure 5.2 • The stabilizer device pushes on the left ventricular (*LV*) wall, restricts local motion, and decreases LV dimensions; their contribution to SV is predominant. Compression of the anterior and lateral walls has more serious hemodynamic consequences than compression of the inferior (posterior) wall. The most profound disturbances are observed during lateral wall exposure for anastomosis on the left circumflex coronary artery (*CX*). LAD, left anterior descending coronary artery; MR, mitral regurgitation; MV, mitral valve; RCA, right coronary artery; RV, right ventricle; RVOT, right ventricular outflow obstruction; TC, tricuspid valve.

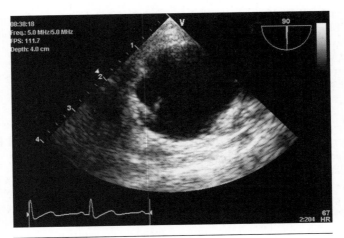

Figure 5.3 • Upper esophageal short axis view of the aortic arch demonstrating a protruding atheroma (grade V) at 7 o'clock.

exposure of the heart is necessary for internal defibrillation or when cardioversion is limited.[1] For this particular patient, intra-operative transesophageal echocardiography (TEE) would allow not only monitoring of volume status and evaluation of cardiac performance, but also examination of the aorta for the presence of atheromas. When interpreting hemodynamic data, the position of the heart must be taken into account. Surgical manipulation of the heart changes its relationship to the ECG electrodes, making it difficult to interpret the ST segments. Similarly, surgical maneuvers affect pulmonary artery catheter readings. Distortion of the heart, particularly verticalization, causes elevations in right atrial and pulmonary wedge pressures[8]. The vertical position of the heart, along with the interposition of air between the heart and esophagus, reduces the quality of TEE images during OPCAB procedures. However, most TEE images remain interpretable and are extremely valuable in the diagnosis of new regional wall motion abnormalities, ventricular function, and volume status.

What is the best anesthetic plan for this patient?

Most commonly, a conventional general anesthetic technique is used during OPCAB procedures.[1] Because the postoperative course is accelerated in the majority of OPCAB patients, the anesthetic technique should be tailored to facilitate early tracheal extubation. The agents' duration of action should be considered when choosing opioids, neuromuscular blockers, and hypnotics. Additionally, every effort should be made to avoid hypothermia. Room temperature should be maintained around 24°C, fluids should be warmed, and a heat-moisture exchanger should be included in the ventilator circuit. New generations of circulating water warming mattresses might minimize heat loss. Forced air warmers can be used when saphenous vein harvest is not performed (or after completion). In some centers, thoracic epidural anesthesia/analgesia is used as an adjunct to general anesthesia. Epidural anesthesia reduces myocardial oxygen demand and increases supply by dilating epicardial vessels and improving collateral blood flow. The routine use of antifibrinolytics is not recommended during OPCAB, because of the potential trend toward a hypercoagulable state. "Full heparinization," with an activated clotting time (ACT) above 400 seconds, is not required during OPCAB procedures because patients are not exposed to the foreign surface of the bypass circuit. However, the patient's coagulation system will be activated by local vascular endothelial injury.[6] Therefore, some degree of anticoagulation is required. Heparin in a dose of 100 to 200 units per kilogram is given before dissection of the LIMA targeting an ACT of 250 to 300 seconds.

Can anesthetic management affect patient outcome after OPCAB?

After the LIMA is harvested, the target coronary arteries are prepared for distal anastomoses. The risk of myocardial ischemia is greatest during anastomosis of the least collateralized vessel, whereas highly collateralized vessels are less at risk.[5] The most stenotic artery is therefore usually the first vessel to be revascularized. Before performing the anastomosis, the surgeon may induce a short period of myocardial ischemia by temporarily occluding the target vessel with an elasticized

suture and then allowing the myocardium to be reperfused. This step is believed to induce ischemic preconditioning, in which the myocardium may build up a tolerance to subsequent ischemia. Additionally, the use of volatile anesthetic agents 30 minutes before vessel occlusion may protect the myocardium against ischemia via anesthetic preconditioning. Early clinical data in patients undergoing CABG surgery, however, suggest that high concentrations (2 MAC) of volatile anesthetics are needed to significantly reduce troponin I release.[4] While the coronary artery is occluded, a favorable myocardial oxygen balance is essential. β-Blockers and calcium-channel antagonists are used to decrease heart rate and myocardial contractility, thereby decreasing myocardial oxygen consumption. Vasopressors, such as phenylephrine and norepinephrine, are used to maintain oxygen supply by increasing coronary perfusion pressure. In most patients, a mean arterial pressure of 70 mm Hg or higher is adequate to preserve coronary flow. It is important to remember that, once the target vessel is opened, the surgical anastomosis must be completed despite any hemodynamic derangements. The surgeon might consider placing a temporary coronary artery shunt.

What hemodynamic changes should the anesthesiologist be prepared to treat/prevent?

During coronary artery bypass graft anastomosis, the anesthesiologist must manage the hemodynamic changes caused by distortion of the heart. During vertical displacement, the ventricles become positioned above the atria; TEE may reveal an increase in atrial size and a decrease in ventricular size (Fig. 5.4). Because blood must now flow against gravity and resistance, atrial filling pressures must be maintained at a higher level to preserve ventricular filling. In addition, the

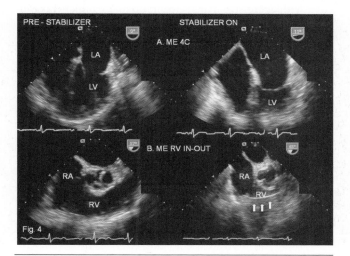

Figure 5.4 • Cardiac chamber compression with application of a stabilizer device (STABILIZER ON) for off-pump coronary artery bypass. **(A)** In the midesophageal four-chamber (ME 4C) view, application of the stabilizer device results in compression of the left ventricular (*LV*) cavity and elongation of the left atrium (*LA*). **(B)** The right ventricle (*RV*) is compressed during application of the stabilizer for construction of the right coronary arterial bypass graft. Notice the near elimination of the RV cavity at end-diastole (*arrows*). RA, right atrium.

heart may be compressed within the chest during vertical and lateral displacement. The right ventricle may become wedged between the left ventricle and the right pericardium, and complete right ventricular outflow obstruction may occur. Volume loading and Trendelenburg positioning serve to increase preload. The surgeon may release the right pericardium to allow adequate space for the right ventricle during this maneuver. Manipulating the heart's position may cause mitral regurgitation. Rotation and verticalization of the heart distorts the mitral valve annulus, causing it to twist and fold over on itself.[3] TEE evaluation may reveal new (or more severe) regurgitation. Large "V" waves may appear on the pulmonary artery catheter tracing. Abnormal mitral valves are more prone to distortion and are more likely to become functionally stenotic during cardiac manipulations for OPCAB. This phenomenon is also seen with distortion of the tricuspid valve and less often with the aortic valve. Stabilizing the epicardium during coronary artery anastomosis causes local distortion of the ventricle. The immobilizing device pushes on the myocardium and restricts wall motion. Because the anterior and lateral walls supply a major portion of stroke volume, their compression causes more severe reduction in cardiac output than when other portions of the ventricle are compressed. The most extreme hemodynamic compromise occurs during CX anastomosis, in which the heart is significantly elevated and perfusion of the lateral wall is compromised. Bradycardia is common during surgical manipulation, particularly during RCA anastomosis. Complete atrioventricular block can occur. The surgeon should consider placing temporary pacemaker wires before occluding the RCA. Additionally, a defibrillator/cardioverter should be available for the treatment of malignant arrhythmias.

What are the indications for conversion to CPB?

Even with aggressive management, up to 5% of patients cannot tolerate the hemodynamic alterations caused by OPCAB. A cardiac index <1.5 liters/minute per m^2, mean arterial pressure <50 mm Hg, or a mixed venous saturation <60% may not be tolerated for more than 15 minutes. Persistent ST elevations >2 mm or malignant ventricular arrhythmias also indicate the need for conversion from an OPCAB to surgery using CPB.[12] A "dry" CPB machine, as well as a perfusion team, should be available during all OPCAB procedures.

What hemodynamic abnormalities occur after reperfusion of the bypassed vessel?

Reperfusion injury may produce significant ECG changes, such as T-wave inversions or arrhythmias, during the first 30 minutes after coronary revascularization. Ventricular function should be evaluated after reperfusion with TEE. Persistent regional wall motion abnormalities predict poor postoperative outcome. Signs of continuing regional ischemia or poor flow through the bypass graft should prompt surgical intervention.

Should heparin be reversed at the end of the case?

Because patients are not fully heparinized during OPCAB procedures, protamine reversal is not always required. Some institutions believe that the risk of a hypercoagulable state

after OPCAB might increase the risk for early bypass graft thrombosis. Most centers, however, use protamine to reduce the risk of postoperative bleeding and transfusions.

Are patient outcomes affected by undergoing OPCAB versus on-pump CABG procedures?

In the immediate postoperative period, OPCAB patients experience a slightly accelerated recovery. They generally have less postoperative bleeding and receive fewer blood transfusions.[10] Preserving pulsatile blood flow, as well as avoiding hypothermia during OPCAB procedures might further contribute to accelerated recovery. The duration of hospitalization in the intensive care unit, as well as the overall hospital length of stay, is shortened with OPCAB surgery compared with traditional CABG surgery.[9,11] Hospital costs are therefore lower in the OPCAB patients. At 1 year, coronary angiography has demonstrated similar graft patency rates in OPCAB and on-pump CABG patients when experienced surgeons perform the surgery.[9,11] Five years postoperatively, rates of myocardial infarction, repeat coronary revascularization, stroke, and mortality are similar in both groups.[13] In low-risk patients, rates of neurocognitive dysfunction are similar in both OPCAB and on-pump patients. However, patients at high risk for poor neurologic outcome may benefit from OPCAB procedures.[7]

KEY MESSAGES

1. Patients with severe atherosclerosis of the ascending aorta benefit from OPCAB because aortic cross clamping is not necessary.

2. During OPCAB, "full" heparinization (ACT >400 seconds) is not required because patients are not exposed to the foreign surface of the CPB circuit. However, the patient's coagulation system will be activated by local vascular endothelial injury. Therefore, some degree of anticoagulation is required. Heparin in a dose of 100 to 200 units per kilogram is given before dissecting the LIMA targeting an ACT of 250 to 300 seconds.

3. Following OPCAB, persistent regional wall motion abnormalities are predictive of poor postoperative outcome.

4. Five years postoperatively, rates of myocardial infarction, repeat coronary revascularization, stroke, and mortality are similar among patients who undergo CABG on or off bypass.

QUESTIONS

1. What surgical approaches are used to perform OPCAB?

Answer: There are two: (a) the MIDCAB approach involves a small left thoracotomy incision, through which the LIMA is anastomosed to the target vessel (usually the LAD) and (b) the typical OPCAB in which multiple

CABGs are constructed is performed via a median sternotomy.

2. What is the role of antifibrinolytic therapy in OPCAB?

Answer: The routine use of antifibrinolytics is not recommended during OPCAB, because of the potential trend toward a hypercoagulable state.

3. How does OPCAB compare with CABG with CPB in terms of graft patency?

Answer: At 1 year, coronary angiography has demonstrated similar graft patency rates in OPCAB and on-pump CABG patients when surgery is performed by experienced surgeons.

References

1. Chassot PG, van der Linden P, Zaugg M, et al. Off-pump coronary artery bypass surgery: physiology and anaesthetic management. Br J Anaesth 2004; 92:400–413.
2. Gayes JM. The minimally invasive cardiac surgery voyage. J Cardiothorac Vasc Anesth 1999;13:119–122.
3. George SJ, Al-Ruzzeh S, Amrani M, et al. Mitral annulus distortion during beating heart surgery: a potential cause for hemodynamic disturbance—a three-dimensional echocardiography reconstruction study. Ann Thorac Surg 2002;73:1424–1430.
4. Julier K, da Silva R, Garcia C, et al. Preconditioning by sevoflurane decreases biochemical markers for myocardial and renal dysfunction in coronary artery bypass graft surgery: a double-blinded, placebo-controlled, multicenter study. Anesthesiology 2003;98:1415–1427.
5. Koh TW, Carr-White GS, DeSouza C, et al. Effect of coronary occlusion on left ventricular function with and without collateral supply during beating heart coronary artery surgery. Heart 1999;81:285–291.
6. Mariani MA, Gu J, Boonstra PW, et al. Procoagulant activity after off-pump coronary operation: is the current anticoagulation adequate? Ann Thorac Surg 1999;67:1370–1375.
7. Mark DB, Newman MF. Protecting the brain in coronary artery bypass graft surgery. JAMA 2002;287:1448–1450.
8. Mishra M, Malhotra R, Mishra A, et al. Hemodynamic changes during displacement of the beating heart using epicardial stabilization for off-pump coronary artery bypass graft surgery. J Cardiothorac Vasc Anesth 2002;16:685–690.
9. Nathoe HM, van Dijk D, Jansen EWL, et al. A comparison of on-pump and off-pump coronary bypass surgery in low-risk patients. NEJM 2003;348:394–402.
10. Nuttall GA, Erchul DT, Haight TJ, et al. A comparison of bleeding and transfusion in patients who undergo coronary artery bypass grafting via sternotomy with and without cardiopulmonary bypass. J Cardiothorac Vasc Anesth 2003;17:447–451.
11. Puskas JD, Williams WH, Duke PG, et al. Off-pump vs conventional coronary artery bypass grafting: early and 1-year graft patency, cost and quality-of-life outcomes. JAMA 2004;291:1841–1849.
12. Raja SG, Dreyfus GD. Off-pump coronary artery bypass surgery: to do or not to do? Current best available evidence. J Cardiothorac Vasc Anesth 2004;18:486–505.
13. Van Dijk D, Spoor M Hijman R, et al. Cognitive and cardiac outcomes 5 years after off-pump vs on-pump coronary artery bypass graft surgery. JAMA 2007;297:701–708.

CHAPTER 6

Aprotinin and Antifibrinolytics in Cardiac Surgery

Michelle Isac

CASE FORMAT: STEP BY STEP

A 79-year-old, 62-kg (body mass index, 22) female presented to the emergency department with severe chest pain and new ST-segment elevation in the inferior leads. She was referred for urgent cardiac catheterization. Angiography confirmed complete occlusion of the right coronary artery (RCA) as well as significant disease of the circumflex artery. The culprit RCA lesion was not amenable to percutaneous coronary intervention (PCI), and the patient was referred for urgent coronary artery bypass grafting (CABG).

Two years before this admission, the patient had undergone a PCI of the left anterior descending (LAD) artery with a drug-eluting stent. Her other medical history includes hypertension and hyperlipidemia for which she was receiving metoprolol and simvastatin. She is also receiving clopidogrel and aspirin since her PCI 2 years ago. Her temperature is 36.9°C; blood pressure, 135/76 mm Hg; heart rate, 65 beats per minute; and her respiratory rate, 18 breaths per minute. The patient's preoperative hemoglobin is 12.6 g/dL, platelet count, 253,000; international normalized ratio, 1.1; and prothrombin time, 29 seconds. Electrolytes, blood urea nitrogen, and creatinine are normal.

Why is cardiac surgery associated with bleeding?

Surgery involving cardiopulmonary bypass (CPB) is associated with complex alterations to the hemostatic system resulting from hypothermia, hemodilution of hemostatic factors, consumption of coagulation factors caused by ongoing thrombin generation, fibrinolysis, platelet consumption and dysfunction, inadequate reversal of heparin, and heparin rebound after its reversal with protamine. In addition, the increasing use of newer anticoagulants such as low-molecular-weight heparins, direct thrombin inhibitors (e.g., hirudin, bivalirudin) and antiplatelet drugs (e.g., glycoprotein IIa/IIIb antagonist, clopidogrel) in patients presenting for cardiac surgery contributes to surgical bleeding.

Is this patient at high risk for perioperative bleeding?

This patient's history suggests that she is at risk for perioperative bleeding. The continued use of clopidogrel is associated with higher rates of bleeding compared with patients not receiving antiplatelet drugs. Several studies have tried to establish risk factors associated with nonsurgical bleeding after cardiac surgery to stratify patients and anticipate adverse outcomes. Identified risk factors include advanced age, female gender, nonelective cases, reoperation, complex surgeries, and smaller body mass index. Prolonged duration of CPB and surgery as well as persistent postoperative hypothermia are further key risk factors.

Before beginning the procedure, the cardiac surgeon, cardiac anesthesiologist, and perfusionist discuss their plans and concerns for this patient. They all agree that this patient is at high risk for perioperative bleeding and that there is a high likelihood that she will need transfusion of platelets after CPB because of her recent use of antiplatelet drugs. The blood bank is alerted to ensure that an adequate supply of packed red blood cells, fresh frozen plasma, and platelets is available.

Why is prevention of bleeding important in cardiac surgery?

Perioperative bleeding results in risk for blood transfusion and re-exploration of the mediastinum because of continued bleeding or tamponade. Perioperative bleeding further results in transfusion of packed red blood cells and hemostatic factors. Blood transfusion is associated with infectious and noninfectious complications. The risk for viral transmission from massive transfusion has markedly decreased as a result of improved screening methods, although the risk for transmission of infectious agents persists (particularly, hepatitis C). Transmission of bacterial pathogens from packed red blood cells, and particularly platelet transfusion, is a higher risk than viral transmission. Other pertinent risks associated with blood transfusion include transfusion-related acute lung injury, volume overload, and hemolytic and nonhemolytic transfusion reactions. Further, limited supply of blood products necessitates that strategies be implemented to minimize transfusions.

What is the incidence of reoperation in cardiac surgery, and what are its associated risks?

Resternotomy for postoperative bleeding is required in approximately 3% to 6% of cardiac surgical patients. The need for emergency mediastinal re-exploration is associated with increased length of intensive care unit stay, increased requirements for intra-aortic balloon counterpulsation, and increased mortality. Not surprisingly, many of the risk factors for resternotomy following cardiac surgery are the same as the risk factors identified for increased bleeding.

The surgical team has discussed blood conservation strategies for this patient, including the use of antifibrinolytic agents.

What pharmacologic approaches can be employed to reduce bleeding and transfusion requirements?

Fibrinolysis is an important contributor to nonsurgical bleeding after cardiac surgery leading to not only breakdown of thrombus but also further consumption of hemostatic factors. The main pharmacologic treatment for preventing excessive bleeding during cardiac surgery is antifibrinolytic drugs such as tranexamic acid (TXA), epsilon-aminocaproic acid (EACA), and aprotinin. EACA and TXA are synthetic derivatives of the amino acid lysine. Lysine analogs inhibit the process of fibrinolysis by adhering to the lysine-binding site on plasminogen. Binding by lysine is required for the conversion of plasminogen to plasmin. Therefore, binding by these lysine analogs inhibits the formation of plasmin. Normally, plasmin causes fibrinolysis (lysis of clot) by degrading fibrin and fibrinogen. Not only is less plasmin generated, but existing plasmin is also inactivated. In contrast, aprotinin is a serione protease inhibitor which inhibits several important enzymes including plasmin and kallikrein. The exact mechanisms of aprotinin's action, however, are not completely understood.

What is the evidence for the efficacy of antifibrinolytic drugs?

Several prospectively randomized, double-blind, placebo-controlled trials have been performed evaluating the efficacy of antifibrinolytics in cardiac surgery to reduce bleeding and blood transfusion. Many studies have been small, particularly those evaluating lysine analogs and those performing head-to-head comparisons of all three agents. Aprotinin has been the most well-studied agent. Several adequately powered, multicenter studies have established the efficacy of aprotinin to reduce bleeding, blood transfusion, and mediastinal re-exploration for bleeding after cardiac surgery compared with placebo, particularly for complex cardiac surgeries or reoperations. These studies supported approval of aprotinin by the U.S. Food and Drug Administration for the indication of reducing bleeding during cardiac surgery.

Similar robust data are not present for TXA or EACA. Nonetheless, multiple studies have reported the efficacy of these agents to reduce bleeding complications of cardiac surgery. These data have been subjected to meta-analysis to enhance the power of the multiple small studies. A recent Cochrane review of antifibrinolytic drugs evaluated 51 trials showing that aprotinin use led to less chest tube drainage, fewer blood transfusions, and less need for reoperation for bleeding compared with placebo. Studies comparing TXA with placebo have also shown decreased requirement for blood product administration and mediastinal drainage but not mediastinal reexploration for bleeding. These results suggest that TXA results in savings of approximately one unit of allogeneic blood from being transfused compared with placebo. The amount of blood loss was reduced by approximately 300 mL with TXA use. Risk for reoperation was not affected by TXA. The small number of studies examining EACA in cardiac surgery has shown that its use was associated with a relative 35% reduction in the need for allogeneic blood transfusion. The use of EACA resulted in a blood loss reduction of approximately 230 mL (intraoperatively) and 200 mL (postoperatively). Studies directly comparing EACA to TXA showed little difference between the two agents in terms of volume of blood transfused or reoperation for bleeding.

The cardiac anesthesiologist expressed concern about the safety of antifibrinolytics but agreed that the benefits in this high-risk patient likely outweighed the risks.

What are the risks associated with antifibrinolytics in cardiac surgery?

Although the efficacy of aprotinin and the lysine analogs have been established, the safety of these agents in high-risk patients is more controversial. The safety of aprotinin, in particular, has been the focus of debate. Prospectively randomized, placebo-controlled studies have supported this agent's safety. These data, in fact, suggest aprotinin use was associated with a lowered risk for perioperative stroke compared with placebo. Aprotinin use is associated with a transient increase in serum creatinine that might reflect its effect on the proximal renal tubules. Because it is a bovine protein, allergic reactions to aprotinin are an established risk including fatal anaphylactic reactions. This risk has led to the use of a test dose, which can also trigger a severe response. Recent exposure (less than 1 year) is known to increase the likelihood of suffering from hypersensitivity reactions. For this reason, it is recommended that aprotinin should be used in settings where CPB can be established quickly.

Considering the mechanism of action of antifibrinolytic agents, it seems logical to expect they may increase the risk of thrombotic complications of surgery. The meta-analysis by the Cochrane Collaboration (which analyzed 211 randomized controlled trials) did not show increased risk of mortality, stroke, myocardial infarction, or deep vein thrombosis with aprotinin, TXA, or EACA. There was an increased trend toward renal dysfunction in the group receiving aprotinin, but this was not statistically significant.

The use of drugs during the well-controlled setting of a clinical trial might not adequately represent their safety profile compared with their widespread clinical use after approval. Of particular concern is attention to anticoagulation. Aprotinin prolongs the celite activated clotting time (ACT) regardless of the appropriate heparinization level. The use of a kaolin-based ACT, thus, is necessary when aprotinin is used and/or targeting higher levels of the ACT during surgery (>750 s). Moreover, in the "real world," other hemostatic agents might be coadministered with aprotinin in bleeding patients. The combined use of lysine analogs with aprotinin can result in intense inhibition of fibrinolysis. Further, the use of recombinant factor VIIa with aprotinin might promote prothrombotic complications. The safety of aprotinin was recently questioned in a recent retrospective analysis of data obtained in a multicenter study. This analysis suggested that patients receiving aprotinin during cardiac surgery had a higher risk for myocardial infarction, stroke, renal dysfunction, and death compared with lysine analog antifibrinolytics. The retrospective study design cannot exclude treatment bias whereby patients given aprotinin were at a higher risk for adverse outcomes regardless of antifibrinolytic treatment. Further, analysis of other large mostly single-center databases has not confirmed these findings.

At this time, a large prospectively randomized, double-blinded multicenter trial comparing aprotinin, TXA, and EACA in patients undergoing cardiac surgery was halted because of higher rates of adverse events in the aprotinin group. The details of this trial are pending. Nonetheless, in light of these recent developments and on the basis of other data reported from analysis of outcomes from a large administrative database, the U.S. Food and Drug Administration has requested a marketing suspension of aprotinin until the data can be reviewed.

> After discussing all the options, the surgical team decided that TXA would be used for this procedure. The patient had an otherwise uneventful procedure receiving two saphenous vein bypass grafts to the circumflex and right coronary arteries. The duration of CPB was 36 minutes, and aortic cross-clamp time was 58 minutes. Heparin was adequately reversed with protamine with a final ACT of 121 seconds. After ample surgical hemostasis was achieved, the sternum was closed, and the patient was brought to the cardiac surgical intensive care unit. Chest tube output was closely monitored for 24 hours with only minimal drainage. The patient was discharged home on postoperative day 5 following an uncomplicated recovery.

KEY MESSAGES

1. The main pharmacologic treatment for preventing excessive bleeding during cardiac surgery is antifibrinolytic drugs such as TXA, EACA, and aprotinin.

2. Lysine analogs inhibit the process of fibrinolysis by adhering to the lysine-binding site on plasminogen.

3. Aprotinin is a serine protease inhibitor inhibiting several important enzymes including plasmin and kallikrein.

4. The safety of aprotinin was recently questioned in a recent retrospective data analysis obtained in a multicenter study. This analysis suggested that patients receiving aprotinin during cardiac surgery had a higher risk for myocardial infarction, stroke, renal dysfunction, and death compared with lysine analog antifibrinolytics.

QUESTIONS

1. **What is the incidence of reoperation in cardiac surgery?**

   Answer: Resternotomy for postoperative bleeding is required in approximately 3% to 6% of cardiac surgical patients.

2. **What is the principal mechanism of action of EACA?**

   Answer: EACA is a synthetic derivative of the amino acid lysine. Lysine analogs inhibit the process of fibrinolysis by adhering to the lysine binding site on plasminogen.

3. **Is aprotinin nephrotoxic?**

   Answer: Aprotinin use is associated with transient increase in serum creatinine levels that might reflect its effect on the proximal renal tubules.

References

1. Henry DA, Charles PA, Moxey AJ, et al. Anti-fibrinolytic use for minimizing perioperative allogeneic blood transfusion. Cochrane Database Syst Rev 2007(4):CD001886.
2. Karthik S, Grayson AD, McCarron EE, et al. Re-exploration for bleeding after coronary artery bypass surgery: risk factors, outcomes, and the effect of time delay. Ann Thorac Surg 2004;78:527–534.
3. Mangano DT, Tudor IC, Dietzel C. The risk associated with aprotinin in cardiac surgery. N Engl J Med 2006;354:353–365.
4. Mannucci PM, Levi M. Prevention and treatment of major blood loss. N Engl J Med 2007; 356:2301–2311.
5. Dietrich W, Busley R, Boulesteix A. Effects of aprotinin dosage on renal function. Anesthesiology 2008;108:189–198.
6. Hogue CW, London MJ. Aprotinin use during cardiac surgery: a new or continuing controversy? Anesth Analg 2006;103:1067–1070.
7. Despotis GJ, Hogue CW Jr. Pathophysiology, prevention and treatment of bleeding after cardiac surgery: a primer for cardiologist and an update for the cardiothoracic team. Am J Cardiol 1999;83:15B–30B.

CHAPTER 7

The Use of Recombinant Factor VIIa in Cardiac Surgery

Jay K. Levin

CASE FORMAT: REFLECTION

A 73-year-old female presented for aortic and mitral valve replacement surgery. Over the previous 6 months, she had noticed increasing dyspnea with activity and occasional chest pain. Preoperative echocardiography demonstrated severe aortic stenosis and moderate-to-severe mitral regurgitation. Ten years previously, she had undergone uncomplicated coronary bypass grafting. Recent coronary angiography demonstrated that her bypass grafts were patent and that no new significant coronary artery stenosis had developed. After an otherwise uncomplicated operation and separation from cardiopulmonary bypass (CPB), significant bleeding occurred despite having achieved her baseline-activated clotting time by protamine administration. No obvious cause of surgical bleeding was evident. Although the patient remained hemodynamically stable, blood drained continuously from the chest tube even after administering four units of fresh frozen plasma. The anesthesiologist considered administration of recombinant factor VIIa (rFVIIa).

DISCUSSION

Often multifactorial, postbypass coagulopathy presents a challenge in managing cardiac surgical patients especially after "re-do surgery" (with repeat sternotomy) or prolonged CPB.[1] Causative factors include preoperative antiplatelet therapy, residual heparin effect, hypothermia, a relative and absolute decrease in platelet number and function, fibrinolysis, and a decrease in coagulation factors and function.

What is the initial management of post-CPB bleeding?

Management of excessive bleeding after CPB requires an evaluation of the cause(s) including those of surgical origin. Immediate responses include management of hypothermia and/or administration of additional protamine as indicated (by temperature and activated clotting time measurement, respectively). Estimation of platelet count and performing coagulation studies are indicated. On-site coagulation testing such as thromboelastography provides a relatively fast and reliable, but nonspecific, assessment of coagulation status including coagulation factor deficiency, platelet dysfunction, and fibrinolysis.

Mechanism of Action of rFVIIa

In 1988, rFVIIa was administered to a patient with hemophilia A undergoing synovectomy.[2] Patients with hemophilia exposed to allogenic blood factors often have inhibitory antibodies to coagulation factors VIII and IX, limiting their effectiveness in the treatment of acute hemorrhage. FVIIa combines with tissue factor released by injured cells and initiates fibrin formation by activating factors IX and X.[3] When administered in doses that achieve supraphysiologic concentrations, rFVIIa can increase thrombin synthesis directly, and the resulting products are particularly resistant to degradation by plasmin.[4]

What are the Indications for rFVIIa?

The current approved indications for administering rFVIIa include the treatment of bleeding in hemophiliac patients with inhibitors to factor VIII, congenital factor VII deficiency, and Glanzmann's thrombasthenia. rFVIIa has been used off-label for excessive nonsurgical bleeding after trauma, liver resection and transplant, prostatectomy, intra-abdominal hemorrhage, intracerebral hemorrhage, and cardiac surgery.

Off-label administration of rFVIIa to cardiac surgical patients?

The widespread administration of rFVIIa to patients undergoing cardiac surgery[5–10] is based on early case reports showing remarkable reduction in bleeding after CPB following complicated coronary artery bypass grafting, ventricular assist device placement, and repeat sternotomy. One case report described the use of rFVIIa to reverse lepirudin anticoagulation following CPB for a patient with a history of heparin-induced thrombocytopenia. Another case report described administration of rFVIIa following CPB in a patient with a history of anaphylactic reaction to protamine. Several retrospective studies have shown rFVIIa to be efficacious in managing refractory bleeding post-CPB, decreasing blood loss, normalizing coagulation factors, and decreasing the need for further blood product administration. One case series showed an immediate decrease in postoperative bleeding but no change in the volume of allogenic blood transfused during the first 24 hours postoperatively.

The currently available prospective, randomized, placebo-controlled trials of rFVIIa after cardiac surgery are limited by small numbers of patients studied. In a study of 10 patients undergoing complex cardiac surgery with CPB, the use of rFVIIa was shown to decrease transfusion of allogenic blood products and a tendency toward reduced blood loss. Aprotinin was administered to both groups of patients. In a study evaluating pediatric cardiac surgical patients, rFVIIa failed to decrease blood loss or transfusion requirements. Thus, a large prospective, randomized, placebo-controlled trial examining the efficacy of rFVIIa to decrease bleeding and blood transfusion after cardiac surgery is needed.

The optimal dose of rFVIIa to decrease bleeding while not increasing the risk of adverse events is yet to be elucidated. Reported doses range from 25 to 195 μg/kg (90 μg/kg is used most commonly). rFVIIa, 40 μg/kg, was successful in stabilizing uncontrolled bleeding after cardiac surgery.[8] A dose-finding study for rFVIIa in this setting is also required.

Risk of Thromboembolic Events

Prothrombotic adverse effects are the major concern with the use of rFVIIa. In low concentrations, rFVIIa activates thrombin formation at sites of tissue factor exposure. At greater concentrations, generated thrombin can diffuse from the sites of vascular injury and could initiate intravascular thrombosis. Normally, naturally occurring anticoagulant proteins such as antithrombin III inactivate excessive thrombin formation. After acute illness or surgery with CPB, however, antithrombin III concentrations are decreased, predisposing to intravascular thrombosis.

Several of the retrospective studies and prospective, randomized, blinded, placebo-controlled studies that reported on the efficacy of rFVIIa for excessive bleeding after cardiac surgery reported safety end points, showing no increase in thromboembolic events. Two case reports (patients with hemophilia after lung transplantation) describe likely thrombotic events in patients receiving rFVIIa. Thus the safety of rFVIIa when used in the setting of perioperative bleeding has not been established.

KEY MESSAGES

1. Nonsurgical bleeding after cardiac surgery is usually multifactorial in origin.

2. When administered in doses that achieve supraphysiological concentrations, rFVIIa increases thrombin synthesis directly.

3. Currently approved indications for rFVIIa include the treatment of bleeding in patients with hemophilia with inhibitors to factor VIII, congenital factor VII deficiency, and Glanzmann's thrombasthenia.

4. The safety of rFVIIa in the setting of perioperative bleeding has not been established.

QUESTIONS

1. What is the physiologic role of FVII in coagulation?

Answer: In its activated form, FVIIa combines with tissue factor released by injured cells and initiates fibrin formation by activating factors IX and X.

2. What are the currently approved indications for administration of FVIIa?

Answer: Currently approved indications for rFVIIa include the treatment of bleeding in hemophiliac patients with inhibitors to factor VIII, congenital factor VII deficiency, and Glanzmann's thrombasthenia.

3. What dose of FVIIa might be administered to a patient bleeding excessively after cardiac surgery?

Answer: Reported doses range from 25 to 195 μg/kg; doses of 90 μg/kg have been used most commonly.

References

1. Marietta M, Facchini L, Pedrazzi P, et al. Pathophysiology of bleeding in surgery. Transplantation Proceedings 2006;38: 812–814.
2. Hedner U, Glazer S, Pingel K, et al. Successful use of recombinant factor VIIa in a patient with severe hemophilia A during synovectomy. Lancet 1988;2:1193.
3. Despotis GJ, Avidan MS, Hogue CW Jr. Mechanisms and attenuation of hemostatic activation during extracorporeal circulation. Ann Thorac Surg 2001;72(5):1821–1831.
4. Weiskopf RB. Recombinant-activated coagulation factor VIIa (NovoSeven®): current development. Vox Sanguinis 2007;92: 281–288.
5. Filsoufi F, Castillo JG, Rahmanian PB, et al. Effective management of refractory postcardiotomy bleeding with the use of recombinant activated factor VII. Ann Thorac Surg 2006;82:1779–1783.
6. Raivio P, Suojaranta-Ylinen R, Kuitunen AH. Recombinant factor VIIa in the treatment of postoperative hemorrhage after cardiac surgery. Ann Thoracic Surg 2005;80:66–71.
7. Heise D, Braeuer A, Quintel M. Recombinant activated factor VII (NovoSeven®) in patients with ventricular assist devices: case report and review of the literature. J Cardiothorac Surg2007;2:47.
8. van de Garde EMW, Bras LJ, Heijmen RH, et al. Low-dose recombinant factor VIIa in the management of uncontrolled postoperative hemorrhage in cardiac surgery patients. J Carthor Vasc Anes 2006;20:573–575.
9. von Heymann C, Redlich U, Jain U, et al. Recombinant activated factor VII for refractory bleeding after cardiac surgery—a retrospective analysis of safety and efficacy. Crit Care Med 2005;33:2241–2246.
10. Bishop CV, Renwick WEP, Hogan C, et al. Recombinant activated factor VII: treating postoperative hemorrhage in cardiac surgery. Ann Thorac Surg 2006;81:875–879.

CHAPTER 8

Postoperative Neuropathy After Cardiac Surgery

Ioanna Apostolidou and Jason S. Johnson

CASE FORMAT: REFLECTION

A 56-year-old, 112-kg, 170-cm male with three-vessel coronary artery disease, hypertension, and type 2 diabetes mellitus presented for coronary artery bypass grafting surgery. The patient's symptoms included chest pain with exertion that was relieved with rest. His current medications were metformin, lisinopril, and metoprolol. He was a nonsmoker, used alcohol socially, and was employed as a data analyst.

The patient's vital signs were as follows: temperature, 37.2°C; blood pressure, 142/86 mm Hg; heart rate, 64 beats per minute; and respiratory rate, 14 breaths per minute. Physical examination showed an obese male with clear bilateral breath sounds and a regular heart rate with no murmur. There was no carotid bruit.

Preoperative laboratory findings revealed normal chemistry, cholesterol, and blood cell counts. Preoperative electrocardiogram readings showed left ventricular hypertrophy but was otherwise normal. At stress exercise testing, significant ST depression occurred in the lateral leads, and subsequent coronary angiogram readings demonstrated 80% stenosis in the left anterior descending artery and 90% stenosis in the circumflex artery and right coronary artery. Ventricular function was normal as were valve anatomy and function.

After induction of anesthesia using etomidate, fentanyl, midazolam, and rocuronium, the patient's airway was secured with an endotracheal tube. A 20-gauge left radial arterial catheter was inserted. A pulmonary artery catheter was advanced in the pulmonary artery via a 9-F introducer sheath (multiaccess catheter) inserted in the right internal jugular vein under ultrasound guidance. The patient's arms were placed at his side in a neutral forearm position, and elbows, forearms, and hands were padded with foam pads. A balanced anesthesia technique was used for anesthesia maintenance with isoflurane, fentanyl, rocuronium, and midazolam.

The surgical technique entailed a median sternotomy with sternal retractors placed to facilitate left internal mammary artery dissection. Saphenous vein grafts were used for the remaining grafts. Total cardiopulmonary bypass time was 2 hours. The patient's heart function was restored without inotropic support, and separation from cardiopulmonary bypass was accomplished without difficulty. Intraoperative fluids consisted of one liter 5% albumin and three liters of Lactated Ringer's solution. The total operative time was 6 hours. The patient was brought to the intensive care unit and received a nitroglycerin infusion of 0.5 µg/kg per minute, while mechanical ventilation was maintained. No intraoperative complications were noted, and the patient's trachea was extubated 4 hours after admission to the intensive care unit.

On the first postoperative day, the patient complained of right-hand numbness and grip strength weakness. Upon further evaluation, sensory loss was detected at the ulnar side of the wrist as well as the dorsal and palmar surfaces of the fifth and medial half of the fourth finger. The patient's hand had a claw-shaped appearance at rest. Tests of motor function showed weakness of flexion of the second to fifth fingers. The appearance of the elbow was normal. An ulnar neuropathy was diagnosed. A physical therapist was consulted to evaluate the patient. By the third postoperative day, the patient had approximately 50% return of strength to the hand but continued to have numbness.

On the fifth postoperative day, the patient was referred to the neurology service for further evaluation. Electromyography (EMG) was performed and showed a pattern consistent with long-standing carpal tunnel compression. On further questioning, the patient recalled occasional numbness in his hands after working long hours at the computer. Over the course of 3 months, the patient's symptoms returned to their preoperative level, with full recovery of hand motor function; he was referred to a hand specialist for treatment of his carpal tunnel disease.

CASE DISCUSSION

Perioperative Peripheral Nerve Injury

Although peripheral nerve injury (PNI) is not a life-threatening complication, it can bring significant distress to the patient and anesthesia provider and can result in short-term, or rarely in long-term, disability. Consequently, PNI poses a major risk for medical practice liability. Perioperative nerve damage was the second major injury (16%) from the ASA Closed Claims Database following death (32%). Ulnar neuropathy is the most frequent nerve injury (28%) followed by brachial plexus (20%), lumbosacral (16%), and spinal cord (13%) neuropathies.[1,2]

The mechanism of perioperative neuropathies is incompletely understood. Although improper patient positioning causing nerve compression, stretching, and ischemia, direct trauma or metabolic derangements can lead to nerve injuries, in the majority of the reported cases, patient positioning is unrelated to the injury, and an explicit mechanism was not identified.[3–5]

PNI can present with sensory, motor, or mixed deficits of the area supplied by the affected nerve. Isolated sensory deficits are usually transient and typically resolve in days or weeks without any intervention. Motor deficits are more serious and the patient should be referred to a neurology department for further evaluation and management. Persistent sensory deficits lasting more than 5 days should also be referred to neurology.

Nerve conduction studies and EMG can help in defining the type of nerve injury (axonal, demyelination, or mixed), its distribution (proximal, distal, symmetric, asymmetric), and the severity and degree of motor or sensory involvement.[6]

Peripheral Nerve Injuries Following Cardiac Surgery

Various PNIs can be a complication of cardiac surgery.[7,8] Brachial plexus neuropathies, phrenic nerve injuries, saphenous neuropathy, recurrent laryngeal nerve injuries, sympathetic chain disturbance with resultant Horner's syndrome, and optic neuropathy have been described.

BRACHIAL PLEXUS

The frequency of brachial plexus injury is estimated at 2% to 18%. It is usually caused by stretching or trauma of the lower roots (C8-T1) resulting in ulnar neuropathy.[9] Excessive sternal opening and cephalad placement of the sternal retractor during sternotomy as well as asymmetric retraction during internal mammary artery dissection along with first rib fracture can cause compression and stretching of the brachial plexus (Fig. 8.1). More commonly, the plexus becomes stretched between a fixed position within its fascial plane and proximally fixed origins. Prolonged stretching of the plexus interferes with axonal transport and leads to transient neuropraxia. Somatosensory-evoked potential studies of the plexus demonstrated greater than 50% amplitude reduction after placement of sternal retractors.[10] Risk factors that may worsen the injury or lead to permanent symptoms include pre-existing neurologic injury such as cubital or carpal tunnel entrapment and advanced age. This scenario was described as the "double-crush" phenomenon in which two injuries to any single nerve will present with significant symptoms, whereas either injury by itself would be asymptomatic. Smoking, diabetes mellitus, height, and weight do not correlate well with risk. Male patients seem to be at a slightly greater risk than females to have permanent symptoms.[7,8] Symptoms vary with the location and severity of injury.

PHRENIC NERVE AND RECURRENT LARYNGEAL NERVE

Injury of the phrenic nerve and recurrent laryngeal nerve, respectively, are two well-known potential complications of cardiac surgery.[11,12] Topical hypothermia with ice slush and/or cardioplegia has been implicated as the principal cause. Sternal retraction, internal mammary artery harvesting, and central venous catheterization have been also related to nerve dysfunction. Unsuccessful attempts of transesophageal echocardiography probe placement have also been implicated in recurrent laryngeal nerve dysfunction. Phrenic neuropathy causing diaphragmatic dysfunction should be considered in

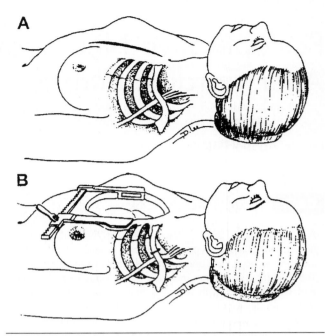

Figure 8.1 • **(A)** Normal course of the brachial plexus as it passes over the first rib. **(B)** Opening the sternum widely causes superior rotation of the first rib that pushes the clavicles into the retroclavicular space leading to stretching of the brachial plexus. (Reproduced with permission from Graham JG, Pye IF, McQueen IN. Brachial plexus injury after median sternotomy. Ann Thorac Surg 1971;4:315–319.)

patients unable to be weaned from mechanical ventilation after cardiac surgery. Similarly, recurrent laryngeal nerve injury may result in postoperative respiratory failure from vocal cord dysfunction. Radiography, ultrasonography, and EMG are currently used diagnostic techniques.

SAPHENOUS NERVE

Saphenous neuralgia can result from harvesting the saphenous vein.[13] Endoscopic vein harvesting techniques may reduce incisional pain, but the benefits on saphenous neuralgia need to be further explored.

OPTIC NERVE

Ischemia of the optic nerve resulting in visual deficits is an infrequent but serious complication of cardiac surgery. Prolonged hypotension, emboli, hemorrhage, and anemia can decrease perfusion to any component of the optical pathway from the retina to the occipital lobe.[2]

Central Venous Catheterization and Nerve Injury

Nerve injury is an infrequent complication of central venous cannulation (<1%). It is caused by direct nerve puncture or compression by a hematoma. Several cases of brachial plexus palsy, phrenic nerve, and recurrent laryngeal nerve injury have been reported after multiple attempts of internal jugular vein or subclavian vein catheterization. The use of ultrasound to facilitate central venous cannulation may reduce the frequency of nerve injury by decreasing the number of venipuncture attempts. The clinical benefits of ultrasound-guided cannulation are greater success rate, fewer attempts, and a lower rate of complications (primarily arterial punctures) when compared with the landmark method.[14] Ultrasound use should be considered in difficult cases such as in patients with distorted anatomy, obesity, and scars at the cannulation site.

Ulnar Neuropathy in Noncardiac Surgery

Ulnar neuropathy (UN) is the most frequent nerve injury reported in the ASA Closed Claims Database.[1] Compression injuries of the ulnar nerve result in immediate symptomatology; however, delayed onset of UN, usually 24 hours after surgery, supports a mechanism other than direct nerve compression as a primary cause in these cases.[5,15] The most common sites of injury are either at the elbow or higher in the brachial plexus course. UN can occur despite careful padding of the upper extremity. Risk factors associated with UN are male gender, body mass index extremes, and hospital stay duration. Symptoms of UN include sensory deficits in the ulnar and palmar aspect of the fifth and the medial half of the fourth digit, handgrip weakness, and fourth and fifth finger clawing from hand muscle imbalance. Pre-existing latent neuropathy conditions may predispose patients to a perioperative UN. This finding is supported by abnormal nerve conduction studies not only of the affected site but also of the contralateral site in a significant proportion of patients.

Prognosis of Peripheral Neuropathies After Cardiac Surgery

The outcome of peripheral neuropathies depends on the type and severity of injury. Most common deficits are transient with complete recovery within 6 to 8 weeks. Rarely, symptoms persist for more than 4 months with slow improvement over time.[7,8,16]

Prevention Strategies and Management of Perioperative Neuropathies

Preventing perioperative neuropathies is a very important part of perioperative care of all surgical patients. Proper patient positioning and padding to avoid direct compression or stretching of the peripheral nerve is of paramount importance especially for prolonged duration procedures. For the upper extremities, avoid pressure over the ulnar groove at the elbow and spiral groove of the humerus and avoid arm abduction greater than 90 degrees in a supine position. For the lower extremities, avoid overextension of the hamstring muscle and avoid pressure of the peroneal nerve at the fibula head. Place protective padding at the pressure nerve sites and use a chest roll in patients in the lateral decubitus position.[17] Peripheral nerve injuries identified in the postoperative period require prompt and thorough evaluation, complete documentation, and close monitoring. If symptoms are severe or persist beyond 1 week postoperatively, a neurologist should evaluate the patient. EMG studies may help to define the type and location of the nerve injury or may reveal a pre-existing condition.

KEY MESSAGES

1. Brachial plexus injuries commonly occur during cardiovascular surgery.

2. All PNIs should be followed closely and referred for further evaluation as appropriate.

3. The majority of PNIs have a good overall prognosis with complete resolution of symptoms within weeks or months of the injury.

4. EMG can identify pre-existing neuropathies if performed early in the evaluation of a perioperative injury.

QUESTIONS

1. Which neuropathies are most commonly encountered during the perioperative period?

   Answer: UN is the most frequently encountered nerve injury (28%) followed by brachial plexus (20%), lumbosacral (16%), and spinal cord (13%) neuropathies.[1,2]

2. Which PNIs are associated with cardiac surgery?

   Answer: Brachial plexus neuropathies, phrenic nerve injuries, saphenous neuropathy, recurrent laryngeal nerve injuries, sympathetic chain disturbance with resultant Horner's syndrome, and optic neuropathy have been described following cardiac surgery.

3. Which peripheral neuropathies are associated with central venous catheterization?

   Answer: Cases of brachial plexus palsy, phrenic nerve, and recurrent laryngeal nerve injury have been reported after multiple attempts at internal jugular vein or subclavian vein catheterization.

References

1. Cheney FW, Domino KB, Caplan RA, Posner KL. Nerve injury associated with anesthesia: a closed claims analysis. Anesthesiology 1999;90:1062–1069.

2. Miller's Anesthesia. 6th Ed. New York: Churchill Livingstone, 2005.

3. Winfree CJ, Kline DG. Intraoperative positioning nerve injuries. Surg Neurol 2005;63:5–18; discussion 18. Review.

4. Warner MA. Perioperative neuropathies. Mayo Clin Proc 1998; 73:567–574.

5. Warner MA, Warner ME, Martin JT. Ulnar neuropathy. Incidence, outcome, and risk factors in sedated or anesthetized patients. Anesthesiology 1994;81:1332–1340.

6. Gooch CL, Weimer LH. The electrodiagnosis of neuropathy: basic principles and common pitfalls. Neurol Clin 2007;25:1–28.

7. Sharma AD, Parmley CL, Sreeram G, et al. Peripheral nerve injuries during cardiac surgery: risk factors, diagnosis, prognosis, and prevention. Anesth Analg 2000; 91:1358–1369.

8. Grocott HP, Clark JA, Homi HM, et al. "Other" neurologic complications after cardiac surgery. Semin Cardiothorac Vasc Anesth 2004;8:213–226.

9. Unlu Y, Velioglu Y, Kocak H, et al. Brachial plexus injury following median sternotomy. Interact Cardiovasc Thorac Surg 2007;6:235–237.

10. Hickey C, Gugino LD, Aglio LS, et al. Intraoperative somato-sensory evoked potential monitoring predicts peripheral nerve injury during cardiac surgery. Anesthesiology 1993;78:29–35.
11. DeVita MA, Robinson LR, Rehder J, et al. Incidence and natural history of phrenic neuropathy occurring during open heart surgery. Chest 1993;103:850–856.
12. Dimopoulou I, Daganou M, Dafni U, et al. Phrenic nerve dysfunction after cardiac operations: electrophysiologic evaluation of risk factors. Chest 1998;113:8–14.
13. Mountney J, Wilkinson GA. Saphenous neuralgia after coronary artery bypass grafting. Eur J Cardiothorac Surg 1999; 16:440–443.
14. Randolph AG, Cook DJ, Gonzales CA. Ultrasound guidance for placement of central venous catheters: a meta-analysis of the literature. Crit Care Med 1996;24:2053–2058.
15. Prielipp RC, Morell RC, Butterworth J. Ulnar nerve injury and perioperative arm positioning. Anesthesiol Clin North Am 2002;20:589–603.
16. Ben-David B, Stahl S. Prognosis of intraoperative brachial plexus injury: a review of 22 cases. Br J Anaesth 1997;79:440–445.
17. Practice advisory for the prevention of perioperative peripheral neuropathies: a report by the American Society of Anesthesiologists Task Force on Prevention of Perioperative Peripheral Neuropathies. Anesthesiology 2000;92:1168–1182.

CHAPTER 9

Postoperative Visual Loss

Laurel E. Moore

CASE FORMAT: REFLECTION

A 57-year-old male with a history of prior lumbar fusion presented for spinal fusion from T12-L4. The patient's past medical history was significant for moderate obesity (body mass index, 30 kg m^2), type 2 diabetes, and well-controlled hypertension. The patient's physical activity was markedly limited by back pain, but recent cardiac testing revealed good left ventricular function and no evidence of myocardial ischemia. Preoperative laboratory data were within normal limits including a hematocrit level of 45%. The patient's preoperative vital signs included a blood pressure of 150/90 mm Hg, heart rate of 75 beats per minute, and oxygen saturation of 96% on room air.

The surgery was prolonged (8 hours) but without significant complications. Mean arterial pressure was maintained within 20% of baseline with the exception of one brief (10-minute) episode of hypotension (mean pressure <60 mm Hg) associated with significant bleeding. The patient's estimated blood loss was 3000 mL. The least recorded hematocrit level was 24%. Replacement fluids included four units packed red blood cells, 6000 mL crystalloid, and 500 mL hydroxyethyl starch. Shortly after extubation in the postanesthesia care unit, the patient complained that he could not see.

CASE DISCUSSION

Visual Loss After Spine Surgery

Postoperative visual loss (POVL) has historically been associated with cardiac surgery and more specifically, with cardiopulmonary bypass. The occurrence of POVL, although fortunately rare, appears to be increasing, particularly in patients undergoing spine surgery.[1] Although temporary postoperative visual changes can occur as a result of corneal abrasions or transient corneal edema from the prone position, true POVL in spine-injured patients has an incidence of 0.1% to 0.2%.[1,2] In 2006, the American Society of Anesthesiologists (ASA) published the findings from its POVL registry of 93 spine-injured patients[1] as well as a practice advisory for POVL for patients undergoing spine surgery.[3]

Relevant Anatomy of the Optic Nerve and Retina

The optic nerve can be described in four segments: (a) the intracranial segment (optic chiasm to the optic canal within the lesser sphenoid wing); (b) the intracanalicular segment (within the optic canal); (c) the posterior or intraorbital segment (optic foramen to the lamina cribrosa); and (d) the anterior or intraocular segment (from the lamina cribrosa to the optic disc). The lamina cribrosa is a perforated membrane overlying the posterior scleral foramen through which the optic nerve and central retinal artery and vein enter the eye.

The retina receives its blood supply from branches of the ophthalmic artery, which is the first branch of the intracranial internal carotid artery. Once the ophthalmic artery passes through the optic foramen, it branches into several vessels including the central retinal artery and a series of posterior ciliary arteries.[4] Both arterial systems are necessary for retinal function and as end vessels, there is the potential for watershed regions at risk for ischemia.[5] The intraorbital optic nerve is supplied by a pial plexus, which in turn, is supplied by branches of the central retinal artery and posterior ciliary arteries.[6] The most anterior portion of the optic nerve is supplied primarily by short posterior ciliary arteries and not the central retinal artery.[5] It is not clear that the blood supply to the optic nerve is autoregulated during episodes of increased intraocular pressure.[7]

Mechanism of Injury

The causes of POVL are multiple and include cerebral cortical infarction, pituitary apoplexy, direct injuries to the eye and visual tracts, and ischemic injuries to the optic nerve and/or retina. The most common of these are ischemic injuries to the visual tracts, which fall into two primary categories: central retinal artery occlusion (CRAO) and ischemic optic neuropathy (ION). ION can be further subdivided into posterior ischemic retinopathy (PION: optic nerve injury posterior to the lamina cribrosa) and anterior ischemic retinopathy (AION: optic nerve injury anterior to the lamina cribrosa). Because of the increasing incidence of blindness following spine surgery, POVL and more specifically, PION have drawn the attention of treating physicians, researchers, and the lay public. CRAO and ION will be discussed separately.

CRAO

CRAO generally presents with painless monocular visual loss following emergence from anesthesia. CRAO may be an important mechanism of POVL after cardiac surgery because of the risk of emboli to the central retinal artery (incidence as high as 4.5%[8]), although ION is also clearly a mechanism of POVL in this setting. It is less common than ION after spine surgery. On fundoscopic examination, patients classically demonstrate retinal pallor with a cherry-red spot at the macula. The pupillary light reflex is reduced or absent in the affected eye.

In terms of mechanism, CRAO can be embolic or effectively produced by increased intraocular pressure limiting perfusion pressure to the retina. Intraocular pressure has been shown to increase in patients in the prone position.[9,10] Perfusion pressure may be further reduced if the patient's orbit is compressed against a head holder (classically a horseshoe head holder) or some other object, the so-called head rest syndrome. Patients may present with marked orbital edema and limited extraocular movements (to complete ophthalmoplegia), as perfusion to the entire orbit including surrounding tissues and extraocular muscles may be compromised.

In the ASA visual loss registry,[1] 10 of 93 POVL patients undergoing spine surgery were determined to have CRAO. In contrast to the 83 patients with ION, the patients with CRAO were less likely to have been pinned using a Mayfield head holder (all were on head rests), procedures were shorter, and there was less blood loss. Furthermore, no patients with CRAO had bilateral injuries unlike 66% of ION patients. Whereas visual loss from CRAO is generally felt to have a better chance of visual recovery than ION, in the ASA registry, there was no difference in outcome between patients with CRAO and ION.

ION

Of the 131 reported cases of visual loss in the ASA POVL registry between 1999 and 2004, 93 (72%) were associated with spine surgery, and 83 (89% of all spine cases) were caused by ION.[1] Clearly, this number is increasing, but whether this is related to more complex surgical procedures, patient factors, or better recognition of POVL is unclear. In any case, ION is a devastating complication without clear etiology, making prevention a challenge for surgeons and anesthesiologists.

Patients with ION present with painless binocular or monocular visual loss, and the severity can range from a field cut to complete loss of light perception. The problem is generally recognized upon emergence from anesthesia but may be delayed for hours. Like CRAO, patients have a reduced or absent pupillary light reflex. External evidence of eye injury is generally absent. In patients with AION, the initial fundoscopic examination reveals an edematous disc, whereas with PION, the initial fundoscopic examination findings are generally normal. Over time, patients with both AION and PION will develop fundoscopic evidence of disc degeneration, and the likelihood of significant visual recovery is poor.

Although it appears easy to explain ION on the basis of vascular disease and reduced oxygen delivery to the optic nerve, the etiology is more complicated. There are reports of ION occurring in patients with normal intraoperative hematocrit levels and perfusion pressures.[11] There are also rare reports of children developing ION,[12] which would imply that there is a population of patients who may be at increased risk for ION based on the anatomy of the blood supply to the optic nerve or lack of autoregulation for this blood supply. In the ASA registry,[1] 66% of patients with ION had bilateral symptoms suggesting that the defect, whatever it is, is global in nature. Certainly, patients have suffered ION without evidence of ischemic injury to other vascular beds (kidney, heart), implying that the visual system may be particularly sensitive to changes in oxygen delivery.

A possible mechanism of ION is an orbital compartment syndrome in which the optic nerve is swollen as a result of increased venous pressure (prone position) or potentially large-volume crystalloid infusion causing tissue edema. This then causes the nerve to be compressed within its sheath or as it enters the orbital fossa or the eye itself.

Limited evidence indicates an association between sildenafil and ION, most commonly in males[13] but also in children.[14] One reference recommends the cessation of sildenafil at least 1 week preoperatively.[15]

Risk Factors for POVL

Although risk factors for atherosclerotic disease such as hypertension, diabetes, and smoking have been put forth as risk factors for POVL (and this certainly seems intuitive), the evidence is less clear. As stated previously, there are clearly certain individuals who for whatever reason are at risk for POVL, but preoperative identification of these individuals is currently not possible. Although intraoperative hypotension and anemia would also appear to place patients at risk for POVL, and these two factors are reported in multiple case reports, they are not necessarily supported by larger samplings. There are reports, however, of POVL improving postoperatively with blood transfusion in the case of anemia[16] and with increased blood pressure.[17]

The two factors that are consistently supported as risk factors for POVL in spine-injured patients include prolonged surgical procedures and large blood loss. In the ASA registry, these are defined as procedures lasting greater than 6 hours and a predicted blood loss of greater than 1 liter.[1] Of the 93 spine-injured patients with POVL, 94% of the procedures lasted 6 hours or longer. Similarly, 82% of POVL patients had an estimated blood loss of 1 liter or greater. It is interesting that despite the fact that women undergo more spinal procedures than men, 72% of cases in the registry were men.

Avoidance of POVL

As the etiologies of POVL are poorly understood, it is impossible to avoid this complication. However, there are a few clear preventive measures that may be taken. First, check the eyes of prone patients on a regular basis, at least every 15 minutes, to ensure that they are clear of pressure of any kind. Particularly for patients on head rests (as opposed to pins), proper initial positioning does not guarantee against subsequent head movement during surgery, causing the orbit to come into contact with the head holder. Furthermore, to optimize retinal or optic nerve perfusion pressure, whenever possible, the head position should be neutral and at or slightly above the level of the heart. In some patients with severe kyphoscoliosis, this optimal positioning may be impossible because of the fixed position of the head on the thorax.

The ASA practice advisory[3] was developed by a small task force of anesthesiologists, spine surgeons (both orthopedic and neurosurgical), and neuro-ophthalmologists who evaluated current data and surveyed practicing anesthesiologists and spine surgeons. The advisory was published to aid in clinical decision making and was not intended to be a formal guideline or standard of practice. Despite this, their review of the subject was comprehensive, and suggestions for care of spine-injured patients were thoughtful. A summary of their suggestions is as follows:

1. Although there are preoperative medical conditions such as anemia, atherosclerotic disease, and obesity, which *may*

be associated with POVL, at present, these cannot be considered predisposing conditions.

2. Factors that place patients as high risk for POVL include prolonged procedures (greater than 6.5 hours) and procedures involving large blood loss (average 45% of estimated blood volume).

3. Although there was agreement among consultants and subspecialty physicians that deliberate hypotension should be avoided in high-risk patients (with or without well-controlled hypertension), there was a split opinion whether induced hypotension should be used in patients without chronic hypertension. In the end, there were inadequate data to recommend against the use of deliberate hypotension. The advisory does recommend continuous blood pressure measurement in high-risk patients.

4. Regarding minimal acceptable hemoglobin levels, again, there was significant variation in the opinions of consultants and subspecialty physicians. The average minimal acceptable hemoglobin level as stated by those surveyed was 9.4 g/dL. The task force could determine no lower limit for hemoglobin concentration that has clearly been associated with the development of POVL.

5. In patients with significant blood loss, it was advised that colloids should be used in conjunction with crystalloids.

6. Although there was a consensus among neuroanesthesiologists that the prolonged use of α-agonists may reduce perfusion pressure to the optic nerve, there were inadequate data to formulate an advisory on this topic.

7. Staged surgical procedures should be considered in high-risk patients.

8. With regard to postoperative management of the patient with POVL, although all groups agree that there is no proven treatment for ION, they also agree that anemia should be treated, blood pressure increased, and oxygen administered. In patients suspected of having POVL, urgent ophthalmologic consultation should be obtained, and magnetic resonance imaging should be considered to rule out intracranial causes of blindness.

9. Preoperative discussion of POVL should be considered for patients at high risk (prolonged procedure, anticipated large blood loss).

Management of POVL

The patient presented in this case had at least two risk factors for POVL: he underwent an 8-hour procedure in the prone position and lost approximately 50% of his blood volume. Whether his history of hypertension or diabetes contributed to his risk is unclear. There were also episodes of reduced blood pressure intraoperatively, but this association with POVL is unclear.

There is no proven treatment for POVL. However, several steps should be taken urgently for this patient including rapidly increasing his blood pressure to at least his baseline value and ensuring that his hemoglobin level is within a reasonable range (9.0 g/dL or greater). Ophthalmologic consultation should be obtained immediately, and a fundoscopic examination should be performed in an effort to evaluate what type of injury may be present. Magnetic resonance imaging scans should be obtained.

In conclusion, POVL is a devastating complication following spine surgery with an outcome that is generally poor. The incidence of CRAO may be reduced with close attention to the orbit intraoperatively, but ION is more sinister in its etiology and thus more difficult to prevent. Information available to us is limited because of the very rare incidence of this complication, and single-institution prospective studies are essentially impossible. Furthermore, there is currently no animal model for POVL. Until more data on the mechanisms of POVL are available, staged procedures, obsessive attention to the eyes of prone patients, and frequent consideration of oxygen delivery to the optic nerve and retina are the best preventive measures available.

KEY MESSAGES

1. The most common causes of POVL are ischemic injuries to the visual tracts, which fall into two primary categories: CRAO and ION.

2. In patients undergoing spine surgery, prolonged surgical procedures and large blood loss are risk factors for POVL.

3. Although the incidence of CRAO can be decreased with close attention to the orbit intraoperatively, ION is more sinister in its etiology and thus more difficult to prevent.

QUESTIONS

1. What is the incidence of POVL in patients who have undergone spine surgery?

   Answer: True POVL in spine-injured patients has an incidence of 0.1% to 0.2%.

2. What are the anatomic segments of the optic nerve?

   Answer:
   a. The intracranial segment (optic chiasm to the optic canal within the lesser sphenoid wing)
   b. The intracanalicular segment (within the optic canal)
   c. The posterior or intraorbital segment (optic foramen to the lamina cribrosa)
   d. The anterior or intraocular segment (from the lamina cribrosa to the optic disc)

3. What are the likely mechanisms underlying POVL?

   Answer: These include cerebral cortical infarction, pituitary apoplexy, direct injuries to the eye and visual tracts, and ischemic injuries to the optic nerve and/or retina.

References

1. Lee L, Roth S, Posner K, et al. The American Society of Anesthesiologists Postoperative Visual Loss Registry. Anesthesiology 2006;105:652–659.
2. Myers MA, Hamilton SR, Bogosian AJ, et al. Visual loss as a complication of spine surgery: a review of 37 cases. Spine 1997;22:1325–1329.
3. Practice Advisory for Perioperative Visual Loss Associated with Spine Surgery: a Report by the American Society of

Anesthesiologists Task Force on Perioperative Blindness. Anesthesiology 2006;104:1319–1328.

4. Hyman C. The concept of end arteries and flow diversion. Invest Ophthalmol 1965;4:1000–1003.

5. Williams EL, Hart WM, Tempelhoff R. Postoperative ischemic optic neuropathy. Anesth Analg 1995;80:1018–1029.

6. Steele EJ, Blunt MJ. The blood supply of the optic nerve and chiasma in man. JANA 1956;90:486–493.

7. Pillunat LE, Anderson DR, Knighton RW, et al. Autoregulation of human optic nerve head circulation in response to increased intraocular pressure. Exp Eye Res 1997;64:737–744.

8. Shaw PJ, Bates D, Cartlidge NE, et al. Neuro-ophthalmological complications of coronary artery bypass graft surgery. Acta Neurol Scand 1987;76:1–7.

9. Walick KS, Kragh J, Ward J, Crawford J. Changes in intraocular pressure due to surgical positioning. Spine 2007;32:2591–2595.

10. Cheng MA, Todorov A, Tempelhoff R, et al. The effect of prone positioning on intraocular pressure in anesthetized patients. Anesthesiology 2001;95;1351–1355.

11. Ho VT, Newman N, Song S, et al. Ischemic optic neuropathy following spine surgery. J Neurosurg Anesthesiol 2005;17:38–44.

12. Chutorian AM, Winterkorn JM, Geffner M. Anterior ischemic optic neuropathy in children: case reports and review of the literature. Pediatr Neurol 2002;26:358–364.

13. Danish-Meyer HV, Levin LA. Erectile dysfunction drugs and risk of anterior ischaemic optic neuropathy: casual or causal association? Br J Opthalmol 2007;91:1551–1555.

14. Sivaswamy L, Vanstavern GP. Ischemic optic neuropathy in a child. Pediatr Neurol 2007;37:371–372.

15. Fodale V, DiPietro R, Santamaria S. Viagra, surgery and anesthesia: a dangerous cocktail with a risk of blindness. Medical Hypotheses 2007;68:880–882.

16. Kawasaki A, Purvin V. Recovery of postoperative visual loss following treatment of severe anemia. Clin Experiment Ophthalmol 2006;34:497–499.

17. Connolly SE, Gordon KB, Horton JC. Salvage of vision after hypotension-induced ischemic optic neuropathy. Am J Opthalmol 1994;117:235–242.

CHAPTER 10

Postoperative Cognitive Dysfunction

Charles W. Hogue

CASE FORMAT: REFLECTION

A 75-year-old male had undergone an otherwise success-ful coronary artery bypass graft (CABG) surgery with aor-tic valve replacement 1 month prior to attendance at his postoperative clinic. His medical history included hyperten-sion, non–insulin-dependent diabetes mellitus, and several episodes of congestive heart failure in the month before his surgery. He was married, had retired as a factory worker, and was physically active until the onset of his current ill-ness. His recent cardiac operation included 140 minutes of cardiopulmonary bypass (CPB), transfusion of two units of packed red blood cells, 18 hours of hospitalization in the intensive care unit, and 7 days of total postoperative hos-pitalization. The patient had a 1-day episode of atrial fib-rillation on postoperative day 2 that converted to sinus rhythm with intravenous amiodarone. During his clinic visit, his wife and daughter were concerned that he seemed for-getful since surgery and his ability to concentrate, such as for reading the newspaper, had noticeably declined.

His vital signs were as follows: temperature, 36.9°C; blood pressure, 155/70 mm Hg; heart rate, 68 beats per minute; and respiratory rate, 20 breaths per minute. The patient's physical examination was unremarkable, and his medications included aspirin, warfarin, amiodarone, and atorvastatin. Twelve-lead electrocardiogram readings showed sinus rhythm, and laboratory results were accept-able. Physical examination, including a comprehensive neurologic exam, was normal. The patient was oriented to person, place, and time. He could repeat 7 numbers after a delay of 5 minutes with mild difficulty. His sensorium ap-peared normal, but he did admit that he had not felt "him-self" since surgery. The plan was to discontinue warfarin and amiodarone.

CASE DISCUSSION

Cerebral Complications of Cardiac Surgery

Clinically, perioperative cerebral injury has a range of mani-festations that includes its most notable form, ischemic stroke. Perioperative stroke occurs in 1.5% to 5.2% of patients after cardiac surgery.[1,2] The range in reported incidences depends on the patient populations (e.g., patient age and risk status, types of procedures), diagnostic definitions, and the intensity of clinical surveillance. Contemporary studies using sensitive brain magnetic resonance imaging with diffusion-weighted imaging report that as many as 45% of patients who have un-dergone cardiac surgery have new ischemic brain lesions that are often clinically undetected. Hemorrhagic stroke is unusual as a primary cause of cerebral injury after cardiac surgery.

Postoperative Cognitive Dysfunction After Cardiac Surgery

Postoperative cognitive dysfunction is another manifestation of brain injury from cardiac surgery that may be less clinically obvious yet more frequent, affecting 20% to 30% of patients 1 month after surgery.[1–3] This form of brain injury is detected by administering a battery of psychometric tests typically be-fore and after surgery. These tests evaluate a broad range of brain areas subserving attention, short- and long-term mem-ory, visuomotor function, and other cognitive domains. In some instances, cognitive dysfunction may be noticed by fam-ily members who detect mild changes in the patient's person-ality, attention, memory, or even the perceptions that their family member "is not the same after surgery."

MECHANISMS

It is generally believed that all forms of brain injury from cardiac surgery (i.e., stroke, delirium, and neurocognitive dys-function) arise from a similar mechanism and that the ultimate manifestation depends on the extent and location of brain injury (e.g., global vs. regional, motor cortex vs. areas subserving cog-nition). This theory, however, is based on indirect data and has not been conclusively proven. In general, perioperative brain in-jury results from cerebral embolism or cerebral hypoperfusion that is exacerbated by inflammatory processes induced by CPB and/or ischemia-reperfusion injury. Abnormal endothelial functions resulting from ischemic damage and inflammatory processes leading to impaired microcirculatory flow likely con-tribute to subsequent injury. Cerebral emboli are often arbitrar-ily classified as macro- and microembolism. Examples of the former include atheroembolism arising from an atherosclerotic ascending aorta. The important role of atherosclerosis of the as-cending aorta in brain injury has led to the practice of epiaortic ultrasound scanning before surgical manipulations of the aorta.[1] This method is more sensitive than palpation and trans-esophageal echocardiography for identifying aortic atheroma allowing the surgeon to choose alternate sites for cannulations and cross clamping. When atherosclerosis is severe, alternate surgical plans (e.g., different site of cannulation, off-pump surgery, etc.) may be necessary. There are many sources of microemboli including air entrained into the circulation or the

CPB circuit, particulate material arising from the operative field, microthrombus, and lipid emboli. The latter are believed to arise from pericardial fat that is aspirated with cardiotomy suction during CABG surgery and then returned to the CPB reservoir unfiltered. Some centers advocate first processing shed pericardial blood with a cell saver before returning the blood to the CPB reservoir. The latter method was found to reduce the frequency of postoperative neurocognitive dysfunction in one study but not confirmed in another.

RISK FACTORS

Some risk factors for stroke and postoperative neurocognitive dysfunction overlap, yet others are distinct. Patient age, atherosclerosis of the ascending aorta, prior stroke, diabetes, hypertension, peripheral vascular disease, duration of CPB, and postoperative atrial fibrillation are common risk factors for stroke and postoperative neurocognitive dysfunction.[1–3] The patient's level of education is inversely related to risk for cognitive dysfunction. An explanation for this relationship is not clear, but higher levels of education might identify individuals who are more proficient at taking psychometric tests or those with more cerebral reserve and are thus capable of tolerating an acute insult to the brain. Genetic susceptibility has been further identified to be associated with cerebral complications from cardiac surgery, but genotypes associated with stroke and neurocognitive dysfunction appear distinct.[1] Candidate genes include those associated with inflammatory cytokines and neuronal reparative pathways. It is hypothesized that abnormal secretion of inflammatory mediators during and after surgery or defective neuronal reparative processes might promote susceptibility to brain injury. Several prospectively randomized trials have reported that there is no difference in the frequency of cerebral outcomes between patients undergoing CABG surgery with or without CPB (off-pump surgery).[1] Other factors found to be associated with cerebral injury include cerebral hyperthermia caused by excessive rewarming after hypothermic CPB and low nadir hematocrit during CPB ($<21\%$ to 24%). Although hyperglycemia is implicated as worsening cerebral injury, there is no evidence to date that aggressive insulin treatment during surgery leads to a lower rate of stroke, encephalopathy, or neurocognitive dysfunction.

Methodologic limitations to psychometric testing include test-retest or practice effect whereby individuals undergoing psychometric testing score higher on repeated testing because of familiarization with testing methodology.[4,5] The statistical approach for defining cognitive decline varies between studies, and the approach chosen affects the ultimate frequency of the complications. There is no accepted standard for defining neurocognitive dysfunction. The often-used definition of a 20% decline in two or more psychometric tests after surgery from baseline has been challenged on the basis that there is often correlation between the results of many psychometric tests. Thus, if two test results are correlated, decrements on these tests might identify the same cognitive defect rather than distinct areas of dysfunction. Principal component analysis in which tests that correlate are grouped into general domains, and cognitive decline defined as a standard deviation decline from baseline overcomes this limitation.

Perhaps a larger limitation of psychometric testing as a means for detecting brain injury from cardiac surgery is its insensitivity and nonspecificity in an aging surgical population.[4] Many patients might have pre-existing cognitive deficits before surgery such that they are incapable of further decrements of a magnitude necessary to show a standard deviation decline. This "basement effect" might overlook cognitive decrements that have profound importance to an elderly patient already functioning at a low cognitive level. At the same time, factors other than brain injury per se might lead to a false-positive diagnosis of neurocognitive dysfunction. Depression, pain, and chronic illness might all lead to low psychometric test results in the absence of cerebral injury during surgery.[7]

ASSOCIATED OUTCOMES

Perioperative cerebral complications are an important source of patient morbidity and mortality. The chance of operative death for patients suffering a new stroke is greater than 10-fold higher than for patients who have not suffered a stroke ($>20\%$ vs. $\sim1\%$ to 2%).[1–3] Stroke, after cardiac surgery is, in fact, the second most common cause of operative death after left ventricular failure. Cerebral complications are further linked to high hospital costs, admission to a secondary health care facility after surgery, high hospital readmission rates, and impaired quality of life.

The prognosis for patients with postoperative neurocognitive dysfunction has now been examined in several longitudinal studies. In a seminal investigation, investigators from Duke University found that neurocognitive dysfunction after CABG surgery predicted further cognitive decrement over a 5-year period.[3] Subsequent study by a team from Johns Hopkins University compared long-term cognitive function in patients recovering from CABG surgery with that of control subjects with coronary artery disease who were medically managed (plus/minus percutaneous coronary artery intervention).[6] These investigators found that the rates of long-term cognitive decline were no different in CABG surgical patients than controls over a 3-year period. These investigators are now reporting similar results after a 6-year follow-up period. The emerging data suggest that many patients with neurocognitive dysfunction after CABG surgery recover after 3 to 6 months. Further cognitive decline appears more related to the natural progression of cerebrovascular disease than the cardiac surgical procedure.

DELIRIUM

Postoperative delirium (as distinguished from emergence delirium) is a disturbance of consciousness or awareness of the environment accompanied by a decreased ability to focus, sustain, or shift attention. Other features may include decrement in cognition (disorientation, reduced memory) or a perceptual disturbance (delusions or hallucinations) that is not caused by pre-existing dementia. Delirium is acute in onset developing over hours to days, and the course may fluctuate throughout the day. Delirium can be categorized into hypoactive, hyperactive, or mixed forms. Hypoactive delirium might be mistaken for depression or dementia. The frequency of delirium depends on the definitions, patient population, and type of surgery. Reported incidences after cardiac surgery range from 20% to 65% of patients and after hip surgery, 16% to 65%, particularly elderly patients and those undergoing CPB.[8] Delirium may be transient, or it may be associated with longer-term decrements in cognition, long-term disability, mortality, loss of independence, admission to a nursing home, and high health resource utilization. The etiology of delirium is unknown, but it may involve similar factors as those leading to postoperative neurocognitive dysfunction. Other factors implicated to be associated with the condition include perioperative stress responses including systemic inflammatory response to surgery, abnormalities of brain cholinergic or norepinephrine neurotransmitter pathways, metabolic abnormalities, electrolyte abnormality, cerebral edema, hypoxia, or infections. Pre-existing patient factors, pain, and medications (e.g., benzodiazepines, drugs with central anticholinergic effects, corticosteroids, and some antibiotics) are suggested to increase susceptibility to postoperative delirium.[8] Acute or chronic substance abuse is further implicated. Data derived mostly from observational studies suggest a link between meperidine use in elderly patients and delirium. Although the data are presently insufficient, there currently does not appear to be an association among other analgesics and risk for delirium. Interventions that may improve or prevent delirium include frequently providing the patient with orientation cues such as a clock, calendar, and list of hospital staff. Physical exercise, visual aids, cognitive stimulation, regular daily routines, and sleep cycles are further measures.

Postoperative Cognitive Dysfunction After Noncardiac Surgery

Cognitive dysfunction has been reported after noncardiac surgery mostly in elderly patients. Overall, the incidence in the immediate postoperative period might be as high as 25%, but this rate declines to roughly 10% by 3 months postoperatively.[8,9] The available evidence suggests that by 1 year, cognitive performance in most patients has returned to that expected for a matched control group not undergoing surgery. As with cardiac surgery, the detection of cognitive dysfunction after noncardiac surgery depends on baseline cognitive state and thus requires paired administration of a psychometric testing battery. Generalized cognitive tests such as the Mini-Mental Exam are mostly insensitive for detecting cognitive dysfunction. There is no signal test for this purpose, as a comprehensive battery is necessary to fully assess the broad range of cognitive domains that might be affected by surgery. Of note, the type of anesthesia, regional versus general, does not seem to influence the incidence of postoperative neurocognitive dysfunction.

KEY MESSAGES

1. Perioperative stroke occurs in 1.5% to 5.2% of patients after cardiac surgery.

2. Postoperative cognitive dysfunction affects 20% to 30% of patients 1 month after cardiac surgery.

3. Patient age, atherosclerosis of the ascending aorta, prior stroke, diabetes, hypertension, peripheral vascular disease, duration of CPB, and postoperative atrial fibrillation, are common risk factors for stroke and postoperative neurocognitive dysfunction after cardiac surgery.

4. Operative death for patients suffering a new stroke is greater than 10-fold higher than for patients who have not suffered a stroke (>20% vs. ~1% to 2%).

QUESTIONS

1. What is the incidence of POCD after noncardiac surgery?

   Answer: After noncardiac surgery, the incidence of POCD in the immediate postoperative period may be as high as 25%, but this rate declines to roughly 10% by 3 months postoperatively.

2. What is delirium?

   Answer: Delirium (as distinguished from emergence delirium) is a disturbance of consciousness or awareness of the environment accompanied by a decreased ability to focus, sustain, or shift attention. Other features may include decrement in cognition (disorientation, reduced memory) or a perceptual disturbance (delusions or hallucinations) that is not caused by pre-existing dementia.

3. How can postoperative cognitive function be formally assessed?

   Answer: It can be assessed by administering a battery of psychometric tests typically before and after surgery. These tests evaluate a broad range of brain areas subserving attention, short- and long-term memory, visuomotor function, and other cognitive domains.

References

1. Hogue CW, Palin CA, Arrowsmith JE. Cardiopulmonary bypass management and neurologic outcomes: an evidence-based appraisal of current practices. Anesth Analg 2006;103: 21–37.
2. Roach GW, Kanchuger M, Mora-Mangano C, et al. Adverse cerebral outcomes after coronary bypass surgery. N Engl J Med 1996;335:1857–1863.
3. Newman MF, Kirchner JL, Phillips-Bute B, et al. Longitudinal assessment of neurocognitive function after coronary artery bypass surgery. N Engl J Med 2001;344:395–402.
4. Selnes OA, Pham L, Zeger S, McKhann GM. Defining cognitive change after CABG: decline versus normal variability. Ann Thorac Surg 2006;82:388–390.
5. Van Dijk D, Keizer AM, Diephuis, JC, et al. Neurocognitive dysfunction after coronary artery bypass surgery: a systematic review. J Thorac Cardiovasc Surg 2000;120:632–639.
6. Selnes OA, Grega MA, Borowicz LM, et al. Cognitive changes with coronary artery disease: a prospective study of coronary artery bypass graft patients and nonsurgical controls. Ann Thorac Surg 2003;75:1377–1386.
7. Fong HK, Sands LP, Leung JM. The role of postoperative analgesia in delirium and cognitive decline in elderly patients: a systematic review. Anesth Analg 2006;102:1255–1266.
8. Newman S, Stygall J, Hirani S, et al. Postoperative cognitive dysfunction after noncardiac surgery. A systematic review. Anesthesiology 2007;106:572–590.
9. Silverstein JH, Timberger M, Reich DL, Uysal S. Central nervous system dysfunction after noncardiac surgery and anesthesia in the elderly. Anesthesiology 2007;106:622–628.

CHAPTER 11

Perioperative Myocardial Infarction

Joshua D. Stearns

CASE FORMAT: STEP BY STEP

A 74-year-old female presented for a right femoral-popliteal arterial bypass. Her medical history was significant for hypertension, peripheral vascular disease, an 80 pack-year history of tobacco use, and recently diagnosed diabetes mellitus. The patient had undergone a cholecystectomy 20 years previously under general anesthesia without incident. Her current medications included lisinopril, glyburide, oxycodone and acetaminophen, and daily aspirin. Preoperative electrocardiogram (ECG) readings revealed normal sinus rhythm at 72 beats per minute and left ventricular hypertrophy by voltage criteria. The patient's preoperative hemoglobin level was 12.5 mg/dL, and her serum creatinine level was 1.3 mg/dL. The planned anesthetic technique was general endotracheal anesthesia with propofol induction and maintenance with fentanyl, nitrous oxide, and isoflurane along with vecuronium for muscle relaxation. Invasive arterial monitoring was utilized.

Initially, the patient tolerated the procedure well without evidence of myocardial ischemia by ECG monitoring (leads II and V5 and ST-segment analysis). An hour and a half into the procedure, however, and following approximately 800 mL of blood loss, the patient's heart rate increased to 110 beats per minute and there was evidence of ST-segment elevation in ECG lead II. Multiple lead analysis showed ST-segment elevation in leads II, III, and aVF. The patient's blood pressure slowly decreased from 135/85 mm Hg to 90/60 mm Hg over several minutes.

What measures should be have been taken at this point to limit myocardial ischemia?

The treatment of myocardial ischemia is aimed at improving the balance between myocardial oxygen (O_2) supply versus demand. Nitrous oxide should have been discontinued, and the patient should have been administered 100% O_2. Her blood pressure should have been increased by intravascular volume replacement and by administering a vasoconstricting agent such as phenylephrine. Avoiding drugs with β-adrenergic effects (e.g., ephedrine, epinephrine, or norepinephrine) is advisable to prevent further tachycardia and increased myocardial O_2 demand. A short-acting β-blocker (e.g., esmolol) should have been considered to lessen the patient's heart rate. The target heart rate should be close to the patient's baseline or the lowest rate that is hemodynamically tolerated. The patient's arterial blood gas, hemoglobin, and electrolytes should have been measured. In light of the preoperative hemoglobin level and the

amount of blood loss, it was likely that the patient would need a transfusion of packed red blood cells. If these initial measures did not lead to an increase in blood pressure, a reduction in heart rate, and resolution of the ST-segment changes, the patient may have been experiencing left ventricular dysfunction or cardiogenic shock secondary to myocardial ischemia.

What mechanism of myocardial ischemia was most likely in this patient?

The etiology of perioperative myocardial ischemia is often multifactorial. In this patient's situation, the presence of tachycardia, blood loss, and likely reduced hemoglobin concentration, suggests that the underlying mechanism for myocardial ischemia was myocardial O_2 supply/demand mismatch. Hypovolemia leads to reflex tachycardia increasing myocardial O_2 demand. At the same time, lessened blood O_2 carrying capacity from reduced hemoglobin compromises myocardial O_2 supply. Hypotension in this case might have resulted from reduced cardiac preload or reduced stroke volume from myocardial ischemia.

What other mechanisms are implicated in perioperative myocardial ischemia/infarction?

Many episodes of myocardial ischemia occur despite a normal heart rate and blood pressure. The latter episodes result from reduced coronary artery blood flow often caused by a ruptured atherosclerotic plaque leading to platelet activation and release of vasoactive substances, thrombus formation, and partial or complete arterial obstruction. Atherosclerotic plaque disruption can occur in patients with only modest angiographic evidence for coronary artery stenosis. Furthermore, a stable coronary artery plaque can acutely transform to a plaque that is vulnerable to fissuring or frank rupture caused by localized inflammation or shear stresses resulting from sympathetic activation or rheologic factors. Patients with extant coronary plaque may be at additional risk for acute coronary syndromes as a result of the multiple stresses associated with surgery.[1]

What is the definition of myocardial infarction?

The World Health Organization uses the following criteria for diagnosis of a myocardial infarction (MI). Two of the following must be present: (a) typical ischemic chest pain; (b) elevated serum creatine kinase (CK-MB enzyme); and/or (c) typical ECG findings including the development or presence of pathologic Q waves.[1]

In 2000, however, the European Society of Cardiology and the American College of Cardiology (ACC) revised the formal definition of an MI incorporating the use of increasingly sensitive biochemical assays such as troponin I and T for the diagnosis (information to follow).[2]

Do perioperative MIs present in a fashion consistent with the World Health Organization's definition of MI?

Most often, perioperative MI is not accompanied by typical chest pain caused by residual anesthetics, analgesic drugs, or sedation, especially in the setting of patients who remain intubated postoperatively. In addition, perioperative MI often manifests few of the classic ECG findings such as ST-segment elevation or Q waves.[1] As a result, the use of biochemical markers of myocardial injury often provides the most definitive diagnosis of perioperative MI. According to one study, 12% of patients developed elevated cardiac troponin T (cTnT) levels, while only 3% exhibited characteristics that confirmed perioperative MI by the World Health Organization definition.[3]

Which biochemical markers are commonly used in the diagnosis of perioperative MI?

Biochemical markers for detecting myocardial injury include serum creatine kinase (CK-MB) and cTnT or troponin I (cTnI) assays. Cardiac troponins are both specific and sensitive for detecting myocardial injury and appear to provide improved detection of MI as compared to CK-MB levels.

What threshold levels of CK-MB and cardiac troponins are diagnostic of perioperative MI?

CK-MB is not specific for cardiac tissue; thus, interpreting elevations in this isoenzyme is confounded perioperatively by other sources (e.g., muscle injury). Cardiac troponins are specific for the heart, but they are also released because of myocardial ischemia that does not necessarily lead to actual myocyte necrosis. There is much debate, therefore, as to the specific cut-off values that can be used to define an MI in the perioperative setting. Several studies suggest that even small elevations of cardiac troponins in the perioperative period identify some myocardial injury.[4] These elevations and the accompanying myocardial injury may be implications for both short- and long-term mortality. Over time, the threshold values have decreased suggesting that there is an association between small troponin elevations and cardiac outcome. Laboratory cut-offs for diagnoses differ from institution to institution. An increase in CK-MB $>10\%$ (upper limit of normal $= 170$ IU), cTn-I >1.5 ng/mL, or cTn-T >0.1 ng/mL have been shown to be independent predictors of mortality from cardiac events at 1-year and 5-year follow-up for patients undergoing vascular surgery.[4]

What are the pharmacologic treatment options for patients diagnosed with a perioperative MI?

Medical therapy for perioperative MI is directed based toward rectifying myocardial O_2 demand/supply mismatch. Myocardial O_2 demand is reduced by the judicious use of β-blockers while ensuring myocardial perfusion pressure. Certainly, the most well-studied and used pharmacologic preventive treatment for perioperative myocardial ischemia or perioperative MI is β-blocker therapy. Several studies have shown reduced adverse cardiac events for patients in the perioperative setting, especially in patients considered at high risk for coronary heart disease. Patients considered high risk include those with risk factors such as diabetes mellitus and hypertension as well as patients who have been shown to exhibit "inducible" myocardial ischemia by exercise or pharmacologic stress testing. (Table 11.1). Furthermore, the initiation of β-blockers days or weeks in advance of surgery appears to provide greater benefit (a target heart rate of <65 beats per minute is optimal).

TABLE 11.1 ACC/AHA Recommendations for Perioperative Use of β-Blockers Based on Published Randomized Clinical Trials

Surgery	No clinical risk factors	One or more clinical risk factors	Coronary heart disease or high cardiac risk	Patients currently taking β-blockers
Vascular	Class IIb, level of evidence = B	Class IIa, level of evidence = B	Patients found to have myocardial ischemia on preoperative testing: class I, level of evidence = B; patients without ischemia or not previous test: class IIa, level of evidence = B	Class I, level of evidence = B
Intermediate risk	Insufficient data	Class IIb, level of evidence = C	Class IIa, level of evidence = B	Class I, level of evidence = C
Low risk	Insufficient data	Insufficient data	Insufficient data	Class I, level of evidence = C

ACC, American College of Cardiology; AHA, American Heart Institute.
Adapted from Fleisher LA, Beckman JA, Brown KA, et al. ACC/AHA 2007 guidelines on perioperative cardiovascular evaluation and care for noncardiac surgery: a report of the American College of Cardiology/American Heart Association Task Force on Practice Guidelines (Writing Committee to Revise the 2002 Guidelines on Perioperative Cardiovascular Evaluation for Noncardiac Surgery). Circulation 2007;116:e418–499.

Aspirin has been shown to be beneficial in the setting of acute MI. Both its anti-inflammatory effects and antiplatelet aggregation effects appear to play a role in the reduction of thrombotic activity characteristic of the plaque rupture mechanism for MI. The benefits of aspirin may be increased in the perioperative setting because of the accompanying inflammatory response to surgery. A meta-analysis of perioperative use of aspirin identified an almost 50% reduction of postoperative acute MI when administered with a dose of 325 mg or less.[5] The relative benefits of aspirin (given via a gastric tube or rectally) for secondary prevention of myocardial injury will outweigh the minimal risk of enhanced bleeding for most surgical procedures.

Heparin has been a mainstay for the treatment of acute MI; however, in the postoperative setting, the advantages of unfractionated heparin, other anticoagulants (such as low-molecular-weight heparin or direct thrombin inhibitors such as bivalirudin), and antiplatelet drugs must be considered in reference to the risks of bleeding from the surgical wound. Antiplatelet drugs commonly used include clopidogrel and glycoprotein IIb/IIIa inhibitors.[6] The use of anticoagulants and/or antiplatelet drugs should be initiated with the consultation of a cardiologist. This consultation should address other potential therapies such as angiotensin-converting enzyme inhibitors might be further considered particularly for anterior MI or in the setting of left ventricular dysfunction. Increasing interest has been placed on the use of statins (3-hydroxy-3-methylglutaryl coenzyme A reductase inhibitors) in the prevention of MI. Their use in the acute setting of an MI is unclear, although initial data suggest that statins confer benefits when administered in the acute setting.

α-2 Adrenoceptor agonists such as clonidine and dexmedetomidine may have benefits if used prior to surgery; however, the slow onset of effect of α-2 adrenoceptor agonists may limit their value in the treatment of an identified MI. Nitroglycerin use for coronary dilatation may be of benefit if hemodynamics are stable and if there is ongoing evidence by ECG of ischemia.[7]

What potential interventions should be considered as treatment for ongoing ischemia or infarction?

Placement of an intra-aortic balloon pump should be considered for refractory or recalcitrant myocardial ischemia. The definitive treatment of an acute MI is coronary artery reperfusion. Thrombolytic therapy is contraindicated because of the recent surgical incision and may be less effective than percutaneous coronary artery interventions (PCI). Early consultation with an invasive cardiologist is mandatory when there is an acute MI. Prompt transfer of the patient to the coronary catheterization laboratory for coronary angiography and possible coronary artery angioplasty with or without stent placement may rescue compromised myocardium.[7]

According to the ACC/American Heart Association Guidelines for Perioperative Cardiovascular Evaluation for Noncardiac Surgery, what would be an appropriate preoperative strategy for evaluating cardiovascular risk in the patient presented in this case?

The ACC/American Heart Association (AHA) Guidelines stratify perioperative cardiac risk and specify the appropriate

TABLE 11.2 Cardiac Conditions That Should Have Further Evaluation in Advance of Surgical Procedure

1. Unstable coronary syndrome—unstable or severe angina
2. Decompensated congestive heart failure—NY class IV
3. Malignant arrhythmias including
   i) High-grade atrioventricular block
      a) Mobitz type II AV block
      b) Third-degree AV block
   ii) Supraventricular tachycardia
      c) Atrial fibrillation with rapid ventricular response
      d) Symptomatic bradycardia
      e) Symptomatic ventricular arrhythmias
   iii) New-onset ventricular tachycardia
4. Severe valvular disease
   i) Severe aortic stenosis
   ii) Severe mitral stenosis

Adapted from Fleisher LA, Beckman JA, Brown KA, et al. ACC/AHA 2007 guidelines on perioperative cardiovascular evaluation and care for noncardiac surgery: a report of the American College of Cardiology/American Heart Association Task Force on Practice Guidelines (Writing Committee to Revise the 2002 Guidelines on Perioperative Cardiovascular Evaluation for Noncardiac Surgery). Circulation 2007; 116:e418–499.

preoperative cardiac evaluation based on three components. First, active evidence of cardiac disease and/or of clinical risk factors helps determine proper cardiac evaluation (Tables 11.2 and 11.3). Patients demonstrating existing cardiac disease (major risk factors) should have further cardiac evaluation before surgery, whereas those presenting with clinical risk factors may or may not require further testing. Previous guidelines stratified clinical risk factors into mild-, intermediate-, and high-risk; however, the most recent ACC/AHA guidelines have replaced that stratification with a list of clinical risk factors (Table 11.3). Second, an evaluation of a patient's functional capacity is considered. Third, the type of surgery is factored into the algorithm with high- (e.g., vascular), intermediate-, and low-risk being assigned to each surgery (Table 11.4). According to the latest update, the presented patient had one clinical risk factor (diabetes mellitus) and was undergoing a high-risk procedure (vascular surgery). The case described does not, however, describe the patient's functional capacity. Nevertheless, the algorithm offers the practitioner the option of considering further cardiac evaluation or proceeding with the case using perioperative β-blockers.[8]

What role does preoperative coronary revascularization play in the reduction of perioperative MI?

PCI

PCI includes both coronary angioplasty with or without the use of intraluminal stents. The routine use of these interven-

TABLE 11.3 Clinical Risk Factors for Perioperative Cardiac Events

1. History of ischemic cardiac disease
2. History of compensated or previous heart failure
3. History of cerebrovascular disease
4. Diabetes mellitus
5. Renal insufficiency

Adapted from Fleisher LA, Beckman JA, Brown KA, et al. ACC/AHA 2007 guidelines on perioperative cardiovascular evaluation and care for noncardiac surgery: a report of the American College of Cardiology/American Heart Association Task Force on Practice Guidelines (Writing Committee to Revise the 2002 Guidelines on Perioperative Cardiovascular Evaluation for Noncardiac Surgery). Circulation 2007; 116:e418–499.

tions in advance of an elective surgery is heavily debated. To date, no randomized trials to evaluate the efficacy of preoperative percutaneous transluminal coronary angioplasty for reducing perioperative MI have been conducted. Several retrospective cohort studies have examined patient populations who underwent percutaneous transluminal coronary angioplasty in an effort to ameliorate symptomatic angina and/or to reduce perioperative risk of myocardial ischemia. Overall, the three studies reported a low incidence of perioperative MI and/or perioperative cardiac death.[9–11] Unfortunately, no comparison groups were analyzed.

The placement of coronary artery stents, either bare metal or drug eluting, prior to surgery introduces the need for antiplatelet drug therapy with aspirin and clopidogrel to avoid intrastent thrombosis. The optimum duration of dual antiplatelet drug therapy after PCI with intracoronary stent placement is currently under debate. However, a widely used antithrombotic strategy should include the use of clopidogrel for 6 weeks with concomitant aspirin that should be continued for life. Stent manufacturers recommend that clopidogrel should be continued for at least 3 months with sirolimus-eluting stents and 6 months with paclitaxel-eluting stents.[12] Despite these recommendations, more recent experience suggests that dual antiplatelet therapy is needed for longer than 1 year after insertion of a drug-eluting stent. Elective surgery should be delayed if the patient has not received an adequate duration of dual antiplatelet drug therapy. The optimum management of patients requiring surgery during the window of mandatory dual antiplatelet drug therapy is not known. Consultation with a cardiologist should be made, and consider glycoprotein IIb/IIIa drug use while clopidogrel is stopped. Because of this management dilemma, the prophylactic use of PCI with stents as a strategy to reduce cardiac risk in the perioperative period is not well supported by the literature. If PCI with stenting has taken place in advance of surgery, an interval of at least 6 weeks should take place before surgery. In the case of drug-eluting stents, a minimum of 12 months should be considered[8] (Fig. 11.1).

Surgical Coronary Revascularization

Revascularization by coronary artery bypass grafting has been proposed and used as a means to reduce cardiovascular risk in high-risk patients undergoing noncardiac surgery. However, the Coronary Artery Revascularization Prophylaxis trial demonstrated that coronary artery revascularization prior to elective vascular surgery conferred no long-term outcome benefits.[13] As such, the decision to use coronary revascularization before elective surgery should be based on the same criteria for the use of coronary artery bypass grafting in patients not scheduled to undergo noncardiac surgery.

TABLE 11.4 Cardiac Risk Stratification Based on Type of Surgery

Risk Stratification (Risk of Cardiac Events)	Types of Procedures
Vascular (>5%)	Aortic and other major vascular surgery
	Peripheral vascular surgery
Intermediate risk (1% to 5%)	Intraperitoneal and intrathoracic surgery
	Carotid endarterectomy
	Head and neck surgery
	Orthopedic surgery
	Prostate surgery
Low risk (<1%)	Endoscopic procedures
	Superficial procedures
	Cataract surgery
	Breast surgery
	Ambulatory surgery

Adapted from Fleisher LA, Beckman JA, Brown KA, et al. ACC/AHA 2007 guidelines on perioperative cardiovascular evaluation and care for noncardiac surgery: a report of the American College of Cardiology/American Heart Association Task Force on Practice Guidelines (Writing Committee to Revise the 2002 Guidelines on Perioperative Cardiovascular Evaluation for Noncardiac Surgery). Circulation 2007; 116:e418–499.

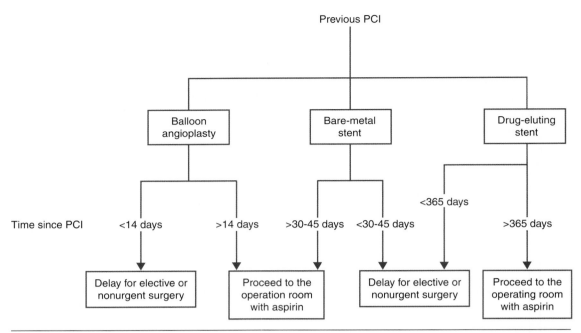

Figure 11.1 • ACC/AHA Proposed Guidelines, Based on Expert Opinion, for Management of Patients with Recent Percutaneous Coronary Interventions Requiring Noncardiac Surgery. (Reproduced with permission from Fleisher LA, Beckman JA, Brown KA, et al. ACC/AHA 2007 guidelines on perioperative cardiovascular evaluation and care for noncardiac surgery: a report of the American College of Cardiology/American Heart Association Task Force on Practice Guidelines [Writing Committee to Revise the 2002 Guidelines on Perioperative Cardiovascular Evaluation for Noncardiac Surgery]. Circulation 2007;116:e418–499.)

KEY MESSAGES

1. Perioperative MI leads to significant morbidity and mortality and costs the health care system billions of dollars each year.

2. Perioperative MI is proposed to have two basic yet often overlapping mechanisms: (a) myocardial O_2 supply/demand mismatch and (b) ruptured coronary plaque or associated thrombus leading to coronary occlusion.

3. Perioperative MI is most commonly diagnosed by the presence of elevated cardiac enzymes because the usual cardiac symptoms are typically masked by anesthetic and analgesic drugs and also because it frequently occurs with few or none of the classic ECG findings.

4. Perioperative β-blocker use has been shown to be the most effective medical therapy for reducing perioperative MI—especially in high-risk patients, including those undergoing vascular surgery.

5. Perioperative use of aspirin and statin drugs may also reduce the risk of PMI.

QUESTIONS

1. Which biochemical markers are commonly used in the diagnosis of perioperative MI?

   Answer: Biochemical markers for detecting myocardial injury include CK-MB and cTnT or troponin I (cTnI) assays. Cardiac troponins are both specific and sensitive for detecting myocardial injury and appear to provide improved detection of MI as compared to CK-MB levels.

2. What limitations apply to interpreting elevations in biomarkers of myocardial injury?

   Answer: CK-MB is not specific for cardiac tissue; thus, interpreting elevations in this isoenzyme is confounded perioperatively by other sources (e.g., muscle injury). Cardiac troponins are specific for the heart, but they are also released because of myocardial ischemia that does not necessarily lead to actual myocyte necrosis.

3. Why is aspirin administration indicated in the setting of acute MI?

   Answer: Both its anti-inflammatory effects and antiplatelet aggregation effects appear to play a role in the reduction of thrombotic activity characteristic of the plaque rupture mechanism for MI.

References

1. Priebe HJ. Perioperative myocardial infarction—aetiology and prevention. Br J Anaesth 2005;95:3–19.
2. Alpert JS, Thygesen K, Antman E, Bassand JP. Myocardial infarction redefined—a consensus document of The Joint European Society of Cardiology/American College of Cardiology Committee for the redefinition of myocardial infarction. J Am Coll Cardiol 2000;36:959–969.
3. Kim LJ, Martinez EA, Faraday N, et al. Cardiac troponin I predicts short-term mortality in vascular surgery patients. Circulation 2002;106:2366–2371.
4. Landesberg G, Mosseri M, Zahger D, et al. Association of cardiac troponin, CK-MB, and postoperative myocardial ischemia with long-term survival after major vascular surgery. J Am Coll Cardiol 2003;42:1547–1554.
5. Robless P, Mikhailidis DP, Stansby G. Systematic review of antiplatelet therapy for the prevention of myocardial infarction, stroke or vascular death in patients with peripheral vascular disease. Br J Surg 2001;88:787.
6. Ramanath VS, Eagle KA. Evidence-based medical therapy of patients with acute coronary syndromes. Am J Cardiovasc Drugs 2007;7:95–116.
7. Hogue CW Jr, Stamos T, Winters KJ, et al. Acute myocardial infarction during lung volume reduction surgery Anesth Analg 1999;88:332–334.
8. Fleisher LA, Beckman JA, Brown KA, et al. ACC/AHA 2007 guidelines on perioperative cardiovascular evaluation and care for noncardiac surgery: a report of the American College of Cardiology/American Heart Association Task Force on Practice Guidelines (Writing Committee to Revise the 2002 Guidelines on Perioperative Cardiovascular Evaluation for Noncardiac Surgery). Circulation 2007;116:e418–499.
9. Allen JR, Helling TS, Hartzler GO. Operative procedures not involving the heart after percutaneous transluminal coronary angioplasty. Surg Gynecol Obstet 1991;173:285.
10. Elmore JR, Hallett JW Jr, Gibbons RJ, et al. Myocardial revascularization before abdominal aortic aneurysmorrhaphy: effect of coronary angioplasty. Mayo Clin Proc 1993;68:637.
11. Gottlieb A, Banoub M, Sprung J, et al. Perioperative cardiovascular morbidity in patients with coronary artery disease undergoing vascular surgery after percutaneous transluminal coronary angioplasty. J Cardiothorac Vasc Anesth 1998;12:501.
12. Howard-Alpe GM, de Bono J, Hudsmith L, et al. Coronary artery stents and non-cardiac surgery. Br J Anaesthesia 2007;98:560–574.
13. McFalls EO, Ward HB, Moritz TE, et al. Coronary-artery revascularization before elective major vascular surgery. N Engl J Med 2004;351:2795–2804.

Heparin-Induced Thrombocytopenia

Roy Kan

FORMAT: STEP BY STEP

A 56-year-old woman with hypertension and hyperlipidemia presented to the emergency department with congestive heart failure. A cardiology evaluation revealed triple-vessel coronary artery disease with marked global left ventricular hypokinesia (left ventricular ejection fraction, 15%). The patient underwent urgent coronary artery bypass surgery during which intravenous (IV) heparin 30,000 U was administered for cardiopulmonary bypass (CPB). Her platelet count prior to surgery was 180,000/μL.

The patient continued to do poorly after coronary revascularization with low cardiac output despite large doses of dobutamine and milrinone. The patient underwent placement of a biventricular assist device on the next day, during which IV heparin was administered again. There was a progressive decline in platelet count from 98/μL prior to the biventricular assist device placement to 36/μL 3 days later.

What causes thrombocytopenia?

In general, the etiology of thrombocytopenia includes hemodilution from infusion of fluids or blood products, increased platelet destruction, or reduced platelet production by the bone marrow. Increased platelet destruction may result from nonimmune causes (e.g., sepsis, disseminated intravascular coagulation, or thrombotic thrombocytopenic purpura) or from immune causes (e.g., posttransfusion purpura or idiopathic thrombocytopenic purpura). Drugs that can lead to immune-mediated thrombocytopenia include heparin, quinine, quinidine, sulfa drugs, vancomycin, and others. Platelet production by the marrow may be affected by disease conditions (e.g., aplastic anemia, leukemia, myelodysplasia) or drugs (e.g., cytotoxic agents, alcohol).

Given the association with heparin use in this case, the diagnosis of heparin-induced thrombocytopenia (HIT) must be actively excluded.

Heparin therapy was discontinued and replaced with lepirudin. Laboratory testing for heparin platelet factor 4 (PF4) complex antibodies was positive for HIT.

What is HIT?

HIT is classified into two types. HIT type I is also known as *nonimmune heparin-associated thrombocytopenia*. It is the more benign of the two forms of HIT characterized by a typ-ical onset time of 4 days after heparin exposure, a platelet nadir of 100,000 to 150,000/μL, and a recovery time of 1 to 3 days with minimal complications. It has an estimated incidence of 5% to 30%. HIT type I is caused by platelet microaggregation and subsequent sequestration in the spleen. It is not associated with heparin-dependent antibodies. Heparin administration should be continued despite the low platelet count.

HIT type II is an immune-mediated syndrome caused by an antibody to the heparin-PF4 complex. It is a disorder initiated by an immunologic response to heparin exposure and is characterized by an absolute or relative thrombocytopenia that paradoxically increases the risk of thrombosis, leading to life-threatening complications.

An estimated 600,000 new cases of HIT type II occur in the United States every year with thromboembolic complications occurring in approximately 300,000 patients and death in approximately 90,000 patients. Health care costs from HIT type II complications in cardiac surgery alone are estimated to be approximately $300 million USD.

What is the pathophysiology of type II HIT?

The pathogenesis of HIT has been thoroughly reviewed. The administration of heparin in susceptible patients leads to heparin binding to PF4 on the platelet membrane. The formation of heparin-PF4 complexes changes the conformation of PF4 exposing epitopes that allow its recognition and binding by immunoglobulin G (IgG). The platelets, in turn, are activated by the Fc domain of the IgG. A positive feedback loop is created whereby activated platelets release microparticles that promote thrombin formation, which, in turn, fuels further platelet activation. Activated platelets also release PF4, which leads to immune complex production. The resultant thrombocytopenia and thrombin generation produces a prothrombotic state, which is exacerbated by the antibody-mediated endothelial injury and tissue factor production.

The Iceberg Model of HIT proposed by Warkentin suggests that thrombocytopenia and associated thrombosis only occurs in a small subset of patients with platelet-activating antiheparin/PF4 antibodies. It has been estimated that about 7% to 50% of heparin-treated patients generate heparin-PF4 HIT antibodies.[2] HIT antibodies circulate only temporarily, with a median half-life of 85 days by antigenic assay. These antibodies may be clinically significant because the presence and concentration, regardless of thrombocytopenia, are associated with increased morbidity or mortality in various clinical settings, such as acute coronary syndromes, hemodialysis, and cardiovascular or orthopedic surgery.

Both unfractionated and low-molecular-weight heparin can cause type II HIT, but the risk is higher with the former, particularly when given intravenously or in high doses. The use of both porcine and bovine can result in type II HIT, but the risk is higher with the latter.

High-risk groups for type II HIT include orthopedic patients given postoperative heparin as well as cardiac transplant and neurosurgery patients (11% and 15%, respectively). Other risk factors for HIT include high-titer, IgG HIT antibodies and female gender.

What are the clinical manifestations and complications of type II HIT?

Type II HIT has three clinical presentations: (a) latent phase in which antibodies are present without thrombocytopenia, (b) HIT whereby antibodies are present with thrombocytopenia, and (c) heparin-induced thrombocytopenia-thrombosis (HITT) in which antibodies are present with thrombocytopenia and thrombosis.

Of the patients who develop latent type II HIT with IgG seroconversion, 30% to 50% will develop thrombocytopenia. Of these patients, 30% to 80% will demonstrate isolated thrombotic events, of which 0.01% to 0.1% will experience multiple thromboses or white clot syndrome. Bleeding is rare despite the severity of the thrombocytopenia. Approximately 10% of patients with HIT and thrombosis require a limb amputation. The mortality rate is approximately 20% to 30%.

Platelet counts of 20,000 to 150,000/μL are seen typically 5 to 10 days after exposure to heparin. A fall in platelet count of more than 50% is considered to be diagnostic. In patients with elevated baseline platelet counts, a 50% or greater decrease without falling below a normal platelet level may be observed. The platelet counts usually return to normal levels in 5 to 10 days after heparin is stopped.

Rapid-onset HIT leads to reduced platelet counts within minutes to hours of heparin exposure. This tends to occur in patients with preformed heparin-PF4 antibodies from a previous heparin exposure within the prior 3 months. The platelet count should be determined immediately for comparison with a pre-bolus count.

HIT can sometimes present days to weeks after heparin has been stopped. This scenario, known as *delayed-onset HIT*, is less common than the more rapid presentations of HIT but should be considered if a recently hospitalized, heparin-treated patient presents with thrombosis.

Up to 50% of patients with isolated HIT (thrombocytopenia with no evidence of thrombosis) develop clinical evidence of thrombosis despite cessation of heparin within the first week if no alternative anticoagulant is started. Clinical thrombosis may manifest as:

1. Venous thrombosis (30% to 70%)
   a. Deep vein thrombosis
   b. Pulmonary embolism
   c. Adrenal vein thrombosis, leading to adrenal necrosis
   d. Cerebral sinus venous thrombosis
   e. Venous limb gangrene

2. Arterial thrombosis (15% to 30%)
   a. Limb artery thrombosis
   b. Stroke
   c. Myocardial infarction
3. Skin lesions at heparin injection site (10%)
   a. Skin necrosis
   b. Erythematous plaques
4. Acute reaction after IV bolus of heparin (10%)
5. Disseminated intravascular coagulation (10%)

How is HIT diagnosed?

HIT should be suspected whenever the platelet count decreases by 50%, or when new thrombosis occurs 5 to 14 days after the start of heparin therapy. Routine platelet count monitoring, including a pre-heparin value, is recommended for most heparin-treated patients. For patients with suspected HIT, laboratory testing is recommended, but because of its high thrombotic risk, treatment for such patients should not be withheld while waiting for laboratory results. Clinical scoring systems may be used to estimate the probability of HIT. An example of such a scoring system is the "Four Ts" (for timing, thrombocytopenia, thrombosis, and oTher sequelae). A score of 0, 1, or 2 is assigned depending on the onset time and severity of thrombocytopenia, the presence of thrombotic manifestations, as well as the absence of other causes of thrombocytopenia. An overall score greater than 6 is highly suggestive for HIT.

Laboratory testing for HIT antibodies may be divided into antigenic and functional testing. Antigenic tests include enzyme-linked immunosorbent assay and rapid particle gel immunoassay that detect antibodies to heparin-PF4 complexes or complexes of PF4 and other polyanions. Commercial enzyme-linked immunosorbent assay, which detect IgG, IgM, and IgA, are sensitive for detecting antibodies but are not specific for HIT. Measurement of only IgG antibodies enhances clinical specificity, whereas antibody titer based on the optical density can be more informative. Higher-titer antibodies are associated with increased thrombotic risk. Antibody titers by gel particle immunoassay correlate with clinical likelihood scores in suspected HIT.

Functional tests include the ^{14}C-serotonin release assay and the platelet aggregation test. The platelet aggregation test measures platelet aggregation resulting from IgG in the serum or plasma of an HIT patient given heparin. It has a high specificity of 90%, is simple to perform, and is widely available. However, the sensitivity of this test is poor, although this can be improved by using washed platelets. The serotonin release assay measures serotonin released from aggregated platelets from HIT. Although this test has high sensitivity and specificity, it requires the use of radioactive reagents and is technically demanding and time consuming to perform.

What is the treatment for HIT?

When HIT is suspected, all forms of heparins should be immediately stopped while awaiting laboratory confirmation of the diagnosis. Avoid using "flush" solutions containing heparin including dialysate fluid and central venous or pulmonary catheters with heparin coatings. Low-molecular-weight heparins should be avoided because of possible cross-reaction with heparin-PF4 antibodies to exacerbate HIT.

Serial monitoring of platelet counts is mandatory as is vigilant monitoring for thrombotic manifestations of HIT. Prophylactic platelet transfusion is not recommended, as it may increase the risk of thrombosis.

Heparin should be avoided, if possible, for as long as heparin-PF4 antibody testing is positive, although a longer heparin-free period is often preferred because of the availability of safe, effective alternative anticoagulants and uncertainty regarding the risk of recurrence on heparin re-exposure. The British Committee for Standards in Hematology recommends the use of nonheparin anticoagulation for most patients requiring anticoagulation with previous HIT.

Alternative anticoagulant coverage is used to prevent thrombotic complications. However, warfarin should not be used as the initial, sole anticoagulant therapy because of its slow onset of action. In addition, the protein C and protein S deficiency induced by warfarin can cause microvascular thrombosis resulting in coumarin-induced venous limb gangrene. If warfarin has already been started when HIT is recognized, vitamin K should be given to reverse the effects of warfarin and to minimize the risk of warfarin-induced limb gangrene or skin necrosis. Warfarin may be introduced at a later stage when platelet levels have normalized and when overlapping alternative anticoagulants are at therapeutic levels. Parenteral and oral anticoagulants should overlap for at least 5 days, with a therapeutic international normalized ratio achieved for at least 2 days before the parenteral anticoagulant is stopped.

Given the time course for thrombotic risk in HIT, nonheparin anticoagulation should be maintained for at least 1 month with a longer duration warranted if HIT-associated thrombosis occurred. Available agents include direct thrombin inhibitors such as lepirudin, bivalirudin, or argatroban. Consideration is given to the pharmacokinetic profile and route of elimination of each agent (Table 12.1). There are no agents currently available to reverse the anticoagulant effects of direct thrombin inhibitors.

An alternative to the direct thrombin inhibitors is danaparoid, a glycosaminoglycan derived from porcine intestine that has been used safely and effectively in critically ill patients with HIT. Fondaparinux is a novel anticoagulant that is modeled after the antithrombin-binding pentasaccharide region of heparin. It has anti-Xa and anti-IXa activity that does not cross-react with HIT antibodies. Although it is approved in the United States and elsewhere for prophylaxis and treatment of venous thromboembolism, the usefulness of fondaparinux for the treatment of type II HIT has not been established.

The usefulness of antiplatelet agents has not been established. Aspirin has only marginal therapeutic benefit because of its variable inhibition of platelet activation by HIT antibodies. Although the prostacyclin analog, iloprost, has been used to treat patients with type II HIT undergoing CPB surgery in combination with heparin, its use has been limited by severe hypotension. The role of ADP inhibitors such as ticlopidine and clopidogrel in the treatment of HIT has not been evaluated.

An emergency heart transplant was arranged for this patient. What are the drugs available for anticoagulation during cardiac transplant?

For patients with current or previous HIT who require cardiac surgery, the surgery should be delayed, if possible, until heparin-PF4 antibodies are negative. In patients with acute HIT undergoing cardiac surgery, direct thrombin inhibition is preferred over heparin or danaparoid. Of the direct thrombin inhibitors available, bivalirudin is preferred over lepirudin, as the former is least organ dependent for its metabolism and is not associated with anaphylaxis from lepirudin re-exposure. Appropriate dosing of the direct thrombin inhibitors during cardiac surgery has not been established, however, and no direct thrombin inhibitor is approved for use in this setting.

The most appropriate method for anticoagulation monitoring during CPB when direct thrombin inhibitors are used is not clear. The activated clotting time is affected by many variables

TABLE 12.1 Drugs for Nonheparin Anticoagulation

	Lepirudin	Argatroban	Bivalirudin	Danaparoid	Fondaparinux
Drug type	DTI	DTI	DTI	Heparinoid	FXa inhibitor
Clearance	Renal	Hepatic	Renal, Enzymic	Renal	Renal
Half-life	80 min	40 min	36 min	7 h	15 h
Cross-reactivity with HIT antibodies	No	No	No	Minimal	Negligible
Monitoring	ECT or aPTT	ACT or aPTT	ACT or aPTT	Anti-FXa	Not required
Target aPTT	1.5–2.5 baseline	1.5–3 baseline	1.5–2.5 baseline	NA	NA
Effect on INR	Yes	Yes	Yes	No	No
Approved in HIT	Yes	Yes	Yes (for PCI)	Yes (no in USA)	No

ACT, activated clotting time; aPTT, activated partial thromboplastin time; DTI, direct thrombin inhibitors; ECT, ecarin clotting time; INR, international normalized ratio; NA, not applicable; PCI, percutaneous coronary intervention.

in addition to thrombin inhibition, including hemodilution, thrombocytopenia, and hypothermia. The activated clotting time, thus, is a poor monitor of thrombin inhibition or the effectiveness of anticoagulation. Thromboelastography has been used to monitor both clot initiation and clot strength during cardiac surgery with direct thrombin inhibition. The ecarin clotting time has been used for monitoring lepirudin and bivalirudin during cardiac surgery, but this is not a commercially available test in the United States.

Cardiotomy suction blood should be processed in a cell saver that uses citrate and not heparin for anticoagulation. Care must be taken to administer additional bivalirudin into the CPB reservoir after separation from bypass to ensure anticoagulation while the blood is recirculated.

KEY MESSAGES

1. An estimated 600,000 new cases of type II HIT occur in the United States every year with thromboembolic complications occurring in approximately 300,000 patients, and death in approximately 90,000 patients.

2. The administration of heparin in susceptible patients leads to heparin binding to PF4 on the platelet membrane. The formation of heparin-PF4 complexes changes the conformation of PF4 exposing epitopes that allow its recognition and binding by IgG.

3. Type II HIT has three clinical presentations: (a) latent phase in which antibodies are present without thrombocytopenia, (b) HIT whereby antibodies are present with thrombocytopenia, and (c) HITT in which antibodies are present with thrombocytopenia and thrombosis.

4. When alternative anticoagulant coverage is used to prevent thrombotic complications, warfarin should not be administered as the initial, sole anticoagulant therapy because of its slow onset of action.

QUESTIONS

1. How is HIT classified?

   Answer: HIT is classified into two types. Type I HIT, also known as *nonimmune heparin-associated thrombocytopenia* is caused by platelet microaggregation and subsequent sequestration in the spleen. Type II HIT is an immune-mediated syndrome caused by an antibody to the heparin-PF4 complex.

2. What are the clinical manifestations and complications of type II HIT?

   Answer: Type II HIT has three clinical presentations: (a) latent phase in which antibodies are present without thrombocytopenia, (b) HIT whereby antibodies are present with thrombocytopenia, and (c) HITT in which antibodies are present with thrombocytopenia and thrombosis.

3. How is HIT antibody detected?

   Answer: Laboratory testing for HIT antibody is classified as antigenic or functional testing. Antigenic tests include enzyme-linked immunosorbent assay and rapid particle gel immunoassay that detect antibodies to heparin-PF4 complexes or complexes of PF4 and other polyanions. Functional tests include the ^{14}C-serotonin release assay and the platelet aggregation test.

References

1. Keeling D, Davidson S, Watson S, the Haemostasis and Thrombosis Task Force of the British Committee for Standards in Haematology (2006). The management of heparin-induced thrombocytopenia. Br J Haematol 2007;133:259–269.
2. Warkentin TE. Heparin-induced thrombocytopenia. Hematol Oncol Clin North Am 2007;21:589–607.
3. Levy JH, Tanaka KA, Hursting MJ. Reducing thrombotic complications in the perioperative setting: an update on heparin-induced thrombocytopenia. Anesth Analg 2007;105:570–582.
4. Keeling D, Davidson S, Watson H. The management of heparin-induced thrombocytopenia. Br J Haematol 2006;133:259–269.
5. Warkentin TE, Greinacher A. Heparin-induced thrombocytopenia: recognition, treatment, and prevention. Chest 2004;126: S311–S337.

CHAPTER 13

Hypertonic Saline Resuscitation

David M. Rothenberg

CASE FORMAT: REFLECTION

A 33-year-old male presented to the emergency department having sustained a closed head injury and blunt abdominal trauma following a motor vehicle collision. He had suffered loss of consciousness at the scene but was now awake and complaining of neck and abdominal pain. His past medical and surgical histories were unremarkable. He was taking no medications and had no known allergies. He denied alcohol, tobacco, or drug use. The patient's vital signs were as follows: blood pressure, 90/60 mm Hg; heart rate, 110 beats per minute; respiratory rate, 24 breaths per minute; and his temperature was 36.5°C.

On physical examination, the patient was oriented to person only, and a left sixth cranial nerve palsy was demonstrated. Posterior neck tenderness was elicited, the lungs were clear to auscultation, his abdomen was distended, rebound tenderness was present, and bowel sounds were diminished.

Following administration of 3 liters of normal saline (at the scene and in the emergency department), laboratory results were as follows: hemoglobin, 9.6 gm dL^{-1}; white blood cell count, 13,000/mm^3; Na^+, 145 mEq/L; K^+, 3.6 mEq/L; HCO_3^-, 18 mEq/L; Cl^-, 110 mEq/L; creatinine, 1.4 mg%; and blood urea nitrogen, 31 mg%. Abdominal paracentesis was positive for blood. A chest radiograph revealed possible free air under the diaphragm. The patient's computerized tomography (CT) scan of the head and neck demonstrated bilateral frontal lobe contusions with a moderate-sized right frontal parietal subdural hematoma (Fig. 13.1) but a normal cervical spine. A perforated cecum was seen on abdominal CT.

The patient underwent exploratory laparotomy, drainage of the subdural hematoma, and insertion of an external ventricular drain and intracranial pressure monitor. He received a total of 6 liters of intravenous normal saline, 500 mL of human albumin, and 2 units of packed red blood cells. Forty-eight hours later, he remained comatose, and the CT scan of his head revealed diffuse cerebral edema. On the third postoperative day, he developed oliguria and was noted to have intra-abdominal pressures of 35 mm Hg.

CASE DISCUSSION

Intravascular volume resuscitation in the setting of traumatic head injury, polytrauma, and severe burns is controversial not only in terms of targeted hemodynamic end points but also in terms of quantity and nature of fluid administration. Given that the extracellular space is four to five times larger than the plasma volume, large volume, isotonic crystalloid resuscitation is often required for trauma or burn patients to re-establish circulatory stability. Trauma, burns, or major surgery lead invariably to an obligatory loss of fluid into the intracellular or so-called third space compartment and an increase in the ratio of extracellular to plasma volume. Progressive brain swelling, increases in lung water, intra-abdominal hypertension, as well as immunologic and microcirculatory dysfunction can develop. The use of low-volume, hypertonic solutions may decrease the risk of these adverse events by restoring circulation and decreasing third space fluid sequestration, while preventing or minimizing the incidence of cerebral and pulmonary edema and abdominal compartment syndrome.

Traumatic Brain Injury

Cerebral edema and intracranial hypertension often develop from traumatic brain injury (TBI) and are associated with poor outcome. Osmotherapy with mannitol remains the most widely recommended mode of treatment. However, experimental data indicate that hypertonic saline (HTS) (3%, 7.5%, 23.4%) can be as effective in reducing intracranial pressure and may have a longer duration of action. Prospective, randomized human trials assessing the use of HTS in patients with TBI, however, are limited. Vailet et al. evaluated 7.5% HTS versus mannitol in 20 patients with TBI and intracranial hypertension refractory to conventional therapy and found HTS to be more effective.[1] Cooper et al. compared a prehospital bolus of 250 mL of 7.5% HTS versus Lactated Ringer's solution in victims of traumatic brain injury.[2] Although there were no outcome differences between groups, patients in the HTS group had a prolonged period of sustained elevation in cerebral perfusion pressure, consistent with the aforementioned experimental studies. Although experimental and clinical data validate the effectiveness of HTS in reducing ICP, data proving improved outcomes are lacking.[3] A significant confounding variable is that the majority of patients studied also suffered from polytrauma, thus making it more difficult to differentiate the etiologies of morbidity and mortality.

Acute Lung Injury/Adult Respiratory Syndrome/Immunomodulation

Acute lung injury and adult respiratory distress syndrome occur in as many as 40% of patients suffering from polytraumatic injuries. A cascade of inflammatory mediators released following the sequestration of activated polymorphonuclear neutrophils

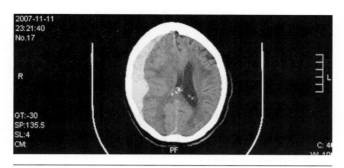

Figure 13.1 • A right-sided frontoparietal subdural hematoma with ventricular compression and evidence of increased intracranial pressure.

within the microcirculation of the lung is purported to be an important mechanism by which secondary injury occurs in the setting of trauma and hemorrhagic shock. Experimental studies have shown HTS-mediated immunomodulation, which suggests a role in mitigating the inflammatory process. Junger and colleagues found HTS (7.5% sodium chloride, 4 mL/kg) enhanced T-cell function in vitro and cell-mediated immune function in vivo in a murine model of hemorrhagic shock.[4] HTS also protected animals by improving survival from sepsis. Rizoli et al. noted a beneficial effect of HTS (4 mL/kg of 7.5% sodium chloride) in significantly reduced transpulmonary albumin leak, bronchioalveolar lavage fluid neutrophil counts, and the degree of histopathologic lung injury, when compared to Lactated Ringer's solution resuscitation in a rodent model of hemorrhagic shock.[5]

Secondary Abdominal Compartment Syndrome

Abdominal compartment syndrome is defined as the presence of sustained intra-abdominal pressure elevation ≥20 mm Hg with or without abdominal perfusion pressure <50 mm Hg and associated with new-onset single or multiorgan system failure. Abdominal compartment syndrome can occur as a result of primary abdominal trauma or surgery or secondary to massive fluid resuscitation-induced visceral edema in nontrauma or burn patients, particularly in the setting of shock. The gut is prone to ischemia-reperfusion injury, and the subsequent increase in microvascular permeability leads to large quantities of free intraperitoneal fluid and subsequent intra-abdominal hypertension. Intra-abdominal hypertension and secondary abdominal compartment syndrome significantly

decrease cardiac output by diminishing preload and increasing systemic vascular resistance. Unintended intra-abdominal hypertension can also impair respiratory, renal, gastrointestinal, and hepatic function and lead to multiorgan system failure. Aggressive crystalloid fluid resuscitation in an attempt to counter these pathophysiologic changes often contributes to the development of abdominal compartment syndrome and has been termed "futile crystalloid preloading." Some studies have suggested that more than 6 liters of crystalloid fluids within the first 24 hours of resuscitation of critically ill patients may result in a higher incidence of abdominal compartment syndrome and multiorgan system failure.[6] In this regard, it has been suggested that the use of HTS may be advantageous in minimizing intra-abdominal hypertension. Oda et al. compared the administration of hypertonic lactated saline versus standard Lactated Ringer's solution in patients who sustained burn injuries of greater than 40% of their body surface areas and found a significant decrease in the incidence of intra-abdominal hypertension and secondary abdominal compartment syndrome.[7] Improvements in oxygenation were also noted. Despite these preliminary findings, further randomized controlled studies are necessary before definitive recommendations can be made regarding the use of HTS to prevent secondary abdominal compartment syndrome.

Types and Methods of Hypertonic Saline Administration

HTS tends to mobilize intracellular water, reduced cellular edema, and reduced overall volume requirements during resuscitation. Plasma volume is expanded, cardiac output is increased, and overall oxygen delivery is improved all relatively rapidly when compared with isotonic saline resuscitation. The most often used formulation of hypertonic solution is a combination of 7.5% sodium chloride (2400 mOsm/L saline) and 6% dextran 70, a colloid solution that exerts two to three times the colloid osmotic pressure of an equal concentration of human albumin. An infusion of 4 to 6 mL/kg over several hours appears to be safe and effective. Bolus doses of 250 mL of 7.5% sodium chloride over 10 to 15 minutes also appear to be well tolerated in clinical studies.[8] Table 13.1 details the characteristics of the most commonly administered HTS solutions.

Complications of HTS Administration

HTS resuscitation can be associated with hyperosmolarity and hypernatremia. Serum osmolarity levels greater than 320 mOsm/L have been associated with acute renal failure during the use of mannitol; data are lacking regarding HTS

TABLE 13.1 HTS Characteristics

HTS (%)	Na1/Cl⁻ (mEq/L)	Osmolality (mOsm/L)	Maximum Infusion Rate
3	513	1030	100 mL/hr
5	855	1710	100 mL/hr
7.5	1282	2400	250 mL (bolus)
23.4	4000	8000	NA

HTS, hypertonic saline solution.

and these complications. Central pontine myelinolysis is a complication of the rapid correction of extracellular serum sodium levels in the setting of hypotonic hyponatremia. Retrospective studies, however, have failed to demonstrate central pontine myelinolysis either by magnetic resonance imaging or at postmortem examination. Other concerns with HTS administration include rebound intracranial hypertension and hyperchloremic metabolic acidosis.[9]

In conclusion, the use of HTS may offer a novel approach in caring for patients with traumatic brain injury, polytrauma, or burn injuries; however, its use must be tempered by the lack of clinically relevant outcome data. Current randomized, controlled trials may offer further insight into this type of therapy.[10]

KEY MESSAGES

1. HTS can be of benefit in the management of traumatic brain injury by decreasing intracranial pressure.

2. Massive crystalloid resuscitation may result in a secondary abdominal compartment syndrome that can be mitigated by the use of HTS solutions.

3. Complications of HTS administration may include hyperchloremic metabolic acidosis, hyperosmolarity, and rebound intracranial hypertension.

QUESTIONS

1. Hypertonic saline resuscitation for a patient with traumatic brain injury may result in which of the following complications?
   A. Central pontine myelinolysis
   B. Cerebral edema
   C. Cerebral artery vasospasm
   D. Rebound intracranial hypertension
   E. Diabetes insipidus

   Answer: D

2. A 33-year-old male receives hypertonic saline resuscitation following a 50% body surface area thermal injury. Which of the following physiologic parameters may be expected to decrease when compared to standard therapy with isotonic crystalloid solutions?
   A. Intra-abdominal pressure
   B. PaO_2/fiO_2 ratio
   C. Urine output
   D. Cardiac output
   E. Gastric pH

   Answer: A

3. Which of the following serum electrolyte abnormalities is more likely to occur when large volume fluid resuscitation is performed with Lactated Ringer's solution rather than with small volume hypertonic saline?
   A. Hypomagnesemia
   B. Hypocalcemia
   C. Hypokalemia
   D. Hyponatremia
   E. Hypochloremia

   Answer: D

References

1. Vialet R, Albanese J, Thomachot L, et al. Isovolume hypertonic solutes (sodium chloride or mannitol) in the treatment of refractory posttraumatic intracranial hypertension: 2 mL/kg 7.5% saline is more effective than 2 mL/kg 20% mannitol. Crit Care Med 2003;31:1683–1687.
2. Cooper DJ, Myles PS, McDermott FT, et al. Prehospital hypertonic saline resuscitation of patients with hypotension and severe traumatic brain injury: a randomized controlled trial. JAMA 2004;291:1350–1357.
3. White H, Cook D, Venkatesh B. The use of hypertonic saline for treating intracranial hypertension after traumatic brain injury. Anesth Anal 2006;102:1836–1846.
4. Junger WG, Coimbra R, Liu FC, et al. Hypertonic saline resuscitation: a tool to modulate immune function in trauma patients? Shock 1997;8:235–241.
5. Rizoli SB, Kapus A, Fan J, et al. Immunomodulatory effects of hypertonic resuscitation on the development of lung inflammation following hemorrhagic shock. J Immunol 1998;161: 6288–6296.
6. Kirkpatrick AW, Balogh Z, Ball CG, et al. The secondary abdominal compartment syndrome: iatrogenic or unavoidable? J Am Coll Surg 2006;202:668–679.
7. Oda J, Ueyama M, Yamashita K, et al. Hypertonic lactated saline resuscitation reduces the risk of abdominal compartment syndrome in severely burned patients. J Trauma 2006;60:64–71.
8. Kramer GC. Hypertonic resuscitation: physiologic mechanisms and recommendations for trauma care. J Trauma 2003;54: S89–S99.
9. Bunn F, Roberts I, Tasker R. Hypertonic versus isotonic crystalloid for fluid resuscitation in critically ill patients. Cochrane Database Syst Rev 2008.
10. Brasel KJ, Bulger E, Cook AJ, et al. Hypertonic resuscitation: design and implementation of a prehospital intervention trial. J Am Coll Surg 2008;206:222–232.

CHAPTER 14

Preoperative Liver Function Test Abnormalities

David M. Rothenberg

CASE FORMAT: REFLECTION

A 39-year-old, 6-ft, 80-kg man presented for repair of his left anterior cruciate ligament following a skiing injury. The patient's past medical history was significant only for hypertension treated with hydrochlorothiazide. His past surgical history included a right inguinal hernia repair performed under inhalational general anesthesia 1 year prior to this admission. His social history included occasional alcohol use but no history of recreational drug use. The patient's vital signs were as follows: blood pressure, 140/90 mm Hg; heart rate, 88 beats per minute; respiratory rate, 12 breaths per minute; and his temperature was normal. The remainder of his physical examination was unremarkable.

The orthopaedic surgeon had ordered an array of laboratory tests including complete blood count, coagulation profile, serum electrolytes, and liver function tests (LFTs). The results of the laboratory tests were within normal limits with the exception of serum aspartate aminotransferase (AST), 65 IU/L (normal range, 10–34 IU/L) and alanine aminotransferase (ALT), 55 IU/L (normal range, 8–37 IU/L). Total bilirubin and alkaline phosphatase levels were within normal limits as was the internationalized normalized ratio (INR).

At the outpatient surgery center, the anesthesiologist was reluctant to perform an anesthetic because of the elevation in LFTs and recommended further workup of the patient's abnormal transaminase results.

DISCUSSION

Patients with asymptomatic elevation in preoperative LFTs pose a dilemma for anesthesiologists in assessing perioperative hepatic risk, as prospective studies addressing this concern are lacking. The preoperative evaluation of risk for the development of postoperative hepatic dysfunction requires not only consideration of the magnitude of LFT abnormalities and whether or not active inflammatory or cholestatic disease exists, but also the nature of the surgical procedure planned.

The first question that must be asked regarding patients with asymptomatic elevation in LFTs is why the tests were initially ordered. Indiscriminate laboratory testing that reveals an increase in LFTs in an otherwise asymptomatic patient often leads to a delay in surgery based on the concern that administering an anesthetic may predispose the patient to postoperative hepatic dysfunction and subsequent morbidity or mortality. Abnormalities in LFTs including ALT, AST, and alkaline phosphatase are present in a small proportion of the general population[1] and in as many as 36% of patients with psychiatric illnesses (in whom alcohol and illicit drug use may be a contributory factor).[2] The overall prevalence of clinically significant liver dysfunction in asymptomatic patients, however, is less than 1%.[3] Therefore, the decision to pursue further costly diagnostic workup is rarely indicated on the basis of laboratory results alone. Rather, the most logical approach to such a patient begins with a targeted history and physical examination eliciting signs and symptoms of active hepatobiliary disease. This includes findings such as right upper quadrant pain or tenderness and history of scleral icterus, pruritus, fatigue, anorexia, nausea, or vomiting. Stigmata of cirrhosis are often self-evident; however, the patient should also be queried regarding a history consistent with chronic hepatitis, Wilson's disease, hemochromatosis, diabetes, as well as a history of previous blood product transfusion. All medications, vitamins, and herbal remedies should be reviewed for potential hepatotoxic adverse effects, and the patient should be further questioned regarding the frequency and pattern of alcohol usage. Finally, a targeted history should also make reference to include illicit drug use, presence of tattoos, consumption of raw seafood, and sexual activity. If a detailed history and physical examination fail to suggest an etiology of the abnormal LFTs, it is reasonable to assume that the initial abnormalities were false positives and the tests should be repeated. Slight elevation in LFTs (less than twice normal values) do not warrant further testing before anesthesia or/and surgery. Greater elevation in LFTs requires a more detailed analysis of each specific abnormality. Abnormal LFTs in otherwise healthy patients can also reflect either a subclinical acute process, such as viral or toxin-mediated hepatitis or a chronic disorder such as chronic hepatitis.

Abnormalities of ALT and AST in combination tend to indicate hepatocellular injury.[4,5] An elevation in ALT greater than AST favors a diagnosis of viral hepatitis; an increase in AST greater than ALT tends to suggest alcohol-mediated hepatic injury. Increases in alkaline phosphatase and serum γ-glutamyltransferase indicate hepatobiliary disease, specifically extrahepatic bile duct obstruction or intrahepatic cholestasis. Further assessment of LFT abnormalities should include assessment of synthetic function. These tests entail measurement of serum bilirubin, albumin, and prothrombin time (as expressed by the INR); the latter being a sensitive index of hepatic synthetic function, often changing within 24 hours of hepatobiliary injury because of impaired synthesis of essential coagulation factors.

At this time, no prospective, randomized controlled trials have been performed to evaluate the perioperative risk of anesthesia or surgery in otherwise asymptomatic patients with

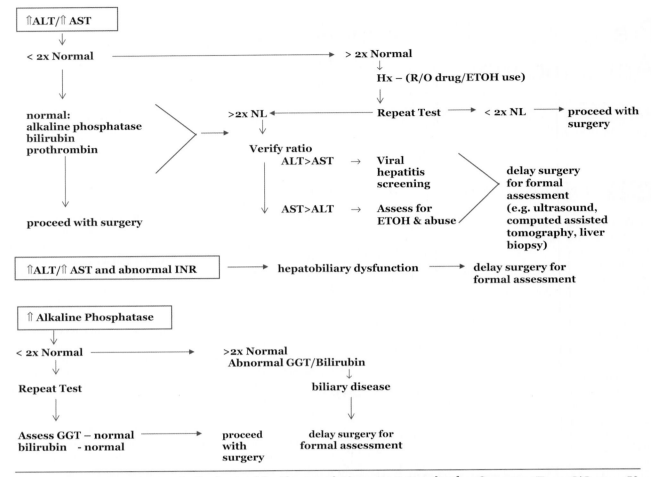

Figure 14.1 • Asymptomatic Patient with Abnormal Liver Test Results for Surgery. (From O'Connor CJ, Rothenberg D, Tumank KJ. Anesthesia and the hepatobiliary system. In Miller's Anesthesia, 6th Ed. New York: Elsevier, 2005.)

elevated LFTs. A suggested approach to such patients is delineated in Figure 14.1.

The preponderance of medical literature regarding perioperative morbidity and mortality in patients with acute hepatitis of any etiology suggests that elective surgery should be delayed until resolution of hepatic dysfunction. Patients with steatosis or steatohepatitis should also probably be considered to be at risk for developing postoperative liver failure, especially if they are to undergo major abdominal surgery. Additionally, patients with chronic hepatitis should be evaluated before elective surgery for any evidence of hepatic synthetic dysfunction. When surgery cannot be delayed or avoided, care must be taken during all phases of surgery to maintain hepatic vascular perfusion and to avoid factors that may precipitate liver failure, hepatic encephalopathy, or both.

Finally, patients with abnormal LFTs and a clinical constellation that is consistent with cirrhosis may be at particular risk for developing postoperative hepatic failure depending on the stage of cirrhosis as well as the type of surgery. Preoperative risk in patients with cirrhosis is often assessed by using the Child-Turcotte-Pugh scoring system (Table 14.1) and occasionally in conjunction with the model for end-stage liver disease scores (Table 14.2). Elective surgery should be considered contraindicated in patients with Child-Turcotte-Pugh classification C. Additionally, it is best to avoid elective

surgery in cirrhotic patients with an elevated INR, hypoalbuminemia, or preoperative infection or encephalopathy.

The actual surgical procedure itself, however, may be the most important risk factor for the development of postoperative hepatic dysfunction.[6] Abdominal surgery per se appears to significantly decrease total hepatic blood flow, particularly in patients with cirrhosis undergoing hepatic resection for hepatocellular carcinoma.[7,8] Cardiothoracic surgery is also associated with a high mortality rate in patients with pre-existing liver dysfunction.[9] Cardiopulmonary bypass may exacerbate pre-existing hepatic dysfunction by a multitude of mechanisms, including hepatic artery and portal venous hypoperfusion, low cardiac output syndrome, micro- or macroembolism, cytokine or oxygen free radical formation, and the influence of vasoactive and anesthetic drugs.

In assessing the patient described in this case, it is important to recognize that the peripheral nature of anterior cruciate ligament surgery imparts a minimal risk for this patient to develop postoperative liver failure, despite the slight elevation in this patient's LFTs. The magnitude of LFT elevation also indicates minimal risk of developing postoperative liver dysfunction and most likely represents either an effect of alcohol use or, less likely, that this is related to a cholestatic effect of hydrochlorothiazide. Repeating the LFTs is indicated primarily to rule out further increases indicative of ongoing or progressive pathology.

TABLE 14.1 Modified Child-Turcotte-Pugh Scoring System

Parameters	Modified Child-Turcotte-Pugh Score*		
	1	2	3
Albumin (g/dL)	>3.5	1.8–3.5	<2.8
Prothrombin time			
Seconds prolonged	<4	4–6	>6
International normalized ratio	<1.7	1.7–2.3	>2.3
Bilirubin (mg/dL)†	<2	2–3	>3
Ascites	Absent	Slight–moderate	Tense
Encephalopathy	None	Grade I–II	Grade III–IV

*Class A, = 5 to 6 points; B, = 7 to 9 points; and C, = 10 to 15 points.
†For cholestatic diseases (e.g., primarily biliary cirrhosis), the bilirubin level is disproportionate to the impairment in hepatic function, and an allowance should be made. For these conditions, assign 1 point for a bilirubin level less than 4 mg/dL, 2 points for a bilirubin level of 4 to 10 mg/dL, and 3 points for a bilirubin level greater than 10 mg/dL. Reproduced with permission from Pugh RNH, Murray-Lyon IM, Dawson JL, et al. Transection of oesophagus for bleeding of oesophageal varices. Br J Surg 1973;60:646–649.

KEY MESSAGES

1. Asymptomatic elevation in LFTs may or may not pose a significant perioperative risk for the patient undergoing anesthesia.

2. Specific LFT abnormalities can indicate the influence of preoperative medications, alcohol use, or active inflammatory disease.

3. Preoperative LFTs should only be considered on patients who present with a history or physical evidence of hepatic dysfunction.

4. The decision to perform surgery and administer anesthesia to patients with abnormal LFTs should be predicated on the nature of the surgery and the magnitude of changes on the LFTs.

TABLE 14.2 MELD Score Calculation

MELD = 3.78 [Ln serum bilirubin (mg/dL)] +
11.2 [Ln INR] + 9.57 [Ln serum creatinine
(mg/dL)] + 6.43

In addition, the following are modifications of the MELD score:

- The maximum score given is 40. All values higher than 40 are given a score of 40.

- If the patient has been dialyzed twice within the last 7 days, the serum creatinine level used should be 4.

- Any value less than 1 is given a value of 1.

INR, internationalized normalized ratio; MELD, end-stage liver disease.

QUESTIONS

1. Which of the following serum levels may be associated with increased perioperative morbidity?
   A. ALT 55 IU/L
   B. Bilirubin 3.6 mg%
   C. INR 1.6
   D. AST 90 IU/L
   E. Alkaline phosphatase 42 mg%
   Answer: D

2. A patient presenting for total hip replacement is noted to have clinical stigmata of cirrhosis including mild ascites. Preoperative laboratory values include a serum albumin level of 2.7 gm%, INR of 2.8, and a serum bilirubin level of 4 mg%. The most appropriate next step in this patient's care should be:
   A. Therapeutic paracentesis
   B. Preoperative plasma transfusion
   C. Delay of surgery
   D. Administration of 5% albumin
   E. Avoidance of inhalational general anesthesia
   Answer: C

3. Which of the following surgeries is associated with an increase in postoperative hepatic dysfunction in a patient with a preoperative history of chronic active hepatitis?
   A. Pneumonectomy
   B. Partial colectomy
   C. Bilateral total knee replacement
   D. Carotid endarterectomy
   E. Total thyroidectomy
   Answer: B

References

1. Kamath PS. Clinical approach to the patient with abnormal liver test results. Mayo Clin Proc 1996;71:1089–1095.
2. Farrell RL, DeColli JA, Chappelka AR. Significance of abnormal liver function studies in psychiatric admissions to military hospitals. Mil Med 1975;140:101–103.
3. Pratt DS, Kaplan MM. Primary care: evaluation of abnormal liver-enzyme results in asymptomatic patients. N Engl J Med 342:2000;1266–1271.
4. Cohn JA, Kaplan MM. The SGOT/SGPT ratio—an indicator of alcoholic liver disease. Dig Dis Sci 1979;24:835–838.
5. Hay JE, Czaja AJ, Rakela J, Ludwig J. The nature of unexplained chronic aminotransferase elevations of a mild to moderate degree in asymptomatic patients. Hepatology 1989;9:193–197.
6. Friedman LS. The risk of surgery in patients with liver disease. Hepatology 1999;29:1617–1623.
7. Mansour A, Watson W, Shayani V, Pickelman J. Abdominal operations in patients with cirrhosis: still a major surgical challenge. Surgery 1997;22:730–736.
8. Ziser A, Plevak DJ, Wiesner RH, et al. Morbidity and mortality in cirrhotic patients undergoing anesthesia and surgery. Anesthesiology 1999;90:42–53.
9. Filsoufi F, Slazberg SP, Rahmanian PB, et al. Early and late outcomes of cardiac surgery in patients with liver cirrhosis. Liver Transpl 2007;13:990–995.

CHAPTER 15

Perioperative Use of Albumin

W. Christopher Croley

A 68-year-old, 60-kg male with a history of hypertension, hypercholesterolemia, and non–insulin-dependent diabetes presented for a left hemicolectomy. The patient was currently taking metoprolol, metformin, and simvastatin. He completed a bowel preparation consisting of clear liquids, a Fleet enema, and 4 liters of GoLYTELY on the day before his procedure. The patient reported a recent history of nausea, vomiting, fatigue, and a 5-kg weight loss. His preoperative assessment revealed the following normal vital signs: blood glucose, 108 mg/dL and hemoglobin, 13 gm/dL. Electrocardiogram readings showed normal sinus rhythm with possible left ventricular hypertrophy. On physical examination, the patient had clear lung fields, normal heart sounds, a Mallampati I airway, and was edentulous.

Preoperatively, the patient had two 16-gauge intravenous (IV) cannulae and a right radial arterial line inserted. Once inside the operating suite, standard monitors were applied and general anesthesia was induced with 180 mg of sodium thiopental, 250 μg of fentanyl, and muscle relaxation was achieved with vecuronium 6 mg. The patient's trachea was easily intubated with a 7.5-mm endotracheal tube. Anesthesia was maintained with fentanyl (3 μg/kg per hour), sevoflurane (inspired 1%–1.5%), and further increments of vecuronium were administered as required. After induction of anesthesia, a right internal jugular triple-lumen catheter was inserted under ultrasound guidance for central venous pressure (CVP) monitoring. His initial CVP was 2 mm Hg. His vital signs remained stable throughout the procedure with mean arterial blood pressures (MAPs) between 60 to 75 mm Hg and CVP values ranging from 1 to 15 mm Hg. Estimated blood loss for the 4-hour procedure was 900 mL. The patient received 4000 mL of Lactated Ringer's solution and 750 mL of 5% human albumin. His trachea was extubated at the end of the procedure, and he was transferred to the surgical intensive care unit for further monitoring. On arrival to the surgical intensive care unit, his vital signs were as follows: heart rate, 105 beats per minute; blood pressure, 85/40 mm Hg with a MAP of 55 mm Hg; respiratory rate, 24 breaths per minute; and CVP, 2 mm Hg. He received an additional 500 mL of 5% human albumin, which increased his CVP to 10 mm Hg and MAP to 70 mm Hg. The patient was monitored in the surgical intensive care unit for 1 day and was then transferred to the general surgical floor. He was discharged home on the seventh postoperative day. On discharge from the hospital, his hemoglobin level was 9 gm/dL, and his creatinine and other laboratory measures were at their baseline values.

CASE DISCUSSION

The debate on crystalloid versus colloid fluid resuscitation continues to elicit strong opinions from clinicians who are forced to deal with volume resuscitation of patients on a daily basis. Although human albumin has been used for more than 60 years, semi-synthetic colloid fluids have only been introduced relatively recently. Albumin and semi-synthetic solutions are available in various concentrations. Although human albumin has been used for many years, there are insufficient data from large clinical trials to demonstrate improvement in morbidity or mortality rates when using human albumin as a resuscitation fluid.

Human albumin preparations contain more than 95% albumin with a uniform molecular size (Table 15.1). The capillary membrane is fairly permeable to small ions (i.e., Na^+ and Cl^-) but is relatively impermeable to larger molecules such as albumin. Therefore, it is postulated that colloids will remain in the intravascular space for a longer period of time than crystalloids. The duration that a colloid will affect plasma volume expansion is a function of the rate of colloid molecule loss from the circulation and by metabolism. Proponents of colloid fluid resuscitation argue that the increased duration of plasma volume expansion and decreased leaking of colloid molecules from the capillary membrane ultimately lead to less tissue edema, which may (in theory at least) benefit patient outcome. Human albumin has several disadvantages not associated with synthetic colloid products because it is a human-derived product (Table 15.2). Some of these disadvantages include expense, risk of transmission of infectious agents, and possible allergic reactions.

The Saline versus Albumin Fluid Evaluation trial is a randomized controlled trial of approximately 7000 patients that compared albumin and saline as resuscitation fluids and showed no difference in outcome between the two groups. This landmark trial is consistent with results of several other trials that have evaluated colloid versus crystalloid for fluid resuscitation and failed to demonstrate a significant mortality benefit.

Despite a lack of evidence demonstrating a clear benefit of colloid over crystalloid, some clinicians continue to use albumin

TABLE 15.1 Composition of Commonly Used Crystalloid Fluids

Solution	Osmolarity (mOsm/L)	Na⁺ (mmol/L)	Cl⁻ (mmol/L)	K⁺ (mmol/L)	Ca⁺⁺ (mmol/L)
0.9% Sodium chloride	308	154	154	-0-	-0-
Lactated Ringer's solution	309	147	156	4.0	2.2
Normasol	280	140	98	5	0

as a preferred resuscitation fluid. It is proposed that large volumes of crystalloid dilute plasma proteins, as well as plasma oncotic pressure, resulting in tissue and pulmonary edema. Clinically, the decrease in oncotic pressure and increase in tissue edema has not been proven to be detrimental in terms of patient mortality (Fig. 15.1).

For patients with limited IV access, albumin or other colloid fluids will expand plasma volume more rapidly than crystalloid and at a lower volume of total fluid infused. Outside of this particular indication, albumin should not be routinely used as a preferred resuscitation fluid because of lack of evidence of improved mortality, increased cost, and possible adverse events associated with administration. Future studies should aim to compare crystalloid versus colloid in terms of meaningful patient outcomes other than mortality. It will require careful systematic evaluation to identify specific clinical scenarios in which one or another type of fluid resuscitation will benefit the patient.

KEY MESSAGES

1. No mortality differences have been shown between patients who receive crystalloid versus colloid fluid for resuscitation in the perioperative period.

2. Human albumin is one of several colloid fluids available for volume resuscitation.

3. Limitations of albumin administration include acquisition cost, possible allergic reactions, and infectious risks.

QUESTIONS

1. You are preparing to transport a 69-year-old female to the endoscopy suite from the intensive care unit for an upper endoscopy when she begins to vomit bright red blood, becomes tachycardic to 140 beats per minute,

TABLE 15.2 Concerns with Human Albumin Administration

- Relatively expensive
- Possible transmission of infectious agents
- Allergic reactions
- Limited supply

and has a weak radial pulse. The patient has one 22-gauge IV in her left forearm, and four units of blood are on hold in the blood bank. The most appropriate initial fluid given the following options would be:

A. 250 mL of 0.9 normal saline

B. 500 mL of dextran

C. 250 mL of 5% human albumin

D. 100 mL of 3% hypertonic saline

Answer: C. This patient has one small-bore IV line and will need rapid volume expansion while blood is ordered from the blood bank and additional IV access is established; 5% albumin will provide greater plasma volume expansion in a shorter period of time than crystalloid. Dextran may have deleterious effects on platelets and worsen bleeding. Hypertonic saline is not indicated for rapid volume expansion during hypovolemic shock.

2. All of the following affect duration of albumin for plasma volume expansion except:

A. Continued resuscitation with 0.9% normal saline

B. Hypoalbuminemia

C. Rate of loss from circulation

D. Metabolism of administered albumin

E. None of the above

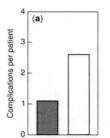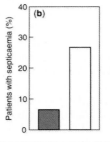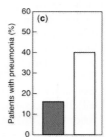

Figure 15.1 • (A) Mean complications per patient and percentage of patients, p value <0.008. Graph (B) depicts the percentage of patients with septicemia, p value <0.04. Graph (C) depicts patients with pneumonia, p value <0.05. These were each randomized controlled trials comparing albumin versus no albumin in patients with hypoalbuminemia that required total parenteral nutrition. Gray, albumin; white, no albumin. (Adapted from Haynes GR, Navickis RJ, Wilkes MM. Albumin administration—what is the evidence of clinical benefit? A systematic review of randomized controlled trial. Eur J Anest 2003;20:771–793.)

Answer: B. Continued resuscitation with 0.9% normal saline will dilute the plasma oncotic pressure and decrease the amount of time that the albumin has an effect on plasma volume expansion; hypoalbuminemia has no correlation with how long the albumin is administered, as resuscitation fluid will remain intravascular.

3. Problems associated with albumin include all of the following except:

A. Increased cost

B. Limited availability of product

C. Potential allergic reactions

D. Potential transmission of infectious organisms

E. Difficulty cross-matching blood after its administration

Answer: E. All answers listed are problems associated with albumin administration.

References

1. Miller RD. Miller's Anesthesia, 6th Ed. Philadelphia: Elsevier, 2005.
2. Boldt J, Schölhorn T, Mayer J, et al. The value of an albumin-based intravascular volume replacement strategy in elderly patients undergoing major abdominal surgery. Anesth Analg 2006;103:191–199.
3. The SAFE Study Investigators. A Comparison of albumin and saline for fluid resuscitation in the intensive care unit. NEJM 2004;350:2247–2256.
4. Vincent JL, Sakr Y, Reinhart K, et al. Is albumin administration in the acutely ill associated with increased mortality? Results of the SOAP study. Critical Care 2005;9:R745–R754.
5. Haynes GR, Navickis RJ, Wilkes MM. Albumin administration—what is the evidence of clinical benefit? A systematic review of randomized controlled trials. Eur J Anesth 2003; 20:771–793.
6. Russell JA, Navickis RJ, Wilkes MM. Albumin versus crystalloid for pump priming in cardiac surgery: meta-analysis of controlled trials. JCVA 2004;18:429–437.
7. Fuhong S, Zhen W, Ying C, et al. Fluid resuscitation in severe sepsis and septic shock: albumin, hydroxyethyl starch, gelatin, or Ringer's Lactate—does it really make a difference? Shock 2007;27:520–526.

CHAPTER 16

Neurologic Complications of Peripheral Nerve Blockade

Christopher J. O'Connor

FORMAT: REFLECTION

A 55-year-old, 90-kg man with a history of hypertension, non–insulin-dependent diabetes mellitus, and shoulder pain presented for right total shoulder arthroplasty. He had previously undergone inguinal hernia repair and an appendectomy without anesthetic complications. His regular medications included metoprolol, valsartan, metformin, and naproxen. The preoperative evaluation identified left ventricular hypertrophy on his electrocardiogram, his nonfasting serum glucose level was 170 mg/dL, and hemoglobin concentration was 12.9 mg/dL. Initially, the patient's vital signs were as follows: blood pressure, 136/80 mm Hg; heart rate, 65 beats per minute; arterial oxygen saturation, 98%; and respiratory rate, 18 breaths per minute. Neurologic function of the operative arm was normal.

The anesthetic plan comprised an interscalene block (to be inserted preoperatively) and a continuous interscalene catheter for postoperative analgesia, in conjunction with general anesthesia and tracheal intubation.

An intravenous catheter was placed in the contralateral arm, and standard monitors were applied. Oxygen was administered at 3 L per minute by nasal cannulae, and incremental doses of midazolam (0.5 mg) and fentanyl (25 mcg) were administered according to the anesthesiologist's clinical judgment. A nerve stimulator was prepared by attaching the grounding lead to a surface electrode, the patient's chest, and a 17-gauge insulated Tuohy needle was primed with local anesthetic. The right side of the patient's neck was prepared using sterile precautions. Local anesthetic (LA) (lidocaine 2%, 2 mL) was injected subcutaneously at the interscalene groove, and the Tuohy needle was advanced until the characteristic musculocutaneous nerve response (biceps muscle contraction) was achieved. Following negative aspiration of the needle for blood, 35 mL of 0.5% ropivacaine with epinephrine (1/10,000) was incrementally injected with serial aspirations after each 3-mL injection. No change in heart rate or sensorium was noted. Following completion of the LA injection and as the interscalene catheter was inserted through the Tuohy needle, the patient's left hand and arm began to twitch, and he became unresponsive to verbal command. The needle was immediately withdrawn, and midazolam (3 mg) was administered, while oxygen (100%) was given using positive-pressure bag/mask ventilation. The twitch-

ing resolved immediately, and within 15 minutes, the patient was once more responsive and oriented. Sensory and motor testing of the right arm and shoulder revealed dense anesthesia.

The patient underwent uncomplicated total shoulder arthroplasty and recovery. Five days later, however, he reported a sensory paresthesiae in the median nerve distribution of his right arm. Nerve conduction studies demonstrated mild conduction disturbance of his right median nerve that resolved completely over 3 weeks. His recovery was otherwise uneventful.

DISCUSSION

Central Nervous System Toxicity

Central nervous system (CNS) toxicity follows vascular absorption or intravascular injection of LA and manifests as a change in the patient's sensorium or mental status, the patient's perception of a metallic taste, tinnitus, or as an overt grand mal seizure. CNS toxicity tends to precede cardiovascular toxicity and is typically short lived. Appropriate management entails administration of small doses of midazolam or sodium thiopental and support of ventilation and oxygenation during the (usually) brief duration of the seizure or altered mental status. If the patient's mental status returns to baseline promptly, and if no injuries are sustained during the event, it is reasonable to proceed with surgery.

Peripheral Nerve Injury

Nerve injury following peripheral nerve blockade (PNB) is gratifyingly uncommon. Published investigations of the incidence of this complication are limited by study design and inconsistent neurodiagnostic follow-up. Moreover, it is often difficult to determine the precise etiology of postoperative neurologic deficits (PNB-related vs. surgical). Despite these limitations, certain conclusions can be drawn. The mechanism of nerve injury after surgery accompanied by PNB can be related to several factors, including block-related events (e.g., needle trauma, intraneural injection [INI],[1,2] and LA neurotoxicity), surgical factors (e.g., surgical trauma, stretch injuries, and the impact of tourniquets, hematomata, compressive dressings, and positioning), and the impact of pre-existing conditions (e.g., bony deformities and peripheral neuropathy).

Needle trauma is probably uncommon, whereas INI appears to be the likely mechanism of block-related nerve injury in most patients. High injection pressures[2] and severe pain on injection indicate INI and subsequent fascicle disruption. The peripheral nerve is a complex structure bounded by the epineurium that encases multiple nerve fascicles surrounded by a perineural layer. Each fascicle contains myelinated neurons that can be damaged by intrafascicular injection of LA. This appears to produce neurologic injury by inducing swelling and edema of the fascicle with subsequent neurovascular compromise and possibly by direct LA toxicity.[3,4] Interestingly, Bigeleisen demonstrated that 81% of patients undergoing ultrasound (US)-guided axillary block had evidence of INI in at least one nerve, with no subsequent evidence of neurologic injury,[3] suggesting that small-volume INI does not produce clinical nerve injury and occurs commonly without a clinically detectable adverse outcome. This finding is borne out by clinicians experienced with US-guided PNB. Although US may facilitate accurate LA deposition around rather than within the nerve, there are no clinical data to validate that assumption. Bigeleisen's findings also imply that injection beneath the perineurium is the probable site of injury from INI.

In addition to block-related injury, surgical factors appear to be especially important in producing neurologic deficits. Experimental data, as well as electrophysiologic studies in patients have shown the compressive and neuronal ischemic effects of excessive tourniquet duration and inflation pressure on peripheral nerves. Horlocker et al.[5] and Fanelli et al.[6] demonstrated that duration of tourniquet inflation and pressures >400 mm Hg, respectively, were associated with an increased incidence of postoperative neurologic deficit after limb surgery. Retractor injury to the femoral nerve during hip arthroplasty, stretch injury of the brachial plexus during shoulder arthroplasty, and peroneal nerve injury related to preoperative valgus deformities and flexion contractures after

knee arthroplasty, are additional mechanisms that can result in postoperative neurologic deficit unrelated to PNB. In fact, Horlocker et al.[7] noted that 89% of neurologic deficits after 1614 axillary blocks were related to the surgical procedure itself, a finding consistent with other clinical reports. In addition, 4% of patients undergoing shoulder arthroplasty sustain brachial plexus injuries in the absence of PNB, again suggesting surgical nerve injury.[8] Candido et al. observed that of the 4.4% of 684 patients experiencing paresthesia after interscalene block for shoulder surgery, 45% were located at the site of the block, and 23% were in the distribution of the greater auricular nerve; more serious distal sensorimotor neuropathies were thus infrequent.[9] Finally, although preoperative neuropathy and nerve localization techniques can be associated with postoperative nerve injury, well-designed prospective studies have failed to show any consistent relationship between diabetes, pre-existing neuropathy, or the use of nerve localization techniques and the incidence of neurologic deficit after PNB.

Most postoperative neurologic complaints manifest within the first 48 hours after surgery. They are typically sensory deficits and usually resolve within 2 to 4 weeks, although rarely, deficits can require up to 9 months for complete recovery. Nerve conduction studies (NCS) and electromyography (EMG) typically reveal conduction delays consistent with neuropraxia, a temporary injury pattern associated with functional recovery. Assessment of neurologic deficits should include a careful neurologic examination, and, in most cases, NCS and EMG. Repeat studies are commonly performed at 4 to 6 weeks, after which clinical assessment appears to suffice in the absence of severe motor deficits.

Determining the incidence of block-related nerve injury is difficult (Tables 16.1 to 16.3). However, prospective analyses of more than 70,000 patients have indicated an incidence of 0.02%. This is likely to be an underestimate caused by self-reporting. Other prospective and retrospective analyses have

TABLE 16.1 Incidence of Neurologic Injury After Peripheral Nerve Blockade: Single-Injection Nerve Block

Author	Patient No.	Study Design	Incidence (F/U Time)	Block Type UE	Block Type LE	Recovery (at mos)
Auroy, 2002	50,223	Pro	0.02% (NS)	All	All	42% (6 mo)
Auroy, 1997	21,278	Pro	0.02% (48 h)	All	All	100%
Fanelli, 1999	3996	Pro	1.7% (1 mo)	ISB, Ax	F-SB	99% (3 mo)
Stan, 1995	1995	Pro	0.2% (? 1 wk)	Ax	—	100% (2 mo)
Klein, 2002	2382	Pro	0.25% (7 d)	All, ISB	F-SB	100% (3 mo)
Horlocker, 1999	1614	Retro	8.4% (2 wk)	Ax	—	100% (5 mo)
Candido, 2006	693	Pro	8.5% (2 d–1 mo)	ISB	—	97% (4 mo)
Bishop, 2005	568	Retro	2.3% (2 wk)	ISB	—	91% (6 mo)
Giaufre, 1996	1995	Pro	0%	All	All	—

Ax, axillary; F-SB, femoral-sciatic block; F/U, follow-up; ISB, interscalene block; LE, lower extremity; NS, not significant; pro, prospective; retro, retrospective; UE, upper extremity.

TABLE 16.2 Incidence of Neurologic Injury After Peripheral Nerve Blockade: Continuous Catheters

Author	Patient No.	Study Design	Incidence (%)	Block Type UE	Block Type LE	Recovery (at mos)	Comments
Capdevila, 2005	1416	Pro	0.2% (24 h)	All	All	100% (3 mo)	
Borgeat, 2003	700	Pro	8% (10 d)	ISC	—	100% (7 mo)	
Borgeat, 2001	530 (SS+CC)	Pro	14% (10 d)	ISC	—	99% (9 mo)	No difference SS and CC
Swenson, 2006	620	Pro	0.3% (1 wk)	ISC	FIC, SC	100% (2 mo)	
Bergman, 2003	405	Retro	1% (postop)	AxC	—	100%	
Sada, 1983	597	Pro	0.5% (?)	AxC	—	?	
Grant, 2001	228	Pro	0% (1, 7 d)	ISC	?	—	
Singelyn, 1999	446	Pro	0.1% (?)	—	FC	?	
Cuvillon, 2001	211	Pro	0.4% (6 wk)	—	FC	99% (12 mo)	

FC, femoral catheter; FIC, fascia iliaca catheter; F/U, follow-up; ISB, interscalene block; ISC, interscalene catheter; LE, lower extremity; NS, not significant; sc, sciatic catheter; UE, upper extremity.

shown greater complication rates of 0% to 8% after single-injection upper extremity blockade and rates <0.5% for lower extremity blocks. Studies of continuous catheter (CC) techniques have similarly revealed low neurologic injury rates. Capdevila et al.[10] demonstrated a 0.21% incidence of nerve injuries after 1416 upper and lower extremity CC techniques as did Swenson et al.[11] in a similar analysis of 620 CC techniques.

In conclusion, nerve injury can occur after PNB but is infrequent, is typically a transient sensory neuropraxia, and may be related to surgical (rather than block-related) mechanisms.

It may result from INI, a complication that can be minimized by discontinuing injection when either high injection pressures or pain are encountered, and it appears unrelated to the type of nerve localization technique employed. Whether US guidance will decrease the already low incidence of these complications has yet to be determined. It certainly holds promise for visual, real-time assessment of needle placement and LA deposition. Ultimately, as long as needles, nerves, and local anesthetics are in close proximity, the potential for nerve injury will exist.

TABLE 16.3 Pattern and Causality of Nerve Lesions: Single Injection

Author	Injury Pattern/Nerve Involvement	Block Type UE	Block Type LE	Anesthesia vs Surgery Cause
Auroy, 2002	Per neuropathy	All	All	Not specified
Auroy, 1997	Not specified	All	All	Not specified
Fanelli, 1999	Not specified	ISB, Ax	F-SB	Not specified
Stan, 1995	1 ulnar/MC paresthesia	Ax	—	0.2% because of block
Klein, 2002	ISB-RN injury SCB-UN Injury	All, ISB	F-SB	50% clearly surgical
Horlocker, 1999	Pain/numbness: UN (4), RN, MN	Ax	—	88% because of surgery
Candido, 2006	Paresthesia: ISB Site, aur ner, thumb	ISB	—	54% because of block
Bishop, 2005	Sensory neuropathy ulnar 5/10	ISB	—	Not specified
Schroeder, 1996	Not specified	All	—	72% because of surgery

aur ner, auricular nerve; Ax, axillary; blk, block; F-SB, femoral-sciatic block; ISB, interscalene block; LE, lower extremity; MC, musculocutaneous; MN, median nerve; Per, peripheral; RN, radial nerve; UE, upper extremity; UN, ulnar nerve.

KEY MESSAGES

1. Seizures are unpredictable but not uncommon complications of PNB. They are typically brief in duration, have few sequelae, and are easily managed with conservative therapy, including sedative/hypnotics in small doses, supplemental oxygen, and airway support.

2. Serious nerve injury after PNBs is rare and is typically sensory in nature. Such injury may be related to the nerve block itself (i.e., primarily intraneural injection, rarely needle trauma), direct surgical injury, or tourniquet-related nerve ischemia. It usually resolves in 3 to 6 weeks, although rarely sensorimotor lesions can last as long as 9 months.

3. Evaluation of persistent nerve injury after extremity surgery using PNB entails careful clinical assessment within 48 hours of surgery, NCS, EMG, and clinical evaluation at 2 and 6 weeks postoperatively. NCS and EMG help to estimate the severity and location of the lesion and the time course and likelihood of recovery but may not reveal its etiology (e.g., surgery vs. block-related nerve injury).

QUESTIONS

1. The most appropriate evaluation of persistent paresthesia after surgery involving PNB includes:
   A. MRI of the involved extremity
   B. Careful observation for 4 weeks
   C. Somatosensory-evoked potential measurements
   D. EMG and NCS
   E. Surgical re-exploration of the involved limb
   Answer: D.

2. Most postoperative neurologic complaints after PNB and orthopaedic surgery:
   A. Manifest 96 hours after surgery
   B. Resolve within 1 week
   C. Are usually motor deficits
   D. Represent neuropraxia of the involved nerves
   E. Are secondary to the nerve block
   Answer: D

3. The mechanism of peripheral nerve injury after PNB and orthopaedic surgery most likely results from:
   A. The use of paresthesia-seeking techniques
   B. Needle trauma
   C. The compressive effects of dressings
   D. Local anesthetic toxicity
   E. Surgical factors
   Answer: E

References

1. Hadzic A, Dilberovic F, Shah S, et al. Combination of intraneural injection and high injection pressure leads to fascicular injury and neurologic deficits in dogs. Reg Anesth Pain Med 2004;29:417–423.
2. Kaufman B, Nystrom E, Nath S, et al. Debilitating chronic pain syndromes after presumed intraneural injection. Pain 2000;85:283–286.
3. Bigeleisen P. Nerve puncture and apparent intraneural injection during ultrasound-guided axillary block does not invariably result in neurologic injury. Anesthesiology 2006;105:779–783.
4. Borgeat A. Regional anesthesia, intraneural injection, and nerve injury. Anesthesiology 2006;105:647–648.
5. Horlocker T, Hebl JR, Gali B, et al. Anesthetic, patient, and surgical risk factors for neurologic complications after prolonged total tourniquet time during total knee arthroplasty. Anesth Analg 2006;102:950–955.
6. Fanelli G, Casati A, Garancini P, et al. Nerve stimulator and multiple injection technique for upper and lower limb blockade: failure rate, patient acceptance, neurologic complications. Anesth Analg 1999;88:847–852.
7. Horlocker T, Kufner RP, Bishop AT, et al. The risk of persistent paresthesia is not increased with repeated axillary block. Anesth Analg 1999;88:382–387.
8. Lynch N, Cofield RH, Silbert PL, et al. Neurologic complications after total shoulder arthroplasty. J Shoulder Elbow Surg 1996;5:53–61.
9. Candido K, Sukhani R, Doty R Jr, et al. Neurologic sequelae after interscalene brachial plexus block for shoulder/upper arm surgery: the association of patient, anesthetic, and surgical factors to the incidence and clinical course. Anesth Analg 2005;100:1489–1495.
10. Capdevila X, Pirat P, Bringuier S, et al. Continuous peripheral nerve blocks in hospital wards after orthopedic surgery: a multicenter prospective analysis of the quality of postoperative analgesia and complications in 1,416 patients. Anesthesiology 2005;103:921–923.
11. Swenson JD, Bay N, Loose E, et al. Outpatient management of continuous peripheral nerve catheters placed using ultrasound guidance: an experience in 620 patients. Anesth Analg 2006;103:1436–1443.

CHAPTER 17

Peripheral Nerve Block Versus Epidural Analgesia for Total Knee Arthroplasty

Asokumar Buvanendran

CASE FORMAT: REFLECTION

A 62-year-old, 5'10" male weighing 122 kg presented to the anesthesia preoperative clinic 2 weeks before scheduled right total knee arthroplasty (TKA) for osteoarthritis. He expressed major concerns regarding postoperative pain control and recollected severe postoperative pain from his previous left TKA with poor range of motion currently in addition to chronic pain of his left knee. The patient's past medical history was significant only for hypertension and sleep apnea. His medications included metoprolol and nonsteroidal anti-inflammatory drugs (NSAIDs); the latter had been discontinued 1 week before his visit to the preanesthesia clinic because of concerns regarding perioperative bleeding. He had a continuous positive airway pressure (CPAP) machine, which he used most nights. The remaining history, physical examination, and diagnostic workup did not indicate cardiac disease. Physical examination revealed an obese, cooperative patient with a Mallampati class III airway and normal vital signs.

The patient was very concerned about stopping the NSAID, as it was the only drug providing him with pain relief for his right knee arthritis. He was willing to discuss any option that would provide him with adequate pain relief and also a better functional outcome than that following his previous TKR.

CASE DISCUSSION

TKA is a very effective treatment modality for severe chronic osteoarthritis of the knee. This procedure has become increasingly common over the past 2 decades.[1] In 2002 alone, more than 350,000 primary unilateral TKAs were performed.[1] This number has escalated to about 441,000 in 2004 and is expected to increase to 3.5 million by 2030.[1] This dramatic rise in the utilization rate for TKA can be attributed to an increasing elderly population and increased usage because of advances in surgical, anesthetic, and analgesic techniques. These advances have collectively contributed to decreased blood loss, less postoperative pain, a shorter duration of hospital stay, and improved functional outcome. The duration of hospital stay after TKA has decreased from an average of 7 to 10 days in the early 1990s to an average of 2 to 4 days currently.[2] The remainder of this discussion addresses the anesthetic management of this challenging patient.

Neuraxial Anesthesia and Analgesia

Although general anesthesia is still practiced in many hospitals for joint replacement, this trend is gradually decreasing as clinical studies have shown a greater incidence of adverse effects associated with general anesthesia and intravenous opioids compared with regional anesthesia/analgesia.[3] TKA is associated with severe postoperative pain, which interferes with early mobility and physical therapy, thereby affecting both short- and long-term patient outcomes. With the widespread use of regional anesthetic techniques, combined spinal epidural anesthesia followed by continuous and patient-controlled epidural analgesia has become a common anesthetic/analgesic procedure for joint replacement surgeries. Epidural analgesia has been shown to reduce postoperative blood loss, provide superior pain control, and improve postoperative functional outcome in comparison with intravenous patient-controlled analgesia.[4] Epidural analgesic solutions that are commonly used include opioids such as fentanyl, local anesthetics such as bupivacaine (many hospitals currently use ropivacaine because of its preferential sensory blockade properties and cardiovascular safety), or a combination of the two. Common adverse effects associated with epidural analgesia include hypotension, urinary retention, pruritus, nausea, vomiting, and headache. Significant intraoperative hypotension can lead to postoperative nausea and vomiting and can also be associated with decreased postoperative cognitive function. This may be detrimental to initiation of early physical therapy, which is crucial for improved knee range of motion. Serious adverse effects such as epidural hematoma and the associated nerve damage, respiratory depression, and infection have also been reported.

If the patient in the case presented consents to neuraxial anesthesia, a reasonable approach would be to perform combined spinal epidural using bupivacaine (10–15 mg) and fentanyl 25 μg for the spinal anesthetic because of their synergistic analgesia. Given this patient's history of sleep apnea, caution is advisable as administration of opioids intrathecally can trigger respiratory depression. Administration of a short-acting opioid intrathecally can be safe but requires appropriate monitoring postoperatively. In addition, this patient should receive an appropriate multimodal regimen (Table 17.1). Postoperative analgesia can be maintained with a local anesthetic alone or in combination with clonidine (α_2-agonist at low doses) as an adjuvant, thereby avoiding narcotics as the additive in the epidural mixture because of his history of sleep apnea. The patient should be monitored while using CPAP for respiratory parameters. As the patient undergoes rehabilitation, the epidural solution can be titrated to provide analgesia.

TABLE 17.1 Recommended Multimodal Drugs

Drug	Preoperative and Intraoperative	Postoperative
Acetaminophen	1000 mg	500–1000 mg three times daily
COX-2 inhibitor: celecoxib	400 mg 2 hours before surgery	200 mg twice per day
Ketamine	20–70 mg IV	
Gabapentin or pregabalin	600 mg or 100 mg respectively	300 or 75 twice per day
Clonidine	100 μg PNB	
Clonidine	10 μg via epidural	

IV, intravenous; PNB, peripheral nerve blockade.

The epidural catheter can be removed on the third postoperative day or earlier depending on his achievement of discharge criteria set by the physiotherapist. The subject of deep vein thrombosis (DVT) prophylaxis for joint arthroplasty is controversial with some authorities advocating aspirin alone, especially for patients undergoing minimally invasive joint replacement.

The risk of developing a hematoma in the epidural space is greater in patients who receive low-molecular-weight heparin (LMWH) postoperatively for DVT prophylaxis, especially after surgery involving the lower limbs.[9,10] The dramatic increase in the use of LMWH in the early 2000s for DVT prophylaxis influenced the movement toward peripheral nerve blockade (PNB) (and use of continuous catheter techniques) for pain after orthopaedic procedures. Thus, the use of LMWH and other anticoagulants has been an important determinant of how postoperative analgesia is provided after total joint replacement.

PNB

PNB of the major nerves supplying the lower extremities has emerged as a good alternative technique to an epidural for providing postoperative analgesia following procedures on the lower limb, especially in view of the current anticoagulation guidelines. PNB can be achieved by "single-shot" blockade or by continuous infusion. For lower limb surgeries, a femoral nerve block, a sciatic nerve block, an obturator nerve block, or a "three-in-one" block can be performed. Femoral nerve blocks are most commonly used for knee arthroplasties, either alone or in combination with a sciatic nerve block. After completion of the femoral nerve block, the patient is turned laterally for placement of a sciatic perineural catheter using a gluteal approach. Anatomically, an obturator nerve block in combination with a femoral nerve block provides superior analgesia compared with femoral plus sciatic nerve block. Performing an effective obturator nerve block is challenging. A "three-in-one" block is intended to block the lateral femoral cutaneous, the femoral, and the obturator nerves using a single injection.

Several studies have compared the analgesic efficacy and incidence of adverse effects of PNBs (femoral alone or femoral plus sciatic) versus epidural analgesia. In a systematic review of studies that compared the two techniques, Fowler et al. concluded that the analgesic efficacy of epidural and PNB techniques was similar but that the incidence of adverse effects (hypotension, urinary retention, and nerve injury) was less for PNB.[5] Nerve injuries associated with PNB present much less patient morbidity than a neuraxial injury. The review also evaluated the potential benefit of combining a sciatic block with a femoral block and concluded that there was no additional benefit.[5] Although the lumbar plexus block has greater consistency with regard to blocking the obturator nerve compared to the infrainguinal femoral block (three-in-one), it is unclear as to whether there is any benefit in adding the obturator block.[6] The incidence of quadriceps weakness with PNBs is greater and can therefore interfere with early mobilization of the patient, but there appears to be no difference in rehabilitative outcomes for the two groups at the time of discharge.[6] Only limited evidence exists on whether continuous femoral nerve block is more effective than a single-shot femoral block. In one randomized trial by Salinas et al., continuous femoral block (vs. single shot) lessened pain scores and increased opioid consumption significantly; however, the duration of hospital stay and functional outcome did not differ between the two groups.[7] Although the mechanism is not clear,[8] the addition of clonidine 100 μg to PNB leads to prolongation of analgesic effect.

In the case presented herein, a reasonable alternative approach would be to insert femoral nerve and sciatic nerve catheters preoperatively. This combination could be used to provide adequate anesthesia for TKA either alone or with a mini-dose single-dose of spinal anesthetic. The local anesthetic concentration in the two peripheral catheters should be low so that patients can participate actively in their physiotherapy. It is also important to administer neuronal blockade as one element of a multimodal regimen that is adjusted in response to patient recovery throughout the perioperative period.

Opioids and Obstructive Sleep Apnea

A known or presumptive diagnosis of obstructive sleep apnea (OSA) in a patient scheduled for surgery can influence the choice of anesthetic as well as postoperative analgesic management. In every obese adult patient, preoperative assessment should include questions on nocturnal snoring, and/or

TABLE 17.2 Screening Questions for Sleep Apnea

- Do you snore excessively?
- Is your sleep refreshing?
- Do you have periods when you stop breathing while sleeping?

snorting and/or apnea, and daytime sleepiness (Table 17.2). Patients with OSA are particularly sensitive to the depressant effects of opioids, sedatives, and tranquilizers.[11,12] Opioids have been shown to increase the effects of sleep and decrease arousal mechanisms. In a patient without OSA, the ensuing hypoxemia and hypercarbia after the use of opioids and other sedatives trigger carotid and brainstem chemoreceptors to increase respiratory drive. In individuals with OSA, however, this physiologic response is vulnerable to the effects of opioids and other sedatives. In these patients, it is recommended that opioid analgesia should be avoided, and a multimodal analgesic regimen, which includes regional analgesia, should be used during the postoperative period.[13] It is important that such patients (as in the case described) continue their CPAP settings during the perioperative period, and oxygen saturation should be monitored continuously. Given the severity of postoperative pain associated with TKA, judicious administration of opioids may be necessary even in the presence of a functioning PNB.

Multimodal Analgesia for TKA

Tissue inflammation resulting from surgery triggers the production of prostaglandins (PG). Prostaglandins, particularly PGE_2, mediate pain by sensitizing the peripheral nociceptors to mechanical and chemical mediators of pain. Prostaglandins have also been shown to play a role in central sensitization. One isoenzyme of cyclooxygenase (COX-2) is primarily responsible for the production of PGE_2. Selective COX-2 inhibitors decrease postoperative inflammation and pain and improve the overall functional outcome in patients after TKA.[14,15] Unlike other NSAIDs, selective COX-2 inhibitors such as celecoxib, do not compromise hemostasis; therefore, patients can continue to take celecoxib until the day of surgery and continue this regimen into the postoperative period. This presents one solution to the concerns expressed by the patient in this case. Discontinuing NSAIDs before surgery can lead to increased preoperative pain (osteoarthritis flare-up), and in turn, to increased postoperative pain scores. Patients who discontinue NSAIDs should be started on COX-2 inhibitors before surgery and for 10 to 14 days (for suggested doses, see Table 17.1) postoperatively until the inflammatory response to surgery has resolved. Pregabalin is an α_2-δ ligand that can act in synergy with COX-2 inhibitors to decrease postoperative hyperalgesia. Randomized controlled trials conducted in the perioperative setting in orthopaedic populations, both with gabapentin and pregabalin, have demonstrated an opioid-sparing effect (10%–20%). However, neither of these drugs alone or in combination can completely replace opioids for pri-

mary analgesia. Nevertheless, they are valuable elements of a multimodal approach to postoperative pain management. In addition, the use of pregabalin or gabapentin may decrease the incidence of chronic pain developing after knee surgery[1] (as in the case described). Patients who already have chronic pain from a previous surgery and are undergoing another surgical procedure are at a greater risk of developing an adverse outcome. Therefore, the perioperative physician should make every attempt to attenuate the surgical response, both humeral and neuronal, so that the patient can have an improved outcome. Other agents that could be used in the perioperative period for this patient include a round-the-clock regimen of acetaminophen (not exceeding 4 g/day), magnesium (N-methyl-D-aspartate antagonist), and vitamin C (antioxidant).

SUMMARY

Patients undergoing TKA should be offered a COX-2 inhibitor until the day of surgery to relieve pain from osteoarthritis. A multimodal analgesic regimen should be applied and adjusted during the perioperative period.[16] Postoperative management should include either a femoral nerve catheter or an epidural to optimize analgesia, so that patients can undergo aggressive physical therapy for an improved functional outcome.

KEY MESSAGES

1. Postoperative analgesia for patients undergoing TKA is vital for improved long-term outcome. Either PNB or an epidural can safely be instituted.

2. Patients with OSA present a significant challenge to anesthesiologists, and caution needs to be exercised in administering opioids and sedatives.

3. Acute postoperative pain is associated with an increased likelihood of developing chronic pain. It is likely that an effective multimodal analgesic regimen including neuraxial or PNB decreases the incidence of persistent postsurgical pain.

QUESTIONS

1. Which of the following statements is true?
   A. Poor postoperative pain control surgery will lead to good outcome.
   B. Opioids can be safely administered in patients with sleep apnea.
   C. Excellent postoperative pain control has been associated with improved functional outcomes.
   D. PNBs should not be performed in orthopaedic patients.
   Answer: C

2. Pregabalin acts at which receptor?
   A. N-methyl-D-aspartate receptor
   B. Aminobutyric acid receptor
   C. $\alpha 2 - \delta$ subunit of calcium channel
   D. Inhibits prostaglandins
   E. Acts at the α_2 channel
   Answer: C

3. Obese patients need to be asked the following questions except:
   A. History of snoring
   B. History of waking up in the night
   C. History of lethargy early in the morning and falling sleep during the day
   D. Do not bring the CPAP machine they use at home to the hospital
   Answer: D

References

1. Mahomed NN, Barrett J, Katz JN, et al. Epidemiology of total knee replacement in the United States Medicare population. JBJS 2005;87:1222–1228.
2. National Hospital Discharge Survey, 1991–2004. The U.S. Department of Health and Human Services.
3. Chu CPW, Yap JCCM, Chen PP. Postoperative outcome in Chinese patients having primary total knee arthroplasty under general anesthesia/intravenous patient controlled analgesia compared to spinal-epidural anesthesia/analgesia. Hong Kong Med J 2006;12:442–447.
4. Choi PT, Bhandari M, Scott J, Douketis J. Epidural analgesia for pain relief following hip or knee replacement. Cochrane Database Systematic Review. 2003;(3):CD003071.
5. Fowler SJ, Symons J, Sabato S, Myles PS. Epidural analgesia compared with peripheral nerve blockade after major knee sur-gery: a systematic review and meta-analysis of randomized trials. Br J Anaesth 2008;100:154–164.
6. Campbell A, McCormick M, McKinlay K, Scott NB. Epidural vs. lumbar plexus infusions following total knee arthroplasty: randomized controlled trial. Eur J Anesthesiol 2008;1–6.
7. Salinas FV, Liu SS, Mulroy MF. The effect of single-injection femoral nerve block versus continuous femoral nerve block after total knee arthroplasty on hospital length of stay and long-term functional recovery within an established clinical pathway. Anesth Analg 2006;102:1234–1239.
8. Kroin JS, Buvanendran A, Beck DR, et al. Clonidine prolongation of lidocaine analgesia after sciatic nerve block in rats is mediated via the hyperpolarization activated cation current, not by alpha-adrenoreceptors. Anesthesiology 2004;101:488–494.
9. Checketts MR, Wildsmith JAW. Central nerve block and thromboprophylaxis—is there a problem? Br J Anaesth 1999;82: 164–167.
10. Horlocker TT, Wedel DJ, Benzon H, et al. Regional anesthesia in the anticoagulated patient: defining the risks. Reg Anesth Pain Med 2003;28:172–197.
11. Harrison MK, Childs A, Carson PE. Incidence of undiagnosed sleep apnea in patients scheduled for elective total joint arthroplasty. J Arthroplast 2003;18:1044–1047.
12. Practice Guidelines for the perioperative management of patients with obstructive sleep apnea. Anesthesiology 2006;104: 1081–1093.
13. Benumof JL. Obstructive sleep apnea in the adult obese patient: implications for airway management. Anesthesiol Clin N Amer 2002;20:789–811.
14. Buvanendran A, Kroin JS, Berger RA, et al. Up-regulation of prostaglandin E2 and interleukins in the central nervous system and peripheral tissue during and after surgery in humans. Anesthesiology 2006;104: 403–410.
15. Buvanendran A, Kroin JS, Tuman KJ, et al. Effects of perioperative administration of a selective cyclooxygenase 2 inhibitor on pain management and recovery of function after knee replacement: a randomized controlled trial. JAMA 2003;290:2411–2418.
16. Reuben SS, Buvanendran A. Preventing the development of chronic pain after orthopedic surgery with preventive multimodal analgesic techniques. JBJS 2007;89:1343–1358.

CHAPTER 18

Paravertebral Nerve Blockade for Thoracic Surgery

Adrienne Wells

FORMAT: REFLECTION

A 72-year-old, 65-kg female with a history of dyspnea, productive cough, and fatigue presented for a left lower lobectomy for lung cancer. Her medical history was significant for a 90 pack-year smoking history, coronary artery stent placement following an acute myocardial infarction 3 months previously, and obstructive lung disease. Her medications included metoprolol, salmeterol/fluticasone inhaler, lovastatin, aspirin, and clopidogrel.

Preoperative evaluation revealed a frail elderly woman who was sitting up in bed, receiving oxygen by nasal cannulae. She was slightly dyspneic but able to complete sentences and carry on a conversation. Her airway examination was normal, but lung auscultation revealed coarse breath sounds throughout and decreased breath sounds at the left base. The patient's heart sounds were normal, and the results of her laboratory tests were within normal limits, except for hemoglobin concentration (16 gm/dL) and carbon dioxide content of 34 mEq/dL. Her echocardiogram showed evidence of an old inferior myocardial infarction. Her pulmonary function tests demonstrated significant obstructive disease, and SpO_2 on 4 liters of oxygen via nasal cannula was 97%. The decision was made to include a regional technique as part of her plan for postoperative analgesia. Because she may have had impaired hemostatic function caused by concomitant aspirin and clopidogrel therapy, it was decided to provide continuous paravertebral blockade (PVB) with a local anesthetic/opioid combination.

The patient arrived in the operating room with a large-bore intravenous cannula and an arterial cannula in place. After application of standard monitors, she was then placed in a sitting position, and the paravertebral space at T8–T9 was identified. A loss-of-resistance technique was used, and the paravertebral space was found at a depth of 3.5 cm from the skin. An epidural catheter was advanced easily, and the test dose was negative. Fifteen milliliters of a 0.25% ropivacaine solution was administered via the catheter, and an infusion 0.2% of ropivacaine was started at 5 mL per hour.

A double-lumen endobronchial tube was placed, and the patient's left lung was deflated to facilitate surgical access and one-lung ventilation. Her SpO_2 decreased despite administration of 100% oxygen. Positive end-expiratory pressure was administered to the dependent lung, and continuous positive airway pressure was applied to the nondependent lung, resulting in improvement in SpO_2 (to 96%). A left lower lobectomy and mediastinal node dissection were performed uneventfully.

CASE DISCUSSION

Changes in Respiratory Function After Thoracotomy

Following thoracic surgery, characteristic respiratory abnormalities include a restrictive defect with severely reduced vital capacity and functional residual capacity. This decreased inspiratory capacity, limits the patient's ability to cough effectively, and increases the risk of atelectasis. Full return to preoperative values may not be seen for several weeks after surgery. Patients, such as the one presented in this case, who have pre-existing respiratory dysfunction and a long smoking history, are at greatest risk for postoperative pulmonary complications.

Both thoracic epidural analgesia (TEA) and PVB have been shown to preserve postoperative lung function. Some evidence suggests that the protective effect of PVB outweighs that of TEA. Figure 18.1 compares the proportionate preservation of lung function with different analgesic options.

Postthoracotomy Pain

Postthoracotomy pain is mediated by nociceptive output via three different nerve pathways: the intercostal, phrenic, and vagus nerves. Elevated catecholamine levels are observed, and the sympathetic nervous system is also activated. Effective pain control without respiratory depression is the major goal postoperatively and can be accomplished using either TEA or PVB.[1-3] It has been suggested that PVB may be unique because it can modulate the neuroendocrine stress response and abolish evoked potentials to thoracic dermatomal stimulation.

TEA

Long considered the gold standard for the treatment of postthoracotomy pain and still practiced exclusively in many institutions, TEA is an effective means of pain control in this setting. Unfortunately, TEA results in a bilateral sympathectomy, which can produce hypotension. In turn, this can require a reduction in the rate of the epidural infusion of local anesthetics and result in inadequate analgesia. Urinary retention can also occur. TEA has several limitations, with active anticoagulation considered an absolute rather than a relative contraindication. Because this patient had been treated with clopidogrel 3 days before surgery, she was still considered to have a potential impairment in hemostasis. The clinically accepted time for cessation of clopidogrel therapy before using a central neuraxial technique is 5 to 7 days, although

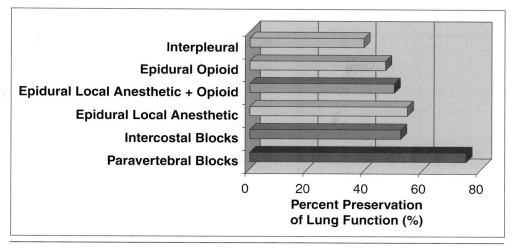

Figure 18.1 • Comparison of Paravertebral Blockade and Thoracic Epidural Analgesia for the Treatment of Postthoracotomy Pain. This figure demonstrates better efficacy of paravertebral blockade in preserving lung function after thoracotomy compared with a variety of other analgesia modalities. (Data from Richardson J, Sabanathan S, Shah R. Post-thoracotomy spirometric lung function: the effect of analgesia. A review. J Cardiovasc Surg 1999:40:445–456.)

this recommendation is largely empiric and based on the time required for full return of normal platelet function.

PVB

First described in 1905, PVB remains underutilized. The paravertebral space is defined anterolaterally by the parietal pleura, posteriorly by the superior costotransverse ligaments, medially by the vertebrae, and superiorly and inferiorly by the heads of the ribs. The paravertebral space, like the epidural space, communicates both superiorly and inferiorly. Local anesthetic injected here will produce a unilateral somatic and sympathetic block.[1,4] Because this block is unilateral, paravertebral catheters generally produce less hypotension than TEA. Limited data suggest that PVB is more effective than TEA in preserving lung function after thoracotomy[5] (Fig. 18.2). Although the absolute contraindications for PVB are similar to those for TEA, anticoagulation is a relative contraindication. There are few vessels in the paravertebral space, and a paravertebral hematoma has fewer potential neurologic complications than a thoracic epidural hematoma.

Technique for PVB

Paravertebral catheter placement involves a loss-of-resistance technique, similar to that of thoracic epidural catheter placement. With the patient in the sitting position, the desired thoracic level is identified. A mark should be made 2.5 cm lateral to the midpoint of the spinous process, and a 17-gauge Tuohy needle is advanced slowly until the transverse process is contacted (Fig. 18.3). The needle should then be redirected in a caudad fashion until a loss of resistance is felt, typically at 1 cm beyond the transverse process. The catheter should be threaded no more than 4 cm into the space for an adult and 2 to 3 cm for a child. This decreases the likelihood that

the catheter tip advances along the course of an intercostal nerve root. Test dosing is the same as for thoracic epidural placement.

CONCLUSION

In summary, postthoracotomy pain is an important and often difficult problem to manage. TEA and PVB are both useful techniques for providing postoperative analgesia. The lesser incidence of hypotension, decreased stress response, unilateral blockade, and potentially better preserved pulmonary function than with TEA, make continuous PVB an attractive option, especially for patients with abnormal hemostatic function.

KEY MESSAGES

1. Preoperative respiratory dysfunction may be associated with significant impairment of postoperative pulmonary function after thoracotomy and lung resection.

2. The etiology of postthoracotomy pain is multifactorial and involves both nociceptive and neuropathic pathways.

3. TEA or PVB can decrease respiratory depression associated with opioid use and can improve postoperative respiratory function.

4. Paravertebral catheter placement is technically straightforward and produces unilateral anesthesia and analgesia, compared with the bilateral effects of TEA.

A

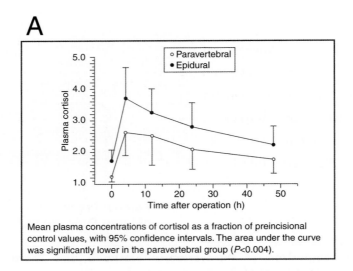

Mean plasma concentrations of cortisol as a fraction of preincisional control values, with 95% confidence intervals. The area under the curve was significantly lower in the paravertebral group ($P<0.004$).

B

C

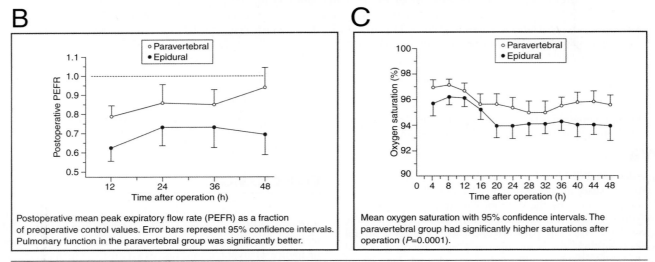

Postoperative mean peak expiratory flow rate (PEFR) as a fraction of preoperative control values. Error bars represent 95% confidence intervals. Pulmonary function in the paravertebral group was significantly better.

Mean oxygen saturation with 95% confidence intervals. The paravertebral group had significantly higher saturations after operation ($P=0.0001$).

Figure 18.2 • Graph A Shows the Lower Cortisol Levels Seen with Paravertebral Blockade Compared with Thoracic Epidural Analgesia After Thoracotomy. Graphs B and C show the improvement in spirometric values and oxygen saturation levels in patients treated with paravertebral blockade. (Reproduced with permission from Richardson J, Sabanathan S, Jones J, et al. A prospective, randomized comparison of preoperative and continuous balanced epidural or paravertebral bupivacaine on post-thoracotomy pain, pulmonary function and stress responses. Br J Anaesth 1999;83:387–392.)

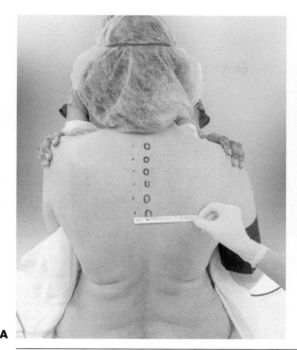
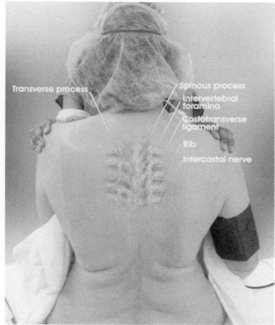

Figure 18.3 • Technique of Thoracic Paravertebral Blockade. (From Hadzic A, Vloka JD. Peripheral nerve blocks: principles and practice New York: McGrawHill, 2004.)

QUESTIONS

1. Thoracic PVB:
   A. Produces a bilateral thoracic sympathectomy
   B. Produces more hypotension than thoracic epidural blockade
   C. Is associated with improved postthoracotomy analgesia
   D. Is inferior to intercostal blocks for postthoracotomy analgesia
   E. Involves a noncontinuous space at the thoracic level

   Answer: C

2. Which of the following is the most important property of TEA?
   A. Effective postoperative analgesia
   B. Absence of urinary retention
   C. Bilateral sympathectomy
   D. Motor blockade
   E. Alteration of cortisol levels

   Answer: A

3. Ideal performance of thoracic PVB includes:
   A. Passage of catheters 6 cm into the paravertebral space in adults
   B. Palpation of the ipsilateral transverse process
   C. Needle insertion 2.5 cm lateral to the spinous process
   D. Performance in the lateral position
   E. Needle advancement 3 cm beyond the transverse process

   Answer: C

References

1. Richardson J, Lonqvist PA. Thoracic paravertebral block. Br J Anaesth 1998;81:230–238.
2. Richardson J, Sabanathan S, Shah R. Post-thoracotomy spirometric lung function: the effect of analgesia. J Cardiovasc Surg 1999:40:445–456.
3. Craig D. Postoperative recovery of pulmonary function. Anesth Analg 1981;60:46–51.
4. Saito T, Den S, Cheema SPS, et al. A single injection, multisegmental paravertebral block extension of somatosensory and sympathetic block in volunteers. Acta Anaesthesiol Scand 2001; 45:30–33.
5. Richardson J, Sabanathan S, Jones J, et al. A prospective, randomized comparison of preoperative and continuous balanced epidural or paravertebral bupivacaine on post-thoracotomy pain, pulmonary function and stress responses. Br J Anaesth 1999; 83:387–392.

CHAPTER 19

Carotid Artery Stenosis

Christopher J. O'Connor

CASE FORMAT: REFLECTION

An 82-year-old woman presented for carotid artery stenting (CAS) because of several recent transient ischemic attacks and a 70% restenosis of the left internal carotid artery. She had undergone a left carotid endarterectomy (CEA) 4 years previously. Her history was remarkable for hypertension, hypercholesterolemia, and coronary artery disease with prior stenting of her left anterior descending and circumflex coronary arteries 2 years ago. Her medications included metoprolol, lisinopril, simvastatin, clopidogrel, and aspirin. Her previous CEA had been performed under general anesthesia maintained using a remifentanil infusion, nitrous oxide, and low concentrations of sevoflurane. She had recently presented with several episodes of amaurosis fugax. Carotid ultrasound and digital subtraction angiography studies confirmed a 70% restenosis of her left carotid artery. CAS was selected as the operative procedure to dilate and stent the stenotic vessel. Using intravenous (IV) sedation and infiltration with local anesthetic to expose her right femoral artery, carotid angioplasty and stenting were performed using a cerebral protection device to minimize distal embolization of atherosclerotic debris. After successful completion of CAS, the patient was transferred to the intensive care unit for monitoring with stable vital signs. Two hours after the procedure, she abruptly developed right-sided leg and arm weakness. A heparin infusion was started and continued for 48 hours; oral aspirin and clopidogrel therapy was maintained. Three days postoperatively, she underwent right groin exploration for drainage of a femoral hematoma and also required transfusion of two units of packed red blood cells. The patient was eventually discharged from the hospital to a nursing facility 10 days after CAS.

CASE DISCUSSION

CEA is a well-validated procedure for managing symptomatic and asymptomatic carotid artery stenosis. Several studies have shown that CEA is superior to medical treatment for symptomatic patients with a stenosis of >60%, provided that centers performing CEA do so with a low rate of morbidity and mortality.[1–3] The Joint Committee of the Society for Vascular Surgery has determined that institutions performing this surgery should have a combined stroke mortality rate of <3% for asymptomatic patients, <5% for symptomatic patients, and <7% for those with a prior stroke. CAS and transluminal balloon angioplasty of the carotid artery was introduced as a minimally invasive approach to carotid stenosis that would avoid the risks associated with surgery and general anesthesia in high-risk patients. CAS avoids a neck incision that can lead to cranial nerve injuries or postoperative wound infections. However, the efficacy of CAS versus CEA in decreasing subsequent neurologic morbidity had not been determined when CAS was introduced. Several recent studies and meta-analyses[4–7] indicate that CEA can be performed safely with a lesser risk (compared with CAS) of stroke or death at 3 and 6 months postoperatively. Many surgeons consider CEA to be the "gold standard" for the treatment of carotid stenosis in both low- and high-risk patients.

CEA

CEA entails a longitudinal arteriotomy of the involved vessel after cross clamping of the internal carotid artery. The plaque is removed by cephalad extension of the endarterectomy plane until all of the plaque has been removed. To decrease the incidence of restenosis, many surgeons perform CEA (and several have shown superior results) with patch angioplasty. Either a piece of autologous vein or synthetic material is used to close the arteriotomy. Patch angioplasty significantly decreases the risk of perioperative stroke or death, the risk of perioperative restenosis, and the long-term risk of restenosis.

Anesthetic goals during CEA are to prevent stroke and perioperative myocardial infarction (MI) by optimizing intraoperative cerebral and myocardial perfusion. Although adequate cerebral perfusion can be maintained during the period of carotid clamping from the contralateral carotid artery via the Circle of Willis, 10% to 15% of the time, clamping will lead to symptomatic hemispheric ischemia.

The optimal anesthetic for CEA has yet to be determined (Table 19.1). The use of regional anesthesia—comprising deep or superficial cervical plexus block, local anesthetic infiltration, or a combination of these—has been advocated to decrease the incidence of perioperative MI, maintain intraoperative hemodynamic stability, reduce the duration of hospitalization, and reduce costs. However, none of these contentions has ever been firmly established in large-scale, randomized trials. It has been suggested that the response of the awake patient during carotid clamping represents the "gold standard" for neurologic monitoring in that patients can reliably display signs of cerebral ischemia during the period of carotid clamping. Although this may be true, it has yet to be borne out by any evidence base

TABLE 19.1 A Comparison of the Advantages and Disadvantages of Regional Versus General Anesthesia for Carotid Endarterectomy

Technique	Advantages	Disadvantages
Regional	Less intraoperative hypotension	More intraoperative hypertension
	Simple nerve block	Unfamiliarity for surgical team
	Intubation not required	Challenging airway control if GA needed
	Sensitive neurologic monitor	Sedation may obscure neurologic monitoring
	Avoids postoperative somnolence of GA	Patient discomfort if cerebral ischemia develops
	Shorter hospitalization, lower cost, fewer CV complications	Sedation-induced hypoxemia may increase cerebral ischemia
	Provides postoperative analgesia	Need to convert to GA
General	Reliable airway control	Intubation required
	Secure control of $PaCO_2$, PaO_2	More intraoperative hemodynamic changes
	Possible neuroprotective effects of anesthetics	Delayed emergence may obscure diagnosis of new cerebral event

CV, cardiovascular; GA, general anesthesia.

data. In addition, technical factors may limit the use of regional anesthesia. These include the presence of a short, obese neck; a high carotid bifurcation or tortuous arteries; and patients who are anxious or agitated. In the United States, more than 90% of CEAs are performed on patients under general anesthesia. It is likely that until the superiority of one technique over another has been established, most clinicians will continue to choose general anesthesia for CEA.

A variety of monitors/methods have been used to assess the adequacy of cerebral perfusion during CEA. These include electroencephalography or somatosensory-evoked potentials, transcranial Doppler, and stump pressure measurement. None of these methods is infallible, and they cannot reliably detect intraoperative cerebral ischemia or predict postoperative stroke. Stump pressure measurements and cerebral oximetry yield low rates of sensitivity and specificity for the detection of cerebral ischemia. Transcranial Doppler monitoring is technically more demanding (e.g., maintenance of angle of insonation) and inconsistent in acquiring blood flow signals. However, 16-lead electroencephalography monitoring is a reliable and valid neurologic monitor during CEA. Ultimately, the choice of intraoperative monitor may be less critical than surgical factors, because cerebral ischemia during the period of carotid clamping is an uncommon cause of perioperative stroke. Most neurologic injuries occur secondary to perioperative thromboembolic events (as in the case described).

CAS

CAS (Fig. 19.1) was originally introduced as a minimally invasive approach to managing carotid stenosis that would avoid

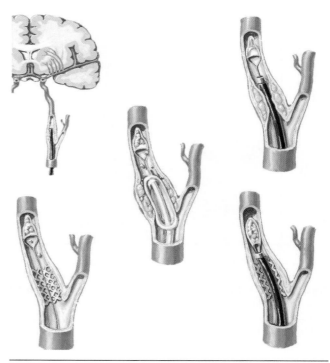

Figure 19.1 • The Technique of Carotid Artery Angioplasty and Stenting.

the risks of surgery and general anesthesia in high-risk patients. CAS is currently approved only for patients in clinical trials evaluating the efficacy of CAS. It was advocated for the high-risk patient with clinically significant cardiac (severe ischemic disease or significant congestive heart failure) or pulmonary disease, very advanced patient age (>80 years), or those with certain anatomic factors that make CEA more difficult. However, current evidence indicates that CAS has a greater 30-day death or stroke rate and greater 1-year stroke and death rates compared with CEA (Fig. 19.2). In addition, CAS appears superior only in the setting of conditions that render surgery technically difficult, such as restenosis after prior CEA (as in the patient in this case), prior radical neck surgery, previous neck radiation, and in selected patients with severe concurrent cardiopulmonary disease. Currently, carotid

stenting should only be performed in high-volume, specialized centers with experience in CAS, where stenting and angioplasty can be used in selected individuals with specific lesions amenable only to nonoperative treatment. One advantage of CAS compared with CEA is the lesser incidence of cranial nerve injuries (although local complications such as groin hematomas are more common with CAS).

Anesthesia for CAS is usually performed with local anesthetic infiltration, with or without monitored anesthesia care and sedation. Bradycardia can occur at balloon dilation of the carotid artery; this can typically be managed with balloon deflation and administration of IV anticholinergic agents. The use of cerebral protection devices—either umbrellas or balloon devices to trap embolic material—has lessened the incidence of procedural-related cerebral ischemic events.

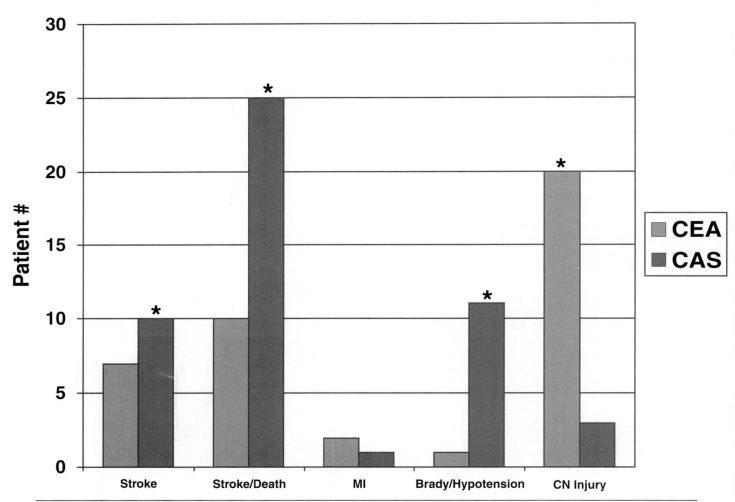

Figure 19.2 • Data Comparing Outcomes Between CAS and CEA. It is apparent that the incidence of stroke or combined stroke and death are lower in patients undergoing CEA compared with CAS. It is also clear that the incidence of myocardial infarction—expected to be lower with the less-invasive approach of CAS—was no different between the two groups. In contrast, hypotension and bradycardia were higher in the CAS group. Cranial nerve injuries were higher in the CEA group, as expected. CAS, carotid artery stenting; CEA, carotid endarterectomy; CN, cranial nerve; MI, myocardial infarction. * $p < 0.05$. (Data from Mas JL, Chatellier G, Beyssen B, et al. Endarterectomy versus stenting in patients with symptomatic severe carotid stenosis. N Engl J Med 2006;355: 1660–1671.)

KEY MESSAGES

1. Overall, CEA appears to be associated with a lesser risk of stroke, MI, and death when compared with CAS.

2. Based on currently available evidence, CAS should be reserved for high-risk patients with severe concomitant cardiac disease or anatomic conditions that render surgery technically difficult, such as restenosis after prior CEA, prior radical neck surgery, or previous radiation to the neck.

3. CEA is commonly performed on patients with general anesthesia, although many patients can be managed safely with IV sedation and combined superficial/deep cervical plexus blocks. In contrast, CAS is primarily performed on patients who receive IV sedation and local infiltration with a local anesthetic.

QUESTIONS

1. As compared with CEA, CAS is most often associated with:
   A. Lower incidence of local complications
   B. More frequent nonfatal strokes
   C. Intraoperative hypotension
   D. Lower rates of perioperative MI
   E. Fewer cranial nerve injuries

   Answer: B

2. Regional anesthesia for CEA:
   A. Is associated with higher hospital costs than general anesthesia
   B. Results in lower perioperative stroke rates than general anesthesia
   C. Is best achieved with a superficial cervical plexus block
   D. Has a high conversion rate to general anesthesia
   E. Allows for communication with the patient during carotid occlusion

   Answer: E

3. Which of the following is most likely to detect cerebral ischemia during carotid occlusion?
   A. Stump pressure measurement
   B. Cerebral oximetry
   C. Sixteen-lead electroencephalography analysis
   D. Transjugular venous oxygen saturation
   E. Motor-evoked potentials

   Answer: C

References

1. Abbruzzese TA, Cambria RP. Contemporary management of carotid stenosis: carotid endarterectomy is here to stay. Perspect Vasc Surg Endovasc Ther 2007;248–256.
2. Biggs KL, Moore WS. Current trends in managing carotid artery disease. Surg Clin North Am 2007;995–1016.
3. Flanigan DP, Flanigan ME, Dorne AL, et al. Long-term results of 442 consecutive, standardized carotid endarterectomy procedure in standard-risk and high-risk patients. J Vasc Surg 2007;46:876–882.
4. Luebke T, Aleksic M, Brunkwall J. Meta-analysis of randomized trials comparing carotid endarterectomy and endovascular treatment. Eur J Vasc Endovas Surg 2007;34:470–479.
5. Mas JL, Chatellier G, Beyssen B, et al. Endarterectomy versus stenting in patients with symptomatic severe carotid stenosis. N Engl J Med 2006;355:1660–1671.
6. Naylor AR. What is the current status of angioplasty vs. endarterectomy in patients with asymptomatic carotid artery disease? J Cardiovasc Surg 2007;48:161–180.
7. Rothwell PM. Current status of carotid endarterectomy and stenting for symptomatic carotid stenosis. Cerebrovasc Dis 2007;24(suppl 1):116–125.

CHAPTER 20

Postpneumonectomy Pulmonary Edema

Nanhi Mitter

CASE FORMAT: STEP BY STEP

A 72-year-old, 5'8", 60-kg man with a history of hypertension, benign prostatic hypertrophy, and hyperlipidemia presented with progressive dyspnea, cough, and recent (2-month) weight loss of 7 kg. Bronchoscopy and mediastinoscopy confirmed the diagnosis of non-small cell carcinoma, and he was scheduled to undergo a right pneumonectomy.

The patient was currently smoking two packs of cigarettes per day and had an 80-pack year smoking history. His pulmonary function tests revealed a decreased forced expiratory volume/forced vital capacity (60% predicted) and a reversible component to his bronchospasm. His medications included fluticasone/salmeterol, aspirin, simvastatin, metoprolol, and amlodipine. He was not using home oxygen therapy.

On preoperative evaluation, the patient seemed comfortable with a normal airway examination and diminished breath sounds over the right lung field. His vital signs were as follows: blood pressure, 150/84 mm Hg; heart rate, 70 beats per minute; respiratory rate, 20 breaths per minute; and SpO₂, 90% to 94% on room air. His room air blood gas revealed pH, 7.34; pCO₂, 56 mm Hg, and pO₂, 98 mm Hg. The patient's preoperative cardiac evaluation revealed left ventricular hypertrophy on electrocardiogram and normal left ventricular ejection fraction on echocardiography. He had not experienced chest pain but described fatigue and shortness of breath on minimal exertion, which he attributed to his lung disease. Preoperative investigations revealed a hemoglobin concentration of 17 g/dL (all other parameters were normal).

After a 16-gauge intravenous and an arterial catheter were inserted, the patient was taken to the operating room where an epidural catheter was introduced at the T8 level. After a test dose was administered via the epidural catheter, two 5-mL increments of 2% lidocaine with epinephrine (1:200,000) were administered. An infusion of bupivacaine (0.125%) and fentanyl (10 mcg/mL) was commenced and continued throughout the case. The patient's trachea was intubated using a left-sided 37 F double-lumen tube (DLT). A central venous catheter was inserted into the right internal jugular vein. Upon institution of one-lung ventilation (OLV), the patient's oxygen saturation decreased from 99% to 92% over 15 minutes.

What is the appropriate initial response to the decrease in SpO₂?

Possible etiologies of hypoxemia during OLV include malposition of the DLT, bronchospasm, low FiO₂, dependent lung atelectasis, and secretions. The anesthesiologist should confirm the patient is receiving an FiO₂ of 1.0 and establish that the DLT is correctly positioned. It would be reasonable to apply suction to the ventilated lung and administer a bronchodilator such as albuterol. CPAD to the non-ventilated lung would be the next step to improve oxygenation.

Following these maneuvers, the patient's SpO₂ increased to 96%. Surgery proceeded, and while the surgeon was dissecting the pulmonary artery, severe hemorrhage ensued, and an acute blood loss of 2 liters (over 5 minutes) was observed. Two units of packed red blood cells were administered, and the arterial blood gas revealed a metabolic acidosis (pH = 7.30) with a hemoglobin level of 7 g/dL. The patient's central venous pressure was 5 mm Hg, blood pressure was 100/50 mm Hg, and his heart rate measured 110 beats per minute.

Are patients undergoing pneumonectomy at risk of "fluid overload"?

Excess intraoperative fluids may play a role in the development of post-pneumonectomy pulmonary edema. In the face of global hypoperfusion, however, as evidenced by metabolic acidosis and the observed hemodynamic instability, fluid resuscitation takes priority.

The anesthesiologist administered another two units of packed red blood cells. The surgeon controlled the bleeding, and 2 hours later, the right lung was resected, and the patient's chest was closed. The total blood loss was estimated to be 3 liters and the results of the patient's blood gas analysis and hemoglobin concentration had normalized. He had received a total of 4 units of packed red blood cells and 1 liter of crystalloid; his vital signs were also normal. Upon auscultation of his left lung, mild expiratory wheeze was audible.

After complete reversal of neuromuscular blockade and administration of albuterol (by metered dose inhaler with extension), the patient's trachea was extubated, and 40% oxygen was administered by Venturi face mask. The patient was admitted to the ICU postoperatively; his chest radiograph (CXR) upon arrival revealed mild pulmonary congestion in his left lung field and an absent right lung.

The patient's ICU course was uneventful. On the second postoperative day, he was transferred to the ward but experienced mild dyspnea 1 day later. He continued to complain of progressive dyspnea, and his SpO₂ gradually decreased from

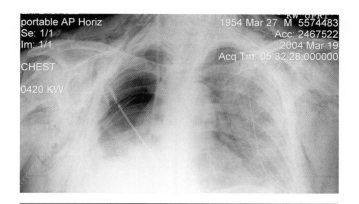

Figure 20.1 • In the patient's postoperative day 3 chest x-ray, note the pulmonary edema pattern in the left lung and the normal cardiac silhouette, suggesting an acute lung injury pattern.

97% on a 50% oxygen face mask to 90% over the course of his third postoperative day. A CXR revealed pulmonary edema in the left lung field (Fig. 20.1). Blood gas analysis revealed PaO_2 to be 60 mm Hg.

What are the risk factors for postoperative pulmonary edema?

The risk factors for postpneumonectomy pulmonary edema are listed in Table 20.1.[1–6]

What are the options for ventilatory management of this patient?

At this point, the options for ventilatory management include noninvasive ventilation, transfer to the ICU for closer monitoring, or immediate tracheal intubation and transfer to the ICU.

In light of the pneumonectomy, fluid administration, CXR, and arterial blood gas results, it was decided to reintubate the patient's trachea and transfer him to the ICU. This decision was made to avoid further hypoxemia given that the clinical picture was consistent with hydrostatic pulmonary edema or acute lung injury. Over the next few hours, the patient's oxygenation improved, and he was successfully weaned from the ventilator on postoperative day 5. The remainder of his postoperative course was uneventful.

TABLE 20.1 Predictors of Postpneumonectomy Pulmonary Complications

1. Right pneumonectomy
2. Excessive perioperative fluid administration
3. Increased intraoperative ventilation pressures
4. Preoperative alcohol abuse
5. Decreased postoperative predicted DLCO (diffusing capacity of the lung)
6. Radiation therapy

KEY MESSAGES

1. Patients undergoing pneumonectomy are at risk for postoperative pulmonary dysfunction from interstitial edema, atelectasis, and restrictive respiratory patterns caused by inadequate analgesia.

2. Risk factors for postpneumonectomy pulmonary edema include excess intraoperative fluid administration, prior chest irradiation, right pneumonectomy, and possibly preoperative alcohol use and high intraoperative ventilatory pressures.

3. The management of postpneumonectomy pulmonary edema is largely supportive, including supplementary oxygen, mechanical ventilatory support if necessary, diuresis, and aggressive pulmonary toilet.

QUESTIONS

1. Which of the following statements are true?
   A. Patients undergoing a right pneumonectomy have no added risk for postoperative pulmonary edema.
   B. All patients undergoing a pneumonectomy should have pulmonary function tests completed preoperatively.
   C. Hypoxic pulmonary vasoconstriction should be maximized in the dependent lung.
   D. All patients should be ventilated with high lung volumes (10–12 mL/kg). This is the only way to ensure that atelectasis will not develop.
   E. None of the above
   Answer: B

2. Which of the following statements is false regarding management of hypoxemia during OLV?
   A. The bronchial cuff of the DLT when visualized with a fiberoptic bronchoscope should be about 1 cm above the carina.
   B. During OLV, positive end-expiratory pressure to the dependent, ventilated lung may worsen the shunt.
   C. During OLV, constant positive airway pressure to the nondependent, nonventilated lung may improve oxygenation.
   D. High tidal volumes may injure alveoli in the ventilated lung.
   E. An FiO_2 of 1.0 should be used.
   Answer: A

3. Which of the following are risk factors for the development of postpneumonectomy pulmonary edema?
   A. Right pneumonectomy
   B. A history of breast cancer
   C. Large volumes of intraoperative fluid
   D. A and C
   E. None of the above
   Answer: D

References

1. Alam N, Park BJ, Wilton A, et al. Incidence and risk factors for lung injury after lung cancer resection. Ann Thorac Surg 2007; 84:1085–1091.
2. Bapoje SR, Whitaker JF, Schulz T, et al. Preoperative evaluation of the patient with pulmonary disease Chest 2007;132:1637–1645.
3. Licker M, de Perrot M, Spiliopoulos A, et al. Risk factors for acute lung injury after thoracic surgery for lung cancer. Anesth Analg 2003;97:1558–1565.
4. Dulu A, Pastores SM, Park B, et al. Prevalence and mortality of acute lung injury and ARDS after lung resection. Chest 2006; 130:73–78.
5. Leo F, Scanagatta P, Baglio P, et al. The risk of pneumonectomy over the age of 70: a case-control study. Eur J Cardiothorac Surg 2007;31:779–782.
6. Dancewica M, Kowalewski J, Peplinski J. Factors associated with perioperative complications after pneumonectomy for primary carcinoma of the lung. Interact Cardio Vasc Thorac Surg 2006;5:97–100.

CHAPTER 21

Perioperative Antiplatelet Therapy

Nanhi Mitter

CASE FORMAT: REFLECTION

A 62-year-old female with a history of coronary artery disease, hyperlipidemia, and hypertension presented with vaginal bleeding and was scheduled for a total abdominal hysterectomy and bilateral salpingo-oophorectomy. Unfortunately, 3 days before she was due to undergo this operation, she experienced substernal chest pain radiating to her jaw. She was taken to the emergency department where her electrocardiogram readings (Fig. 21.1) and cardiac enzymes were consistent with an ST-segment elevation myocardial infarction (MI). She underwent emergency coronary angiography, which revealed 99% occlusion of the left circumflex artery. An angioplasty was performed, a bare metal stent (BMS) was placed across the lesion, and normal flow was re-established. She was admitted to the coronary care unit, and after an uneventful recovery was discharged home 5 days later.

The patient's total abdominal hysterectomy and bilateral salpingo-oophorectomy had been canceled and was rescheduled for 4 weeks after her ST-segment elevation MI. On preoperative evaluation for the re-scheduled procedure, she was noted to be taking metoprolol, hydrochlorothiazide, simvastatin, and aspirin. She had stopped taking clopidogrel 7 days previously but had continued to take aspirin. She had stopped smoking 3 years previously, and her alcohol consumption was minimal. With the exception of hemoglobin concentration 8.9 g/dL, all of her laboratory values were within normal limits. Since her ST-segment elevation MI, she had been asymptomatic and had been able to walk on a treadmill without difficulty. She appeared nervous but otherwise healthy. The patient's vital signs were as follows: temperature, 37.0°C; blood pressure, 120/71 mm Hg; heart rate, 62 beats per minute; respiratory rate, 18 beats per minute; and room air oxygen saturation, 99%. Her physical examination was unremarkable, and the upper airway was evaluated as normal.

After standard ASA monitors were applied and the arterial and venous cannulae were inserted, anesthesia was induced, and the patient's trachea was intubated uneventfully. A triple-lumen catheter was inserted in her right internal jugular vein, and her central venous pressure (CVP) was monitored continuously. Two hours into the procedure, blood loss was estimated to be 1 liter, the patient became tachycardic and hypotensive, and her CVP was 3 mm Hg. Arterial blood gas analysis revealed metabolic acidosis, and the patient's hemoglobin concentration was 6.6 g/dL. Two units of

packed red blood cells and 50 mL of 8.4% sodium bicarbonate were administered rapidly, and hyperventilation was instituted. Despite aggressive fluid resuscitation, the patient remained hypotensive (mean arterial pressure 40–45 mm Hg) with a CVP of 3 mm Hg. A transesophageal echocardiographic probe was inserted and revealed no regional wall motion abnormalities. After transfusion of two further units of packed red blood cells, the patient's hemodynamic parameters normalized. The surgery continued without further incident. At the end of the procedure, her CVP was 11 mm Hg. A repeat arterial blood gas analysis revealed a normal pH and a hemoglobin level of 11g/dL. The patient's trachea was extubated, and she was transferred to the ICU where a cardiac evaluation was normal.

CASE DISCUSSION

Percutaneous coronary interventions (PCI) generally should not be performed as a preoperative step to prevent adverse cardiovascular events for patients undergoing noncardiac surgery unless they present with an acute coronary syndrome. Patients who present with an acute coronary syndrome and who require subsequent noncardiac surgery require special evaluation and manipulation of their medical therapy.[1] The type of intervention—percutaneous transcoronary angioplasty versus coronary artery stenting—should be planned considering the choice of dual-antiplatelet therapy (DAT), risk of bleeding, and the nature and timing of surgery.

Using the guidelines outlined in Table 21.1 will help with planning for surgery.

Current recommendations regarding DAT include the use of aspirin and a thienopyridine agent. DAT is initiated because upon balloon inflation or stent deployment, the endothelium of the coronary artery is denuded. Normally, the endothelium functions to inhibit platelet aggregation along the vessel wall. Without the endothelium present, pharmacologic agents such as aspirin and a thienopyridine agent must provide for the platelet inhibitory function until the endothelium resumes this role.

In the setting of balloon angioplasty (BA) and BMS, the endothelium develops after 4 to 6 weeks; hence DAT is no longer necessary and is subsequently discontinued.[2] After a period of time, however, late stent restenosis of the BMS can lead to MI or even death, and therefore, drug-eluting stents (DES) have become widely used. There are two types of DES—the sirolimus-eluting stent and the paclitaxel-eluting

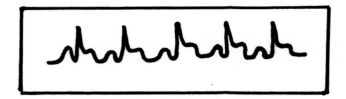

Figure 21.1 • The patient's electrocardiogram reading reveals an ST-segment elevation myocardial infarction.

stent. These stents are impregnated with chemotactic agents that help to prevent re-endothelialization that leads to late stent restenosis. Because these stents prevent re-endothelialization, DAT is mandated to prevent acute thrombosis of the stent for longer periods of time compared with BMS or balloon angioplasty.

In patients who have undergone balloon angioplasty, performing noncardiac surgery within the first 2 weeks may be unsafe because of residual injury from recent vessel manipulation. Performing surgery between 2 to 4 weeks is ideal because of theoretical vessel healing and the low risk of restenosis at the site, which is most common after 8 weeks. Patients should be treated with DAT for 4 to 6 weeks.[2–4]

In patients undergoing stenting with BMS, the risk of acute thrombosis is greatest in the first 2 weeks, and the risk for restenosis is greatest >12 weeks. Therefore, the ideal time for noncardiac surgery after BMS is 4 to 6 weeks, as it is rare for thrombosis to occur during this interval because of at least partial endothelialization of the BMS. DAT should be continued for 1 month when BMS are used and in some cases longer.[4]

In patients undergoing stenting with DES, the current recommendation is to delay elective surgery until the patient has completed the appropriate course of DAT. In the event of urgent or emergent surgery when the thienopyridine therapy must be discontinued, then, if at all possible, the aspirin should be continued perioperatively, and the thienopyridine therapy should be restarted as soon as possible.

In this case, the patient had a BMS placed and underwent surgery after 4 weeks. Although this is the ideal time to perform surgery in patients with BMS, the risk of acute stent thrombosis (albeit rare, <0.1% in most case series) and reinfarction is present.[1,5]

Invasive monitoring such as a transesophageal echocardiogram can be helpful in these patients to differentiate between intrinsic cardiac etiology (i.e., in-stent restenosis manifesting as regional wall motion abnormalities) versus extrinsic factors that may lead to hemodynamic instability (i.e., hypovolemia secondary to acute blood loss or to bowel preparation). High-risk patients can be managed by optimizing the myocardial oxygen supply/demand ratio. Methods to achieve this goal include but are not limited to avoiding tachycardia, providing adequate analgesia in the preoperative setting, optimizing oxygenation and ventilation, avoiding alkalosis and acidosis, avoiding anemia, aggressive fluid resuscitation, perioperative β-blockade, and statin use. Finally, postoperative management may include ICU admission and close follow-up.

KEY MESSAGES

1. Preoperative management of a patient who has had a recent acute MI but needs urgent noncardiac surgery requires special consideration with respect to anticoagulation and the type of revascularization procedure to be performed.

2. Antiplatelet therapy is necessary in patients undergoing PCI because of denuding of the endothelium from balloon deployment or the device used. The American College of Cardiology and the American Heart Association recommend varying durations for DAT depending on the type of coronary intervention.

3. For patients who have had a DES placed, continuation of both clopidogrel and aspirin in the perioperative period is recommended. If clopidogrel needs to be stopped, aspirin should be continued throughout the perioperative period.

TABLE 21.1 Recommendations Regarding Time Frame for Surgical Intervention After Revascularization

Mode of Revascularization	Unsafe	Safe Period	Unsafe
BA	<2 weeks	>2 weeks	
BMS	<4–6 weeks	4–6 weeks	>12 weeks
DES	<1 year	After 1 year	

This table demonstrates "safe" and "unsafe" time periods for patients undergoing elective noncardiac surgery after a revascularization procedure. The decision regarding timing of surgery should be ultimately made by the anesthesiologist, surgeon, cardiologist, internist, and patient involved. Data based on the American College of Cardiology/American Heart Association 2007 guidelines.
BA, balloon angioplasty; BMS, bare metal stent; DES, drug-eluting stent.

QUESTIONS

1. Which of the following drug combinations are used as DAT for patients undergoing PCI?

   A. Aspirin and clopidogrel

   B. Lovenox and clopidogrel

   C. Coumadin and clopidogrel

   D. Coumadin and aspirin

   Answer: A

2. Which of the following is a true statement regarding antiplatelet therapy (AT) in patients who have undergone PCI?

   A. The patients are placed on AT because they are at risk for stroke after PCI.

   B. In patients undergoing PCI with DES, only 3 months of aspirin are necessary for AT.

   C. Patients need AT after PCI because in the process of balloon or stent deployment, the endothelium is denuded—the normal endothelium is necessary to prevent platelet aggregation.

   D. Patients only need AT if they are having a stent placed.

   Answer: C

3. Which of the following statements is/are correct?

   A. All patients who have symptomatic coronary artery disease should undergo revascularization just so that they can have their elective surgery.

   B. It is recommended to wait 4 to 6 weeks after patients have had a BMS placed before proceeding with surgery.

   C. Only 6 weeks of DAT are necessary for patients who have had placement of a DES.

   D. Elective surgery can be performed without incident in patients after BA within the first 2 weeks of the PCI.

   Answer: B

References

1. Fleisher LA, Beckman JA, Brown KA, Calkins H, et al. ACC/AHA 2007 Guidelines on Perioperative Cardiovascular Evaluation and Care for Noncardiac Surgery: Executive Summary. A Report of the ACC/AHA Task Force on Practice Guidelines. Circulation 2007;116: 1971–1996.

2. Brilakis ES, Orford JL, Fasseas P, et al. Outcome of patients undergoing balloon angioplasty in the two months prior to noncardiac surgery. Am J Cardiol 2005;96:512–514.

3. Leibowitz D, Cohen M, Planer D, et al. Comparison of cardiovascular risk of noncardiac surgery following coronary angioplasty with versus without stenting. Am J Cardiol 2006;97: 1188–1191.

4. King SB, Smith SC, Hirshfeld JW, Morrison DA, et al. 2007 Focused Update of the ACC/AHA/SCAI 2005 Guideline Update for Percutaneous Coronary Intervention. A Report of the ACC/AHA Task Force on Practice Guidelines: 2007 Writing Group to Review New Evidence and Update the ACC/AHA/ SCAI 2005 Guideline for Percutaneous Coronary Intervention, Writing on Behalf of the 2005 Writing Committee. Circulation 2008;117:261–295.

5. Chen MS, John JM, Chew DP, et al. Bare metal stent restenosis is not a benign clinical entity. Am Heart J 2006;151:1260–1264.

CHAPTER 22

Intraoperative Blood Conservation Strategies

W. Christopher Croley

CASE FORMAT: REFLECTION

A 14-year-old, 50-kg female presented for spine surgery. She was an otherwise healthy teenager who had undergone previous back surgery for scoliosis. She reported taking ibuprofen "occasionally" for back pain. Physical examination was unremarkable except for severe thoracic scoliosis. Her preoperative hemoglobin concentration was 13 g/dL, and all other laboratory values were within normal limits.

The patient was scheduled to undergo an estimated 6-hour procedure in the prone position. Her parents were present in the preoperative holding area and expressed their concern with her preoperative hemoglobin concentration and the possible need for a blood transfusion perioperatively. Several strategies were discussed with the patient and her parents.

A decision was made jointly to use acute normovolemic hemodilution before starting the case, cell saver intraoperatively, and blood transfusion only if signs of decreased oxygen carrying capacity were demonstrated.

Two 16-gauge peripheral intravenous catheters were inserted while the patient was in the holding area. In the operating room, standard ASA monitors were placed, and general anesthesia was induced with sufentanil (1 mcg/kg), propofol (2 mg/kg), and rocuronium (0.6 mg/kg). After induction of general anesthesia, tracheal intubation was readily accomplished with a 7.0-mm oral endotracheal tube. An 18-gauge right radial arterial line was inserted for blood pressure monitoring, blood sampling, and to facilitate normovolemic hemodilution. Anesthesia was maintained with a sufentanil infusion at 0.3 mcg/kg per hour, sevoflurane (inspired concentration 1.5%–2%), and a 50:50 mixture of nitrous oxide/oxygen. Motor-evoked potentials were monitored; therefore, no additional neuromuscular blocking agent was used.

Utilizing strict aseptic technique, 500 mL of blood was collected using the arterial cannula in a citrate-phosphate-dextrose containing bag. Simultaneously, 500 mL of 6% hetastarch was administered intravenously. The patient was hemodynamically stable throughout the procedure. Approximately 4.5 hours into the surgery, the estimated blood loss was 900 mL, and the surgeon was starting to close. Using the products of cell salvage collected intraoperatively, 300 mL was administered. The patient's trachea was extubated at the end of the procedure, and she was transferred to the recovery room with stable vital signs. Her postoperative hemoglobin concentration was 10 g/dL. She was discharged home on the third postoperative day, at which time her hemoglobin concentration was 9 g/dL. The patient and her family were very happy that she did not require allogeneic blood during her hospitalization.

Infectious risks, immunosuppression, limited availability, and acquisition costs are legitimate concerns of clinicians responsible for transfusion of blood products. These concerns cause those responsible for perioperative care to continually evaluate and implement therapies to reduce perioperative blood loss and thereby minimize the need for allogeneic blood transfusion. Numerous mechanical, pharmacologic, and physiologic strategies have been identified to decrease blood transfusion.[1–5] Several of these strategies can be used in combination in a single case.

Preoperative autologous blood donation (ABD) is one technique that can be used.[6,7] This procedure entails patients donating their own blood, which is then stored for transfusion at a later date. This process must be initiated several weeks in advance of anticipated need to allow time for restoration of intravascular volume as well as preparation of the donated blood. Patients can donate every 72 hours, and the last donation should be at least 72 hours before a scheduled procedure. ABD is contraindicated in patients with anemia (hemoglobin <11 g/dL or hematocrit levels <33% before each donation). Problems associated with this technique include mislabeling blood products, bacterial contamination of stored units, and the costs associated with collection and administration. Costs associated with preoperative ABD can be 50% to 70% greater than similar techniques of acute normovolemic hemodilution and cell salvage (Table 22.1).

Acute normovolemic hemodilution (ANH) is the process of removing whole blood while simultaneously infusing crystalloid or colloid fluid to maintain intravascular volume. This is an effective, low-cost means of intraoperative blood conservation that is underutilized. Blood is collected in citrate-phosphate-dextrose-containing bags at the beginning of the procedure and stored in the operating room, at room temperature, for up to 8 hours. Collection bags are numbered by the order in which they were collected and are then transfused in the reverse order. This means the first bag collected, which (theoretically at least) has a greater red blood cell mass and greater concentration of clotting factors, is transfused last. Because this product is not collected and stored off-site, risks of clerical errors and processing of the blood are greatly reduced. ANH is also a more cost-effective method of decreasing perioperative blood transfusion requirements. Platelets and clotting factors are usually

TABLE 22.1 Contraindications to Autologous Blood Donation

- Anemia (hemoglobin <11 g/dL)
- Infection or risk of bacteremia
- Angina
- Recent myocardial infarction
- Uncontrolled seizure disorders

TABLE 22.2 Overview of Pharmacologic Agents

Antifibrinolytic Agents	Aminocaproic acid
	Tranexamic acid
Topical Agents	Thrombin
	Gelatin sponges
	Fibrin
Procoagulant Drugs	Desmopressin

Adapted from Porte RJ, Leebeek FWG. Pharmacological strategies to decrease transfusion requirements in patients undergoing surgery. Drugs 2002;62:2193–2211.

well preserved with this method because the blood is stored at room temperature and then transfused within a relatively short time. Relatively few studies have examined the practice of ANH. A small number of prospective, randomized studies have been completed and represent ANH as equivalent to preoperative autologous donation in reducing the need for allogeneic blood transfusions.

Cell salvage and reinfusion is another commonly used method for autologous blood procurement and can be done intraoperatively or postoperatively. Cell salvage techniques involve devices that collect blood as it is lost and facilitate its subsequent retransfusion. Red blood cells collected in this manner are commonly filtered through a microaggregate filter before transfusion to remove tissue debris and blood clots. The function of red blood cells from salvage techniques appears to be similar to that of allogeneic red blood cells. This technique cannot be used if topical procoagulants (e.g., topical thrombin) are present in the surgical field from which the blood is being recovered. Salvaged blood often undergoes a washing procedure using saline solutions to remove some inflammatory mediators (e.g., cytokines). Unwashed salvaged blood has a greater incidence of hypotension, hyperthermia, and pulmonary edema when reinfused than washed blood. Other risks associated with cell salvage include air emboli, infection, and coagulation derangements.

Induced hypotension is an anesthetic technique that can be used to minimize intraoperative blood loss.[8] This technique has been well described, primarily in the orthopaedic literature, where it has been shown that blood loss can be reduced by 30% to 50% when using a hypotensive or regional (spinal or epidural) technique. Induced hypotension involves lowering the mean arterial pressure to 50–55 mm Hg, using either sympathectomy associated with neuraxial anesthesia or vasoactive agents (e.g., esmolol, nicardipine, nitroprusside). Hypoperfusion is the obvious concern when deliberately lessening the patient's blood pressure. This technique should be used cautiously in patients with altered autoregulatory mechanisms (e.g., hypertension) and those susceptible to ischemic complications (e.g., coronary artery disease, renal insufficiency, diabetes). It should also be noted that induced hypotension and ANH are sometimes used in combination. Using this combination increases the risk of decreased oxygen delivery.

Pharmacologic methods that can decrease the need for perioperative blood transfusion (but not necessarily intraoperative blood loss) include preoperative administration of erythropoietin and/or intraoperative administration of antifibrinolytic agents such as aprotinin, ε-aminocaproic acid, or tranexamic acid.[9] Erythropoietin is a glycoprotein hormone that stimulates red blood cell production. Numerous studies of or-

thopaedic patients undergoing hip or knee arthroplasty have shown a decreased requirement for perioperative blood transfusion when erythropoietin has been administered several weeks before surgery. Some studies have shown generation of substantial (up to 1102 mL) red blood cell production, when exogenous erythropoietin has been administered. Antifibrinolytic agents should be considered when there is an imbalance between coagulation and fibrinolysis. Other pharmacologic aids that help control perioperative blood loss include topical agents (e.g., thrombin) and procoagulant drugs such as desmopressin (Table 22.2).

There are numerous methods (some outlined previously) for minimizing intraoperative blood loss and decreasing perioperative allogeneic blood transfusion requirements. To date, none of these methods has been shown to decrease the duration of hospital stay. In view of the multiplicity of methods available, it is important for institutions to establish and implement transfusion guidelines with appropriate transfusion thresholds and individualized to each patient (Table 22.3). The techniques discussed in this case can be used alone or in combination and should be tailored to meet the needs of each patient.

TABLE 22.3 Examples of Blood Transfusion Indications

Patient with acute blood loss >20% of blood volume: Transfuse

Hemoglobin/hematocrit <10 g/dL or 30%, ask:

- History of coronary artery disease
- History of stroke
- History of valvular heart disease
- Syncope
- Tachycardia
- Angina
- Hypoxemia
- Mental status changes
- Electrocardiogram changes
- Decreased mixed venous oxygenation

If yes to any → Consider transfusion

KEY MESSAGES

1. Blood transfusion risks can often be minimized if strategies are used to avoid allogeneic blood transfusion.

2. Perioperative blood conservation requires collaboration and planning by members of the surgical and anesthesia teams.

3. Multiple techniques may need to be combined to minimize perioperative blood loss and decrease the need for allogeneic blood transfusion. Examples of blood conservation techniques include acute normovolemic hemodilution, controlled hypotension, ABD, and cell salvage/reinfusion.

4. ABD as well as donor-directed blood donation can still pose some risks that are associated with banked blood from anonymous donors.

QUESTIONS

1. When comparing ABD toANH as blood conservation strategies, ABD:

   A. Is more cost-effective than ANH

   B. Is more efficacious than ANH

   C. Produces better preservation of platelet function than ANH

   D. Is less likely to be associated with clinical errors than ANH

   E. Results in bacterial contamination of blood more often than ANH

   Answer: E

2. The most efficacious of the following techniques to reduce perioperative blood transfusion is:

   A. Acute normovolemic hemodilution

   B. Autologous blood donation

   C. Induced hypotension

   D. Intraoperative antifibrinolytic drug use

   E. Lowered transfusion thresholds

   Answer: E

3. Which of the following patient conditions is most likely to contradict the use of autologous blood donation?

   A. A history of congestive heart failure

   B. Preoperative anemia

   C. Insulin-dependent diabetes mellitus

   D. Moderate aortic stenosis

   E. A history of a prior stroke

   Answer: B

References

1. Bridgens JP, Evans CR, Dobson PMS, et al. Intraoperative red blood-cell salvage in revision hip surgery. A case-matched study. J Bone Joint Surg Am2007;89:270–275.

2. Carless P, Moxey A, O'Connell D, et al. Autologous transfusion techniques: a systematic review of their efficacy. Transfusion Medicine 2004;14:123–144.

3. Dutton RP. Controlled hypotension for spinal surgery. Eur Spine J 2004;13:S66–S71.

4. Goodnough LT. Blood and blood conservation: a national perspective. J Cardiothor Vasc Anes 2004;4:6s–11s.

5. Goodnough LT. Rationale for blood conservation. Surgical Infections 2005;6:3s–8s.

6. Keating EM, Callaghan JJ, Ranawat AS, et al. A randomized, parallel-group, open-label trial of recombinant human erythropoietin vs. preoperative autologous donation in primary total joint arthroplasty. J Arthroplasty 2007;22:325–333.

7. Park JO, Gonen M, D'Angelica MI, et al. Autologous versus allogeneic transfusions: no difference in perioperative outcome after partial hepatectomy. J Gastrointest Surg 2007;11:1286–1293.

8. Lim YJ, Kim CS, Bahk JH, et al. Clinical trial of esmolol-induced controlled hypotension with or without acute normovolemic hemodilution in spinal surgery. Acta Anaesthesiol Scand 2003;47:74–78.

9. Porte RJ, Leebeek FWG. Pharmacological strategies to decrease transfusion requirements in patients undergoing surgery. Drugs 2002;62:2193–2211.

CHAPTER 23

Transfusion Thresholds and Intraoperative Coagulopathy

Anthony Hennessy

FORMAT: REFLECTION

A 69-year old, 70-kg man was admitted to hospital on the day before planned revision hip arthroplasty. He had undergone an ipsilateral total hip replacement 6 years previously. This hip had caused him severe pain and disability for the preceding 4 months. Four years previously, he had suffered "a small heart attack" for which he spent 5 days in a distant hospital. He had not experienced angina since then and described good exercise tolerance, playing a round of golf 3 days a week up to 4 months previously when his mobility had deteriorated. He was taking aspirin 75 mg a day, which he had discontinued 7 days previously as per his surgeon's request. The patient was also taking bisoprolol 10 mg daily and pravastatin 20 mg daily.

The patient's clinical examination was unremarkable: blood pressure, 135/81 mm Hg (mean arterial pressure, [MAP] 95 mm Hg); electrocardiogram (ECG) showed sinus bradycardia at 58 beats per minute (BPM) with no other abnormality; chest radiograph was normal; hemoglobin (Hb) level, 12.1 g/dL; and other laboratory results were within normal limits. The blood bank made four units of cross-matched packed red blood cells (PRBC) available on request.

A 20-gauge radial arterial cannula, a 14-gauge intravenous cannula, and a triple-lumen central venous catheter were inserted, and administration of Hartmann's solution (1 L) was started preoperatively. A combined spinal epidural was placed at L3 to L4 using an 18-gauge Tuohy needle and a 27-gauge pencil point spinal needle. Isobaric bupivacaine 0.5% (2 mL) was injected intrathecally followed by bupivacaine 0.5% (5 mL) epidurally producing a satisfactory sensory block to T10. Midazolam 2 mg was administered; oxygen (O$_2$) at 28% via face mask was applied, a temperature-monitoring urinary catheter was inserted, and the patient was draped and prepared for surgery. Surgery commenced with O$_2$ saturations of 97%, heart rate 68 BPM, and the patient's MAP was 71 mm Hg.

The anesthetist calculated a maximal allowable blood loss (MABL) to a minimum Hb of 8 g/dL based on the patient's stable ischemic heart disease using the formula:

$$MABL = \left[\frac{(\text{initial Hb} - \text{minimum allowable Hb})}{\text{initial Hb}} \right] \times (\text{weight in kg})$$

$$\times (\text{mL of blood per kg body weight}).$$

$$\left(\frac{12.1 - 8.0}{12.1} \right) \times 70 \times 72 = MABL \text{ of } 1708 \text{ mL}.$$

An extended incision was required, as surgical access was difficult. Despite careful surgical technique, the patient bled at a steady rate, losing 600 mL of blood during the first hour. Ephedrine 6 mg × 2 was administered to maintain MAP >70 mm Hg during that time. Removing the old prosthesis and cement with exposure of cancellous acetabular and femoral bone led to ongoing hemorrhage despite packing of the femur.

After 2 hours of surgery, the patient's estimated blood loss was 1300 mL. He had received 2 L of Hartmann's solution with 500 mL of colloid and five aliquots of ephedrine (each 6 mg) to maintain MAP >70 mm Hg and urine output >50 mL per hour. An epidural bolus of bupivacaine 0.5% 5 mL had been administered to maintain adequate sensory block. The patient's SpO$_2$ was 97%, his heart rate was 82 BPM, and ECG ST monitoring was unchanged. His core temperature was 35.9°C. Arterial blood gas analysis demonstrated the patient's Hb level was 9.1 g/dL, and his serum lactate level was 3.1 mmol/L. Having decided that a transfusion threshold of 8.0 g/dL was reasonable, the anesthetist requested two units of PRBCs and decided to recheck the Hb in 1 hour. Surgeons described the patient as "oozy" and murmured about the aspirin effect. A coagulation screen was dispatched to the laboratory.

The patient required aliquots of ephedrine with greater frequency over the following 30 minutes to maintain MAP >70 mm Hg, and the anesthetist decided to transfuse the two units of PRBC, as there was ongoing hemorrhage.

After reconstruction of the acetabular cup using bone graft, wires, and an acetabular cage, reaming commenced on the femur with a visible increase in blood loss.

The patient's MAP decreased to 55 mm Hg, his heart rate increased to 88 BPM, and his core temperature decreased to 35.3°C. The anesthetist administered 100 μg aliquots of phenylephrine to maintain the patient's MAP >60 mm Hg.

Repeat analysis showed that the patient's Hb concentration was 7.7 g/dL, and his serum lactate levels were 5.8 mmol/L. The anesthetist requested and transfused two further units of PRBC and ordered four more (he was informed that those would be available in 1 hour). The results of the coagulation screen were telephoned to the operating room: the international normalized ratio was 1.7, and the activated partial thromboplastin time was 41 seconds.

Two units of fresh frozen plasma were transfused. The femoral shaft required bone graft before insertion of the femoral prosthesis, which was eventually accomplished after

3 hours. The surgery continued with measurement and fitting of the femoral component requiring one change followed by closure. The total blood loss was estimated to be 2110 mL.

The patient was transferred to the postanesthetic care unit. His vital signs were stable as follows: MAP, 61 mm Hg; SpO$_2$, 97%; heart rate, 91 BPM; and a temperature of 35.1°C. He complained of feeling cold and was shivering. One hour postoperatively, Hb concentration was 8.7 g/dL, international normalized ratio was 1.9, and activated partial thromboplastin time was 44 seconds. There was ongoing loss in the drains. One unit of PRBC was transfused, and two additional units of fresh frozen plasma and one unit of cryoprecipitate were administered.

The patient developed chest pain with ST depression on ECG during the night and required transfer to the coronary care unit. He remained there for 3 days during which T-wave inversion on ECG and an increase in serum troponin levels were diagnostic of a subendocardial myocardial infarct.

CASE DISCUSSION

Revision hip arthroplasty is performed commonly, as primary hip arthroplasty is associated with a 10% failure rate by 10 years. Reasons for failure include aseptic loosening, instability, and infection. Removing the implanted prosthesis and exposing cancellous bone of both the acetabulum and femur leads to prolonged exposure of, and bleeding from the medullary vasculature. The associated blood loss is substantial, as the mean intraoperative blood loss was 2249 mL (range, 900–5600 mL) by one estimate.[1]

The World Health Organization defines anemia as a Hb level <13 g/dL.[2] In general, for patients undergoing noncardiac surgery, preoperative anemia is associated with a poor postoperative outcome. A large recent retrospective study showed a 1.6% increase in 30-day postoperative mortality for each percentage-point increase or decrease in the hematocrit value from normal.[3] Mild degrees of anemia have been associated with worse outcomes in patients with ischemic heart disease.[4] Early preoperative screening for elective surgery and intervention to investigate anemia and optimize Hb levels would reduce transfusion and improve outcome. Thirty days before surgery is an appropriate time for screening to allow for optimization.[5] A combination of appropriate investigations and therapy using iron, folate, vitamin B$_{12}$, and erythropoietin can be used. Commonly used erythropoietin regimens include[6] 600 units/kg weekly × four doses 300 units/kg for 15 days.

Preoperative autologous blood donation is useful in decreasing allogenic transfusion exposure but requires rigorous organization and planning to be of value.[7] There is a risk of adverse reactions to and infections from blood storage. It is probably not the optimal management for a patient with ischemic heart disease such as in the case discussed. This type of treatment would not outweigh the benefits of Hb optimization with erythropoietin.

Antifibrinolytic Therapy

Aprotinin has been used with success in decreasing blood loss in orthopaedic surgery including spine, hip, and knee surgery. Aprotinin decreases the systemic inflammatory response, fib-rinolysis, and thrombin generation, resulting in less allogeneic blood transfusion and less bleeding. For revision or bilateral hip arthroplasty, blood loss is decreased through the administration of aprotinin by 25% to 50% in various studies.[8] There are concerns about adverse thrombogenic and renal effects of aprotinin.[9] A recent prospective randomized controlled trial in patients undergoing high-risk cardiac surgery has shown an excess mortality rate in patients who received aprotinin compared with those who received tranexamic acid or aminocaproic acid.[10] The excess mortality occurred despite a greater decrease in blood loss in the aprotinin group.

Tranexamic acid inhibits fibrinolysis by blocking the lysine binding sites of plasminogen to fibrin. Studies have shown a reduction in blood loss of 43% to 54% in patients undergoing knee surgery.[11] Conclusive evaluation of potential prothrombotic adverse effects and demonstration of beneficial effects on reducing blood loss in orthopaedic surgery are required before the routine use of tranexamic acid can be recommended for hip revision arthroplasty.

Intraoperative Blood Salvage

Perioperative red cell salvage and filtration, combined with appropriate washing of red blood cells and retransfusion is an appropriate therapy to decrease allogenic transfusion provided that infection and malignancy have been excluded. The available evidence supports its use when the expected blood loss is >1500 mL. Adverse effects include transmission of infection and possibly worsening of coagulopathy.[12] Use of a blood salvage system in the case discussed would have decreased the patient's exposure to allogenic transfusion and the risks of associated adverse effects.

Transfusion Thresholds/Maximal Allowable Blood Loss with Coexisting Ischemic Heart Disease

Calculating a maximal allowable blood loss for an individual patient is useful and is usually based on a formula first popularized by Gross.[13] Selecting the initial Hb as the denominator results in a conservative estimate of MABL. Variations using mathematical modeling with different hemoglobin or hematocrit values and incorporating ongoing hemodilution and cell salvage have been reported.[14]

The Transfusion Requirement in Critical Care trial has produced excellent prospective data on transfusion requirements in chronic stable critical care patients.[15] The trial excluded patients with active hemorrhage and other acute hemodynamic insults. The outcome was no worse in the group for whom a transfusion threshold was 7.0 g/dL as compared with that for whom the threshold was 9.0 g/dL. The only patient subgroup with evidence of poorer outcome in the lower threshold arm was patients with known ischemic heart disease.

These data cannot be extrapolated to calculate MABL in the hemorrhaging patient. Similarly, the use of these hemoglobin values to rigidly define transfusion thresholds intraoperatively would not be appropriate. O$_2$ consumption and utilization are markedly different in patients with intraoperative hemodynamic stress and hemorrhage compared with recovering stable critical care patients.

The poorer outcome of patients with unstable ischemic heart disease in the lower threshold group in the Transfusion Requirement in Critical Care trial may be relevant to the management of the patient described in this case. It is difficult to define the point at which O_2 consumption/extraction by myocardial tissue is maximal and can only be improved by augmenting the O_2 carrying capacity.

The best evidence currently available supports the following:

- Hb >10 g/dL: Transfusion is unlikely to be useful.
- Hb <7 g/dL: Transfusion is likely to be useful.

Between these levels, the decision to transfuse should be based on the rate of blood loss and ongoing loss supported by laboratory and clinical evidence of inadequate tissue oxygenation.

Maximal allowable blood loss and Hb thresholds are very useful for guidance at the outset but are difficult to apply satisfactorily in patients with ongoing substantial hemorrhage. The rate of early blood loss, the identified risk of perioperative acute coronary syndrome, and the known complexity and duration of this surgery should have prompted an earlier intervention to optimize O_2 carrying capacity.

Intraoperative Hypothermia

Mild perioperative hypothermia (<1°C) increases blood loss by approximately 16% (4%–26%) and increases the relative risk for transfusion by approximately 22% (3%–37%).[16] Maintaining perioperative normothermia decreases blood loss and transfusion requirement by clinically important amounts.[16] Shivering will increase O_2 consumption contributing further to tissue hypoxia and critical organ ischemia. Aggressive intraoperative warming reduces blood loss during hip arthroplasty.[17] Perioperative hypothermia also adversely affects wound healing.[18] In the case discussed, development of intraoperative hypothermia was the most preventable factor that contributed to the adverse patient outcome.

Perioperative Coagulopathy

Coagulopathy can develop in patients with substantial hemorrhage as a result of hemodilution, hypothermia, administration of fractionated blood products, and disseminated intravascular coagulation.

The decision when and if to discontinue antiplatelet medication or other anticoagulants is important and difficult. This case highlights these difficulties, as discontinuing antiplatelet medication increases the risk of postoperative myocardial infarction by a factor of three, and continuation will increase hemorrhage volume by a factor of 1.5. In the elective setting, multidisciplinary assessment of the risk/benefit ratio for each individual patient will be necessary to optimize outcome and minimize risk in the perioperative period.[19]

Intraoperative and postoperative management of potential or actual coagulopathy includes (a) visual assessment of the surgical field for microvascular bleeding and laboratory monitoring for coagulopathy, (b) transfusion of platelets, (c) transfusion of fresh frozen plasma, (d) transfusion of cryoprecipitate, (e) administration of drugs to treat excessive bleeding (e.g., desmopressin, topical hemostatics), and (f) recombinant activated factor VII.

The American Society of Anesthesiologists guidelines state that, in a patient with ongoing bleeding:

1. Platelets should be administered when the count is <50,000 cells/mm^3.

2. Fresh frozen plasma should be administered when the international normalized ratio or activated partial thromboplastin time is elevated.

3. Cryoprecipitate should be administered when fibrinogen concentrations are <80 mg/dL (2.3 umol/L).

These guidelines also indicate that recombinant activated factor VII is an appropriate rescue drug when traditional, well-tested options have been exhausted.[20]

Development of coagulopathy in the case described herein was multifactorial. Observation of the surgical field and communication with the surgical team would have led to earlier awareness of the need for intervention.

KEY MESSAGES

1. Anemia requires investigation and treatment before major elective surgery.

2. Estimates of transfusion thresholds, maximum allowable blood loss, and rates of ongoing blood loss should be used to guide transfusion.

3. Intraoperative red cell salvage can reduce allogenic transfusion.

4. Preoperative consideration should be given to aggressive maintenance of intraoperative normothermia.

5. In the operative setting, abnormal excessive bleeding or "ooze" can provide early evidence of coagulopathy.

QUESTIONS

1. **What is the result of choosing "initial Hg" as the denominator when calculating MABL?**

   Answer: A conservative (small) estimate of MABL results.

2. **At what level of anticipated blood loss in intraoperative cell salvage viable?**

   Answer: 1500 mL

3. **What is the effect of mild intraoperative hypothermia (<1°C) on blood loss?**

   Answer: It substantially increases intraoperative blood loss (approximately 16%).

References

1. Blackley HR, Davis AM, Hutchison CR, et al. Proximal femoral allografts for reconstruction of bone stock in revision arthroplasty of the hip. JBJS Am 2001;83:346–54.
2. DeMaeyer E, Adiels-Yagman M. The prevalence of anaemia in the world. World Health Stat Q 1985;38:302–316.
3. Wu WC, Schifftner TL, Henderson WG, et al. Preoperative hematocrit levels and postoperative outcomes in older patients undergoing noncardiac surgery. JAMA 2007;297: 2481–2488.
4. Lee PC, Kini AS, Ahsan C, et al. Anemia is an independent predictor of mortality after percutaneous coronary intervention. J Am Coll Cardiol 2004;44:541–546.

5. Goodnough LT, Shander A, Spivak JL, et al. Detection, evaluation and management of anemia in the elective surgical patient. Anesth Analg 2005;101:1858–1861.

6. Feagan BG, Wong CJ, Kirkley A, et al. Erythropoietin with iron supplementation to prevent allogeneic blood transfusion in total hip joint arthroplasty: a randomized controlled trial. Ann Intern Med 2000;133:845–854.

7. Forgie MA, Wells PS, Laupacis A, et al. Preoperative autologous donation decreases allogeneic transfusion but increases exposure to all red blood cell transfusion: results of a meta-analysis. International Study of Perioperative Transfusion (ISPOT) Investigators. Arch Intern Med 1998;158:610–616.

8. Murkin JM, Shannon NA, Bourne RB, et al. Aprotinin decreases blood loss in patients undergoing revision or bilateral total hip arthroplasty. Anesth Analg 1995;80:343–348.

9. Mangano DT, Tudor IC, Dietzel C, et al. The risk associated with aprotinin in cardiac surgery. N Engl J Med 2006;354:353–365.

10. Fergusson DA, Hebert PC, Mazer CD, et al. A comparison of aprotinin and lysine analogues in high-risk cardiac surgery. N Engl J Med 2008;358:2319–2331.

11. Jansen AJ, Andreica S, Claeys M, et al. Use of tranexamic acid for an effective blood conservation strategy after total knee arthroplasty. Br J Anaesth 1999;83:596–601.

12. Scottish Intercollegiate Guidelines Network. Perioperative blood transfusion for elective surgery. Blood sparing strategies. Available at: http://www.sign.ac.uk/guidelines. Accessed March 5, 2009.

13. Gross JB. Estimating allowable blood loss: corrected for dilution. Anesthesiology. 1983;58:277–280.

14. Waters JH, Lee JS, Karafa MT. A mathematical model of cell salvage efficiency. Anesth Analg 2002;95:1312–1317.

15. Hébert PC, Wells G, Blajchman MA, et al. A multicenter, randomized, controlled clinical trial of transfusion requirements in critical care. N Engl J Med 1999;340:409–417.

16. Rajagopalan S, Mascha E, Na J, et al. The effects of mild perioperative hypothermia on blood loss and transfusion requirement. Anesthesiology 2008;108:71–77.

17. Winkler M, Akça O, Birkenberg B, et al. Aggressive warming reduces blood loss during hip arthroplasty. Anesth Analg 2000;9:978–984.

18. Kurz A, Sessler DI, Lenhardt R, et al. Perioperative normothermia to reduce the incidence of surgical-wound infection and shorten hospitalization. N Engl J Med 1996;334:1209–1215.

19. Chassot PG, Delabays A, Spahn DR. Perioperative antiplatelet therapy: the case for continuing therapy in patients at risk of myocardial infarction Br J Anaesth 2007;99:316–328.

20. Practice Guidelines for Perioperative Blood Transfusion and Adjuvant Therapies: An Updated Report by the American Society of Anaesthesiologists Task Force on Perioperative Blood Transfusion and Adjuvant Therapies. October 2005. Available at: www.asahq.org. Accessed March 5, 2009.

CHAPTER 24

Anesthesia for Bariatric Surgery

Christopher J. O'Connor

CASE FORMAT: REFLECTION

A 44-year-old, 5' 11", 170-kg man (body mass index [BMI], 52) with a history of hypertension, obstructive sleep apnea (OSA), and non–insulin-dependent diabetes mellitus presented for laparoscopic gastric bypass surgery. His medications included metoprolol, pioglitazone, and hydrochlorothiazide. He had a continuous positive airway pressure (CPAP) machine at home but rarely used it. His preoperative assessment was remarkable for a serum glucose level of 200 mg/dL, an electrocardiogram showing left ventricular hypertrophy and right heart strain, and an echocardiogram revealing moderate tricuspid regurgitation, right ventricular hypertrophy, and estimated peak systolic pulmonary artery pressure of 45 mm Hg. The patient's left ventricular function was normal. Physical examination revealed a morbidly obese man with clear lungs, normal heart tones, and a Mallampati grade III airway with a "thick neck" and limited cervical extension. It was noted that venous access would be difficult to secure. Baseline room air arterial oxygen saturation was 94%.

The patient was scheduled to undergo a laparoscopic gastric bypass procedure. A 22 guage intravenous line was placed with difficulty, and famotidine 20 mg and metoclopramide 20 mg were administered intravenously, with 30 mL of sodium citrate. Midazolam 2 mg was administered intravenously before insertion of a radial arterial catheter. In the operating room, standard monitoring was commenced, and topical anesthesia was applied to the patient's oropharynx. A transtracheal injection of 4% lidocaine was performed, as was an awake fiberoptic intubation. A pulmonary artery catheter was inserted via the right internal jugular vein using ultrasound guidance. After anesthesia induction, intermittent positive pressure was instituted using a tidal volume of 8 mL/kg, respiratory rate of 14 breaths per minutes, 60% inspired oxygen, and 7 cm H_2O positive end-expiratory pressure. Peak airway pressures of 36 cm H_2O were observed. The patient's anesthetic consisted of a neuromuscular blockade with vecuronium, a remifentanil infusion at 0.5 mcg/kg per minute, and 1% to 1.5% inspired sevoflurane. The procedure was completed in 3 hours, with blood loss of 250 mL, and 4.2 liters of Lactated Ringer's solution was used as a fluid replacement. An insulin infusion was used to maintain normoglycemia. At the end of surgery, 60 mg of ketorolac and 4 mg of ondansetron were administered. The patient's trachea was successfully extubated, and he was transferred to the surgical intensive care

unit with a non-rebreather oxygen face mask in place. He remained in the surgical intensive care unit for 24 hours for cardiopulmonary monitoring, glycemic control, and to facilitate the use of CPAP. The patient was discharged home after 5 days but returned after 2 weeks with a suspected pulmonary embolus. This was treated with intravenous heparin and subsequently with subcutaneous low-molecular-weight heparin before being discharged home for the second time.

CASE DISCUSSION

Bariatric surgery has been shown to be more efficacious than any other method of weight reduction, and several studies have shown consistent reductions in weight and the incidence of related comorbidities, as well as overall mortality.[1,9,11,13] There is a significant reduction in the incidence of hyperlipidemia, hypertension, type 2 diabetes, and OSA accompanying the weight loss induced by bariatric surgery.[3] Classification of obesity is shown in Table 24.1.

Bariatric surgery encompasses several types of procedures, broadly classified as either restrictive (gastric banding, vertical-banded gastroplasty, malabsorptive [biliopancreatic diversion]), or combined procedures (gastric bypass) (Fig. 24.1). Restrictive procedures cause weight loss by limiting the stomach's capacity to accommodate food, whereas malabsorptive surgery involves bypass or resection of the stomach and bypass of long segments of the small intestine to reduce the area for nutrient absorption. Gastric bypass is a combined procedure that involves dividing the stomach into a small, proximal pouch and a separate, large, distal nonfunctional remnant. The upper pouch is then attached to the jejunum through a small gastrojejunal anastomosis. The proximally divided jejunum is then reattached to the jejunum 75 to 150 cm below the gastrojejunal anastomosis, thus creating a Roux-en-Y limb.[5] Malabsorptive surgery is effective but causes more severe postoperative metabolic complications, whereas purely restrictive procedures produce less durable weight loss than gastric bypass. Laparoscopic gastric bypass appears to be the most efficacious of all bariatric procedures.

Airway Management

Morbid obesity and OSA, a common comorbid condition, can make mask ventilation difficult. Proper positioning of the obese patient with blankets to elevate the head and shoulders ("ramped" position) has been shown to improve laryngeal exposure. Although some evidence suggests more difficult

TABLE 24.1 Classification of Obesity

Classification	Body Mass Index
Overweight	25 kg/m^2
Obese	30 kg/m^2
Morbidly obese	40 kg/m^2
Super obese	50 kg/m^2

intubation in morbidly obese patients, a study of 100 morbidly obese patients found that neither obesity nor BMI predicted difficult intubation, but rather large neck circumference (a marker of OSA) and a greater Mallampati score were predictive. Obese patients, however, desaturate O_2 more quickly than nonobese individuals after the induction of apnea and general anesthesia; as a result, thorough preoxygenation is essential. Moreover, if there is any question about the potential difficulty of tracheal intubation, an awake intubation technique should be strongly considered.

Just as the approach to tracheal intubation should be approached with caution, the timing and decision regarding extubation should also be managed conservatively. Many clinicians choose postoperative mechanical ventilation in the super obese or for patients undergoing open, rather than laparoscopic, procedures.

Anesthetic Management

Drug pharmacokinetics differ in morbidly obese patients. Propofol dosing can be determined using total body weight, rather than ideal or lean body weight.[16] Because of their lipophilicity, thiopental and benzodiazepines may need to be administered in greater doses to obese than to nonobese patients. Opioid pharmacokinetics are more complex, with limited data

suggesting that remifentanil and fentanyl dosing should be based on ideal body weight, whereas sufentanil dosing can be accurately predicted using total body weight. Neuromuscular blocking drug dosing is more predictable because of the hydrophilic nature of nondepolarizing agents. Both vecuronium and rocuronium should be dosed based on ideal body weight to avoid prolonged neuromuscular blockade. Although all volatile agents can be safely used in morbidly obese patients, desflurane and sevoflurane are associated with more rapid emergence than isoflurane. Dexmedetomidine—a selective α_2-adrenergic agonist—may reduce intraoperative opioid requirements, while also improving intraoperative hemodynamics.[2,4] Epidural analgesia, although technically more difficult to administer in the morbidly obese, improves postoperative analgesia, as does the use of incisional local anesthetic infiltration.[12]

Ultimately, no one anesthetic technique has been shown to be superior to another for morbidly obese patients undergoing bariatric surgery, but the presence of OSA and common sense suggest that anesthetic techniques that employ shorter-acting agents may allow a more prompt recovery, less postoperative respiratory depression, and a more rapid return to baseline respiratory function.

Intraoperative Monitoring

There is little evidence that morbidly obese patients require more intense cardiovascular monitoring during bariatric surgery than nonobese patients.[6] The presence of significant comorbidities should guide the use of more invasive monitors. Patients with pulmonary hypertension, however, such as those with OSA or super obesity, may require the use of a pulmonary artery catheter. Difficulties with peripheral venous access and blood sampling are facilitated by inserting a central venous catheter, often using ultrasound guidance. Finally, it may be necessary to place intra-arterial catheters because of technical difficulties associated with blood pressure cuffs.

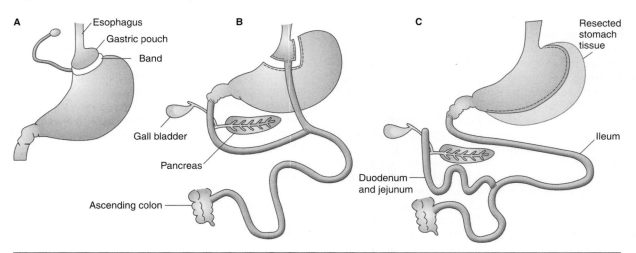

Figure 24.1 • **(A)** Adjustable gastric banding. An inflatable silicone band around the upper stomach partitions it into a ~30-mL proximal pouch and a large, distal remnant, connected through a narrow, nondistensible adjustable constriction. **(B)** Gastric bypass divides the stomach into a small, proximal pouch measuring ~30 mL and a separate, large, distal defunctionalized remnant. The upper pouch is joined to the jejunum through a narrow distensible gastrojejunal anastomosis. The proximally divided jejunum is reattached to the jejunum 75 to 150 cm below the gastrojejunal anastomosis creating a Roux-en-Y limb. **(C)** Biliopancreatic diversion, with or without a pylorus-sparing "duodenal switch" causes malabsorption as pancreatic and biliary secretions are diverted to the distal small intestine approximately 50 cm from the ileocecal valve. Absorption is thus limited to the distal ileum. A "sleeve" gastrectomy is depicted. (From Kral JG, Näslund E. Surgical treatment of obesity. Nature Clinical Practice Endocrinology & Metabolism 2007;3:574–583.)

TABLE 24.2 Risk Factors for Postoperative Complications

- Age >45
- Male gender
- Super obesity (body mass index >50 kg/m^2)
- Pulmonary hypertension
- Obstructive sleep apnea

Patient Outcome

The overall rates of mortality and morbidity associated with bariatric surgery are less than 1% and 15%, respectively, although rates may be greater for open versus laparoscopic procedures and for patients with multiple comorbidities. A variety of risk factors have been identified by multivariate analyses and risk models as predictive of mortality. These include male gender, age >45 years, BMI >50 kg/m^2, and the presence of OSA/pulmonary hypertension (Table 24.2).[7,8] Postoperative mortality appears to be secondary to pulmonary embolism/deep venous thrombosis, intra-abdominal leaks/sepsis, and myocardial infarction. Other nonfatal complications include wound infection, pneumonia, ventral hernias, nutritional deficiencies, and surgical events related to a given procedure (e.g., pouch enlargement, band slippage).

CONCLUSION

For morbidly obese patients, bariatric surgery is an effective method of weight reduction that decreases the incidence of comorbidities as well as long-term mortality.

KEY MESSAGES

1. Morbidly obese patients have a high incidence of comorbidities, including diabetes mellitus, hypertension, OSA, gastroesophageal reflux disease, and pulmonary hypertension/right heart dysfunction.

2. Important anesthetic considerations include selective use of special monitors (often intra-arterial and central venous catheters), conservative airway management, insulin therapy to maintain normoglycemia, and the use of short-acting anesthetic agents.

3. Intraoperative ventilatory management should employ high-inspired oxygen concentrations and 5 to 10 cm H$_2$O-positive end-expiratory pressure. Postoperative care should include aggressive cardiopulmonary monitoring for select patients with significant comorbidities and the use of CPAP for patients with OSA.

4. Perioperative management and postoperative morbidity and mortality are related to several risk factors, as well as the preoperative BMI, and super-obese patients (BMI >60) have the greatest incidence of complications.

QUESTIONS

1. The incidence of which of the following conditions is least reduced by bariatric surgery?
   A. Hypertension
   B. Coronary artery disease
   C. Diabetes mellitus
   D. Hyperlipidemia
   E. Sleep apnea

   Answer: B

2. Which of the following medications should dosing be based on total body weight?
   A. Fentanyl
   B. Rocuronium
   C. Propofol
   D. Remifentanil
   E. Vecuronium

   Answer: C

3. Which of the following patient characteristics increases morbidity and mortality after bariatric surgery?
   A. > Female gender
   B. BMI >40 kg/m^2
   C. Age >40 years
   D. OSA
   E. Presence of diabetes mellitus

   Answer: D

References

1. Adfams TD, Gress RE, Smith SC, et. Al. Long-term mortality after gastric bypass surgery. NEJM 2007;357:753–761.
2. Bakhamees HS, El-Halafawy YM, El-Kerdawy HM, et al. Effects of dexmedetomidine in morbidly obese patients undergoing laparoscopic gastric bypass. Middle East J Anesthesiol 2007;19:537–551.
3. Dixon JB, O'Brien PE, Playfair J, et al. Adjustable gastric banding and conventional therapy for type II diabetes. JAMA 2008;299:316–323.
4. Hofer RE, Sprung J, Sarr MG, et al. Anesthesia for a patient with morbid obesity using dexmedetomidine without narcotics. Can J Anesth 2005;52:176–180.
5. Kral JG, Näslund E. Surgical treatment of obesity. Nature Clinical Practice Endocrinology & Metabolism 2007;3:574–583.
6. Kurubsa R, Koche LS, and Murr MM. Preoperative assessment and perioperative care of patients undergoing bariatric surgery. Med Clin N Am 2007;90:339–351.
7. Levi D, Goodman ER, Patel M, et al. Critical care of the obese and bariatric surgical patient. Crit Care Clin 2003;19:11–31.
8. Leykin Y, Pellis T, Del Mestro E, et al. Anesthetic management of morbidly obese and super-morbidly obese patients undergoing bariatric operations: hospital course and outcomes. Obesity Surgery 2006;16:1563–1569.
9. Livingston EH. Obesity, mortality, and bariatric surgery rates. JAMA 2007;298:2406–2408.

10. Passannante A, Rock P. Anesthetic management of patients with obesity and sleep apnea. Anesthesiol Clin North Am 2005;23: 479–491.

11. Omalu BI, Ives DG, Buhari AM, et al. Death rates and causes of death after bariatric surgery for Pennsylvania residents, 1995 to 2004. JAMA 2007;142:923–928.

12. Schumann R, Shikora S, Weiss JM, et al. A comparison of multimodal perioperative analgesia to epidural pain management after gastric bypass surgery. Anesth Analg 2003;96:469–474.

13. Sjöström L, Narbro K, Sjöström CD, et al. Effects of bariatric surgery on mortality in Swedish obese subjects. NEJM 2007;357:741–752.

CHAPTER 25

Vasopressin and Resuscitation

Stephen F. Dierdorf

CASE FORMAT: REFLECTION

A 75-year-old, 95-kg male patient with a 4-day history of worsening abdominal pain presented for an emergency laparotomy for a suspected perforated duodenal ulcer. His coexisting medical conditions included hypertension treated with daily losartan 100 mg and coronary artery disease. He underwent coronary artery bypass grafting at age 72 and has been free of cardiac symptoms since.

The preoperative assessment performed in the emergency department showed a patient in obvious discomfort with a blood pressure of 100/60 mm Hg, heart rate of 110 beats per minute, and a respiratory rate of 28 breaths per minute. His temperature was 39°C. The patient was receiving supplemental oxygen via nasal cannula at 4 liters per minute, and arterial saturation by pulse oximetry was 96%. There had been no urine output since arrival at the hospital. Laboratory results obtained upon admission to the emergency department were as follows: hemoglobin, 15 g/dL; hematocrit level, 45%; serum potassium, 4.3 mEq/L; sodium, 140 mEq/L; bicarbonate, 18; blood urea nitrogen, 35; and creatinine, 1.0. The echocardiogram readings showed first-degree atrioventricular block with normal QRS morphology. The patient was taken to the operating room for exploratory laparotomy, and standard monitors were applied. After preoxygenation and pretreatment with 2 mg cis-atracurium, anesthesia was induced with propofol 100 mg. Succinylcholine 160 mg was administered to facilitate tracheal intubation, which was performed without difficulty with an 8-mm inner diameter tracheal tube. Soon after induction, the patient's blood pressure decreased to 60/20 mm Hg, and his heart rate increased to 140 beats per minute (BPM). ST depression appeared in the inferior leads on the surface echocardiogram. Immediate treatment consisted of the intravenous infusion of norepinephrine at 5 μg per minute, increasing to 30 μg per minute, the administration of 1500 mL of Lactated Ringer's solution, and 500 mL of 5% albumin. Despite this treatment, the patient's blood pressure continued to decline, his blood pressure became unmeasurable, and his heart rate decreased to 55 beats per minute. Epinephrine 1 mg was administered intravenously. The patient's heart rate increased to 120 BPM, and his blood pressure increased to 30/15 mm Hg. A second dose of epinephrine 1 mg increased his heart rate to 160 BPM and produced frequent premature ventricular contractions leading to ventricular tachycardia and ventricular fibrillation.

DC countershock was unsuccessful and asystole developed. Forty units of intravenously administered vasopressin resulted in spontaneous cardiac activity and an increase in blood pressure to 60/30 mm Hg. During the next 5 minutes, 500 mL of 5% albumin was administered, and a continuous vasopressin infusion at 0.2 units per minute was initiated. The patient's heart rate and blood pressure stabilized at 90 BPM and 100/50 mm Hg, respectively.

CASE DISCUSSION

This case is representative of the course of anesthesia for an elderly patient with significant preoperative physiologic derangement. The cause of clinically significant hypotension during anesthesia is not always clear, and there are many treatment options. Ideally, a definitive cause for the hypotension can be elucidated, and specific therapy can then be instituted. The goal of resuscitation is restoring vital organ perfusion and function. In some cases, the presumptive diagnosis is accurate, but therapy is controversial. The controversy surrounding resuscitation concerns the role of vasopressors and volume expansion: Is one better than the other, or is combination therapy better? Clinical studies of cardiac arrest are difficult because of the large number of variables and the lack of a matched control group. Animal models of cardiac arrest and shock have been developed, but the ability to translate those findings to real-world patients is unknown. The vasopressors most frequently used for resuscitation from cardiac arrest have been epinephrine and norepinephrine. Although the vasoconstrictive effects of vasopressin have been known for more than 100 years, it was not until the mid-1990s that vasopressin garnered much scientific attention for resuscitation.

Vasopressin, an antidiuretic hormone, is a naturally occurring nonapeptide synthesized in the hypothalamus and stored and secreted by the posterior pituitary. Vasopressin release is triggered by increased plasma osmolarity, decreased blood pressure, and decreased cardiac filling (hypovolemia). Three vasopressin receptors have been identified: V_1 mediates vasoconstriction, V_2 acts on the renal collecting tubules and causes water retention, and V_3 mediates corticotrophin release in the central nervous system. Stimulation of V_1 receptors on vascular smooth muscle cells mobilizes intracellular calcium and increases extracellular calcium influx, thereby causing vasoconstriction (Table 25.1).[1,2] The metabolic effects of vasopressin are mediated via V_2 and V_3 receptors and can influence a large number of physiologic systems.

TABLE 25.1 Vasopressin Receptors and Effects

Receptor	Effector Site	Effect
V_1	Vascular smooth muscle	Vasoconstriction
	Platelets	Aggregation
	Brain	Baroreflex mediation
V_2	Renal collecting duct cells	Antidiuresis
V_3	Anterior pituitary	ACTH secretion

ACTH, adrenocorticotropic hormone.

The metabolic effects of vasopressin in critically ill humans, however, have not been extensively studied. Current knowledge suggests that vasopressin does not alter glucose, lactate, or electrolyte levels; may reduce oxygen demand; and preserves pulmonary arterial endothelial function.[3] The plasma half-life of vasopressin is 4 to 20 minutes. Terlipressin is a synthetic analog of vasopressin with a half-life of 6 hours. Vasopressin contributes little to blood pressure control during normal physiologic conditions. When other compensatory mechanisms are not effective, vasopressin becomes an important mechanism for normalizing hemodynamics. Metabolic acidosis attenuates the effects of catecholamines. The vasoactive effects of vasopressin, however, are unaffected by acidosis. Vasopressin may be more effective than catecholamines if acidosis is present or when catecholamines become ineffective. Low-dose vasopressin may produce vasodilation in the coronary and cerebral arterial beds and increase myocardial blood flow (Table 25.2).[4]

There are five different scenarios for which vasopressin may be efficacious: (a) cardiac arrest, (b) vasodilatory shock, (c) anaphylactic shock, (d) hemorrhagic shock, and (e) during liver transplantation.

Cardiac Arrest   Despite early reports of success in a small number of patients suffering cardiac arrest in 1996, subsequent human and animal research has not fully clarified the role of vasopressin for resuscitation.[5–9] Epinephrine has been the mainstay of pharmacologic therapy for cardiac arrest for decades. Vasopressin may offer some advantages in patients

with asystole, and a combination of epinephrine (1 mg) and vasopressin (40 units) may be better than either drug alone. Current recommendations are that vasopressin (40 units) may be substituted for the first or second dose of epinephrine (1 mg) during cardiac arrest. The outcome from out-of-hospital cardiac arrest is very poor, and survival rates worldwide average 6%. Survival rates from out-of-hospital witnessed ventricular fibrillation have, however, been reported to be as high as 74%. This success is predicated on laypersons trained in cardiopulmonary resuscitation and the immediate availability of defibrillators. Patients in the operating room are well monitored, and adverse events can be detected early and managed with highly controlled interventions.

Septic Shock   The cornerstones of therapy for vasodilatory or septic shock have been antibiotics, volume resuscitation, and catecholamines. The key to improved survival in patients with septic shock is rapid intervention. Current recommendations for the treatment of septic shock include administration of antibiotics and volume resuscitation to maintain a central venous pressure of 8 to 12 mm Hg and a mean arterial blood pressure of 65 mm Hg or greater. If volume administration does not produce the desired hemodynamic responses, norepinephrine and dopamine are the vasoactive drugs of choice.[10] In cases of septic shock refractory to catecholamines or at doses that cause side effects such as tachydysrhythmia, vasopressin increases blood pressure and permits a reduction in catecholamine doses. Vasopressin in high doses can cause mesenteric vasoconstriction to the point of intestinal ischemia. In low doses, vasopressin appears to improve gastrointestinal perfusion. A continuous vasopressin infusion may be preferable to intermittent bolus doses of the longer-acting terlipressin to reduce the likelihood of mesenteric vasoconstriction and gastrointestinal ischemia.

Anaphylactic Shock   Recommended therapy for anaphylactic shock is fluid administration and epinephrine. Vasopressin has been shown to completely reverse histamine-induced vasodilation, whereas epinephrine results in only partial reversal. Until further definitive evidence exists, vasopressin is a reasonable choice when epinephrine fails to produce hemodynamic stability.[11]

Hemorrhagic Shock   The goals of resuscitation from hemorrhagic shock have been to restore circulating blood volume to preserve or improve vital organ perfusion and function. There is increasing evidence in animal models that volume resuscitation alone produces a worse outcome than limited volume resuscitation in combination with vasopressin or norepinephrine.[12] The precise mechanism of improved outcome with vasopressin remains to be elucidated. Proposed mechanisms include vasopressin-induced vasoconstriction shifting blood from the wound site and an increase in circulating vasopressin levels from depleted endogenous stores. Successful resuscitation with vasopressin may be dose dependent. Low-dose vasopressin may improve hemodynamics while avoiding the deleterious effects of organ ischemia from high doses of vasopressin.

Liver Transplantation   Patients with liver failure have multisystem disease, and the development of hepatorenal syndrome

TABLE 25.2 Vasopressin Doses

	Condition	Dose
Vasopressin	Cardiac arrest	0.5 units/kg (bolus)
	Hypotension	0.00002–0.002 units/kg per minute
Terlipressin	Hypotension	1 mg intravenously (repeat every 4–6 hours)

is a poor prognostic indicator. Low-dose vasopressin infusions may increase renal blood flow and have been used with some success in treating hypotension immediately after liver transplant. At present, research data are insufficient to determine the role of vasopressin in patients with liver failure.

Intraoperative Hypotension Patients receiving long-term therapy with angiotensin-converting enzyme inhibitors or angiotensin receptor blockers are more likely to develop hypotension during anesthesia. This hypotension may be resistant to treatment with catecholamines and volume expansion. The vasoconstrictive effect of vasopressin is independent of catecholamine and angiotensin receptors. Vasopressin has been shown to be effective for the treatment of hypotension in patients receiving those drugs.[13]

The use of vasopressin for patients with severe hypotension and shock is controversial. In milieu of the shock state, vascular smooth muscle may be less sensitive to, and even refractory to the effects of catecholamine. For patients who respond poorly to catecholamines, vasopressin provides another therapeutic option. Continued research should better define the role of vasopressin.

SUMMARY

Hypovolemia and sepsis contributed to the intraoperative shock that occurred with the patient described in this case. Volume resuscitation does not always correct the hemodynamic instability caused by septic or hemorrhagic shock. Excessive fluid administration may, in fact, worsen the outcome. It is not always possible to know the patient's balance between endogenous substances and intravascular volume that results in hemodynamic stability. Choices to be made in this situation include how much and what type of fluid to administer and which, if any, vasoactive drugs should be given. Norepinephrine and epinephrine have been used for decades to treat hypotension and shock. Patients unresponsive to these drugs may develop side effects that offset the benefits as the dosages are increased. Vasopressin is a naturally occurring vasoactive substance that may be deficient in some patients and may require replacement therapy. Vasopressin in combination with catecholamines may improve the hemodynamic profile and permit a dose reduction of the catecholamines. The initial enthusiasm regarding vasopressin for resuscitation has been tempered by subsequent research. Vasopressin has a different mechanism of action at the cellular level than catecholamines, and the two different drugs may be complementary. If epinephrine administration fails to achieve the desired effect, vasopressin is the next best choice. Although the advantages of vasopressin as compared with other vasopressors for the treatment of shock are not yet clear, the timing of intervention may be critical.[14,15] The anesthesiologist can potentially intervene with effective treatment at the very early stages of shock, thus increasing the likelihood of a successful outcome. More selective uses of vasopressin in the operating room include treatment for anaphylactic shock, vasodilatory shock after cardiopulmonary bypass, and refractory hypotension in patients receiving angiotensin-converting enzyme inhibitors or angiotensin receptor blockers.

KEY MESSAGES

1. There are multiple causes of intraoperative hypotension and shock.
2. Vasopressin is effective for managing intraoperative hypotension caused by several factors.
3. Vasopressin complements epinephrine for resuscitation following cardiac arrest.
4. Successful resuscitation depends on early multimodal treatment.

QUESTIONS

1. By what mechanism does vasopressin cause vasoconstriction?

   Answer: Vasopressin stimulates vasopressin-1 receptors. Activation of these receptors increases calcium movement into vascular smooth muscle and results in vasoconstriction.

2. How does the effect of vasopressin differ from the effect of epinephrine when used for the treatment of cardiac arrest?

   Answer: Vasopressin is effective in an acidotic milieu; whereas, the effect of epinephrine is attenuated by acidosis. Vasopressin does not cause tachycardia.

3. Does treatment with vasopressin produce a better outcome from cardiac arrest than treatment with epinephrine?

   Answer: Despite initial reports of the efficacy of vasopressin for treatment of cardiac arrest, other studies have not confirmed the superiority of vasopressin. Nonetheless, vasopressin may be effective when epinephrine fails.

References

1. Treschan TA, Peters J. The vasopressin system. Anesthesiology 2006;105:599–612.
2. Barrett LK, Singer M, Clapp LH. Vasopressin: mechanisms of action on the vasculature in health and in septic shock. Crit Care Med 2007;35:33–40.
3. Dunser MW, Westphal M. Arginine vasopressin in vasodilatory shock: effects on metabolism and beyond. Curr Opin Anesthesiol 2008;21:122–127.
4. Jochberger S, Wenzel V, Dunser MW. Arginine vasopressin as a rescue vasopressor agent in the operating room. Curr Opin Anaesthesiol 2005;18:396–404.
5. Lindner KH, Prengel AW, Brinkmann A, et al. Vasopressin in refractory cardiac arrest. Ann Intern Med 1996;124:1061–1064.
6. Wyer PC, Perera P, Jin Z, et al. Vasopressin or epinephrine for out-of-hospital cardiac arrest. Ann Emerg Med 2006;48: 86–97.
7. Aung K, Htay T. Vasopressin for cardiac arrest. Arch Intern Med 2005;165:17–24.
8. Ali B, Zafari AM. Narrative review: cardiopulmonary resuscitation and emergency cardiovascular care: review of the current guidelines. Ann Intern Med 2007;147:171–179.

9. Hazinski MF, Nadkarni VM, Hickey RO, et al. Major changes in the 2005 AHA guidelines for CPR and ECC: reaching the tipping point for change. Circulation 2005;112:IV206–211.

10. Dellinger RP, Levy MM, Carlet JM, et al. Surviving sepsis campaign: international guidelines for management of severe sepsis and septic shock: 2008. Crit Care Med 2008;36:296–227.

11. Levy JH, Adkinson NF. Anaphylaxis during cardiac surgery: implications for clinicians. Anesth Analg 2008;106:392–403.

12. Stadlbauer KH, Wagner-Berger HG, Raedler C, et al. Vasopressin, but not fluid resuscitation, enhances survival in a liver trauma model with uncontrolled and otherwise lethal hemorrhagic shock in pigs. Anesthesiology 2003;98:699–704.

13. Wheeler AD, Turchiano K, Tobias JD. A case of refractory intraoperative hypotension treated with vasopressin infusion. J Clin Anesth 2008;20:139–142.

14. Bellomo R, Wan L, May C. Vasoactive drugs and acute liver injury. Crit Care Med 2008;36(Suppl):S179–S186.

15. Patel BM, Chittock DR, Russell JA, Walley KR. Beneficial effects of short-term vasopressin infusion during severe septic shock. Anesthesiology 2002;96:576–582.

CHAPTER 26

Anesthesia and Hypertension

Stephen F. Dierdorf

FORMAT: STEP BY STEP

A 56-year-old, 5'6", 127-kg male presented for resection of a right upper lung lobe mass via a right thoracotomy. The patient had a 3-month history of a dry cough. A chest radiograph and subsequent chest computed tomography scan revealed a 4-cm mass in the upper lobe of the right lung. Past surgical history included a right inguinal hernia repair at 18 years and a laparoscopic cholecystectomy at 46 years. The patient was diagnosed with hypertension at 47 years of age, and treatment at the time of surgery included an angiotensin receptor blocker (losartan) and an angiotensin-converting enzyme (ACE) inhibitor (lisinopril). During the past 4 years, his blood pressure had been labile and difficult to control. At times, a β-adrenergic blocker (metoprolol) was added to the treatment regimen. He had not taken metoprolol during the 3 months prior to surgery. The patient had a 5-year history of sleep apnea and used a continuous positive airway pressure machine at night. Physical examination revealed an obese male with no evidence of respiratory distress. The patient's blood pressure was 165/105 mm Hg, and his heart rate was 82 beats per minute. His laboratory testing values were as follows: hemoglobin level, 14.5; hematocrit, 43; sodium, 141 mEq/L; potassium, 4.3 mEq/L; fasting glucose, 83 mg/dL; creatinine, 1.0 mg/dL; and blood urea nitrogen, 10. The preoperative room air arterial blood gas was PaO_2, 82; $PaCO_2$ 41; pH, 7.39, and base excess, 0. The patient's resting echocardiogram reading was normal. A preoperative transthoracic echocardiogram showed concentric left ventricular hypertrophy, an enlarged left atrium, and grade I diastolic dysfunction (impaired relaxation).

What is the pathogenesis and treatment of hypertension?

Hypertension is one of the most common disorders in the adult population of developed countries, and the incidence is 30% in some parts of the world. The increase in the incidence of hypertension in the last 50 years has been dramatic. The precise cause of this increase is not known parallels the increase in the incidence of obesity. Obesity causes physiologic derangements such as sympathetic nervous system activation, insulin resistance, endothelial dysfunction, and increased aldosterone levels, all of which promote hypertension. Whether the two conditions are causally related or coincidentally related remains to be determined.

Although there are well-known specific causes of hypertension such as pheochromocytoma, primary aldosteronism, renovascular disease, and coarctation of the aorta, the specific cause of hypertension in most patients is unknown (essential hypertension). There are several mechanisms by which renal dysfunction causes hypertension: (a) reduced glomerular filtration rate that limits sodium excretion, (b) humoral disorders that increase sodium reabsorption, and (c) renal ischemia. Recently, it has been suggested that prolonged ingestion of fructose increases uric acid production, which in turn, activates the renin-angiotensin system, thereby increasing blood pressure.[1] More research will be required to fully delineate the different mechanisms that cause hypertension with the hope of developing specific treatment plans.

The traditional definition of hypertension is blood pressure greater than 140/90 mm Hg. The correlation between blood pressure and the incidence of myocardial ischemia and stroke is so strong that the definition of hypertension has been modified, and individuals with blood pressure greater that 120/80 but less than 140/90 mm Hg are considered to have pre-hypertension. Treatment of prehypertensive patients decreases the likelihood of ischemic heart disease.[2]

As more data have accumulated regarding the effects of different antihypertensive drugs on patient outcome, improved recommendations for treatment have developed. The ACE inhibitors and angiotensin receptor blockers (ARB) have been shown to be effective for a wide range of patients. Thiazide diuretics and calcium channel blockers are generally indicated for the initial treatment of uncomplicated hypertension. β-Adrenergic blockers are no longer considered to be a first line antihypertensive but are indicated for patients with ischemic heart disease and heart failure.[3,4] Therapy may also be guided by monitoring the effects of antihypertensives on secondary cardiac effects such as left ventricular hypertrophy with echocardiography.[5] Patients with hypertension are a very heterogeneous group, and therapy directed at reducing the impact of hypertension on end-organ function in an individual patient would be desirable (Tables 26.1 and 26.2).

Should the patient's surgery be postponed because of elevated blood pressure?

The risks of anesthesia and surgery in a patient with hypertension include myocardial ischemia, stroke, renal dysfunction, and intraoperative blood pressure lability. Blood flow to most critical organs is autoregulated across a wide range of blood pressures. Chronically hypertensive patients can have altered autoregulatory responses, but it is difficult in an individual

TABLE 26.1 Types of Hypertension

Type	Blood Pressure (mm Hg)
Normal	120/80
Prehypertension	130/85
Mild hypertension	140/90
Moderate hypertension	160/100
Severe hypertension	180/110
Very severe hypertension	210/120
Isolated systolic hypertension	Systolic blood pressure >140 mm Hg, diastolic blood pressure <90 mm Hg
Pulse pressure hypertension	Pulse pressure >65 mm Hg

TABLE 26.2 Treatment Recommendations for Hypertension

<55 years of age	ACEI
	ARBs
If additional therapy required, add CCB or diuretics	
>55 years of age	CCBs
(African descent, any age)	Diuretics (thiazide)

If additional therapy is required, add an ACEI or ARB.
β-adrenergic blockers may be required for patients with ischemic heart disease or heart failure. Other antihypertensive drugs that may be required for treatment of resistant hypertension are spironolactone, vasodilators (hydralazine), and α-2 adrenergic agonists (clonidine). ACEI, angiotensin-converting enzyme inhibitor; ARB, angiotensin receptor blocker; CCB, calcium channel blocker.

patient to precisely define those altered autoregulatory responses. As anesthetics typically reduce blood pressure, the concern in hypertensive patients is whether the decrease in blood pressure reduces vital organ perfusion.

Studies performed in the 1960s and 1970s indicated that there was a significant perioperative risk of cardiac dysrhythmias and myocardial ischemia in hypertensive patients. Many of these patients, however, were not receiving any antihypertensive therapy. Most hypertensive patients today are receiving treatment, and the perioperative risks may not be as prevalent. The addition of many parenteral antihypertensive drugs for perioperative use has increased the anesthesiologist's ability to control blood pressure intraoperatively.

Current guidelines state that elective surgery in a patient with a blood pressure of 180/110 mm Hg or greater should have surgery postponed until better blood pressure control has been instituted. If urgent or emergent surgery is required, control can be instituted with rapid-acting antihypertensives.[6] These recommendations are based on the review of a number of studies that could not show a significant correlation between hypertension and adverse perioperative cardiac events. Despite liberalization of blood pressure values for surgery, patients with hypertension-induced end-organ damage such as ischemic heart disease, heart failure, renal disease, and cerebrovascular disease have an increased risk of adverse perioperative events.[7] Appropriate preoperative evaluation and perioperative management of these disorders is subsequently required.

As the patient's blood pressure was less than 180/110 mm Hg, and the evidence of end-organ damage was mild (diastolic dysfunction, left ventricular hypertrophy), it was decided to proceed with the surgery. The fact that the lung mass was most likely malignant conveyed some urgency for the surgery. The patient agreed to the insertion of a thoracic epidural catheter before induction for postoperative pain management. Sedation for epidural catheter insertion was achieved with the intravenous administration of 2 mg of midazolam and 50 mcg of fentanyl. After sedation, the patient's blood pressure

decreased to 135/85 mm Hg. A thoracic epidural catheter was placed without difficulty at T5.

What are the goals for perioperative management of the patient with hypertension?

An accurate assessment of preoperative blood pressure is required so that perioperative blood pressure targets can be established. Anxiety (white coat hypertension) causes an elevation in blood pressure that does not accurately reflect the patient's steady state blood pressure. A review of serial blood pressure measurements from the medical records of the patient's primary care physician will provide a better blood pressure baseline. Blood pressure can be reduced with preoperative sedation and alleviation of anxiety. After the patient's "normal" blood pressure has been established, the goal during the perioperative period is to maintain blood pressure within 20% of normal. Postoperative analgesia with regional anesthesia may improve outcome after major surgery in hypertensive patients.[8] For the patient described in this case, a continuous thoracic epidural was selected as the technique of choice for postoperative analgesia. After establishing that the patient's normal blood pressure was 135/85 mm Hg (mean, 100 mm Hg), a target goal with a mean blood pressure of 80 to 100 mm Hg would be desirable.

Anesthesia was induced with propofol 1.5 mg/kg and rocuronium 0.8 mg/kg followed by positive pressure ventilation by mask with oxygen in sevoflurane followed by tracheal intubation with a 41-F left-sided double-lumen tube. After laryngoscopy and intubation, the patient's blood pressure was 210/120 mm Hg, and his heart rate was 94 beats per minute.

Do patients with hypertension have intraoperative cardiovascular lability?

Hypertensive patients have a more active response to laryngoscopy and frequently demonstrate marked increases in blood pressure. The hypertensive response is more pronounced with prolonged laryngoscopy times. This response may be attenuated with a number of different drugs such as β-blockers, opioids, dexmedetomidine, and vasodilators. Aggressive treatment may, however, result in hypotension. Whether blood pressure and heart rate lability influence outcome and whether outcome is worse in hypertensive patients is a complex issue. There is some evidence that tachycardia and hypertension are associated with adverse outcomes in patients undergoing prolonged surgery.[9] Whether better intraoperative control would have improved outcome is unknown. Today's anesthesiologist is much better equipped with a variety of drugs to control intraoperative hemodynamics than the anesthesiologist of 30 years ago.

Intravenous metoprolol was administered in incremental dosages of 1 mg (total dosage, 3 mg) to reduce the patient's heart rate, which declined to 71 beats per minute. His blood pressure decreased to 180/100 mm Hg. Intravenous nicardipine was administered in 1-mg increments (total dosage, 2 mg), and his blood pressure decreased to 125/75 mm Hg. Fifteen minutes after induction, the patient's blood pressure decreased to 80/50 mm Hg, and he did not respond well to ephedrine and phenylephrine.

Does treatment of hypertension with ACE inhibitors and ARBs increase the likelihood of intraoperative hypotension?

Postinduction hypotension is more likely to occur in hypertensive patients treated with angiotensin receptor blockers as compared with hypertensive patients treated with β-adrenergic blockers or calcium channel blockers. Hypotension in this group of patients typically responds poorly to ephedrine and phenylephrine and is more responsive to vasopressin or terlipressin.[10] Whether angiotensin II antagonists and ACE inhibitors should be discontinued 24 hours before surgery is controversial.[11] This choice may be impractical and may lead to other unanticipated side effects. Such a recommendation is reminiscent of the recommendation for the discontinuation of β-adrenergic blockers preoperatively in the 1970s. A more rational approach may be to administer vasopressin initially or as soon as ephedrine and phenylephrine have proved ineffective.

A typical scenario in patients with hypertension is a significant increase in blood pressure with laryngoscopy that is treated with β-adrenergic blockers, vasodilators, or an increased inhaled concentration of volatile anesthetic. Aggressive treatment of post-laryngoscopy hypertension may result in hypotension once the stimulant effect of laryngoscopy has dissipated. The risk of hypotension may be reduced by the use of short-acting antihypertensives and somewhat less aggressive treatment.

Although this patient did not exhibit isolated systolic hypertension, do elderly patients with this condition have an increased perioperative risk?

The aging process produces changes in the walls of large arteries that increase the stiffness and rigidity of the blood vessels. The loss of elasticity in the aorta causes an increase in systolic pressure, a decrease in diastolic pressure, and a subsequent increase in pulse pressure. Although the treatment of isolated systolic hypertension (ISH) was controversial, it is now accepted that there is an increased risk of morbidity and mortality from ISH and that treatment is indicated.[12] Treatment of elderly

patients with ISH, however, can be challenging and must be done with caution. An aggressive reduction of blood pressure can cause myocardial ischemia or cerebrovascular insufficiency.

Younger patients may exhibit systolic hypertension and an increased pulse pressure that has been termed *pulse pressure hypertension* (PPH). Although the causative mechanisms for PPH may be different from ISH, there is an increased risk of adverse postoperative cerebral and renal outcomes in patients with PPH.[13] Whether elective surgery should be postponed in patients with PPH or ISH remains to be determined.[14]

KEY MESSAGES

1. Elective surgery in a patient with a blood pressure of 180/110 mm Hg or greater should have surgery postponed.

2. Intraoperative control of hemodynamics in hypertensive patients may be challenging.[15]

3. Postinduction hypotension is more likely to occur in hypertensive patients treated with angiotensin receptor blockers compared with hypertensive patients treated with β-adrenergic blockers or calcium channel blockers.

4. Aggressive treatment of post-laryngoscopy hypertension may result in hypotension once the stimulant effect of laryngoscopy has dissipated.

QUESTIONS

1. What are the risks of anesthesia and surgery for patients with poorly controlled hypertension?

   Answer: Risks include myocardial infarction, stroke, cardiac dysrhythmias, renal dysfunction, and perioperative blood pressure lability.

2. Why are β-adrenergic blockers no longer considered to be first line anti-hypertensive drugs?

   Answer: Angiotensin receptor blockers (ARB) have been shown to be effective anti-hypertensives without the side effects of β-blockers, such as bradycardia, exercise and cold intolerance, and peripheral vasoconstriction.

3. What is the most effective treatment of intraoperative refractory hypotension in patients receiving preoperative angiotensin receptor blockers (ARB) and/or angiotensin converting enzyme (ACE) inhibitors?

   Answer: Some patients receiving ARBs or ACE inhibitors can develop significant intraoperative hypotension. Vasopressin is more effective than ephedrine and/or phenyephrine.

References

1. Johnson RJ, Feig DI, Nakagawa T, et al. Pathogenesis of essential hypertension: historical paradigms and modern insights. J Hypertens 2008;26:381–391.

2. Rosendorff C, Black HR, Cannon CP, et al. Treatment of hypertension in the prevention and management of ischemic heart disease. Circulation 2007;115:2761–2788.

3. Higgins B, Williams B. Pharmacological management of hypertension. Clin Med 2007;7:612–616.

4. Trewet CLB, Ernst ME. Resistant hypertension: identifying causes and optimizing treatment regimens: South Med J 2008; 101:166–173.

5. Davila DF, Donis JH, Odreman R, et al. Patterns of left ventricular hypertrophy in essential hypertension: should echocardiography guide the pharmacological treatment? Int J Cardiol 2008; 124:134–138.

6. Eagle KA, Berger PB, Calkins H, et al. ACC/AHA guideline update for perioperative cardiovascular evaluation for noncardiac surgery—executive summary. Anesth Analg 2002;94: 1052–1064.

7. Hanada S, Kawakami H, Goto T, Morita S. Hypertension and anesthesia. Curr Opin Anaesthesiol 2006;19:315–319.

8. Tziavrangos E, Schug SA. Regional anaesthesia and perioperative outcome. Curr Opin Anaesthesiol 2006;19:521–525.

9. Reich DL, Bennett-Guerrero E, Bodian CA, et al. Intraoperative tachycardia and hypertension are independently associated with adverse outcome in noncardiac surgery of long duration. Anesth Analg 2002;95:273–277.

10. Brabant SM, Bertrand M, Eyraud D, et al. The hemodynamic effects of anesthetic induction in vascular surgical patients chronically treated with angiotensin II receptor antagonists. Anesth Analg 1999;1388–1392.

11. Bertrand M, Godet G, Meersschaert K, et al. Should angiotensin II antagonists be discontinued before surgery? Anesth Analg 2001;92:26–30.

12. Duprez DA. Systolic hypertension in the elderly: addressing an unmet need. Am J Med 2008;121:179–184.

13. Aronson S, Fontes ML. Hypertension: a new look at an old problem. Curr Opin Anaesthesiol 2006;19:59–64.

14. Prys-Roberts C. Isolated systolic hypertension: pressure on the anaesthetist? (editorial) Anaesthesia 2001;56:505–510.

15. Howell SJ, Sear JW, Foex P. Hypertension, hypertensive heart disease and perioperative cardiac risk. Br J Anaesth 2004;92: 570–583.

CHAPTER 27

Pharmacologic Myocardial Preconditioning

John Vullo

FORMAT: STEP BY STEP

A 73-year-old, 86-kg female presented for three-vessel off-pump coronary artery bypass grafting. She had been experiencing exertional angina and dyspnea increasing in severity for the 3 months before scheduled surgery. Coronary angiography revealed 90% occlusion of the right coronary artery and 70% occlusion of the left anterior descending and circumflex arteries. Her electrocardiogram demonstrated nonspecific ST-T waves changes and first-degree atrioventricular block (PR interval, 0.24). Transthoracic echocardiography showed inferior wall hypokinesis, impaired left ventricular relaxation, an enlarged left atrium, mild mitral regurgitation, and an ejection fraction of 45%. The patient had long-standing hypertension treated with daily valsartan and hydrochlorothiazide. Other medications included atenolol, simvastatin, and an over-the-counter-medication for heartburn.

The patient's past surgical history included a cholecystectomy at 32 years of age and an abdominal hysterectomy at 68 years of age without known anesthetic complications.

The physical examination, including airway evaluation, was not remarkable. The patient's vital signs were as follows: blood pressure, 152/84 mm Hg; heart rate, 76 beats per minute; and respiratory rate, 16 breaths per minute. Room air arterial oxygen saturation by pulse oximetry was 95%. The laboratory testing values were as follows: hematocrit level, 38; hemoglobin level, 12.7 g/dL; creatinine, 1.0; potassium, 4.2; and sodium, 138.

The patient asked if anything could be done before her surgery to improve her cardiac outcome.

What are the primary determinants of myocardial oxygen supply and demand?

Myocardial oxygen supply is determined by coronary blood flow and arterial oxygen content. Oxygen content is regulated by arterial oxygen saturation, oxygen tension, and hemoglobin as defined by the equation:

$$CaO_2 = 1.34 \times \text{hemoglobin} \times O_2 \text{ saturation} + 0.0031 \times PaO_2$$

Coronary blood flow occurs as a result of the pressure differential between aortic diastolic pressure and left ventricular end-diastolic pressure. An increase in left ventricular end-diastolic pressure or a decrease in aortic diastolic pressure can significantly decrease coronary blood flow and myocardial oxygen supply. Two other important causes of decreased coronary blood flow are coronary artery stenosis and coronary artery spasm. Myocardial oxygen demand is dependent on heart rate, left ventricular contractility, and myocardial wall stress, as determined by afterload. The heart requires a 50% increase in blood flow for a doubling of any of these factors.

What medications can be used to improve the balance between myocardial oxygen supply and demand?

Treatment of coronary artery disease must be individualized for each patient to provide medical and revascularization treatments that optimize myocardial oxygen supply and demand while preserving left ventricular function.[1-3]

There are several medications that can favorably influence myocardial oxygen supply and demand. Nitrosovasodilators can decrease left ventricular pressures, decrease left ventricular afterload by decreasing systolic pressure, and increase coronary circulation through direct coronary artery and arteriolar dilation or reversal of spasm. β-Adrenergic blockers directly reduce myocardial oxygen consumption and improve coronary blood flow by prolonging the diastolic filling time. Calcium channel blockers decrease myocardial contractility and reverse coronary artery spasm. Ranolazine, a late sodium channel blocker, reduces diastolic wall stress, and antithrombotic agents maintain coronary artery patency by platelet inhibition. Statin drugs, generally used to reduce lipid levels, have also been found to reduce inflammation and oxidative stress.[4]

There are several clinical studies suggesting the efficacy of different medications that may reduce perioperative cardiac risk. Many of these studies lack the power to justify broad recommendations for the entire surgical population. The anesthesiologist must carefully evaluate each patient and individualize the anesthetic for each patient.

The enthusiasm for perioperative β-adrenergic blocker therapy has been tempered by the outcomes of the recently published results of the PeriOperative ISchemic Evaluation trial, which showed a decrease in the perioperative myocardial infarction rate but an increased risk of death and stroke in patients receiving long-acting metoprolol.[5]

How did the patient's preoperative medical problems influence the selection of perioperative monitors?

The patient had significant coronary artery disease and long-standing hypertension with less-than-optimal control. The standard intraoperative monitors used included a five-lead continuous electrocardiogram, capnography, and pulse oximetry. An indwelling radial artery catheter, central venous catheter, and a transesophageal echocardiograph (TEE) were also used. A pulmonary artery catheter was not inserted, as the TEE would provide more information about ventricular function, segmental wall motion, and ventricular filling.

What induction drugs should be selected for this patient?

The goals of anesthesia for this patient are to reduce myocardial oxygen demand, provide adequate coronary filling pressure, and preserve left ventricular function. Concerns during induction include the potential for hypotension in a patient with mildly depressed left ventricular function and probable hypovolemia from chronic diuretic therapy. Induction of anesthesia should be performed in a slow, controlled manner by slow intravenous (IV) bolus injection or IV infusion. A BIS-guided IV infusion of propofol would accomplish those goals. Etomidate is a suitable alternative to propofol, although adrenal suppression continues to cause concern about the use of etomidate. Perhaps more important than the actual induction drug is the rapidity with which induction is performed.

Upon arrival in the operating room, a noninvasive blood pressure cuff, electrocardiogram, pulse oximeter, and BIS monitors were applied. Prior to the induction of anesthesia, IV sedation with midazolam (30 μg/kg) and fentanyl (1 μg/kg) was performed. A right radial arterial catheter was inserted with local anesthesia. Induction of anesthesia commenced with a propofol infusion at 600 μg/kg per minute and remifentanil 025 μg/kg per minute until loss of consciousness was confirmed with loss of eyelash reflex and the BIS was 46. Rocuronium (0.8 mg/kg) was administered, and positive pressure was ventilation provided. The patient's trachea was intubated without difficulty with a 7.0-mm inner diameter orotracheal tube. After the tracheal intubation, her blood pressure was 115/75 mm Hg, and her heart rate was 68 beats per minute. The propofol infusion rate was decreased to 100 μg/kg per minute, and the remifentanil infusion rate was decreased to 0.15 μg/kg per minute.

Another anesthesiologist suggested that volatile, inhaled anesthetics produce myocardial ischemic preconditioning. What is ischemic preconditioning?

Myocardial preconditioning is a phenomenon that increases the heart's resistance to a period of ischemia. This protection persists after the intervention has taken place and has been removed. Methods relying on direct cardioprotection cease to provide protection once therapy is withdrawn. Ischemic preconditioning (IPC) was first described by Murry et al. in 1986.[6] IPC is elicited by exposing the heart to a brief episode or episodes of sublethal ischemia. A preconditioned heart that undergoes a subsequent period of prolonged ischemia will develop a much smaller infarct when compared with a nonconditioned heart. There are two phases to IPC, early and late. The early phase develops within minutes of ischemic exposure and lasts for 2 to 4 hours and is very effective for reducing lethal ischemia or infarct size. The late phase takes 24 hours to develop and lasts for 3 to 4 days. The late phase has the unique property of reducing myocardial stunning following reperfusion as well as reducing infarct size. Preconditioning leads to the release of cellular substances including adenosine, bradykinin, and endorphins, which activate G protein-coupled receptors. Multistep processes activate signaling kinases, which maintain mitochondrial adenosine triphosphate (ATP) generation and inhibit apoptosis.[7]

Patients who have had anginal episodes preceding an infarct have better outcomes than those without antecedent angina. Repeated coronary occlusions during cardiac catheterization can decrease subsequent ischemic events for as long as 1 year. Intermittent cross-clamping of the aorta during cardiac surgery before cardiopulmonary bypass seems to provide some cardioprotection.

Can anesthetics precondition the heart?

Many in vitro studies have shown the cardioprotective effects of volatile, inhaled anesthetics including halothane, enflurane, isoflurane, desflurane, and sevoflurane. Isoflurane and sevoflurane have been shown to reduce infarct size even when the volatile agent is discontinued prior to coronary artery occlusion. Proposed mechanisms for anesthetic-induced IPC include preservation of ATP, attenuation of inflammation, and reduced calcium loading. At the intracellular level, volatile anesthetics open mitochondrial ATP-sensitive K^+ (K_{ATP}) channels and in turn, decrease mitochondrial energy consumption during ischemia (Table 27.1). Volatile anesthetics have also been shown to inhibit platelet aggregation, reduce myocardial damage, and decrease the likelihood of apoptosis during reperfusion after ischemia. The release of reactive oxygen species (ROS) during reperfusion depresses myocardial contractility. Volatile anesthetics reduce the release of ROS and attenuate or abolish neutrophil-induced myocardial depression.[8] Opioid agonists such as morphine and remifentanil seem to enhance the protection of the myocardium achieved by anesthetic preconditioning. Studies of propofol and ketamine have produced conflicting results regarding myocardial preconditioning. Midazolam and etomidate do not affect

TABLE 27.1 Proposed Mechanisms of Anesthetic Myocardial Preconditioning
Anti-inflammation
Reduced calcium loading
ROS
Decreased platelet adhesion
Improved ATP synthesis
Decreased neutrophil adhesion
Opening of K_{ATP} channels (mitochondria)

ATP, adenosine triphosphate; K_{ATP}, ATP-sensitive K^+; ROS, decreased reactive oxygen species.

TABLE 27.2 Drugs That Affect Anesthetic Preconditioning

Produce APC

Halothane

Isoflurane

Enflurane

Sevoflurane

Desflurane

Opioids

Flumazenil

Reduce APC

Sulfonylureas

Glitazones

Cyclooxygenase-2 inhibitors

No Effect on APC

Midazolam

Etomidate

Conflicting Evidence

Propofol

Ketamine

APC, anesthetic preconditioning.

K_{ATP} channels and do not produce anesthetic preconditioning (APC) (Table 27.2).

Hyperglycemia and diabetes may block the effects of IPC and APC. Sulfonylureas may also reduce the effectiveness of IPC and APC.

Is APC clinically relevant?

Clinical studies of APC are difficult because of the many confounding variables such as altered hemodynamics, coexisting diseases, concomitant drug administration, and multi-drug anesthetic techniques. Several clinical studies, however, have produced compelling evidence that APC is clinically significant.[9,10] Clinical markers of improved outcome after coronary artery bypass grafting include reductions in the release of creatine kinase MB and troponins I and T, reduced incidence of dysrhythmias, and improved myocardial function.[11,12] It also appears that administration of volatile anesthetics is preferable throughout the intraoperative period rather than selected periods before and after ischemia.[13] In patients undergoing single-vessel off-pump coronary artery bypass grafting, both enflurane and a 5-minute period of ischemia/reperfusion preserved myocardial function and reduced free radical formation compared with a control group.[14]

After induction of anesthesia, the propofol was discontinued, and maintenance anesthesia was provided with remifentanil (0.1 μg/kg per minute) and a sevoflurane-oxygen mixture. During the maintenance phase of anesthesia, the patient's blood pressure was 108/86 mm Hg, and her heart rate was 72 beats per minute. Brief periods of hypotension occurring during the grafting process were treated with intermittent doses of phenylephrine (1–2 μg/kg). After completion of the grafts, TEE showed no regional wall abnormalities and a left ventricular ejection fraction of 50% (Simpson's method). Postoperative sedation was provided with dexmedetomidine 0.5 μg/kg per hour. The patient's trachea was extubated 3 hours after surgery.

There are many concerns for patients with coronary artery disease undergoing cardiac or noncardiac surgery. Optimal preoperative medical management of patients with ischemic disease has not yet been determined. Patients consequently present for surgery with a variety of drug regimens and recommendations from cardiologists. The results of new studies have confounded the attempts of large medical organizations to develop firm guidelines for the testing of patients with coronary artery disease undergoing noncardiac surgery. Frequent revisions of guidelines are required as the results of new studies appear.[15]

Appropriate monitoring of intraoperative cardiac function has been controversial for many years. The wealth of information provided by TEE exceeds what is possible with a pulmonary artery catheter. The TEE is relatively noninvasive, and the development of less expensive and more mobile echo units has increased convenience of use. Ischemic myocardial preconditioning of volatile anesthetics has produced a more balanced approach to anesthesia that uses volatile anesthetics in combination with opioids. The anesthesiologist must continue to develop perioperative management plans tailored to the individual's medical conditions.

KEY MESSAGES

1. The PeriOperative ISchemic Evaluation trial demonstrated a decrease in the perioperative myocardial infarction rate but an increased risk of death and stroke in patients receiving metoprolol in the perioperative period.

2. Volatile anesthetics open mitochondrial K_{ATP} channels and decrease mitochondrial energy consumption during ischemia of the myocardium.

3. Anesthetic preconditioning is likely to be clinically significant.[9,10]

QUESTIONS

1. What are the mechanisms by which anesthetics produce myocardial ischemic preconditioning (IPC)?

   Answer: The mechanisms include anti-inflammation, reduced calcium loading, reduction of reactive oxygen species (ROS), decreased platelet adhesion, and enhanced ATP synthesis.

2. What anesthetics have been shown to produce myocardial IPC?

   Answer: Anesthetics that produce myocardial IPC include isoflurane, sevoflurane, desflurane, and opioids.

3. Are there drugs that inhibit or reduce myocardial IPC?

Answer: Anti-diabetic drugs such as sulfonylureas and glitazones inhibit myocardial IPC.

References

1. Daemen J, Serruys PW. Optimal revascularization strategies for multivessel coronary artery disease. Curr Opin Cardiol 2006;21: 595–601.
2. Banerjee P, Card D. Preserving left ventricular function during percutaneous coronary intervention. J Invasive Cardiol 2007;19: 440–443.
3. Chambers TA, Bagai A, Ivascu N. Current trends in coronary artery disease in women. Curr Opin Anaesth 2007;20:75–82.
4. Feringa HHH, Bax JJ, Poldermans D. Perioperative medical management of ischemic heart disease in patients undergoing noncardiac surgery. Curr Opin Anaesth 2007;20:254–260.
5. POISE Study group. Effects of extended-release metoprolol succinate in patients undergoing non-cardiac-surgery (POISE trial): a randomized controlled trial. Lancet 2008;371: 1839–1847.
6. Murry CE, Jennings RB, Reimer KA. Preconditioning with ischemia: a delay of lethal cell injury in ischemic myocardium. Circulation 1986;74:1124–1136.
7. Shim YH, Kersten JR. Preconditioning, anesthetics, and perioperative medication. Best Pract Res Clin Anaesth 2008;22: 151–165.
8. Tanaka K, Ludwig LM, Kersten JR, et al. Mechanisms of cardioprotection by volatile anesthetics. Anesthesiology 2004;100: 707–721.
9. DeHert SG, Turani F, Mathur S, et al. Cardioprotection with volatile anesthetics: mechanisms and clinical implications. Anesth Analg 2005;100:1584–1593.
10. Bienengraeber MW, Weihrauch D, Kersten JR, et al. Cardioprotection by volatile anesthetics. Vasc Pharmacol 2005;42: 243–252.
11. Bein B, Renner J, Caliebe D, et al. Sevoflurane but not propofol preserves myocardial function during minimally invasive direct coronary artery bypass surgery. Anesth Analg 2005;100:610–616.
12. Cromheecke S, Pepermans V, Hendrickx E, et al. Cardioprotective properties of sevoflurane in patients undergoing aortic valve replacement with cardiopulmonary bypass. Anesth Analg 2006;103:289–296.
13. De Hert SG, Van den Linden PJ, Cromheecke S, et al. Cardioprotective properties of sevoflurane in patients undergoing coronary artery surgery with cardiopulmonary bypass are related to the modalities of its administration. Anesthesiology 2004;101:299–310.
14. Drenger B, Gilon D, Chevion M, et al. Myocardial metabolism altered by ischemic preconditioning and enflurane in off-pump coronary artery surgery. J Cardiothor Vasc Anesth 2008;22:369–376.
15. Gregoratos G, Brett AS. Are the current perioperative risk management strategies for myocardial infarction flawed? Circulation 2008;117:3134–3151.

CHAPTER 28

Predicting Difficult Mask Ventilation

Stephen F. Dierdorf

CASE FORMAT: REFLECTION

A 71-year-old, 5' 10", 106-kg male presented for a left carotid endarterectomy for carotid stenosis. Fifteen years before this procedure, he underwent successful coronary artery bypass surgery and has been free of cardiac symptoms since. He had a history of snoring at night and had intermittently used a continuous positive airway pressure machine. He had smoked one pack of cigarettes per day for 52 years. The patient's medications included metoprolol 50 mg daily and aspirin. His preoperative electrocardiogram reading showed nonspecific ST-T waves changes and sinus rhythm. The patient's blood pressure was 152/84 mm Hg, and his heart rate was 55 beats per minute. His airway examination showed Mallampati grade II, slightly decreased cervical extension, full beard present, and thyromental distance, 5 cm.

Monitors applied prior to induction included an electrocardiogram, a pulse oximeter, noninvasive blood pressure, and a 12-lead electroencephalogram. Anesthesia induction was achieved with midazolam 2 mg, fentanyl 100 μg, and propofol 100 mg. Rocuronium 70 mg was administered for muscle relaxation to facilitate tracheal intubation. After induction, mask ventilation was difficult but improved considerably after insertion of an oropharyngeal airway. Rigid direct laryngoscopy was attempted with a no. 3.5 Macintosh blade; only the tip of the epiglottis could be visualized. The oropharyngeal airway was replaced and mask ventilation continued. Two more attempts at rigid direct laryngoscopy were unsuccessful. Tracheal intubation was successful with a flexible fiberoptic scope and a 7.5-mm inner diameter tracheal tube. The surgical procedure was uneventful. At the conclusion of surgery, neuromuscular blockade was reversed with neostigmine 4 mg and 0.6 mg glycopyrrolate. Sustained tetanus was demonstrated with a peripheral nerve stimulator. The patient began to cough during emergence, and his trachea was extubated to avoid further increases in blood pressure. Arterial oxygen saturation at the time of extubation was 100%. The patient did not resume spontaneous ventilation after extubation, and positive pressure ventilation was not possible. An oropharyngeal airway was inserted, but there was no appreciable ventilation as evidenced by the lack of exhaled carbon dioxide and no chest movement. Arterial oxygen saturation decreased to 92%. An intubating laryngeal mask airway (LMA) was inserted, chest excursion was observed, and exhaled carbon dioxide was detected. Oxygen saturation increased to 99%. After 5 minutes of assisted ventilation, the patient awakened, and the LMA was removed.

DISCUSSION

This case illustrates several important features of airway management. The preoperative airway examination must evaluate several variables, as no single airway examination technique is reliable. Based on the findings for this patient, some difficulty in mask ventilation should have been anticipated. After induction of anesthesia, mask ventilation was difficult, but insertion of an oropharyngeal airway allowed satisfactory mask ventilation. Direct laryngoscopy proved to be difficult, and an alternative intubation technique using flexible fiberoptic laryngoscopy was required. The rapidity and ease with which the anesthesiologist changes from the primary technique to an alternative technique reduces the likelihood of an adverse airway event. At the conclusion of the case, extubation was premature, and mask ventilation was impossible until an intubating LMA was inserted. The importance of the airway during the emergence phase of anesthesia is often overlooked even in patients with known airway difficulty. There is often a desire to extubate patients at a deeper plane of anesthesia after head and neck surgery to avoid bleeding and excessive coughing. Depth of anesthesia is difficult to predict, and deep extubation requires careful planning to avoid serious consequences. If extubation is performed when the patient is not fully awake, there is a risk of laryngospasm and upper airway obstruction, especially in patients with sleep apnea.

Airway management is the single most important task for the anesthesiologist. It is also the greatest source of adverse outcomes in the practice of anesthesia.[1] Considerable research and development of new airway devices and techniques has occurred in the past 15 years. Difficult airway management is usually equated to tracheal intubation. Three notable publications that focused on the broad area of the difficult airway reported the incidence of difficult mask ventilation to be 0.07% to 1.4%.[2–4] Research specifically related to difficult mask ventilation, however, has been sparse. The importance of mask ventilation cannot be overemphasized, as it is the first technique used for ventilation after induction of anesthesia; it is a technique that has changed little in the past decades. A careful analysis of difficult airway management should separate mask ventilation and tracheal intubation, as the alternative techniques used for each are different.

The objective of the preoperative airway examination should be evaluation and assessment of the patient for both mask ventilation and tracheal intubation. Two studies predicted difficulty with mask ventilation in 1.56% to 5% of patients. Impossible mask ventilation occurred with a frequency of 1 in 600 to 1 in 1500 patients.[5,6] Predictive factors for difficult ventilation common to both studies were (a) history of snoring (? sleep apnea), (b) presence of a beard, (c) age greater than 55 to 57 years, and (d) a body mass index >26 to 30 kg/m^2. Other factors reported in the studies but not common to both or measured by both were (a) limited mandibular protrusion, (b) lack of teeth, and (c) a thyromental distance less than 6 cm. Differences in findings among studies may be secondary to variations in the definition of difficult mask ventilation. The American Society of Anesthesiologists Practice Guidelines for Management of the Difficult Airway defines difficult mask ventilation as:

1. It is not possible for the unassisted anesthesiologist when using 100% oxygen to maintain the arterial oxygen saturation greater than 90% in a patient whose arterial oxygen saturation was greater than 90% before induction of anesthesia.
2. It is not possible for the unassisted anesthesiologist to prevent or reverse signs of inadequate ventilation during positive pressure ventilation. Signs of inadequate ventilation include cyanosis, absence of exhaled carbon dioxide, absence of breath sounds and chest movement, and hemodynamic changes associated with hypoxemia and hypercarbia[7] (Table 28.1).

The Difficult Airway Society Guidelines from the United Kingdom focus on unanticipated difficult intubation and have little information concerning mask ventilation.[8] Since the initial publication of the American Society of Anesthesiologists difficult airway guidelines in 1993, subsequent studies of difficult mask ventilation have used more liberal definitions of

TABLE 28.1 Preoperative Airway Evaluation

History

Preoperative respiratory conditions

Smoking

Snoring

Obstructive sleep apnea

Age

Physical Examination

Mallampati classification

Cervical range of motion

Mouth opening

Condition of teeth and bite

Thyromental distance

Presence or absence of a beard

Body mass index

Neck circumference

TABLE 28.2 Grading Scale for Mask Ventilation

Grade 0:	Mask ventilation not attempted
Grade 1:	Ventilation by mask
Grade 2:	Mask ventilation with pharyngeal airway
Grade 3:	Difficult mask ventilation (inadequate, unstable, two-person)
Grade 4:	Unable to mask ventilate

Data from Han R, Tremper KK, Kheterpal S, et al. Grading scale for mask ventilation. Anesthesiology 2004;101:267.

difficult mask ventilation by increasing the lower limit of arterial oxygen saturation (92%) and developing a grading system for mask ventilation. The clinical benefit of a stricter definition of difficult mask ventilation is earlier intervention with an alternative technique, thereby reducing the risk of an adverse outcome (Table 28.2).

Mask ventilation is only one part of airway management. Mask ventilation is, however, of considerable importance, as it is the first technique used after a patient loses consciousness. If ventilation with a face mask is adequate, even if tracheal intubation is difficult, there is time to initiate alternative airway management techniques. Inadequate ventilation resulting in hypoxemia reduces the amount of time available for use of alternative techniques. Airway evaluation predictive of difficult mask ventilation, consequently, is important to permit accessibility to other devices and techniques.

The supralaryngeal airways, most notably the LMA, have led to change in how difficult ventilation is defined. Because supralaryngeal airways are extremely effective for ventilation in difficult situations, the definition of *difficult ventilation* is determined by the inability to establish ventilation with a supralaryngeal airway rather than by face mask. Anesthesiologists must be highly skilled in the use of the LMA, and anesthesia training programs have a responsibility is ensure that each trainee is thoroughly versed in the use of the LMA. There are two learning phases for the LMA. The first phase requires 50 to 75 uses and allows the user to learn the rudiments of the LMA and establish ventilation in healthy patients. The second phase requires several hundred uses to develop skills for reliably managing patients with difficult airways.

SUMMARY

Airway management is the most important task that an anesthesiologist performs. At the conclusion of formal training, anesthesiologists are experts at airway management of healthy patients. True expertise for managing the difficult airway requires considerable experience and skill development. A complete preoperative airway examination is a poor predictor of airway outcome. Preoperative airway evaluation, however, does provide the anesthesiologist with an indicator of what alternative techniques may be required for a specific patient.

The anesthesiologist must be skilled with several alternative techniques and should be able to smoothly and quickly move from one technique to another when the clinical situation arises. Unless there is a specific contraindication, extubation with the patient fully awake can avoid several potential airway problems in patients with a history of obstructive sleep apnea.[10]

KEY MESSAGES

1. The airway examination is a multivariate exercise with poor predictive power.

2. Difficult mask ventilation and difficult intubation are different entities.

3. The anesthesiologist must be skilled in alternative airway techniques.

4. Tracheal extubation has risks similar to those associated with intubation.

QUESTIONS

1. Complications with what organ system contribute to the greatest likelihood of adverse outcomes related to the practice of anesthesia?

   Answer: Respiratory system complications produce the highest incidence of adverse outcomes during the course of anesthesia.

2. What are the predictive factors for difficult mask ventilation?

   Answer: Predictive factors for difficult mask ventilation include a history of snoring, presence of a beard, body mass index of >30, and age greater than 55 years.

3. What is the most appropriate procedure for impossible mask ventilation of a morbidly obese patient?

   Answer: Insertion of a supraglottic airway (e.g., LMA) would be the most appropriate method for ventilation of a morbidly obese patient should mask ventilation fail.

References

1. Cheney FW, Posner KL, Lee LA, et al. Trends in anesthesia-related death and brain damage. Anesthesiology 2006;105:1081–1086.
2. Rose DK, Cohen MM. The airway: problems and predictions in 18,500 patients. Can J Anaesth 1994;41:372–383.
3. El-Ganzouri AR, McCarthy RJ, Tuman KJ, et al. Preoperative risk assessment: predictive value of a multivariate risk index. Anesth Analg 1996;82:1197–1204.
4. Asai T, Koga K, Vaughan RS. Respiratory complications associated with tracheal intubation and extubation. Br J Anaesth 1998;80:767–773.
5. Langeron O, Masso E, Huraux C, et al. Prediction of difficult mask ventilation. Anesthesiology 2000;92:1229–1236.
6. Kheterpal S, Han R, Tremper KK, et al. Incidence and predictors of difficult and impossible mask ventilation. Anesthesiology 2006;105:885–891.
7. Task Force on Guidelines for Management of the Difficult Airway. Practice guidelines for management of the difficult airway. Anesthesiology 1993;78:597–602.
8. Henderson JJ, Popat MT, Latto IP, Pearce AC. Difficult Airway Society guidelines for management of the unanticipated difficult intubation. Anaesthesia 2004;59:675–694.
9. Han R, Tremper KK, Kheterpal S, O'Reilly M. Grading scale for mask ventilation. Anesthesiology 2004;101:267.
10. American Society of Anesthesiologists Task Force on Perioperative Management of Patients with Obstructive Sleep Apnea: practice guidelines for the perioperative management of patients with obstructive sleep apnea. Anesthesiology 2006;104:1081–1093.

CHAPTER 29

Awake Tracheal Intubation

Stephen F. Dierdorf

A 64-year-old, 74-kg male with laryngeal cancer presented for laryngectomy and right radical neck dissection. The patient complained of hoarseness, dysphagia, and dyspnea when supine that had increased in severity over the previous 3 months. He had declined surgery 6 months before the current scheduled surgery. The patient had smoked 2 packs of cigarettes per day for 44 years. The ear, nose, and throat surgeon's consultation noted that there was a large mass originating from the right false vocal cord, and the cross-sectional area of the glottic inlet was reduced by 65%. The mass extended into the anterior tracheal wall, and there was a significant reduction of epiglottic mobility.

The patient's past medical history included an inferior wall myocardial infarct followed by off-pump three-vessel coronary artery bypass grafting at 61 years of age. Since the coronary artery bypass grafting, he had been free of chest pain; however, dyspnea from the laryngeal cancer had restricted his physical activity. An open cholecystectomy had been performed at age 44 without known anesthetic complications. He has had a long-standing history of hypertension treated with angiotensin-converting enzyme inhibitors. The patient's vital signs were as follows: blood pressure, 145/85 mm Hg; heart rate, 84 beats per minute; respiratory rate, 22 breaths per minute; and the room air oxygen saturation was 91%. The preoperative airway examination showed decreased cervical range of motion and decreased mouth opening. There was a hard 8-cm fixed mass in the right neck, and there was stridor with forced inspiration.

How should the patient's airway be managed for anesthesia induction?

The patient had several airway abnormalities such as decreased cervical range of motion, poor mouth opening, and an obstructive laryngeal mass that make awake, tracheal intubation the best option. Induction of general anesthesia before intubation increases the risk of further airway obstruction in a patient that may be difficult to ventilate and perform rigid, direct laryngoscopy for tracheal intubation. Insertion of a supraglottic airway after induction of anesthesia does not guarantee a patent airway in a patient with significant laryngeal pathology. The overall clinical presentation of this patient when integrated with the American Society of Anesthesiologists guidelines for management of the difficult airway leads to the logical recommendation for awake, tracheal intubation.[1]

How should the patient be prepared for awake, tracheal intubation?

Patient preparation begins with a thorough explanation regarding the importance of performing intubation while awake. A frank discussion of the potentially dire consequences of the lost airway after anesthesia induction and the necessity of an awake intubation will do much to convince the patient of the merits of awake intubation. The patient must also be assured that his comfort during the procedure is of paramount importance, and a variety of methods including parenteral sedation and topical and/or regional anesthesia will be used to make him comfortable.

The innervation of the upper airway is extensive and is provided by several nerves. Branches of the trigeminal nerve supply the nasal cavity, and the glossopharyngeal nerve provides sensation to much of the pharynx, while the vagus nerves provide sensory innervation to the larynx via the superior laryngeal nerves. The gag reflex is controlled by the vagus nerves.[2] A single nerve block that provides complete upper airway anesthesia is, consequently, not possible. Techniques for regional anesthesia include glossopharyngeal nerve block (oropharynx), superior laryngeal nerve block (larynx above the vocal cords), and transtracheal block (larynx below the vocal cords). Regional nerve blocks may be technically challenging and less reliable in patients with distorted anatomy secondary to tumor growth and tissue infiltration.

Either the nasal or oral route can be selected for fiberoptic intubation. Unless the procedure specifically requires nasotracheal intubation, the oral route is preferred. Nasal intubation is associated with a higher likelihood of complications such as epistaxis, sinusitis, and bacteremia. Passage of a tracheal tube through the nasal passage is more uncomfortable for the patient because the pressure sensation as the tracheal tube compresses the soft tissue of the nasal passage against bony structures is difficult to attenuate.

After the patient arrived in the preoperative holding area, the anesthesiologist provided a thorough explanation of the plan for awake, tracheal intubation. Glycopyrrolate (0.1 mg intravenous [IV]) was administered. The patient was instructed to slowly and deeply inhale 4% lidocaine via a nebulizer. After inhaling the lidocaine, the patient was transferred to the operating room.

Pharyngeal secretions retard diffusion of the local anesthetics across the membranes of the upper airway. An antisialogogue will dry mucous membranes and improve the quality of topical anesthesia. In comparison to atropine, glycopyrrolate produces comparable drying of secretions with less risk of tachycardia or central nervous system side effects. Inhalation of topical anesthetic will disperse the medication throughout the upper airway. This initial phase of upper airway anesthesia can be done in the holding area without parenteral sedation.

After transfer to the operating room, parenteral sedation was initiated with midazolam (30 μg/kg) and fentanyl (1 μg/kg). An IV infusion of dexmedetomidine (0.7 μg/kg per hour) was begun. Before sedation, the patient's heart rate was 86 beats per minute, and his blood pressure was 150/85 mm Hg. After sedation, his heart rate was 71 beats per minute, and his blood pressure was 120/75 mm Hg.

The level of sedation must be closely monitored to avoid oversedation that increases the likelihood of airway obstruction and apnea. Low-dose midazolam produces amnesia without excessive sedation. Fentanyl provides additional sedation and suppresses the cough reflex. Dexmedetomidine, a short-acting α-2 adrenergic agonist provides sedation without significant respiratory depression.[3,4] Dexmedetomidine can be administered as a continuous infusion (0.7 μg/kg per hour) or as a loading dose (1 μg/kg, ideal body weight). Rapid infusion of dexmedetomidine can cause bradycardia and hypotension. Although sedation techniques have been described for each of these drugs independently, the higher doses of a single drug increase the likelihood of complications. Combining the drugs in lower doses produces a comfortable patient without respiratory depression. To obtain an optimal level of sedation, proper timing of sedative administration and adequate time to achieve effect are required.

After a satisfactory level of sedation has developed, additional topical anesthetic can be applied to the tongue, oropharynx, and hypopharynx. Many different methods can be used that employ commercially available products and dispensing devices.[5] Lidocaine ointment can be applied to the under surface (tongue contact side) of an intubating airway. The airway is slowly advanced over the patient's tongue and into the pharynx; as the ointment is warmed, it liquefies and coats the mucous membranes of the oropharynx and hypopharynx. Once the airway has been inserted to maximal depth and the patient is comfortable, a flexible fiberscope can be passed through the airway, and additional topical anesthetic is instilled through the working channel of the fiberscope (Table 29.1).

Which device or technique should be used for intubation?

Every technique for tracheal intubation has been used for awake intubation. The development of new devices and techniques for intubation in the past 15 years has increased the anesthesiologist's options for intubation of the patient with a difficult airway. Technique selection depends on the type of airway abnormality and the likelihood of success without complications. For this patient with a laryngeal mass, it is valuable to inspect the relationship of the mass to the laryngeal inlet without undue trauma. Blind insertion of any device incurs the risk of trauma to the tumor and displacement of the mass into a more obstructive position. A high-resolution

TABLE 29.1 Patient Preparation for Awake, Tracheal Intubation

Thorough explanation of the purpose

Explanation of the process

Administration of an antisialogogue

Inhalation of local anesthetic

Parenteral sedation

Direct application of topical anesthetic

Insertion of an intubating oral airway

Fiberscope insertion

Fiberscope navigation

Passage of tracheal tube

flexible fiberscope allows the anesthesiologist to visualize the larynx without altering the position of the mass with little risk of trauma. The working channel of the fiberscope provides a route for instillation of additional local anesthetic to the laryngeal inlet and the trachea.[6]

Satisfactory sedation and topical anesthesia of the oropharynx was achieved. An Ovassapian intubating airway was slowly inserted into the oropharynx with minimal discomfort to the patient. A 5.2-mm video bronchoscope with a preloaded 6.0-mm inner diameter tracheal tube was passed through the patient's airway and into the hypopharynx. Oxygen at 4 L/min was insufflated via the working channel. At the level of the epiglottis, 2 mL of 4% lidocaine was injected through the working channel. Instillation of the lidocaine provoked mild coughing; no further advance of the fiberscope was attempted until the coughing subsided. After the patient's coughing ceased, the fiberscope was advanced under the epiglottis and into the glottic inlet where 2 mL of 4% lidocaine was instilled through the working channel. Slight coughing developed that quickly subsided, the fiberscope was advanced into the subglottic region, and another 2 mL of 4% lidocaine was administered via the working channel. No coughing occurred with the final lidocaine instillation, and the fiberscope was advanced into the midtrachea. After confirmation of the fiberscope position in the midtrachea, the well-lubricated tracheal tube was advanced over the fiberscope and into the trachea. The tracheal tube cuff was gently inflated, and tracheal intubation was confirmed by capnograph. General anesthesia was induced with IV propofol and inhaled sevoflurane.

There are two basic types of flexible fiberscopes in clinical use. The older optical type fiberscopes contain an imaging bundle of optical fibers through which the endoscopist views the airway. Optical fiberscopes are limited in resolution, magnification, and field of view by the number of fibers in the imaging bundle and are subject to some optical aberration. A camera can be attached for image display on a monitor. The camera, however, does not alter the resolution or field of view. The second and more modern type of fiberscope, the flexible videoscope, has a charged-coupled device (CCD) chip at the end of the scope that transmits a digital signal to a microprocessor that constructs an image on a monitor. Videoscopes provide high-resolution, wide-angle images that are superior to the images of an optical fiberscope. Videoscopes are preferred for use in patients with upper airway tumors or when there is blood in the airway. The wide-angle field of view displays the laryngeal tumor in relationship to the entire hypopharynx. Proper fiberscope selection to meet the requirements of the clinical situation improves the efficiency and success rate for awake, tracheal intubation.

If the endoscopist is patient and recognizes anatomical landmarks before advancing the fiberscope, this will permit methodic manipulation of the scope and navigation through the airway. Instillation of local anesthetic through the working channel of the fiberscope at the levels of the epiglottis, laryngeal inlet, subglottis, and midtrachea enhances patient comfort and cooperation. If the local anesthetic provokes coughing, the scope should not be advanced until the local anesthetic has taken effect and the coughing has ceased. Oxygen insufflated through the working channel blows secretions away from the end of the fiberscope and reduces lens fogging. Direct observation of the airway pathology provides important diagnostic information that may alter the plan for airway management.

What are the potential complications from awake, fiberoptic tracheal intubation?

The complication rate for awake, fiberoptic tracheal intubation is extremely low.[7] There are sporadic case reports of infrequent complications that may be a result of the endoscopist's inexperience or lack of patient cooperation. Care must be taken to avoid oversedation and apnea that can lead to urgent airway management in a patient with a difficult airway. Local anesthetic toxicity rarely occurs in adult patients, but the local anesthetic dosage must be carefully controlled for young children. Passage of the fiberscope or tracheal tube can provoke laryngospasm and/or bronchoconstriction. Adequate airway anesthesia usually prevents such airway responses. The fiberscope should be gently passed, as forceful insertion may traumatize the airway.

Oxygen insufflation through the working channel of the fiberscope has been reported to cause gastric distention. This is an extremely rare event, although the patient's abdomen should be observed periodically for any evidence of distention (Table 29.2).

TABLE 29.2 Potential Complications of Awake, Tracheal Intubation

Oversedation

Local anesthetic toxicity

Gastric distention

Airway obstruction

Laryngospasm

Bronchoconstriction

Airway trauma

Does the availability of supraglottic airways eliminate the need for awake, tracheal intubation?

There is little doubt that the invention and development of supraglottic airways has reduced the need for awake, tracheal intubation.[8,9] This is especially true for situations in which external abnormalities (e.g., cervical spine abnormalities) limit airway access or in children with congenital airway abnormalities (e.g., Pierre-Robin, Treacher-Collins, Klippel-Feil syndromes). For patients with immediate supralaryngeal or intralaryngeal pathology (e.g., tumors, direct trauma), direct visualization of the lesion provides important information concerning airway management. The need for awake, tracheal intubation is still present for the anesthesiologist, as there are still situations in which awake, tracheal intubation may prevent significant morbidity and mortality.[10,11]

KEY MESSAGES

1. Patient preparation for awake, tracheal intubation begins with a thorough explanation of the importance and need for the procedure.

2. Regional nerve blocks performed to facilitate awake, fiberoptic intubation may be technically challenging and less reliable in patients with distorted anatomy secondary to tumor growth and tissue infiltration.

3. For a patient with a laryngeal mass, it is valuable to inspect the relationship of the mass to the laryngeal inlet without causing undue trauma.

4. Compared with (older) optical fiberscopes, flexible videoscopes are preferred for patients with upper airway tumors or when there is blood in the airway.

QUESTIONS

1. Why does administration of an antisialagogue (e.g. glycopyrrolate) improve the quality of topical airway anesthesia for awake, tracheal intubation?

   Answer: Pharyngeal secretions impede the diffusion of topical anesthetics across mucous membranes. Drying of secretions enhances the quality of topical anesthesia.

2. What cranial nerves provide sensation to the upper airway?

   Answer: Sensory input to the upper airway is supplied by the trigeminal, glossopharyngeal, and vagus nerves.

3. Why do videoendoscopes produce a higher resolution image than optical endoscopes?

   Answer: Resolution and field of view of an image provided by an optical endoscope are determined by the number of fibers in the imaging bundle. A bundle with more fibers produces an image of higher resolution. A videoendoscope uses a CCD chip instead of an optical imaging bundle.

References

1. American Society of Anesthesiologists Task Force on Difficult Airway Management. Practice guidelines for management of the difficult airway. Anesthesiology 2003;98:1269–1277.
2. Simmons ST, Schleich AR. Airway regional anesthesia for awake fiberoptic intubation. Reg Anesth Pain Med 2002;27:180–192.
3. Bergese SD, Khabiri B, Roberts WD, et al. Dexmedetomidine for conscious sedation in difficult awake fiberoptic intubation cases. J Clin Anesth 2007;19:141–144.
4. Gerlach AT, Dasta JF. Dexmedetomidine: an updated review. Ann Pharmacother 2007;41:245–254.
5. Reed AP. preparation of the patient for awake flexible fiberoptic bronchoscopy. Chest 1992;101:244–253.
6. Roberts JT. Preparing to use the flexible fiber-optic laryngoscope. J Clin Anesth 1991;3:64–75.
7. Ovaassapian A. The flexible bronchoscope: a tool for the anesthesiologist. Clin Chest Med 2001;22:281–299.
8. Langeron O, Semjen F, Bourgain J-L, et al. Comparison of the intubating laryngeal mask airway with the fiberoptic intubation in anticipated difficult airway management. Anesthesiology 2001;94:968–972.
9. Joo HS, Kapoor S, Rose DK, et al. The intubating laryngeal mask airway after induction of general anesthesia versus awake fiberoptic intubation in patients with difficult airways. Anesth Analg 2001;92:1342–1346.
10. Biboulet P, Aubas P, Dubourdieu J, et al. Fatal and nonfatal cardiac arrests due to anesthesia. Can J Anaesth 2001;48:326–332.
11. Langeron O, Amour J, Vivien B, et al. Clinical review: management of difficult airways. Critical Care 2006;10:243–247.

CHAPTER 30

Is There a Future for Succinylcholine?

Stephen F. Dierdorf

CASE FORMAT: REFLECTION

A 26-year-old woman presented for an emergency laparoscopic appendectomy. Her medical history is unremarkable, and she has not had previous surgery. She began having abdominal pain 48 hours before admission to the hospital. She had eaten a breakfast of toast and scrambled eggs 2 hours before arrival in the emergency department. Preoperative examination revealed normal upper airway anatomy and normal cardiorespiratory systems. Laboratory measurements including a complete blood count and serum electrolytes were normal other than an elevated white blood count.

The patient's overall health status was very good, and there was nothing in her medical history to suggest any potential interactions between systemic diseases and anesthesia.

The primary consideration is a patient with a full stomach for an emergency procedure. The main goal during the induction period was to intubate the trachea and isolate the airway from the gastrointestinal tract as quickly as possible to minimize the risk of regurgitation and aspiration of gastric contents. The choice of a hypnotic induction drug for this patient was not critical. The selection of a muscle relaxant to facilitate tracheal intubation was a more important choice. Should the choice be succinylcholine or a nondepolarizing muscle relaxant? The advantages of succinylcholine are rapid, predictable onset and short duration of action. For this young woman, the risk of myalgia and the possibility of serious, unpredictable side effects of succinylcholine led to the selection of cisatracurium as the muscle relaxant of choice.

In the operating room, standard preinduction monitors (electrocardiogram, automated blood pressure device, pulse oximeter) were placed. Prior to induction, midazolam 3 mg and fentanyl 100 μg were administered intravenously, and preoxygenation was performed for 3 minutes. Anesthesia induction was performed with propofol 2 mg/kg and cisatracurium 0.1 mg/kg. As soon as the patient was unconscious, an assistant applied cricoid pressure, and positive pressure ventilation with oxygen and sevoflurane was carried out. Two minutes after administration of cisatracurium, direct laryngoscopy was done. After the laryngoscope was inserted, the patient retched, and gastric contents were seen to enter the trachea. The trachea was quickly intubated, and positive pressure ventilation with 100% oxygen was performed. Arterial oxygen saturation declined to 82. Despite

positive pressure ventilation and 5 cm of positive end-expiratory pressure, arterial oxygen saturation remained in the low-to-mid 80s. An arterial blood gas showed a PaO_2 of 62 with an inspired oxygen fraction of 1.0. After the appendectomy was completed, the patient was transferred to the intensive care unit, and mechanical ventilation was continued. She was extubated without difficulty 30 hours after surgery.

DISCUSSION

What is the risk of perioperative pulmonary aspiration?

Older studies report the incidence of aspiration in patients receiving general anesthesia as 1 per 2000 to 3000. A more recent study reported the incidence to be 1 in 7000. Whether this decrease represents a true reduction in the incidence of aspiration is not clear. Aspiration is more likely to occur during emergency surgery and in patients with significant coexisting diseases. Although the overall risk of death from perioperative aspiration is low (1 in 35,000–99,000), patients who do aspirate have a 50% chance of developing a respiratory complication and a 5% to 7% chance of dying. The relative infrequency of perioperative pulmonary aspiration should not allow anesthesiologists to become complacent about its risks.[1,2]

Is there a standardized rapid sequence induction?

The introduction of curare into clinical practice in 1942 ushered in a new era in anesthesiology. Muscle relaxation could then be produced with specific muscle relaxants without having to use high doses of inhaled anesthetics. At that time, curare was used as an adjunct to anesthesia and not specifically for tracheal intubation. The introduction of succinylcholine in the 1950s provided anesthesiologists with a drug that produced rapid, profound muscle relaxation suitable for tracheal intubation. Succinylcholine became central to the evolution of the technique for rapid sequence induction (RSI) to minimize the risk of aspiration pneumonitis in patients with a full stomach. The term *rapid sequence induction* has been defined by the era during which the anesthesiologist trained and was never truly standardized. The classic RSI consisted of preoxygenation for 3 to 5 minutes, pretreatment with a small dose of a nondepolarizing muscle relaxant (prevention of fasciculation and increased intragastric pressure), administration of an induction hypnotic, cricoid pressure as soon as the patient was unconscious, administration of succinylcholine, no positive pressure ventilation by mask, and tracheal intubation. There have been many modifications to this sequence with respect to mask ventilation and type of muscle relaxant. Routine use of the pulse oximeter demonstrated how quickly arterial oxygen saturation can decline in a patient presenting for emergency surgery. Mask ventilation is now often performed when the patient becomes apneic. Cricoid pressure is regarded as optional, as it can provoke retching and emesis and may obstruct the upper airway. Pediatric anesthesiologists have significantly modified the RSI technique by substituting rocuronium for succinylcholine and using gentle positive pressure ventilation.[3] Children with normal pulmonary compliance can be easily ventilated with a peak airway pressure of 10 to 12 cm water. Although the list of side effects from succinylcholine is lengthy, and newer muscle relaxants have challenged its indications, succinylcholine is still widely used inside and outside the operating room to facilitate rapid tracheal intubation.[4]

Are there suitable alternatives to succinylcholine?

There is no doubt that the use of succinylcholine has been restricted with the availability of short-acting nondepolarizing muscle relaxants such as rocuronium and cis-atracurium. To produce rapid profound relaxation with these drugs, however, requires four times the ED_{95} resulting in a long recovery period.

Side effects from succinylcholine began to be recognized soon after its widespread use became common practice. These side effects include prolonged apnea (pseudocholinesterase deficiency), myalgia, rhabdomyolysis, masseter spasm, increased intraocular pressure, increased intragastric pressure, hyperkalemia, bradycardia, and a trigger for malignant hyperthermia. After a cause-and-effect relationship was established between succinylcholine and a side effect, methods to avoid the side effect were aggressively pursued. The ability to prevent or attenuate these side effects has prolonged the use of succinylcholine for many years. Rocuronium has emerged as the most useful of the nondepolarizing muscle relaxants for rapid tracheal intubation if succinylcholine is contraindicated. Although rocuronium compares favorably to succinylcholine regarding rapidity of onset and creating situations favorable for tracheal intubation, the dose of rocuronium (1–1.5 mg/kg) required to produce the best conditions for intubation results in a long duration of action.[5–7] Studies performed in pediatric patients show a more favorable comparison between rocuronium (0.9–1.2 mg/kg) and succinylcholine (1.5 mg/kg) with respect to onset of action and intubation conditions.[8,9] Time to recovery at those doses of rocuronium is 40 to 45 minutes. If rocuronium in higher doses is comparable to succinylcholine, the greatest challenge to succinylcholine use may not be another muscle relaxant, but a reversal drug: sugammadex. Sugammadex is a biologically inactive cyclodextrin that is a highly specific antagonist to rocuronium. If sugammadex proves to be as effective as initial studies indicate, succinylcholine will become used less

TABLE 30.1 Side Effects of Succinylcholine

Fasciculation

Myalgia

Increased intragastric pressure

Increased intraocular pressure

Increased intracranial pressure

Hyperkalemia

Malignant hyperthermia

Bradycardia

Rhabdomyolysis

Masseter spasm

Prolonged apnea (cholinesterase deficiency)

often. Proof of sugammadex's efficacy without significant side effects will only come after widespread clinical use. Rapacuronium was touted as the replacement for succinylcholine, and it was not until the drug was released for general clinical use that rapacuronium-induced bronchospasm was reported with increasing frequency. The frequency and severity of the bronchospasm led to its withdrawal from clinical practice.

What is the role of succinylcholine in modern anesthetic practice?

Succinylcholine has been in continuous clinical use for nearly 60 years. It has been a life-saving drug when rapid tracheal intubation has been required. Although succinylcholine has accumulated an extensive list of minor and major side effects, it is still a valuable muscle relaxant in the anesthesiologist's pharmacologic armamentarium. The most important indications for the use of succinylcholine are RSI and when profound relaxation is required for a short period of time. The indications for succinylcholine depend on several factors relative to the clinical situation and the concern for possible side effects. Absolute contraindications to succinylcholine use include patients with postburn injury, spinal cord transaction, susceptibility to malignant hyperthermia, and patients with primary myopathies. Most other contraindications are relative, and the risk of complications must be weighed against the benefits of rapid tracheal intubation (Table 30.1). There are techniques for reducing the incidence and severity of some of the side effects of succinylcholine. Fasciculation and myalgia may be attenuated by pretreatment with one of several drugs, including lidocaine, nonsteroidal anti-inflammatory medications, or a small dose of nondepolarizing muscle relaxant (Table 30.2).[10]

The future for succinylcholine is unclear. The highly specific antagonist for rocuronium, sugammadex, may make succinylcholine obsolete. Other drugs, however, have failed to relegate succinylcholine to historical annals. The combination of rocuronium and sugammadex will require extensive clinical use before it replaces succinylcholine. Until that time, succinylcholine will still be in use.

TABLE 30.2 Drugs That Reduce Post-Succinylcholine Myalgia

Defasciculating dose of a nondepolarizing muscle relaxant

  Pancuronium, rocuronium, vecuronium, atracurium

  Side effects: blurred vision, heavy eyelids, diplopia, dyspnea

Sodium channel blockers (lidocaine)

  Nonsteroidal anti-inflammatory drugs

  Benzodiazepines (weak effect)

SUMMARY

The patient in this case was undergoing emergency surgery and was considered to have a full stomach and to be at risk for aspiration pneumonia based on the time of her last oral intake and probable delayed gastric emptying from appendicitis.

Cisatracurium is slow and unpredictable in onset compared with succinylcholine and rocuronium. Paralysis was incomplete when direct laryngoscopy was attempted, and the patient retched and vomited. Succinylcholine or rocuronium would have been a better choice for muscle relaxation. Stimulation with a peripheral nerve stimulator before direct laryngoscopy would have undoubtedly shown incomplete paralysis, and aspiration could have been avoided.

KEY MESSAGES

1. Patients requiring emergency surgery are at increased risk for aspiration pneumonitis.

2. There are suitable alternatives for succinylcholine for elective surgery.

3. Succinylcholine may still be the most suitable muscle relaxant for RSI.

4. Positive pressure ventilation should be rapidly instituted after aspiration occurs.

QUESTIONS

1. If succinylcholine is contraindicated for a rapid sequence induction, what muscle relaxant produces satisfactory conditions for tracheal intubation in the shortest period of time?

Answer: Rocuronium has the most rapid onset of effect of the non-depolarizing muscle relaxants currently available for clinical use and is a suitable alternative to succinylcholine.

2. Why are patients with primary myopathies more likely to develop hyperkalemia after the administration of succinylcholine?

Answer: Patients with primary myopathies such as Duchenne muscular dystrophy have abnormal muscle membranes that are fragile and susceptible to damage from depolarization. Disruption of muscle membranes results in the release of large amounts of potassium from the muscle cytoplasm into the circulation.

3. Pretreatment with what types of drugs prevents or attenuates succinylcholine-induced myalgia?

Answer: Pretreatment with a defasciculating does of a non-depolarizing muscle relaxant, lidocaine, or non-steroidal anti-inflammatory drugs has been shown to reduce the incidence of myalgia after succinylcholine.

References

1. Warner MA. Is pulmonary aspiration still an important problem in anesthesia? Curr Opin Anaesthesiol 2000;13:215–218.

2. Sakai T, Planinsic RM, Quinlan JJ, et al. The incidence and outcome of perioperative pulmonary aspiration in a university hospital: a 4-year retrospective analysis. Anesth Anlg 2006;103:941–947.

3. Weiss M, Gerber AC. Rapid sequence induction in children—it's not a matter of time! Pediatr Anesth 2008;18:97–99.

4. Stedeford J, Stoddart P. RSI in pediatric anesthesia—is it used by nonpediatric anesthetists? A survey from south-west England. Pediatr Anesth 2007;17:235–242.

5. Mencke T, Knoll H, Schreiber J-U, et al. Rocuronium is not associated with more vocal cord injuries than succinylcholine after rapid-sequence induction: a randomized, prospective, controlled trial. Anesth Analg 2006;102:943–949.

6. Karcioglu O, Arnold J, Topacoglu H, et al. Succinylcholine or rocuronium? A meta-analysis of the effects on intubation conditions. Int J Clin Pract 2006;12:1638–1646.

7. Sluga M, Ummenhofer W, Studer W, et al. Rocuronium versus succinylcholine for rapid sequence induction of anesthesia and endotracheal intubation: a prospective, randomized trial in emergent cases. Anesth Analg 2005;101:1356–1361.

8. Cheng CAY, Aun CST, Gin T. Comparison of rocuronium and suxamethonium for rapid tracheal intubation in children. Paediatr Anaesth 2002;12:140–145.

9. Zelicof-Paul A, Smith-Lockridge A, Schnadower D, et al. Controversies in rapid sequence intubation in children. Curr Opin Ped 2005;17:355–362.

10. Schreiber J-U, Lysakowski C, Fuchs-Bader T, Tramer MR. Prevention of succinylcholine-induced fasciculation and myalgia. Anesthesiology 2005;103:877–884.

CHAPTER 31

Cuffed Tracheal Tubes for Children

Stephen F. Dierdorf

CASE FORMAT: REFLECTION

A 7-year-old, 35-kg girl presented for repair of an aortic coarctation and ventricular septal defect. Although she was asymptomatic, a systolic heart murmur was detected during a routine physical examination. She is quite active physically while playing competitive soccer and gymnastics. Previous surgery included bilateral myringotomies at 2 years of age as well as a tonsillectomy and adenoidectomy at 4 years of age. The parents reported no complications from previous anesthesia other than nausea and vomiting. The patient's preoperative vital signs were as follows: temperature, 37.0°C; right arm blood pressure, 145/85 mm Hg; right leg blood pressure, 80/50 mm Hg; heart rate, 92 beats per minute; and respiratory rate, 18 breaths per minute. A grade II/VI systolic heart murmur was present. Satisfactory preoperative sedation was achieved with oral midazolam 0.5 mg/kg administered 30 minutes before induction. Anesthesia was induced with sevoflurane in oxygen. After induction, an intravenous catheter was inserted into a vein in the patient's right forearm, and a cannula was inserted into the right radial artery. Muscle relaxation was achieved with 0.5 mg/kg of rocuronium, and the trachea was intubated with a 6.0-mm uncuffed orotracheal tube. Positive pressure ventilation demonstrated a large leak around the tracheal tube (12 cm water [H_2O]). The tracheal tube was replaced with a 6.0-cuffed orotracheal tube; 3 mL of air injected into the pilot balloon produced an air seal. Anesthesia maintenance was performed with nitrous oxide (N_2O) and sevoflurane in oxygen and a continuous infusion of remifentanil 0.3 μg/kg per minute. The surgical procedure and separation from cardiopulmonary bypass were uneventful. The patient was transferred directly to the intensive care unit. She was weaned from mechanical ventilation and extubated 4 hours after admission to the intensive care unit. Thirty minutes after extubation, she developed inspiratory stridor that was not relieved by inhaled racemic epinephrine and intravenous dexamethasone. She was reintubated with a 5.5-mm inner diameter uncuffed tracheal tube. There was no audible leak around the 5.5-mm tracheal tube. Tracheal extubation was attempted 12 hours later with similar results, and the patient was reintubated. An ear, nose, and throat surgeon recommended that microlaryngoscopy and bronchoscopy should be performed under general anesthesia in the operating room. Laryngoscopy and bronchoscopy revealed tracheal wall edema, erythema, and mucosal ulceration at the site of the tracheal tube cuff. The patient was extubated 36 hours after bronchoscopy. Three months after surgery, she presented with dyspnea. Bronchoscopy performed with general anesthesia showed a stenotic area at the midtrachea (Fig. 31.1).

DISCUSSION

What are the advantages of a cuffed tracheal tube?

Cuffed tracheal tubes permit an air seal between the tracheal tube and the tracheal wall. The seal permits controlled positive pressure ventilation without a leak and loss of inspired volume. The leak around an uncuffed tracheal tube is hard to control, and as pulmonary or chest wall compliance decreases, effective ventilation diminishes, and the risk of aspiration of gastric and pharyngeal contents around the tracheal tube increases. Leakage of exhaled carbon dioxide will give a falsely low end-tidal carbon dioxide reading. Other advantages of cuffed tracheal tubes include more reliable low-flow anesthesia, less need for tracheal tube replacement, and reduced operating room pollution with trace anesthetic gases.

Are children more vulnerable to postintubation complications?

The controversy surrounding the use of cuffed tracheal tubes in pediatric patients has persisted for decades.[1] Many pediatric anesthesiologists recommend that cuffed tracheal tubes should not be used in children younger than 8 years of age. This recommendation is based on the anatomy of the child's larynx and trachea. The infant larynx is vertically compact, the epiglottis is short, and the aryepiglottic folds are thick. The glottis is 7 mm in the anteroposterior axis and 4 mm in the lateral axis. The narrowest dimension of the neonatal airway is 4 to 5 mm at the subglottis. The cricoid ring has a thick submucosa with abundant mucus-producing glands. From birth to 3 years of age, there is rapid proportional growth of the larynx. The anatomic relationships of the laryngeal structures are therefore, constant.[2] Tracheal mucosal edema produces a proportionately larger decrease in the cross-sectional area of the child's trachea compared with the adult. Tracheal wall pressure exceeding 30 cm H_2O in adults may compromise perfusion of the tracheal wall causing ischemia and permanent tracheal damage. Tracheal perfusion pressure in young children is undoubtedly

113

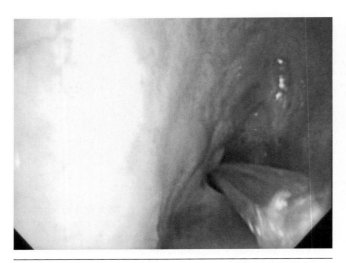

Figure 31.1 • Endoscopic View of Tracheal Stenosis.

TABLE 31.1 Impact of Airway Edema on Cross-Sectional Area

Adult			
Cricoid diameter (mm)	Area	Area (1-mm edema)	Decrease
20	31.4 mm^3	25.4 mm^3	19%
Infant			
5	19.6 mm^3	7.06 mm^3	61%

less than for the adult. The air leak test is commonly used to determine optimal tracheal tube fit. If a leak is present at 25 cm H$_2$O, fewer postoperative adverse respiratory events have been reported.[3] The air leak test, however, may not be as predictive of postextubation stridor in children younger than 7 years of age.[4] N$_2$O can diffuse into the tracheal tube cuff and increase the intracuff pressure to high levels. The rate of diffusion and subsequent pressure increase depends on the surface area for gas exchange, the permeability of the cuff material, and the thickness of the cuff[5] (Table 31.1).

The pediatric airway is vulnerable to injury at three levels: the glottic inlet, the cricoid (subglottis), and the midtrachea. Examination of children after prolonged tracheal intubation frequently reveals damage to the posterior commissure where the tracheal tube usually rests, at the level of the cricoid, and in the trachea from pressure against the tracheal wall. The ideal tracheal tube would be as narrow as possible at the levels of the vocal cords and cricoid, but it would be able to produce an air seal in the trachea. The uncuffed tube that produces a reasonable seal in the trachea may be too large at the level of the glottis and the cricoid. A cuffed tube may be closer to ideal if the cuff is thin, properly fitted for the child's airway, and exerts a low pressure against the tracheal wall at a "just seal" volume or slightly lower.

The consequences of intubation injury can be minor such as hoarseness or more serious, requiring reintubation and long-term therapy. The administration of dexamethasone to reduce mucosal edema and inflammation has been and remains controversial; however, most pediatric anesthesiologists and otolaryngologists use dexamethasone in clinical practice.[6]

Can tracheal tubes be designed specifically for children?

Detailed analyses of currently available tracheal tubes have shown considerable variation among manufacturers regarding depth of insertion, outer wall thickness, cuff position on the tube, and cuff thickness.[7] Most currently available pediatric tracheal tubes lack the careful design and precision manufacturing that might greatly reduce the incidence of postintubation side effects. The relationship between tracheal tube placement and complications is far more complex in children than adults. Most pediatric tracheal tubes are merely smaller versions of adult tracheal tubes, and the design is not based on pediatric anatomy. There is no standardization for pediatric tracheal tubes. Tracheal tube wall thickness and cuff thickness vary among manufacturers and among different tubes from the same manufacturer. Cuff position relative to the tip of the tracheal tube varies greatly. The problems presented by poor design include long cuffs and a substantial increase in outer tracheal tube diameter by thick cuffs.[8] In extreme cases, the proximal cuff may rest at the level of the cricoid or the glottic inlet, while the tip of the tube is in the midtrachea.

The development of a new type of tracheal tube specifically designed for children may herald a new era in pediatric tracheal tubes. The Microcuff Paediatric Tracheal Tube (Microcuff GmbH, Weinheim, Germany) employs a very thin (10 μ) polyurethane low-pressure cuff that is placed distally on the tracheal tube. Intracuff pressures at "just seal" average 11 cm H$_2$O for the Microcuff tube compared with 21 to 36 cm H$_2$O for more conventional tracheal tubes.[9,10] Currently, most of the studies done with this tracheal tube have been published by the same group, and confirmation of these studies is needed. The design of this tracheal tube is theoretically sound and provides a template for other manufacturers to follow.

Routine tracheal tube cuff pressure monitoring or the use of an automated pressure relief valve may be indicated for any cuffed tracheal tube. Precise pressure monitoring eliminates the assumption that pressure is satisfactory.[11]

SUMMARY

This case illustrates several important concepts about tracheal intubation and tracheal tubes in children. Cuffed tracheal tubes in pediatric patients can be used and have several advantages. Great care, however, must be taken to ensure that there is no excessive pressure on the tracheal wall. Arbitrary inflation volumes for tracheal tube cuffs are to be discouraged, as the cuff pressure is unknown. Diffusion of N$_2$O into the cuff can markedly increase the intracuff pressure. It is unfortunate for this patient that she had an excellent surgical result but is left with a serious postintubation complication that will require extensive therapy. The development of pediatric-specific tracheal tubes may reduce the likelihood of complications in the future.

KEY MESSAGES

1. The use of cuffed endotracheal tubes in children is highly controversial.

2. N_2O diffusion into the tracheal tube cuff can markedly increase intracuff pressure and increase the risk of tracheal wall ischemia.

3. The leak test may not predict adverse airway events after extubation.

4. Pediatric tracheal tubes need to be specifically designed for children.

QUESTIONS

1. How does the anatomy of the infant airway at the laryngeal level differ from the anatomy of the adult airway?

   Answer: The adult airway is cylindrical in shape with the narrowest area at the level of the vocal cords. The infant larynx is cone shaped and the narrowest area is at the level of the cricoid cartilage.

2. What is the impact of airway edema on the cross-sectional area of a pediatric airway?

   Answer: Inflammation of the airway lining produces a comparable amount of edema in both adults and children. The reduction in cross-sectional area caused by inflammatory edema can be three to four times greater in the infant as compared to the adult.

3. Does the inhalation of nitrous oxide increase the pressure and volume in a tracheal tube cuff?

   Answer: Nitrous oxide diffuses into air filled cavities much faster than nitrogen can diffuse out of the cavity. If the cavity is non-expandable, the intracavity pressure will increase. The trachea is a relatively rigid tube and the intracuff cuff pressure will increase as nitrous oxide diffuses into the cuff.

References

1. Fine GF, Borland LM. The future of the cuffed endotracheal tube. Pediatr Anesth 2004;14:38–42.

2. Isaacson G. The larynx, trachea, bronchi, lungs, and esophagus. In: Bluestone CD, Stool SE, Alper CM, et al, eds. Pediatric Otolaryngology. 4th Ed. Philadelphia: Saunders, 2003:1361–1370.

3. Suominen P, Taivainen T, Tuomenin N, et al. Optimally fitted tracheal tubes decrease the probability of postextubation adverse events in children undergoing general anesthesia. Pediatr Anesth 2006;16:641–647.

4. Mhanna MJ, Zamel YB, Tichy CM, Duper DM. The "air leak" test around the endotracheal tube, as a predictor of postextubation stridor, is age dependent in children. Crit Care Med 2002; 30:2639–2643.

5. Dullenkopf A, Gerber AC, Weiss M. Nitrous oxide diffusion into tracheal tube cuffs: comparison of five different tracheal tube cuffs. Acta Anaesthesiol Scand 2004;48:1180–1184.

6. Lukkassen MA, Markhorst DG. Does dexamethasone reduce the risk of extubation failure in ventilated children? Arch Dis Child 2006;791–793.

7. Weiss M, Dullenkopf A. Cuffed tracheal tubes in children: past, present, and future. Expert Rev Med Devices 2007;4: 73–82.

8. Weiss M, Dullenkopf A, Gysin C, et al. Shortcomings of cuffed pediatric tracheal tubes. Br J Anaesth 2004;92:78–88.

9. Dullenkopf A, Schmitz A, Gerber AC, Weiss M. Tracheal sealing characteristics of pediatric cuffed tracheal tubes. Pediatr Anesth 2004;14:825–830.

10. Dullenkopf A, Gerber AC, Weiss M. Fit and seal characteristics of a new paediatric tracheal tube with high volume-low pressure polyurethane cuff. Acta Anaesthesiol Scand 2005;49: 232–237.

11. Dullenkopf A, Bernet-Buettiker V, Maino P, Weiss M. Performance of a novel pressure release valve for cuff pressure control in pediatric tracheal tubes. Pediatr Anesth 2006;16: 19–24.

CHAPTER 32

Role of Intraoperative BIS Monitoring

Stephen F. Dierdorf

CASE FORMAT: STEP BY STEP

A 45-year-old, 97-kg male was scheduled to undergo a laparotomy for colon cancer resection. He had a history of mild hypertension that was controlled with 100 mg of losartan per day. He had undergone no prior surgery and had no allergies. The patient's heart rate was 66 beats per minute, and his blood pressure was 124/78 mm Hg. He was concerned about the safety of anesthesia and asked the anesthesiologist a few questions.

How safe is anesthesia, and what monitors will be used during my surgery?

The safety of anesthesia has improved dramatically in the past 30 years. Increased safety can be attributed to increased knowledge of pathophysiology, the introduction of better anesthetic drugs, and the development of more and better monitors. All patients receiving anesthesia are observed with standard monitors such as a continuous electrocardiograph, pulse oximeter, blood pressure cuff, and capnograph. These monitors are considered to be the standard of care by most regulatory and professional anesthesiology organizations. The primary function of these required monitors is the evaluation of cardiorespiratory function during the perioperative period. An optional monitor that may be used is a device that watches neurologic function to monitor effects of the anesthetic and detect cerebral ischemia. Although there are several neurologic monitors available, the BIS monitor (Aspect Medical Systems, Newton, MA) is the most frequently used. Other neurologic monitors in clinical use include the SEDline (Hospira, Lake Forest, IL), the Narcotrend (Schiller AG, Baar, Switzerland), Entropy (GE Healthcare, UK), the Cerebral State Monitor (Danmeter A/S, Odense, Denmark), and the AEP/2 Monitor (Danmeter, Odense, Denmark).

How does the BIS monitor work, and what does it measure?

The electroencephalograph (EEG) measures a complex signal of brain electrical activity. Continuous monitoring of multiple channels of the raw EEG is not practical in the operating room for the anesthesiologist. Signal processing techniques to render the EEG more informative have been developed in recent years. These processing techniques break the EEG signal into a family of sinusoids with three basic elements: amplitude, frequency, and phase angle. Most processing methods analyze power and frequency. Bispectral analysis adds additional information that examines the phase relationships of the sinusoids. The bispectral index is a dimensionless number based on processing of the EEG with bispectral analysis and clinical information. The BIS of the awake patient is 90 to100. Moderate hypnosis is indicated by a number of 60, and deep hypnosis is indicated by 40 (Fig. 32.1).[1–3]

The clinical purpose of BIS monitoring is to determine the level of hypnosis during sedation and general anesthesia with the hope of more precise administration of anesthetic drugs. *Depth of anesthesia* is a difficult term to define and cannot be represented by a single monitor. Depth of anesthesia incorporates hypnosis, analgesia, and reflex responses. The neural function that has gained the most attention with respect to monitoring is intraoperative awareness. Whether routine BIS monitoring reduces the incidence of awareness is controversial.[4,5]

The patient was brought to the operating room. The electrocardiogram, blood pressure cuff, pulse oximeter, and BIS sensor were applied before the induction of anesthesia. Anesthesia was induced with 2.5 mg/kg of propofol, and 0.8 mg/kg of rocuronium was administered to provide muscle relaxation for tracheal intubation. Positive pressure ventilation with sevoflurane in oxygen was provided until muscle relaxation was achieved. Three minutes after the administration of propofol, the patient's blood pressure was 70/45 mm Hg with a heart rate of 58 beats per minute. The BIS was 9.

Can routine BIS monitoring reduce the incidence of hypotension during induction?

Administering an induction drug by an intravenous bolus technique is based on an assumption of how much drug each patient will require. Variability of individual patient drug response would suggest that such assumptions are not always accurate, and the rate of drug administration may influence hemodynamic responses.[6] A carefully titrated drug administration based on BIS response reduces the risk of a relative drug overdose and subsequent hypotension.[7] A BIS index of less than 40 is frequently associated with hypotension. Slow administration of the induction drug either by small bolus injections or continuous infusion to a BIS index of 50 produces a satisfactory level of anesthesia with less decrease in blood pressure and heart rate. This is especially evident in geriatric patients.

The sevoflurane concentration was decreased, and 5 mg of ephedrine was given intravenously. Within 2 minutes, the patient's blood pressure increased to 105/70 mm Hg, and the BIS increased to 50.

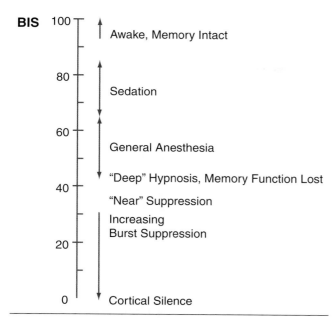

Figure 32.1 • **The Bispectral Index Scale.**

TABLE 32.1 Perioperative Neural Monitors

BIS monitor

SEDLine (Hospira, Lake Forest, IL)

AEP Monitor/2 (Danmeter, Odense, Denmark)

Entropy (GE Healthcare, UK)

Cerebral State Monitor (Danmeter A/S, Odense, Denmark)

Narcotrend (Schiller AG, Baar, Switzerland)

What BIS number (value) is consistent with adequate hypnosis during the maintenance phase of anesthesia?

There is no precise BIS number that is consistent with an adequate level of hypnosis during anesthesia maintenance. In general, a range of 50 to 60 seems desirable. Titration of maintenance anesthesia with isoflurane to a range of 50 to 60 produces faster recovery in elderly patients.[8] There is concern that consistently low BIS levels (<45) may be associated with adverse outcomes.[9] This study has been highly controversial and requires confirmation. Elderly patients (>60 years) seem to have an increased risk of long-term postoperative cognitive dysfunction after major noncardiac surgery.[10]

Routine BIS monitoring during anesthesia has been shown to reduce anesthetic consumption, time to extubation, nausea and vomiting, and recovery room time.[11,12] Prediction of emergence may be influential in avoiding immediate postoperative respiratory complications. If the patient attains clinical evidence of recovery and the BIS is >90, there seems to be minimal risk of airway obstruction and laryngospasm.

There is considerable anecdotal experience that profound decreases in the BIS index may indicate cerebral ischemia. These case reports describe a variety of clinical scenarios such as cardiac arrest, hypotension, anaphylaxis, or cardiac dysrhythmias that may decrease cerebral perfusion. The BIS level usually decreases to less than 10 but increases if cerebral perfusion returns in a timely manner. Whether the rapid return of the BIS to normal anesthetic ranges after a period of cerebral hypoperfusion has prognostic significance is as yet undetermined.

At the conclusion of surgery, residual neuromuscular blockade was reversed with neostigmine, 0.07 mg/kg and glycopyrrolate, 0.01 mg/kg. Sustained tetanus was demonstrated with a peripheral nerve stimulator. The patient opened his eyes upon command, the BIS was 94, and the trachea was extubated. His immediate postoperative course was normal. An anesthesiology colleague asked whether routine BIS monitoring should be required.

Should routine BIS monitoring be required?

Function of the central nervous system is complex, and currently available monitors are primitive in comparison. The BIS monitor is not the only available neural monitor, and others may offer advantages that have not yet been fully researched. When properly used and interpreted, the BIS monitor can provide information that allows the anesthesiologist to provide improved management of anesthesia. The BIS monitor has been used to a greater extent than any previous neural monitor, but it should most likely be regarded as a first step in the development and clinical application of routine neural monitoring to the practice of anesthesiology.[13,14] The designation of a monitor as a standard monitor introduces an extensive list of regulatory and legal requirements that may imply a greater value to the monitor than it actually has.

Neural monitors of the future should give very specific information about the functional status of the patient's central nervous system and the integrity of cerebral perfusion and metabolism. The development of advanced neural monitors should assist anesthesiologists with actually defining and measuring the depth of anesthesia (Tables 32.1 and 32.2).

TABLE 32.2 Advantages of Routine BIS Monitoring

Reduce incidence of awareness

More predictable emergence

Decreased time to extubation

Less nausea and vomiting

Improved nursing utilization

Teaching tool

KEY MESSAGES

1. The bispectral index is a dimensionless number based on processing of the EEG with bispectral analysis and clinical information.

2. Depth of anesthesia incorporates hypnosis, analgesia, and reflex responses.

3. Routine BIS monitoring during anesthesia has been shown to reduce anesthetic consumption, time to tracheal extubation, nausea and vomiting, and recovery room time.

4. The BIS monitor is not the only available "depth of anesthesia" monitor, and others may offer advantages that have not yet been fully investigated.

QUESTIONS

1. What variables of the electroencephalograph (EEG) does bispectral analysis process?

   Answer: Bispectral evaluates and processes power, amplitude, and phase relationships. This analysis technique evaluates more parameters than most processed EEG programs.

2. What range of BIS values is desired during the maintenance phase of anesthesia?

   Answer: During the maintenance phase of anesthesia, the desired BIS range is 50 to 60. It may not, however, be possible to consistently achieve a specific range in clinical practice.

3. What are the potential benefits of the routine use of the BIS monitor?

   Answer: The goal of monitoring the effects of anesthesia on the central nervous system is to precisely administer the proper amount of anesthetic drug(s) to avoid over or under-dosing. A BIS-guided anesthetic may reduce the incidence of intraoperative hypotension, postoperative nausea and vomiting, immediate postoperative respiratory complications, and reduce recovery time.

References

1. Sigl JC, Chamoun NG. An introduction to bispectral analysis for the electroencephalogram. J Clin Monit 1994;10:392–404.
2. Rosow C, Manberg P. Bispectral index monitoring. Anes Clin N Amer 1998;2:89–107.
3. Johansen JW, Sebel PS. Development and clinical application of electroencephalographic bispectrum monitoring. Anesthesiology 2000;93:1336–1344.
4. Myles PS, Leslie K, McNeil J, et al. Bispectral index monitoring to prevent awareness during anaesthesia: the B-Aware randomized controlled trial. Lancet 2004;363:1757–1763.
5. Avidan MS, Zhang L, Burnside BA, et al. Anesthesia awareness and the bispectral index. N Engl J Med 2008;358: 1097–1108.
6. Zheng D, Upton RN, Martinez AM, et al. The influence of bolus injection rate of propofol on its cardiovascular effects and the peak blood concentrations in sheep. Anesth Analg 1998;86: 1109–1115.
7. Heck M, Kumle B, Boldt J, et al. Electroencephalogram bispectral index predicts hemodynamic and arousal reactions during induction of anesthesia in patients undergoing cardiac surgery. J Cardiothor Vasc Anes 2000;14:693–697.
8. Wong J, Song D, Blanshard H, et al. Titration of isoflurane using BIS index improves early recovery of elderly patients undergoing orthopedic surgeries. Can J Anaesth 2002;49:13–18.
9. Monk TG, Saini V, Weldon BC, Sigl JC. Anesthetic management and one-year mortality after noncardiac surgery. Anesth Analg 2005;100:4–10.
10. Monk TG, Weldon BC, Garvan CW, et al. Predictors of cognitive dysfunction after major noncardiac surgery. Anesthesiology 2008;108:18–30.
11. Liu SS. Effects of bispectral index monitoring on ambulatory anesthesia. Anesthesiology 2004;101:311–315.
12. Punjasawadwong Y, Boonjeungmonkol N, Phongchiewboon A. Bispectral index for improving anaesthetic delivery and postoperative recovery. Cochrane Database Syst Rev 2007 Oct 17;4: CD003843.
13. Bowdle TA. Depth of anesthesia monitoring. Anesthesiology Clin 2006;24:793–822.
14. Bruhn J, Myles PS, Sneyd R, Struys MMRF. Depth of anesthesia monitoring: what's available, what's validated and what's next? Br J Anaesth 2006;97:85–94.

CHAPTER 33

Duchenne Muscular Dystrophy and Volatile Anesthetics

Stephen F. Dierdorf

CASE FORMAT: STEP BY STEP

A 4-year-old, 17-kg male was scheduled for bilateral inguinal hernia repair and a muscle biopsy. His pediatrician suspected that the child had Duchenne muscular dystrophy (DMD). His only prior surgery was strabismus surgery at 2 years of age performed with general anesthesia without any known complications. The suggestion that their child may have muscular dystrophy was recent, and the boy's parents asked the anesthesiologist to tell them about the disease.

What is DMD?

The cytoskeleton of the muscle cell is composed of a complex of proteins such as dystrophin, dystroglycan, sarcoglycan, utrophin, syntrophin, and dystrobrevin (Fig. 33.1). Dystrophin is the largest of the proteins and the most critical component of the dystrophin-glycoprotein complex. This complex links the cell membrane to the contractile elements of the muscle cell and stabilizes the membrane during contraction. Patients with DMD have a mutation in the gene that regulates dystrophin production, and they lack dystrophin. The absence of dystrophin increases the fragility of the muscle membrane rendering it prone to damage and release of intracellular contents into the circulation. Skeletal muscle biopsies from patients with DMD demonstrate various stages of muscle cell necrosis, regeneration, and ultimately replacement of contractile muscle with adipose and fibrotic tissue. DMD is a sex-linked recessive trait that is clinically evident in males. Progressive muscle weakness produces symptoms between the ages of 2 and 5 years with significant limitation of mobility by 12 years of age. Sequential serum creatine kinase (CK) levels reflect the disease's progression. Early in the patient's life, CK levels are elevated. As the patient ages and significant amounts of skeletal muscle have degenerated, CK levels decrease. Although skeletal muscle weakness produces the earliest and most obvious clinical abnormalities, cardiac and smooth muscle are affected as well. Loss of myocardial muscle, as reflected by a progressive decrease in R-wave amplitude on the electrocardiogram with aging, results in dilated cardiomyopathy, dysrhythmias, and mitral regurgitation. Echocardiography with tissue Doppler imaging and myocardial strain measurement can reveal subtle changes in myocardial function before the onset of symptoms.[1,2] Smooth muscle involvement causes gastroparesis, delayed gastric emptying, and an increased risk of aspiration.

Diminished skeletal muscle strength produces an ineffective cough that can lead to retention of pulmonary secretions and pneumonia. Death is secondary to congestive heart failure or pneumonia.

Despite identification of the gene defect that causes DMD more than 20 years ago, the pathophysiology is poorly understood, and specific therapy has remained elusive.[3] Studies of gene therapy in a DMD (*mdx*) mouse model have begun. Corticosteroids increase muscle strength and improve cardiorespiratory function.[4] Afterload reduction with angiotensin-converting enzyme inhibitors can improve cardiac function and increase ejection fraction. β-adrenergic blockers may also be efficacious but may cause cardiac conduction changes.

There are other types of muscular dystrophy (Table 33.1). Becker muscular dystrophy (BMD) most closely resembles DMD. Patients with BMD usually have some dystrophin, and the clinical course is milder with onset of symptoms later (11 years) and a longer life expectancy. BMD patients can develop a severe dilated cardiomyopathy.

The parents reported nothing unusual in their son's medical history, and his only previous anesthetic at age 2 was uneventful.

What information should be obtained from the preoperative evaluation?

Many children with DMD are asymptomatic, and the clinical features may be subtle during the early stages of the disease. First-time parents may be unaware of developmental milestones and are unable to report evidence of delayed motor development. The anesthesiologist must be alert for any signs of skeletal muscle dysfunction such as hypotonia, delayed walking and speech, gait disturbances, or pseudohypertrophy of muscles (gastrocnemius). An elevated CK level may be the first evidence of DMD. A preoperative cardiology consultation and echocardiography are recommended for patients with suspected or known DMD.

The parents were somewhat overwhelmed about the suspected diagnosis of DMD and were also concerned about the likelihood of an adverse event.

What are the risks of anesthesia?

A small (<20 cases) but steady accumulation of case reports of adverse effects in patients with DMD has developed during the past 2 decades.[5] The cases, in varying degrees, show evidence of severe rhabdomyolysis, hyperkalemia, metabolic acidosis, hyperthermia, renal failure, coagulopathy, and frequently death (Table 33.2). The similarity of this clinical complex and

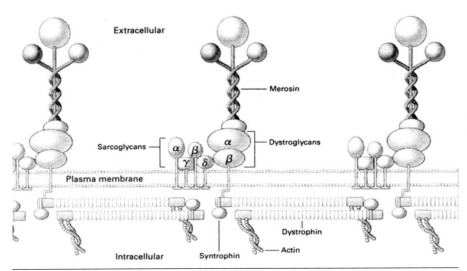

Figure 33.1 • Muscle Cell Cytoskeleton. (Reproduced with permission from Duggan DJ, Gorospe JR, Fanin M, et al. Mutations in the sarcoglycan genes in patients with myopathy. N Engl J Med 1997;336:618–624. Copyright 1997 Massachusetts Medical Society. All rights reserved.)

malignant hyperthermia (MH) led to the suggestion that DMD patients are susceptible to MH. Studies in *mdx* mice have failed to establish any link between DMD and MH. The term applied to the aforementioned clinical complex in patients with DMD is *anesthesia-induced rhabdomyolysis* (AIR). The development of AIR is unpredictable, and many patients with DMD have received volatile anesthetics and succinylcholine without apparent ill effects. The unpredictability of AIR may be related to the timing of the anesthetic exposure relative to the ongoing disease process. Patients who have had a previous uneventful anesthetic may develop AIR during subsequent exposures. AIR can occur during the anesthetic, during early recovery, or during late recovery from anesthesia.[6]

The parents reported that their child is extremely fearful of needles and becomes hysterical when receiving injections. They insisted on an inhalation induction before an intravenous line (IV) is placed.

Twenty-five minutes before the planned induction, 0.5 mg/kg of midazolam in 5 mL of acetaminophen elixir was administered orally for preoperative sedation. After transfer to the operating room, routine monitors were applied. Anesthesia induction was performed with 8% sevoflurane in oxygen. A 22-gauge IV catheter was inserted into a vein on the dorsum of the child's right hand. Rocuronium 0.3 mg/kg was administered, and positive pressure ventilation with 3% sevoflurane in oxygen was performed without difficulty. The patient's trachea was intubated with a 5-mm inner diameter orotracheal tube and surgery commenced. Ten minutes after the start of surgery, the T waves on the electrocardiogram began to peak. The peaked T waves were quickly followed by an increased duration of the QRS complex and ventricular tachycardia. An arterial blood gas sample revealed FiO_2, 1.0; PaO_2, 412; $PaCO_2$, 54; pH, 7.20; BE, -6; and potassium, 9.0 mEq/L. The patient's temperature was 38.2°C. IV lidocaine (1 mg/kg) and bicarbonate (0.5 mEq/kg) were administered without effect, and cardiopulmonary resuscitation was initiated. Calcium gluconate, 20 mg/kg was administered, and the ventricular tachycardia converted to a sinus tachycardia of 140 beats per minute. A Foley catheter was

TABLE 33.1 Types of Muscular Dystrophy
Duchenne
Becker
Emery-Dreifuss
Oculopharyngeal
Fascioscapulohumeral
Congenital
(Ulrich, Walker-Warburg)

TABLE 33.2 Clinical Features of Anesthesia-Induced Rhabdomyolysis
Rhabdomyolysis
Hyperkalemia
Tachycardia
Ventricular dysrhythmias
Metabolic acidosis
Hyperthermia
Renal dysfunction
Coagulopathy

inserted, and the patient's urine was noted to be dark red. Another blood gas sample obtained 30 minutes after the first revealed PaO_2, 402; $PaCO_2$, 45; pH, 7.37; BE, 0; potassium, 4.5 mEq/L; and CK level, 21,500. Tetanic stimulation of the ulnar nerve showed moderate fade. Neostigmine (70 μg/kg) and glycopyrrolate (10 μg/kg) were administered for reversal of neuromuscular blockade. Twenty minutes after the administration of neostigmine, tetanus was sustained, and the trachea was extubated after the child was fully awake. He was transferred to the intensive care unit for close observation. The postoperative course was uneventful, and the patient was discharged to home after 36 hours.

A muscle biopsy performed 1 month after the initial anesthetic was diagnostic for DMD. Anesthesia for the muscle biopsy was performed with IV ketamine, propofol, and remifentanil.

What is the best treatment for AIR?

The most immediate threat to the patient with AIR is acute hyperkalemia, and the plasma potassium level may exceed 12 mEq/L. The characteristic electrocardiogram changes from acute hyperkalemia progress rapidly from peaked T waves to a prolonged QRS complex, to a severely prolonged QRS complex, to ventricular tachycardia, to ventricular fibrillation. The best initial treatment of acute hyperkalemia is IV calcium (20 mg/kg). For the patient with acute transient hyperkalemia seen with AIR, one dose of calcium is generally sufficient. If hyperkalemia persists, another dose of calcium can be administered and an infusion of insulin and glucose begun. The risk of renal dysfunction from deposition of myoglobin in the renal tubules can be reduced with hydration and the administration of mannitol. Serial arterial blood gas measurements are valuable for treatment of acidosis and electrolyte abnormalities.

Are volatile anesthetics contraindicated in patients with DMD?

Whether volatile, inhaled anesthetics are contraindicated in patients with DMD is controversial. The unpredictability of AIR prevents scientifically based recommendations, but the severity of AIR suggests avoidance of volatile anesthetics.[7–9] It can be speculated that younger patients with DMD may be more likely to develop AIR because muscle tissues are undergoing both necrosis and regeneration. Later in life (adolescence) when muscle becomes fibrotic, there may be less likelihood of AIR. The presence of cardiomyopathy, which is more likely in adolescents with DMD, increases the possibility of severe myocardial depression from volatile anesthetics.

The predictability of AIR is unlikely until there is a better understanding of how the pathophysiology of DMD can produce adverse effects from anesthetics. Volatile anesthetics are best avoided but if needed, should be used judiciously, for as short a time as possible, and with alertness for the development of AIR.

Are muscle relaxants contraindicated for patients with DMD?

Succinylcholine is contraindicated for patients with DMD.[10] Nondepolarizing muscle relaxants have been used without

adverse effects. The response to nondepolarizers may, however, be abnormal. Studies with rocuronium indicate that the onset of peak neuromuscular blockade is delayed and that recovery is prolonged.[11,12] Reversal with anticholinesterase inhibitors (neostigmine, pyridostigmine) can generally be achieved, but careful monitoring of neuromuscular function is necessary.

KEY MESSAGES

1. DMD is an insidious disease with subclinical abnormalities that cause changes in skeletal, cardiac, and smooth muscle.

2. Volatile anesthetics can produce life-threatening rhabdomyolysis with acute hyperkalemia, myoglobinuria, and fever that may mimic MH.

3. The best initial therapy of acute hyperkalemia is the administration of IV calcium.

QUESTIONS

1. What is the best immediate therapy for succinylcholine-induced hyperkalemia with cardiac dysrhythmias?

   Answer: The best immediate therapy for succinylcholine-induced hyperkalemia is the intravenous administration of calcium. At the cardiac cell level, calcium is a direct antagonist to potassium. Since the hyperkalemia is transient, one dose of calcium is generally sufficient.

2. What is anesthesia-induced rhabdomyolysis (AIR)?

   Answer: AIR is a clinical complex that occurs in patients with primary myopathies (Duchenne muscular dystrophy) characterized by rhabdomyolysis, acidosis, hyperkalemia, and hyperthermia. AIR can be triggered by succinylcholine and inhaled, volatile anesthetics. Although AIR resembles malignant hyperthermia, AIR is probably a different entity.

3. Why is the muscle membrane of patients with Duchenne muscular dystrophy (DMD) fragile and easily damaged?

   Answer: The cytoskeleton of the muscle membrane is a complex of large proteins that protect and maintain the integrity of the muscle cell. Patients with DMD lack dystrophin a major component of the cytoskeleton. The muscle membrane consequently lacks the strength of normal membranes and can be damaged by excessive depolarization.

References

1. Beynon RP, Ray SG. Cardiac involvement in muscular dystrophies. QJM 2008; 101:337–344.
2. Mori K, Hayabushi Y, Inoue M, et al. Myocardial strain imaging for early detection of cardiac involvement in patients with Duchenne's progressive muscular dystrophy. Echocardiography 2007;24:598–608.

3. Deconinck N, Dan B. Pathophysiology of Duchenne muscular dystrophy: current hypotheses. Pediatr Neurol 2007;36:1–7.

4. Buschby K, Straub V. Nonmolecular treatment for muscular dystrophies. Curr Opin Neurol 2005;18:511–518.

5. Girshin M, Mukherjee Clowney R, Singer LP, et al. The postoperative arrest of a 5 year-old male: an initial presentation of Duchenne's muscular dystrophy. Pediatr Anes 2006;16: 170–173.

6. Phadke A, Broadman LM, Brandom, et al. Postoperative hyperthermia, rhabdomyolysis, critical temperature, and death in a former premature infant after his ninth anesthetic. Anesth Analg 2007;105:977–980.

7. Yemen TA, McClain C. Muscular dystrophy, anesthesia and the safety of inhalational agents revisited, again. Pediatr Anesth 2006; 16:105–108.

8. Hayes J, Veyckemans F, Bissonnette B. Duchenne muscular dystrophy: an old anesthesia problem revisited. Pediatr Anesth 2008; 18:100–106.

9. Lerman J. Inhalation agents in pediatric anesthesia—an update. Curr Opin Anesthesiol 2007;20:221–226.

10. Birnkrant DJ, Panitch HB, Benditt JO, et al. American College of Chest Physicians consensus statement on the respiratory and related management of patients with Duchenne muscular dystrophy undergoing anesthesia or sedation. Chest 2007;132:1977–1986.

11. Wick S, Muenster T, Schmidt J, et al. Onset and duration of rocuronium-induced neuromuscular blockade in patients with Duchenne muscular dystrophy. Anesthesiology 2005;102:915–919.

12. Muenster T, Forst J, Goerlitz P, et al. Reversal of rocuronium-induced neuromuscular blockade in patients with Duchenne muscular dystrophy. Pediatr Anesth 2008;18:252–255.

CHAPTER 34

Anesthesia for Magnetic Resonance Imaging

Stephen F. Dierdorf

FORMAT: STEP BY STEP

A 4-month-old, 4.2-kg male was scheduled for an outpatient cranial magnetic resonance imaging scan (MRI) because of an irregular breathing pattern and possible focal seizures. He was born preterm at 34 weeks postconceptual age and required a stage I Norwood procedure for hypoplastic left heart syndrome. He was discharged to home 2 weeks after surgery and has been feeding and growing well since discharge. The patient's vital signs were as follows: heart rate, 130 beats per minute; blood pressure, 85/54 mm Hg; respiratory rate, 28 breaths per minute; and room air arterial oxygen saturation, 77%. The mother asked the anesthesiologist a few questions as follows.

How does anesthesia for an MRI differ from anesthesia in the operating room?

The physical environment in the MRI suite is much different from the environment in the operating room.[1] Magnetic fields generated in the MRI magnet are quite strong compared with the earth's magnetic field. The gauss (G) and the tesla (T) are units of magnetic field strength. One tesla equals 10,000 gauss. The strength of the earth's magnetic field is 0.6 G. Clinical MR field strengths are 0.5 to 3 T. Magnetic fields of greater than 3 T are used for research, but in coming years, they may be used clinically. The ever-increasing magnetic strengths used for clinical imaging complicate determination of suitability for equipment in the magnetic environment.

The MRI area has been divided into four zones depending on the proximity to the magnet and the strength of the magnetic field (Table 34.1). The intense magnetic field in the MRI suite is not compatible with standard anesthesia machines and monitors. Any magnetic object in the field may become a projectile as the object is drawn into the magnet. Serious injuries have been reported in patients and personnel struck by magnetic objects. A strong handheld magnet (1000 G or greater) should be available for preliminary testing of equipment for potential magnetic attraction. Patients with implanted ferromagnetic objects may be at risk for injury or damage to the device from the strong magnetic field. The current classification places metallic objects into one of three categories: (a) MR safe, (b) MR conditional, and (c) MR unsafe. The safety of MR imaging of patients with implanted cardiovascular devices is controversial. Correct identification of the device and a risk/benefit analysis of the value of the image avoid both an unsafe MRI in some patients and denial of an MRI in other patients. Specific references

and technical information from manufacturers should be consulted to determine suitability for MRI.[2]

The bioeffects of MRI are caused by three different types of electromagnetic radiation: (a) static magnetic field, (b) a gradient magnetic field, and (c) a radiofrequency (RF) electromagnetic field. RF may generate excessive heat in metallic components such as pacemaker leads or thermodilution catheters and melt the conductive components. RF energy can be different in magnetic fields of different strength. Implants that are safe at one field strength may not be safe at lesser or stronger field strengths. Strong magnetic fields can induce small voltages changes in blood, which is electrically conductive. The voltage changes can induce ST- and T-wave changes in the electrocardiogram reading. The physics of the interaction of strong magnetic fields, RF energy, and patients can be complex, and expert analysis by magnetic physicists may be required when safety questions arise.

Factors that make anesthesia for patients in the MRI suite different from the operating room include lack of patient accessibility for airway management, noise level, and the lack of immediately available resuscitation equipment.[3]

Who will be responsible for sedating my child?

Sedation policies and personnel responsible for sedation vary greatly among institutions. The demand for sedation outside the operating room for diagnostic and interventional procedures in children has increased dramatically in the past decade. Although the risk of a serious adverse outcome from sedation is low, the incidence of timely rescue interventions is greater than 1 in 100. This requires the immediate availability of resuscitation equipment and personnel trained in respiratory management.[4] The goal for sedation is a cooperative and comfortable child who can maintain a patent airway with satisfactory ventilation and oxygenation. The line, however, between moderate sedation and deep sedation is not easily defined, and the likelihood of passing into a level of deep sedation is high.[5] Physicians responsible for sedation at different institutions include radiologists, emergency department physicians, critical care physicians, and anesthesiologists. The presence of the anesthesiologist provides an individual with expert airway management skills and someone who can quickly convert to a general anesthetic if sedation fails.

The patient's mother was assured that at this institution, all sedation for imaging procedures is supervised by a pediatric anesthesiologist with the assistance of trained nurses. All patients undergo a thorough preoperative evaluation, and a plan for sedation is developed for each child depending on his or her coexisting problems.

TABLE 34.1 Magnetic Resonance Imaging Zones

Zone I:	Outside the magnetic field. Accessible to the general public
Zone II:	Area between freely accessible area (zone I) and controlled zones III and IV
	Patient and family member movement is supervised. Patient screening is usually done in zone II.
Zone III:	Area where injury can occur if unscreened personnel or patients can incur injuries if noncompatible ferromagnetic objects or equipment are present. Zone III must be strictly restricted.
Zone IV:	Magnetic resonance scanner room. This room must be clearly delineated, and a large red "Magnet On" light must be clearly visible. If cardiopulmonary resuscitation is required in zone IV, MR-trained personnel should stabilize the patient and evacuate to zone II as quickly as feasible.

Is my baby at risk from the contrast agent?

The patient's mother had heard about the potential risks from MRI contrast agents and asked about her infant. Nephrogenic systemic fibrosis (NSF), initially called *nephrogenic fibrosing dermopathy* has been associated with gadolinium-containing MRI contrast agents. NSF is characterized by tissue fibrosis that causes skin thickening and joint contractures. Collagen deposition can also occur in the lung, skeletal muscle, heart, diaphragm, and esophagus. Gadolinium is similar to calcium regarding molecular size and bonding and can displace calcium in a variety of human tissues. Free gadolinium ions interfere with macrophage function and cause premature cell death. Noncomplexed gadolinium is unsuitable for use in humans. Contrast agents complex gadolinium with other molecules that are generally safe for humans with a half-life of 1.3 hours in patients with normal renal function. Patients with chronic renal failure have a gadolinium half-life of 30 to 120 hours. Chronic renal failure with accompanying metabolic acidosis favors dissociation of gadolinium complexes with release of free gadolinium and deposition of gadolinium salts in muscle, skin, liver, and bone. Patients with chronic renal failure appear to be at increased risk for NSF because of decreased gadolinium excretion. Current clinical recommendations are to use alternative contrast agents in patients with chronic renal failure. If gadolinium is absolutely necessary, dialysis can markedly enhance the clearance of gadolinium.[6,7] The risk of NSF is negligible in patients with normal renal function.

What are the options for sedation and anesthesia?

It was explained to the infant's mother that there are several options (Table 34.2). There is no clear advantage to any hypnotic, and the selection of a particular technique depends on the patient's condition and anticipated length of the procedure. Sedation with an oral hypnotic such as chloral hydrate or pentobarbital may provide satisfactory sedation for completion of the MRI. If an intravenous line can be inserted, propofol may be used. An inhalation induction with sevoflurane can be performed followed by intravenous cannulation and laryngeal mask airway insertion or tracheal intubation. The primary goals of sedation or anesthesia for children during an MRI examination are a quiescent infant and minimal risk of cardiopulmonary complications. Sedation with oral hypnotics requires fewer invasive procedures but has a greater likelihood of unacceptable patient movement.[8] After a discussion with the mother, the anesthesiologist decided to sedate the infant with oral chloral hydrate.

Sedation and/or anesthesia for children undergoing diagnostic procedures requires a system that ensures proper preanesthesia evaluation, technique selection, airway management, monitoring, and the presence of a health care provider who can promptly and effectively manage sedation failure and cardiorespiratory complications.[9,10] Because there is a greater risk of adverse outcomes from procedures performed outside the operating room, careful regard for potential complications is important.[11]

TABLE 34.2 Techniques for Sedation for Neuroimaging

Sedation
Oral sedatives
Chloral hydrate
Pentobarbital
Midazolam
Opioids
Intravenous sedatives
Propofol
Dexmedetomidine
General anesthesia
Inhalation anesthesia
Pharyngeal airway
Supraglottic airway
Tracheal intubation
Total intravenous anesthesia
Supraglottic airway
Tracheal intubation

Thirty minutes after the oral administration of 50 mg/kg of chloral hydrate, the infant was not adequately sedated, and an additional 50 mg/kg was given. The patient was ready for the MRI scan 15 minutes after the second dose. The child was sleeping comfortably but could be aroused. The scan, however, had to be stopped after 10 minutes because of excessive patient movement.

What is the plan for failed sedation?

The options for managing the patient when sedation alone fails to produce a satisfactory condition for the MRI scan depend on what system has been developed at the particular institution. At some institutions, the radiologists assume responsibility for sedation protocols and implementation. If sedation fails, the patient is rescheduled for a day when an anesthesiologist is available. If the anesthesiology department operates the system, an anesthesiologist is usually immediately available to provide general anesthesia. There has been no attempt to standardize sedation/anesthesia protocols for MRI examinations. There has been a trend toward institutional development of dedicated sedation teams led by critical care physicians, emergency room physicians, or anesthesiologists.[12]

The infant was removed from the MRI room into an induction room in a zone II area. Because he was still well sedated, a 24-gauge intravenous catheter was inserted into a vein in the dorsum of his right hand. Anesthesia was induced with ketamine 1 mg/kg followed by rocuronium 0.6 mg/kg and positive pressure ventilation provided with 1% sevoflurane in an oxygen-air mixture. The patient's trachea was intubated with a 3.5-mm inner diameter tracheal tube. The monitors were removed, and the infant was transferred to the MRI room that was equipped with an MRI-compatible anesthesia machine. After completion of the scan, the infant was transferred to the induction room for emergence and extubation. Recovery from anesthesia was performed in a recovery area of the MRI suite (zone II).

Considerations for this particular patient include the history of prematurity and the potential effect of sedatives and anesthesia on postanesthesia ventilation and the history of cyanotic heart disease. The effects of sedatives and inhaled anesthetics on postanesthesia respiratory control are variable and difficult to predict in the individual patient. A primary concern is the effect of such drugs on airway patency and respiratory control. Airway patency during the normal awake state occurs because of a complex interaction between the central nervous system and the muscles of the upper airway. Deep sedation interferes with that system and causes airway obstruction at the base of the tongue and the glottic inlet.[13] Standard maneuvers to alleviate airway obstruction, such as chin lift and jaw thrust, do not always alleviate the obstruction, and positive pressure ventilation may be required.[14] Lack of patient accessibility in the MRI unit can delay recognition of obstruction and timely intervention. Capnography permits a rapid diagnosis of hypoventilation. After completion of the study, close monitoring for several hours would be required and overnight observation indicated if there is any concern regarding the risk of apnea. Recovery from a general anesthetic may be faster than recovery from high doses of long-acting sedatives. Children with a history of obesity, sleep apnea, or adenotonsillar hyperplasia have an increased risk of airway obstruction during sedation. General anesthesia with a laryngeal mask airway or tracheal tube would be preferred for patients with those conditions.

The infant has been stable with respect to cardiovascular function and should tolerate sedation or general anesthesia. Inhaled sevoflurane is well tolerated if ventricular function is good (preanesthetic echocardiogram). During an inhalation induction with sevoflurane, the inspired concentration should be slowly increased and must be decreased once controlled ventilation is initiated. Controlled ventilation increases the uptake of inhaled anesthetics and may produce undesired decreases in blood pressure and heart rate.

A recovery area in the immediate vicinity of the MRI suite improves patient flow and operational efficiency. The recovery area can be staffed with recovery room nurses or nurses trained and oriented by the recovery room staff.

KEY MESSAGES

1. In the vicinity of an MRI scanner, patients with implanted ferromagnetic objects may be at risk for injury or damage to the device from the strong magnetic field.

2. Sedation and/or anesthesia for children undergoing diagnostic procedures requires a system that ensures proper preanesthetic evaluation, technique selection, airway management, monitoring, and the presence of a health care provider that can promptly and effectively manage sedation failure and cardiorespiratory complications.

3. There has been a trend toward institutional development of dedicated sedation teams led by critical care physicians, emergency room physicians, or anesthesiologists.

QUESTIONS

1. What is the mechanism by which nephrogenic systemic fibrosis (NSF) occurs after exposure to MRI contrast agents?

   Answer: Gadolinium, the primary MRI contract agent, is similar to calcium with respect to molecular size and bonding and can displace calcium in human tissues and cause fibrosis. Patients with renal failure are more susceptible to NSF because the elimination time for gadolinium is prolonged.

2. What mechanism causes MRI-induced interference with the electrocardiograph (ECG)?

   Answer: The radiofrequency field generated by a strong magnetic field can produce small voltage changes in the blood that cause ST-T wave changes in the ECG.

3. In what zones of the magnetic resonance imaging suite is injury to patients or personnel most likely to occur?

Answer: Injury to patients and personnel can occur in zones III and IV if noncompatible ferromagnetic objects are present. Movement in these areas must be restricted and any objects screened for magnet compatibility.

References

1. Kanal E, Barkovich AJ, Bell C, et al. ACR guidance document for safe MR practices: 2007. AJR 2007;188:1447–1474.
2. Levine GN, Gomes AS, Arai AE, et al. Safety of magnetic resonance imaging in patients with cardiovascular devices. Circulation 2007;116:2878–2891.
3. Gooden CK, Dilos B. Anesthesia for magnetic resonance imaging. Int Anesthesiol Clin 2003;42:29–37.
4. Cravero JP, Bilke GT, Beach M, et al. Incidence and nature of adverse events during pediatric sedation/anesthesia for procedures outside the operating room: report from the pediatric sedation research consortium. Pediatrics 2006;118:1087–1096.
5. Reeves ST, Havidich JE, Tobin DP. Conscious sedation of children with propofol is anything but conscious. Pediatrics 2004;114:e74–e76.
6. Grobner T, Prischl FC. Gadolinium and nephrogenic systemic fibrosis. Kidney International 2007;72:260–264.
7. Kuo PH, Kanal E, Abu-Alfa AK, Cowper SE. Gadolinium-based MR contrast agents and nephrogenic systemic fibrosis. Radiology 2007;242:647–649.
8. Dalal PG, Murray D, Cox T, et al. Sedation and anesthesia protocols used for magnetic resonance imaging studies in infants: provider and pharmacologic considerations. Anesth Analg 2006;103:863–868.
9. Cote CJ, Wilson S. Guidelines for monitoring and management of pediatric patients during and after sedation for diagnostic and therapeutic procedures: an update. Pediatrics 2006;118:2587–2602.
10. Cote CJ, Notterman DA, Karl HW, et al. Adverse sedation events in pediatrics: a critical incident analysis of contributing factors. Pediatrics 2000;105:805–814.
11. Robbertze R, Posner KL, Domino KB. Closed claims review of anesthesia for procedures outside the operating room. Curr Opin Anesthesiol 2006;19:436–442.
12. Cutler KO, Bush AJ, Godambe SA, Gilmore B. The use of a pediatric emergency-staffed sedation service during imaging: a retrospective analysis. Am J Emerg Med 2007;25:654–661.
13. Eastwood PR, Platt PR, Shepherd K, et al. Collapsibility of the upper airway at different concentrations of propofol. Anesthesiology 2005;103:470–477.
14. Meier S, Geiduschek J, Paganoni R, et al. The effect of chin lift, jaw thrust, and continuous positive airway pressure on the size of the glottic opening and on stridor score in anesthetized, spontaneously breathing children. Anesth Analg 2002;94:494–449.

CHAPTER 35

Evidence-Based Prevention of Postoperative Nausea and Vomiting

Richard J. Pollard

CASE FORMAT: STEP BY STEP

A 25-year-old, 5′ 9″, 57-kg triathlete was running on a street when she fell and injured her arm. A distal radial fracture was diagnosed in the emergency department, and an orthopaedic surgeon was consulted. The patient was scheduled for repair of the fracture in the ambulatory surgery center. Intravenous (IV) morphine (6 mg) was administered in the emergency department for analgesia. She was very anxious about the surgery and her subsequent rehabilitation.

The patient had not undergone surgery or anesthesia previously. She did not use tobacco, alcohol, illicit drugs, or nonprescribed drugs. She did have a history of significant motion sickness. Physical examination revealed a lean, athletic-appearing young woman. Her blood pressure was 90/60 mm Hg with a heart rate of 55 beats per minute.

Because the surgeon had a busy clinic and was only available in the late afternoon, the patient was fasting for more than 10 hours. She was very concerned about postoperative nausea and vomiting (PONV) because she remembered that her mother had suffered from this complication.

What is the pathophysiology of PONV?

The underlying mechanisms that cause PONV are complex and involve both mechanical and neurologic processes. The mechanical act of vomiting requires coordination of the respiratory, gastrointestinal, and abdominal muscles. Neurologic control of the mechanical process occurs in the vomiting center located in the lateral reticular formation of the medulla oblongata. This center is in close proximity to the nucleus of the solitary tract in the brainstem and has access to the motor pathways responsible for the act of vomiting. The vomiting reflex involves the gastrointestinal tract and the chemoreceptor trigger zone (CTZ) in the area postrema. Mechanoreceptors and chemoreceptors in the lining of the gut initiate the reflex. These receptors are stimulated by contraction and distention of the gut (mechanoreceptors) or by the presence of noxious materials (chemoreceptors). Once these receptors are activated, signals are sent via the vagus nerve to activate the CTZ. The location of the CTZ in the area postrema allows the CTZ to be activated by chemical stimuli from the blood and cerebrospinal fluid. Other sites can directly affect the vomiting center via separate neurologic connections. These sites include the central nervous system (cerebral cortex, labyrinthine, vi-

sual, and vestibular apparatus) as well as the oropharynx, mediastinum, peritoneum, and genitalia.

The central nervous system has several receptors that can influence nausea and vomiting. The area postrema has large concentrations of dopamine (D_2), opioid, and serotonin ($5HT_3$) receptors. The nucleus tractus solitarius is rich in enkephalins and histaminic (H_1) muscarinic and cholinergic receptors. Neurokinin-1 (NK_1) receptors are found in the nucleus tractus solitarius and in the dorsal motor nucleus of the vagus nerve. Before the surgery, the patient asked the anesthesiologist the following question.

What are my specific risk factors for PONV?

The risk factors for PONV can be categorized as: (a) patient specific, (b) anesthetic, and (c) surgical (Table 35.1). The most important patient-specific factors for PONV are female gender, young age, nonsmoker, and a previous history of PONV or motion sickness. Other patient-specific risk factors include a history of migraine headaches, anxiety, hypovolemia, and an American Society of Anesthesiologists low-risk classification.[1,2] Anesthetic-related risk factors include the use of volatile anesthetics, nitrous oxide (N_2O), intraoperative, or postoperative opioids.[3] The influence of the reversal of nondepolarizing muscle relaxants with neostigmine on PONV is controversial. Earlier studies indicated that reversal with greater than 2.5 mg of neostigmine increased the incidence of PONV. A recent analysis suggests that the association between neostigmine administration and PONV is limited. Duration and type of surgery have been implicated as determinants of PONV. For every 30 minutes of surgical time, there is a predictable 60% increase in subsequent nausea. This means that a baseline risk of 10% is increased to 16% after 30 minutes of surgery and then further increased to >25% after 1 hour of surgery. For adults, there is an increased risk of PONV with intra-abdominal surgery, especially gynecologic and laparoscopic operations. Neurosurgical, ophthalmic, and ear, nose, and throat procedures are also associated with an increased risk of PONV.

Apfel et al. suggested a simplified PONV predictive score that included four factors: (a) female gender, (b) nonsmoker, (c) history of PONV or motion sickness, and (d) the need for postoperative IV opioids.[4] When 0, 1, 2, 3, or 4 risk factors were present, the risk of PONV was 10%, 21%, 39%, 61%, or 79% respectively. This simplified risk stratification enables clinicians to estimate the likelihood of PONV in individual patients and make appropriate adjustments in technique.

Based on Apfel's scoring system, this patient has three risk factors: female gender, non-smoker, and history of

TABLE 35.1 Risk Factors for Postoperative Nausea and Vomiting

Patient Specific	Anesthesia Related	Surgery Related
Female	Volatile gases	Time >30 minutes
Young age	Nitrous oxide	HEENT procedures
Nonsmoker	Intravenous opioids	Major gynecological procedures
Previous PONV	Neostigmine >2.5 mg	Laparoscopy
Motion sickness	**Gastric suctioning**	
Migraines		
Anxiety		
Hypovolemia		
Low American Society of Anesthesiologists status		

Items in regular type are major risk factors. Boldface items are minor risk factors.
HEENT, head ears eyes nose throat; PONV, postoperative nausea and vomiting.

motion sickness. This placed the patient's risk at 61%. The use of preoperative IV opioids, low American Society of Anesthesiologists classification, anxiety, and relative hypovolemia increased that risk.

Do the risks of PONV in children differ from those in adults?

Eberhart et al. applied a multivariate analysis to determine the potential for PONV in children.[5] Risk factors for PONV in children included (a) duration of surgery greater than 30 minutes, (b) age 3 years or older, (c) strabismus surgery, and (4) a history of PONV in the patient, a sibling, or parent. When 0, 1, 2, 3, or 4 risk factors are present, the risk of PONV for the patient was 9%, 10%, 30%, 55%, or 70%, respectively.

The patient requested some form of premedicant that would decrease the likelihood of her developing PONV.

Are there any premedicants that reduce the risk of PONV?

There are at least four receptor systems that influence PONV. Conventional wisdom in the management of patients at risk for PONV advocates the use of a technique that targets different receptor sites (Table 35.2). Multiple studies have shown the efficacy of combination versus single-agent antiemetic prophylaxis.[6,7] Agents used in clinical practice include 5-hydroxytryptamine (5-HT$_3$) receptor antagonists (ondansetron, dolasetron, granisetron, and tropisetron), dexamethasone, and transdermal scopolamine.

The 5-HT$_3$ receptor antagonists are most effective when administered near the conclusion of surgery. These agents are equally effective in reducing the incidence of PONV and are all safe at recommended doses.

The corticosteroid dexamethasone has been shown to be effective as an antiemetic when given at the induction of anesthesia in doses of 4 to 5 mg. The efficacy of dexamethasone is similar to that of the 5-HT$_3$ receptor antagonists.

A transdermal scopolamine patch applied the night before surgery or 4 hours before the end of surgery can significantly reduce the incidence of PONV.[8] The slow onset of effect and side effects such as dry mouth and dizziness, however, may diminish the utility of scopolamine.

Although droperidol is an effective antiemetic, its use has been effectively reduced or discontinued in the United States because of the "black box" warning from the Food and Drug Administration concerning the potential risks of cardiac dysrhythmias.[9]

The NK$_1$ receptor antagonists, such as aprepitant, comprise the newest class of drugs purported to decrease PONV. NK$_1$ receptors are found in the areas of the brain that control the vomiting reflex, and NK$_1$ receptor antagonists may be especially effective in patients with centrally mediated PONV.[10]

Other drugs that have been reported to reduce the incidence of PONV, but have not been rigorously studied as yet are haloperidol, dexmedetomidine, naloxone, and nalmefene.

TABLE 35.2 Antiemetic Drugs

5-HT$_3$ Receptor Antagonists	Anticholinergics
Ondansetron	Scopolamine
Dolasetron	**Antihistamines**
Tropisetron	Dimenhydrinate
Granisetron	**NK$_1$ Receptor antagonists**
	Aprepitant
Corticosteroids	**Phenothiazines**
Dexamethasone	Promethazine
Butyrophenones	
Droperidol	
Haloperidol	

A prophylactic regimen is recommended for patients at moderate to high risk for PONV. Prophylaxis is not generally recommended for low-risk PONV patients; however, because PONV is one of the largest and most costly complications after anesthesia, the anesthesiologist should consider whether the risks and cost of prophylaxis are justified for every patient. It has been shown that patients are willing to pay up to $100 of their own money for completely effective antiemetics. An anesthesiology resident consulted with a senior colleague regarding the best anesthetic technique to prevent PONV in the patient described in this case.

What is the best anesthetic technique to prevent PONV in this patient?

Anesthesia-related risk factors for PONV include the use of volatile inhaled anesthetics, N_2O, intraoperative or postoperative IV opioids, and reversal of nondepolarizing muscle relaxants with neostigmine at doses greater than 2.5 mg. The use of regional anesthesia provides a ninefold decrease in the incidence of PONV in all populations.[11] If general anesthesia is required, using propofol for induction and during maintenance phases of anesthesia decreases the incidence of PONV by 19% during the first 6 postoperative hours. Propofol used in a total IV anesthesia technique reduces the risk of PONV by 25%.

Volatile inhaled anesthetics have been identified as the primary cause of PONV within the first 2 hours after surgery. The incidence of PONV when both volatile anesthetics and N_2O are used may be as high as 59%.[12] Avoidance of N_2O decreases the risk of PONV by 12%.

Whether to use IV narcotics during the perioperative period remains a quandary for anesthesiologists. On one hand, opioids reduce postoperative pain while smoothing intraoperative hemodynamic changes. On the other hand, narcotics increase the risk of PONV. Nonnarcotic analgesics such as nonsteroidal anti-inflammatory drugs and cyclo-oxygenase-2 inhibitors may have a role in reducing the need for opioids and reducing the incidence of PONV. A technique using regional anesthesia or local infiltration anesthesia in conjunction with nonnarcotic analgesics may eliminate the need for perioperative opioids.

Other preventive modalities such as supplemental oxygen or prophylactic orogastric suctioning have not been proven to reduce PONV.

The anesthesiologists agreed that the lowest-risk technique for this patient would be a regional technique such as a brachial plexus block and sedation with propofol with minimal or no opioids. Because the patient expressed a strong preference for general anesthesia, a scopolamine patch was applied at the conclusion of the preoperative interview. Dexamethasone (5 mg) was administered intravenously with the induction of anesthesia and ondansetron (4 mg) administered just before emergence from anesthesia.

Despite this aggressive prophylactic regimen, the patient experienced severe nausea on waking in the postoperative care unit.

Is ondansetron the drug of choice in this case?

There have been very few studies regarding the treatment of patients who have failed antiemetic prophylaxis. The 5-HT$_3$ receptor antagonists have been the most frequently tested medica-

tion in rescue trials. Evidence suggests that in patients who have failed to respond to ondansetron prophylaxis, more ondansetron is no more effective than placebo. Logically, a drug that acts at a different receptor site would be a better choice.[13]

Several days after an otherwise uneventful recovery, the patient asked her anesthesiologist about future treatment options regarding PONV.

In the future, are there nonpharmacological options that might be effective for this patient in the treatment of PONV?

Some nonpharmacologic treatments for PONV may be effective. Techniques such as acupuncture, acupoint stimulation, and transcutaneous nerve stimulation may have antiemetic efficacy comparable to standard treatments. There may be some resistance in clinical practice to utilization of nontraditional therapies; however, some patients are familiar with the techniques and will insist on their use. If patients request such therapy, it would be best to consult a clinician familiar with the techniques.

Although the patient's nausea resolved fully before discharge, she was concerned that the symptoms would return later.

What can the patient expect on discharge from the surgical unit?

Nausea and vomiting occurs in one third of ambulatory surgical patients after discharge from surgery centers. Prophylactic therapy should be administered to patients susceptible to late PONV. The use of longer-acting agents in combination seems to offer the best outcome.[14,15]

KEY MESSAGES

1. Anesthesia-related risk factors for PONV include the use of volatile inhaled anesthetics, N_2O, IV opioids, and reversal of nondepolarizing muscle relaxants with neostigmine at doses greater than 2.5 mg.

2. When 0, 1, 2, 3, or 4 risk factors were present, the incidence of PONV in adults undergoing general anesthesia is 10%, 21%, 39%, 61%, or 79%, respectively.[4]

3. A prophylactic regimen is recommended for patients at moderate to high risk for PONV.

QUESTIONS

1. What are major patient risk factors for postoperative nausea and vomiting?

   Answer: Major risk factors for postoperative nausea include female gender, young age, and a history of motion sickness.

2. What receptors influence postoperative nausea and vomiting?

   Answer: Dopamine, opioid, serotonin, cholinergic, and neurokinin-1 receptors influence nausea and emesis.

These receptors are concentrated in the central nervous system in the areas of the area postrema, the nucleus tractussolitarius, and the motor nucleus of the vagus nerve.

3. **What anesthetic factors increase the likelihood of postoperative nausea?**

Answer: Anesthetic factors that may increase the likelihood of postoperative nausea include the use of volatile, inhaled anesthetics and nitrous oxide, administration of postoperative opioids, and possibly the use of neostigmine to reverse neuromuscular blockade.

References

1. Stadler M, Bardiau F, Seidel L, et al. Difference in risk factors for postoperative nausea and vomiting. Anesthesiology 2003;98: 46–52.
2. Van den Bosch JE, Moons KG, Bonsel GJ, et al. Does measurement of preoperative anxiety have added value for predicting postoperative nausea and vomiting? Anesth Analg 2005;100: 1525–1532.
3. Apfel CC, Kranke P, Katz MH, et al. Volatile anesthetics may be the main cause of early but not delayed postoperative vomiting: a randomized controlled trial of factorial design. Br J Anaesth 2002;88:659–668.
4. Apfel CC, Laara E, Koivuranta M, et al. A simplified risk score for predicting postoperative nausea and vomiting. Anesthesiology 1999;91:693–700.
5. Eberhart LH, Geldner G, Krnake P, et al. The development and validation of a risk score to predict the probability of postoperative vomiting in pediatric patients. Anesth Analg 2004;99: 1630–1637.
6. Henzi I, Walder B, Tramer MR. Dexamethasone for the prevention of postoperative nausea and vomiting. Anesth Analg 2000; 90:186–194.
7. Tramer MR. A rational approach to the control of postoperative nausea and vomiting: evidence from systematic reviews. Part II. Recommendations for prevention and treatment, and research agenda. Acta Anaesth Scand 2001;45:14–19.
8. Kranke P, Morin AM, Roewer N, et al. The efficacy and safety of transdermal scopolamine for the prevention of postoperative nausea and vomiting. Anesth Analg 2002;95:133–143.
9. Habib AS, Gan TJ. The use of droperidol before and after the Food and Drug Administration black box warning: a survey of the members of the Society for Ambulatory Anesthesia. J Clin Anes 2008;20:35–39.
10. Gan TJ, Apfel CC, Kovac A, et al. A randomized, double-blind comparison of the NK1 antagonist, aprepitant, versus ondansetron for the prevention of postoperative nausea and vomiting. Anesth Analg 2007;104:1082–1089.
11. Khalil SN, Farag A, Hanna E, et al. Regional anesthesia combined with avoidance of narcotics may reduce the incidence of postoperative vomiting in children. Middle East J Anesthesiol 2005;18:123–132.
12. Apfel CC, Korttila K, Abdalla M, et al. A factorial trial of six interventions for the prevention of postoperative nausea and vomiting. N Engl J Med 2004;350:2441–2451.
13. Gan TJ, Meyer T, Apfel CC, et al. Consensus guidelines for managing postoperative nausea and vomiting. Anesth Analg 2003;97: 62–71.
14. Gupta A, Wu CL, Elkassabany N, et al. Does the routine prophylactic use of antiemetics affect the incidence of post discharge nausea and vomiting following ambulatory surgery? A systematic review of randomized controlled trials. Anesthesiology 2003; 99:488–495.
15. Gan TJ, Meyer T, Apfel CC, et al. Society for Ambulatory Anesthesia guidelines for the management of postoperative nausea and vomiting. Anesth Analg 2007;105:1615–1628.

Ultrasound Guidance for Central Venous Cannulation

Bryan V. May

CASE FORMAT: STEP BY STEP

An 81-year-old male presented with a 2-hour history of weakness and substernal chest pain caused by moderate physical activity. His medical history was significant for hypertension, chronic atrial fibrillation, multiple transient ischemic attacks, and type 2 diabetes mellitus. A 12-lead electrocardiogram revealed atrial fibrillation with an incomplete right bundle branch block, 2-mm ST depression in leads II, III, and AVF. Physical examination revealed an alert and mildly uncomfortable elderly man. The patient's vital signs were as follows: blood pressure, 164/72 mm Hg; heart rate, 92 beats per minute (irregularly irregular); and respiratory rate, 28 breaths per minute. Chest auscultation revealed no heart murmurs and faint bibasilar rales. The abdominal examination was normal. Cardiac enzymes were consistent with myocardial ischemia (elevated troponin I and creatine kinase MB levels). A transthoracic echocardiogram obtained in the emergency department revealed inferior wall akinesis and a reduced left ventricular ejection fraction (35%). Other transesophageal echocardiogram findings were concentric left ventricular hypertrophy and a small patent foramen ovale with left-to-right shunting. Carotid artery duplex ultrasound showed bilateral high-grade stenosis of both carotid arteries and a partially thrombosed left internal jugular vein. Urgent coronary artery angiography showed significant three-vessel coronary disease that was not amenable to angioplasty or stent placement. The patient was scheduled for emergent coronary artery bypass grafting.

During the brief preoperative interview, it was explained to the patient that after induction of anesthesia and tracheal intubation, a central venous catheter would be inserted into the right internal jugular vein (RIJV), and a catheter would be inserted into the pulmonary artery via the heart. The patient queried the anesthesiologist as to the need for such a catheter and potential complications.

What are the indications for central venous cannulation?

Every year, more than 5 million central venous catheters are inserted into patients in the United States, and 200,000 are inserted into patients in the United Kingdom. Indications include poor peripheral venous access, administration of vasoactive drugs, acute hemodialysis, rapid infusion of large volumes of resuscitation fluids, cardiac pacing, hyperalimentation, and hemodynamic monitoring.[1] In the perioperative period, indications are generally hemodynamic monitoring, infusion of vasoactive drugs, and fluid administration.

What are the complications from central venous catheterization?

The potential complications from central venous cannulation are many and can be fatal (Table 36.1).[2,3] Chronic complications such as infection, thrombosis, or catheter fracture are related to the duration that the catheter is in place and are not common for short-term placement (such as for perioperative use). The nidus for infection, however, can be introduced during the insertion procedure, and every central venous cannulation, whether for short- or long-term placement must be managed with good sterile technique.

Complications that occur during the insertion procedure include hemorrhage (arterial or venous), hematoma formation, inadvertent carotid artery puncture, dysrhythmias, pneumothorax, catheter malposition, perforation of great vessels, pseudoaneurysm formation, arteriovenous fistula, brachial plexus injury, guidewire loss, catheter knotting, and cannulation failure. Operator experience and technique certainly influence the complication rate. Physicians with greater experience (>50 insertions) have a high success rate and a low incidence of complications. Most anesthesiologists have substantial experience with central venous cannulation at the conclusion of their training. Data from the American Society of Anesthesiologists Closed Claims Project indicated that the complications generating litigation included wire/catheter embolism, cardiac tamponade, carotid artery puncture/cannulation, hemothorax, and pneumothorax.[4]

Infection from a central venous catheter site is a serious and potentially lethal complication. Every effort must be made to avoid infection. Adherence to strict sterile technique during catheter insertion is essential. The use of biopatches to cover the insertion site and use of antibiotic-impregnated catheters may also reduce the infection rate; however, emergence of antibiotic-resistant bacteria is of concern. The application of antibiotic ointment to the catheter insertion site has not been shown to reduce the likelihood of infection and can promote fungal colonization of the catheter.[5]

The patient was transported to the operating room for coronary artery bypass grafting. He had a peripheral intra-

TABLE 36.1 Complications of Central Venous Catheterization

Bleeding

Infection

Thrombosis

Carotid artery injury

Stroke

Hematoma formation

Pneumothorax

Hemothorax

Cardiac perforation

Cardiac tamponade

Pseudoaneurysm formation

Arteriovenous fistula

Vertebral artery injury

Dysrhythmias

Catheter fracture

Brachial plexus injury

Horner's syndrome

venous catheter and a right radial arterial line in place. After induction of general anesthesia, a transesophageal echocardiogram probe was inserted, and his right neck was positioned and prepared for central venous cannulation and insertion of a pulmonary artery catheter.

What are the anatomic landmarks for central venous cannulation?

The three veins normally used for central venous cannulation are the internal jugular vein (right vein more frequently than the left), subclavian vein, and the femoral vein. The femoral vein is rarely chosen for hemodynamic monitoring or insertion of a pulmonary artery catheter. There is some controversy as to whether the pressure measured in the femoral vein is a true reflection of central venous pressure, and the distance from the femoral vein insertion site to the pulmonary artery exceeds the length of most pulmonary artery catheters. Femoral vein cannulation is more commonly performed in small children than in adults.

Most anesthesiologists use the RIJV as the insertion site for central venous cannulation. The RIJV has a consistent location in the carotid sheath. It is a relatively short, valveless vessel leading straight to the superior vena cava and the right atrium. Additional advantages include a decreased risk of pneumothorax, as the right lung lies more caudad than the left and avoidance of the left-sided thoracic duct. The central approach to the RIJV is very common and depends on the location of the apex of the triangle formed by the sternal and clavicular heads of the sternocleidomastoid muscle. The internal jugular vein is usually lateral or anterolateral to the carotid artery. The

carotid artery is identified, and the needle is inserted at the apex of the triangle lateral to the carotid artery and directed away from the carotid artery. If the vein is not entered, the needle can be methodically redirected more medially in small increments until the vein is found. The color of the blood can be used to differentiate venous from arterial blood, but this method is not always accurate. If it is uncertain which vessel has been cannulated, a pressure transducer can be attached to the needle or a small-bore catheter for vessel identification.

Anatomic landmarks are easily discernible in patients with well-defined anatomy. Obese patients, those with limited neck mobility, and infants do not have well-defined anatomic landmarks, and techniques dependent on anatomic identification will not be as reliable.

A 22-gauge finder needle was inserted via a central approach (apex of the two heads of the sternocleidomastoid muscle) in an attempt to locate the RIJV; multiple attempts with the finder needle were required to locate this vein. An 18-gauge, 4-inch needle attached to a 5-mL syringe was inserted in the same plane as the finder needle and advanced. Bright red blood was aspirated. After syringe removal, bright red blood pulsated from the needle. The needle was removed, and pressure was applied to the puncture site. Despite the pressure, a hematoma developed on the right side of the patient's neck. With the continued application of pressure, the hematoma stopped expanding. An ultrasound device with a 5-MHz probe was brought to the operating room. Ultrasound imaging of the right neck showed that the RIJV was lying directly on top of the carotid artery. Imaging demonstrated a hematoma surrounding and compressing the RIJV. Although the caliber of the RIJV was decreased by the hematoma, ultrasound guidance facilitated catheterization of the RIJV.

In this case, the patient's RIJV was lying directly above the carotid artery. The finder needle eventually located the RIJV, but the cannulation needle penetrated the RIJV and punctured the carotid artery. Ultrasound guidance allowed prompt identification of the RIJV leading to successful cannulation. Ultrasound imaging to facilitate central venous cannulation was first reported in the anesthesia literature in the 1970s, and many studies have shown the usefulness of ultrasound, especially for the internal jugular vein.[6,7] Broad acceptance by anesthesiologists has been slow to occur. In 2001, the Agency for Healthcare Research and Quality and in 2002, the National Institute for Clinical Excellence recommended ultrasound guidance for elective cannulation of the internal jugular vein in adults and children. This document has had little impact on practicing anesthesiologists. There are several practical reasons that ultrasound guidance for central venous catheter insertion has not become more prevalent. The evidence that ultrasound guidance is clearly superior to traditional anatomic techniques has not been convincing.[8,9] Ultrasound equipment has not been routinely available in every operating room, and delays in finding and preparing the ultrasound machine are considered unjustified if the equipment is unavailable.

How can ultrasound guidance facilitate central venous catheterization of the RIJV?

The two commonly used techniques for ultrasound guidance are static and dynamic (real-time). The static method is relatively quick and requires no sterile preparation of the ultra-

TABLE 36.2 Technique for Dynamic Ultrasound-Guided Central Venous Cannulation

1. Position the patient's head with ultrasound guidance. The head should be rotated to maximize the distance from the carotid artery to the internal jugular vein and maximize the right internal jugular vein's diameter.

2. The cannulation site is prepped and draped in sterile fashion.

3. The ultrasound probe is inserted into a sterile sheath.

4. The internal jugular vein is identified. The jugular vein is easily compressed and should be lateral to the carotid artery, which is round and pulsatile.

5. The internal jugular vein is centered on the ultrasound screen.

6. The puncture needle is inserted at a 45-degree angle along the intercept path with the vein.

7. The accuracy of vessel puncture is determined by ultrasound, blood color, or pressure transduction.

8. The guidewire is threaded into the vein, the vein is dilated, and a catheter is threaded into the vessel.

sound probe. The operator identifies and centers the vein on the ultrasound probe. An indelible mark is placed on the skin to identify the needle insertion point, and a second mark is made distal to the first along the course of the vein. The line determined by the two points guides the operator as to the course of the vein. The probe is removed, and the patient is prepped and draped for cannulation.

The dynamic method requires placing the probe in a sterile sheath after the patient has been prepped and draped (Table 36.2). The operator uses the probe to locate the vein, which is usually lateral to the carotid artery and is easily compressed with pressure on the probe (Figs. 36.1 and 36.2). Once identified, the vein is centered on the ultrasound screen, and the needle is inserted at a 45-degree angle toward the vein along the anticipated intercept path. The needle can be seen as

an echogenic line as it passes through tissue planes. The short axis is generally used to localize the vein and avoid the carotid artery. It may be beneficial to rotate the transducer 90° to the longitudinal plane to better identify the tip of the needle as it approaches the vessel lumen. The dynamic technique is more cumbersome than the static technique and requires practice for a lone operator. An assistant who can hold and manipulate the probe while the operator is inserting the needle can be quite helpful.

The ultrasound probe can be useful for positioning the patient's head. Head rotation can alter the relationship of the internal jugular vein to the carotid artery. Ultrasound imaging can help determine optimal rotation to maximize the distance between the carotid artery and jugular vein and can maximize the vein's diameter.

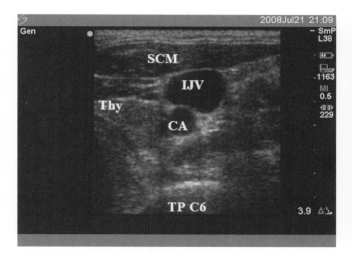

Figure 36.1 • Axial Ultrasound Image of the Left Anterior Neck. The internal jugular vein can be seen lateral to the carotid artery and appears patent when minimal pressure is applied to the ultrasound transducer. CA, carotid artery; IJV, internal jugular vein; Thy, thyroid gland; TP C6, transverse process of sixth cervical vertebra.

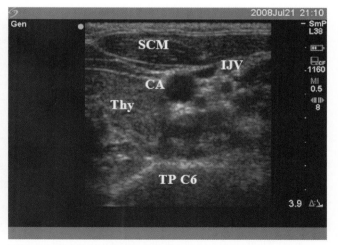

Figure 36.2 • Axial Ultrasound Image of the Left Anterior Neck. Application of pressure to the ultrasound transducer compresses the internal jugular vein, making identification and cannulation difficult. CA, carotid artery; IJV, internal jugular vein; Thy, thyroid gland; TP C6, transverse process of sixth cervical vertebra.

Should ultrasound guidance for central venous cannulation be a standard of care for anesthesiologists?

Declaring a device or technique as a standard of care requires clear evidence of efficacy and ready availability of the device. The evidence to date does not demonstrate clear superiority. Part of the failure to prove that ultrasound guidance is better may be a lack of training with ultrasound guidance. The RIJV is generally easy to recognize with ultrasound, but cannulation is not always easy. The ultrasound image provides a two-dimensional image, but anatomy is three dimensional. It is not always easy to accurately determine the position of the cannulation needle with ultrasound. A standardized, formal teaching program in ultrasound guidance for central venous catheterization may improve performance to the point that a clear difference in insertion efficiency with reduced complications is evident.[10]

Experience is another factor that may make the case for ultrasound guidance less clear. Anesthesiologists are generally very experienced with central venous cannulation using anatomic landmark techniques, and comparative studies with anesthesiologists may be less convincing than with less-experienced practitioners. If anesthesiologists acquire ultrasound guidance skills, it may ultimately prove ultrasound to be a superior technique even in the hands of experienced practitioners.[11]

Ultrasound machines have become more commonplace in the operating room. Stand-alone units as well as transesophageal echocardiogram machines equipped with external probes are often readily available. The development of small high-quality ultrasound units will undoubtedly increase access for the anesthesiologist. Probe selection depends on the patient's size and the depth of the vessel. Better resolution is achieved with a high-frequency ultrasound probe. Tissue penetration, however, decreases with increasing frequency.

The preponderance of evidence suggests that ultrasound guidance will eventually be the standard of care. Anesthesiologists should become skilled with both anatomic landmark and ultrasound-guided central venous catheterization. If anatomic landmark techniques fail, ultrasound may reveal why failure occurred and may provide guidance for successful cannulation.

As anesthesiologists obtain more experience with ultrasound-guided central venous cannulation, the procedure should become more successful, safer, and more efficient.[12]

KEY MESSAGES

1. Indications for central venous line insertion include poor peripheral venous access, administration of vasoactive drugs, acute hemodialysis, rapid infusion of large volumes of resuscitation fluids, cardiac pacing, hyperalimentation, and hemodynamic monitoring.

2. At the level of the apex of the triangle formed by the sternal and clavicular heads of the sternocleidomastoid muscle, the internal jugular vein usually lays lateral or anterolateral to the carotid artery.

3. Applying gentle pressure via the ultrasound probe will compress the internal jugular vein but not the adjacent carotid artery.

QUESTIONS

1. What are the major complications of central venous cannulation via the internal jugular vein?

   Answer: Major complications include hemorrhage, hematoma formation, stroke, perforation of major vessels, and cardiac tamponade.

2. What are the advantages of ultrasound guided cannulation of the internal jugular vein?

   Answer: Ultrasound identification of the internal jugular vein is especially helpful when normal anatomic landmarks are not easily defined. Obese patients, patients with limited cervical mobility, and infants are cases where ultrasound guidance is quite helpful.

3. What is the primary way to differentiate the carotid artery from the internal jugular vein with an ultrasound probe?

   Answer: The carotid artery is round, pulsatile, and relatively non-compressible. The internal jugular vein is generally irregular in shape and easily compressed with the probe.

References

1. Taylor RW, Palagiri AV. Central venous catheterization. Crit Care Med 2007;35:1390–1396.
2. Kusminsky RE. Complications of central venous catheterization. J Am Coll Surg 2007;204:681–696.
3. Garden AL, Laussen PC. An unending supply of "unusual" complications from central venous catheters. Pediatr Anesth 2004;905–909.
4. Domino KB, Bowdle TA, Posner KL, et al. Injuries and liability related to central vascular catheters. Anesthesiology 2004;100:1411–1418.
5. McGee DC, Gould MK. Preventing complications of central venous catheterization. N Engl J Med 2003;348:1123–1133.
6. Randolph AG, Cook DJ, Gonzales CA, et al. Ultrasound guidance for placement of central venous catheters: a meta-analysis of the literature. Crit Care Med 1996;24:2053–2038.
7. Hind D, Calvert N, McWilliams R, et al. Ultrasonic locating devices for central venous cannulation: meta-analysis. BMJ 2003;327:361–367.
8. Grebnik CR, Boyce A, Sinclair ME, et al. NICE guidelines for central venous catheterization in children. Is the evidence base sufficient? Br J Anaesth 2004;92:827–830.
9. Hayashi H, Amano M. Does ultrasound imaging before puncture facilitate internal jugular vein cannulation? Prospective

randomized comparison with landmark-guided puncture in ventilated patients. J Cardiothor Vasc Anesth 2002;16:572–575.

10. Feller-Kopman D. Ultrasound-guided internal jugular access. A proposed standardized approach and implications for training and practice. Chest 2007;132:302–309.

11. Chapman GA, Johnson D, Bodenham AR. Visualisation of needle position using ultrasonography. Anaesthesia 2006;61:148–158.

12. Calvert N, Hind D, McWilliams R, et al. Ultrasound for central venous cannulation: economic evaluation of cost-effectiveness. Anaesthesia 2004;59:1116–1120.

CHAPTER 37

Regional Anesthesia Outcomes

Justin Lane and Brian D. O'Donnell

A 68-year-old man was scheduled for elective repair of an asymptomatic 6.5-cm abdominal aortic aneurysm. He had a myocardial infarction 3 years previously, resulting in endovascular stenting of his left anterior descending and circumflex coronary arteries. He remained asymptomatic of recurring anginal symptoms. The patient was a smoker with a 50 pack-year history but quit after the myocardial infarction. He returned to normal activity, lost weight, and could climb two flights of stairs without difficulty. He had no known drug allergies, and his medications were as follows: aspirin, 75 mg daily; atorvastatin, 10 mg daily; atenolol, 25 mg twice daily; and enalapril, 5 mg daily.

He had a previous uneventful general anesthetic for inguinal hernia repair 10 years ago.

On examination, the patient's vital signs were as follows: temperature, 36.5°C; blood pressure, 125/90 mm Hg; heart rate, 50 beats per minute; and respiratory rate, 16 breaths per minute. His body mass index was 28. Examination of the cardiovascular and respiratory systems was normal. Airway examination revealed Mallampati grade I with normal mouth opening and a four-finger thyromental distance. The patient's electrocardiograph reading revealed sinus rhythm with normal PR and QRS intervals but with voltage evidence of left ventricular hypertrophy (Fig. 37.1). Transthoracic echocardiography was performed and showed mild concentric left ventricular hypertrophy, structurally normal valves with trivial mitral regurgitation, and normal function with an ejection fraction calculated at 58%.

Review of the patient's blood results (Table 37.1) revealed evidence of renal impairment, prompting discontinuation of angiotensin-converting enzyme inhibitor therapy.

How might this patient's preoperative physiological status be optimized?

The American Heart Association/American College of Cardiology 2007 revised guidelines on preoperative assessment of patients undergoing noncardiac surgery[1] stratify this man into a high-risk group with an expected incidence of either cardiac death or nonfatal myocardial infarction of more than 5%. With regard to reducing risk in those with known coronary artery disease, the guidelines ask four questions:

1. What is the amount of myocardium in jeopardy?
2. What is the ischemic threshold, that is, the amount of stress required to produce ischemia?
3. What is the patient's ventricular function?
4. Is the patient on his or her optimal medical regimen?

To answer these questions, the patient's clinical history holds a number of vital pieces of information: (a) he is asymptomatic regarding intercurrent ischemic heart disease; (b) he has excellent exercise tolerance; (c) he is in sinus rhythm, and his ventricular function is normal; (d) he was taking an antiplatelet agent, a β-blocker, an angiotensin-converting enzyme inhibitor, and a statin; and (e) his heart rate and blood pressure are well controlled. The patient received coronary artery stents to the anterior cardiac circulation, and the myocardium supplied by this area is at risk in the event of stent occlusion. However, the American Heart Association/American College of Cardiology states that ". . . because additional coronary restenosis is unlikely to occur more than 8 to 12 months after PCI [percutaneous coronary intervention], it is reasonable to expect ongoing protection against untoward perioperative ischemic complications . . ." The amount of stress that may produce ischemia is uncertain in this patient.

Therefore, whether alterations to medication and further cardiovascular evaluations are necessary must be considered. Continuing antiplatelet therapy with aspirin may contribute to additional blood loss, however, the phenomenon of late stent stenosis following antiplatelet therapy discontinuation justifies continuation in this setting.[2] β-Blockade should be continued in the perioperative period, and the patient's heart rate should be titrated to less than 65 beats per minute.[1,3] Favorable outcomes have been reported with the continuation of statin therapy; discontinuation of long-term statin therapy worsens perioperative cardiac outcomes.[4] Angiotensin-converting enzyme inhibitor therapy was discontinued in this case because of renal impairment. Finally, Polldermans et al[3] report that the further investigation of patients with β-blockade and good heart rate control is unnecessary and delays surgery. In summary, the best available evidence supports the continuation of aspirin, atenolol, and atorvastatin in this man's case, thereby permitting surgery without further cardiac assessment.

What would be the optimal anesthetic plan for this man's open aortic aneurysm repair?

The intraoperative management of this case warrants a number of considerations including appropriate monitoring, choice of anesthesia technique, transfusion threshold, the use of coronary vasodilators, heart rate titration and analgesic technique, to name but a few. Particular attention should be paid to intra- and postoperative pain management.

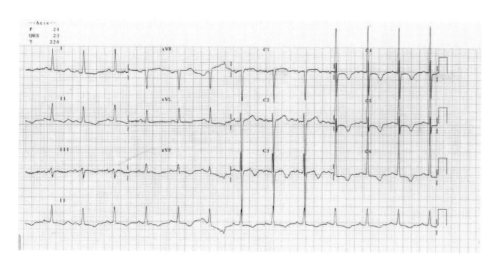

Figure 37.1 • This electrocardiogram shows evidence of left ventricular hypertrophy with the combined S wave in V_3 and the R wave in aVL measuring >28mm (Cornell Criteria [Casale PN, et al. Circulation 1987;75: 565–572]). Also note the associated left ventricular strain pattern, manifest as T-wave inversion, most evident from V_3 to V_6.

The anesthetic plan for this man included the following:

- Invasive monitoring of cardiovascular parameters
- Nitrous oxide-free general anesthesia with endobrachial intubation and positive pressure ventilation
- Epidural catheter placement at the T8 level for intra- and postoperative analgesia using a combination of local anesthetic agent (bupivacaine) and strong opiate (fentanyl)
- High-dependency unit or intensive care unit admission following surgery

What is the rationale for this anesthetic plan?

Monitoring Noninvasive monitoring with an electrocardiogram, SpO_2, and noninvasive blood pressure should be employed as routine. The use of online ST-segment monitoring with electrocardiogram leads placed in either V5 and V4 configuration may facilitate the detection of intraoperative and postoperative myocardial ischemia and infarction.[5] Detecting intraoperative coronary ischemia may facilitate the early administration of coronary vasodilators (nitrates). However, routine use of either ST-segment monitoring or nitrates has not

been associated with improved cardiac outcomes in this patient group.[1] Nitrates may assist in afterload and blood pressure control following placement of the intraoperative aortic cross-clamp.

Invasive blood pressure monitoring is best used during major vascular surgery, facilitating detection of beat-to-beat variation, thus allowing rapid intervention when necessary.[6] The use of central venous cannulae is also recommended in this case to facilitate the administration of vasoactive medications and examine trends in central venous pressure. Pulmonary artery catheters are not routinely recommended and may contribute to patient morbidity.[7]

Anesthesia Technique General anesthesia is the preferred anesthesia modality for open repair of aortic aneurysms. There are no data describing definite benefits regarding the use of specific general anesthetic techniques or agents. Balanced anesthesia with muscle relaxation and multimodal analgesia is advocated. Of particular importance is the maintenance of normal cardiovascular parameters, especially heart rate and blood pressure. Titration of the patient's heart rate to 65 beats per minute or less with β-blockers has been shown to reduce the likelihood of developing cardiovascular complications in the postoperative period.[3]

Nitrous oxide (N_2O) should be avoided in this case for a number of reasons. Myles et al reported an increase in major morbidity in patients undergoing laparotomy using N_2O-based anesthesia. Complications such as postoperative confusion and postoperative nausea and vomiting were also significantly increased after exposure to N_2O.[19] N_2O may also lead to gaseous expansion of intestinal lumen, making access to the retroperitoneum difficult for the surgeon.

Analgesia Effective analgesia is an essential component to balanced anesthesia. It has been described as a fundamental human right.[8] Pain contributes significantly to negative outcomes following surgery. Poor postoperative analgesia has been associated with higher rates of respiratory tract infection[9] and myocardial ischemia,[10,11] prolonged hospital stay, unplanned hospital admission, and increased usage of opiate analgesia.[12] Poor postoperative pain control has also been implicated in increased procedural cost.[13]

TABLE 37.1 Preoperative Blood Results

Parameter	Result
Hemoglobin	16.2 g/dL
Platelet count	425×10^3 per mm^3
White cell count	8.7×10^3 per mm^3
Prothrombin time	12 seconds
Activated partial thromboplastin time	28 seconds
Sodium	148 mEq/L
Potassium	4.3 mEq/L
Urea	8.4 mmol/L
Creatinine	219 mmol/L
Glucose	5.1 mmol/L

At the physiologic level, pain results in alterations to neuroendocrine responses referred to as the *surgical stress response*. The surgical stress results in increased sympathetic activity, which in turn increases heart rate, contractility, and peripheral vascular resistance. This may lead to a reduction in myocardial oxygen supply, thereby precipitating ischemia.

Epidural analgesia provides superior analgesia compared to conventional opiate-based systemic regimens.[9,14,15] Epidural analgesia blunts the surgical stress response and resultant sympathetic stimulation, which may confer a cardioprotective effect. It may also produce vasodilation of epicardial blood vessels, improving myocardial blood flow and preventing myocardial ischemia.[16,17] An epidural catheter placed at the level corresponding to the most proximal dermatome of the surgical incision ensures reliable and predictable analgesia. Appropriate thoracic epidural catheter placement is recommended for major abdominal surgery.[18]

In summary, balanced anesthesia with effective epidural analgesia contributes significantly to improving patient outcome.

A 14-gauge intravenous cannula was placed in the patient's right forearm, and 1 L of Hartmann's solution was administered over 45 minutes. An epidural catheter was placed before induction of general anesthesia at the level of T8. After a negative aspiration test for blood and cerebrospinal fluid, a test dose of 2 mL 0.25% bupivacaine was administered. This dose failed to produce signs consistent with an intrathecal block at 10 minutes. Invasive arterial blood pressure was next established.

General anesthesia was induced using fentanyl (2 μg/kg), propofol (1.5 mg/kg), and vecuronium (0.1 mg/kg). The patient's airway was intubated with an 8.5-mm internal diameter cuffed endotracheal tube, and his lungs were ventilated with 50% oxygen in air to achieve normocarbia. Anesthesia was maintained with sevoflurane titrated to effect. Hemodynamic parameters (heart rate and blood pressure) were kept within 10% of the starting values. Central venous access was established after anesthesia induction. An additional 10 mL of 0.25% bupivacaine was administered into the epidural catheter at this stage.

The intraoperative course was uneventful with an aortic cross-clamp time of 40 minutes. Intravenous glyceryl trinitrate was used to control the patient's blood pressure during the cross-clamp period. Phenylephrine 100-μg bolus doses were used to control blood pressure when the aortic cross-clamp was released. The total estimated blood loss was 750 mL, resulting in a hemoglobin level of 11.2 g/dL at the end of the case. No blood products were administered. Intraoperative analgesia consisted of an epidural infusion of 0.1% bupivacaine with 2 μg/mL of fentanyl at a rate of 8 mL per hour. Intravenous paracetamol 2 g was also administered. Immediately following surgery, the sevoflurane was discontinued, neostigmine and glycopyrrolate neuromuscular block reversal were given, and the trachea was extubated. The patient was transferred to the high-dependency unit where he made an uneventful recovery over the following 48 hours.

How should this man's pain be managed after surgery?

Epidural analgesia should be continued and titrated to effect with a continuous infusion of 0.1% bupivacaine with 2 μg/mL

of fentanyl. Adjuvants, such as paracetamol should be given around the clock (intravenously every 6 hours during the high-dependency unit stay and orally afterward). Nonsteroidal anti-inflammatory drugs should be avoided because of this patient's impaired renal function.

Pain was measured on a verbal rating scale (0–10) at rest and on movement. Zero corresponded to no pain, and 10 corresponded to the worst imaginable pain. Measurement occurred hourly for the first 24 hours and every 4 hours. The epidural infusion was titrated to keep the dynamic pain score at 3 or less at all times. The epidural catheter was removed on the third postoperative day. Removal was timed to be a minimum of 12 hours after and 4 hours before subcutaneous low-molecular-weight heparin (deep venous thrombosis prophylaxis) as per American Society of Regional Anesthesia/European Society of Regional Anesthesia consensus guideline.[20]

In summary, a 68-year-old man with significant comorbidities underwent major aortic surgery to repair an abdominal aortic aneurysm. Continuation of long-standing medication pre-operatively and the use of thoracic epidural analgesia facilitated the safe conduct of anesthesia, blunting the adverse effects of major vascular surgery on the myocardium.

KEY MESSAGES

1. Pain contributes to negative postoperative outcomes following major abdominal surgery such as myocardial ischemia.

2. Epidural analgesia is superior to opiate-based systemic analgesia and attenuates the surgical stress response.

3. Thoracic epidural analgesia, particularly when maintained postoperatively, may help to prevent perioperative myocardial ischemia and infarction.

QUESTIONS

1. What is the role of thoracic epidural analgesia in the prevention of myocardial ischemia in abdominal aortic aneurysm repair?

   Answer: Pain contributes to negative postoperative outcomes following major abdominal surgery such as myocardial ischemia. Neuroendocrine responses and sympathetic activation increase myocardial oxygen demand and reduce supply. Extradural analgesia provides superior pain relief to opiate-based analgesia and attenuates the surgical neuroendocrine stress response. Thoracic epidural analgesia also dilates epicardial blood vessels improving myocardial blood flow. Thus, epidural analgesia may help prevent complications such as postoperative myocardial ischemia and infarction.

2. What are the considerations for removing an epidural catheter in a patient receiving deep vein thrombosis prophylaxis using subcutaneous low-molecular-weight heparin?

Answer: Neuraxial instrumentation in patients receiving low-molecular-weight heparin may increase the risk of extradural hematoma and resultant neurological injury. Neuraxial instrumentation (catheter removal or insertion) should be timed to be a minimum of 12 hours after and 4 hours before administering subcutaneous low-molecular-weight heparin. Published American Society of Regional Anesthesia /European Society of Regional Anesthesia consensus guidelines exist.

3. Why do traditional outcome measures show no difference following regional anesthesia compared with general anesthesia?

Answer: Traditional outcome measures (mortality and major morbidity) show no difference when studied across large patient populations. Although pain has not been considered a traditional outcome, the superiority of regional anesthesia techniques over systemic opioids has been consistently shown. There are proven benefits in certain situations and certain subgroups. The use of neuraxial anesthesia in patients with coronary artery disease undergoing major cardiac or vascular surgery appears beneficial and is more pronounced for thoracic than lumber epidurals and when epidurals are used in the postoperative period.

References

1. Feisher LA, Beckman JA, Brown KA, et al. ACC/AHA 2007 Guidelines on Perioperative Cardiovascular Evaluation and Care for Noncardiac Surgery: a Report of the American College of Cardiology/American Heart Association Task Force on Practice Guidelines (Writing Committee to Revise the 2002 Guidelines on Perioperative Cardiovascular Evaluation for Noncardiac Surgery). Anesth Analg 2008;106:685–712.
2. McFadden EP, Stabile E, Regar E, et al. Late thrombosis in drug-eluting coronary stents after discontinuation of antiplatelet therapy. Lancet 2004;364:1519–1521.
3. Polldermans D, Bax JJ, Schouten O, et al. Should major vascular surgery be delayed because of preoperative cardiac testing in intermediate-risk patients receiving beta-blocker therapy with tight heart rate control? J Am Coll Cardiol 2006;48:964–969.
4. La Manach Y, Godet G, Coriat P, et al. The impact of postoperative discontinuation or continuation of chronic statin therapy on cardiac outcome after major vascular surgery. Anesth Analg 2007;104:1326–1333.
5. Landesberg G, Mosseri M, Wolf, Y et al. Perioperative myocardial ischemia and infarction: identification by continuous 12-lead electrocardiogram with online ST-segment monitoring. Anesthesiology 2002;96:264–270.
6. The Association of Anaesthetists of Great Britain and Ireland. Standards of Monitoring During Anaesthesia and Recovery 4th Ed. Available at: http://www.aagbi.org/publications/guidelines/docs/standardsofmonitoring07.pdf. Accessed May 19, 2008.
7. Practice guidelines for pulmonary artery catheterization: an update report by the American Society of Anesthesiologists Task Force on Pulmonary Artery Catheterization. Anesthesiology 2003;99:988–1014.
8. Brennan F, Carr DB, Cousins M. Pain management: a fundamental human right. Anesth Analg 2007;105: 205–221.
9. Rodgers A, Walker N, Schug S, et al. Reduction of postoperative mortality and morbidity with epidural or spinal anaesthesia: results from overview of randomised trials. BMJ 2000;321:1493.
10. Beattie WS, Badner NH, Choi P. Epidural analgesia reduces postoperative myocardial infarction: a meta-analysis. Anesth Analg 2001;93:853–858.
11. Meissner A, Rolf N, Van Aken H. Thoracic epidural anesthesia and the patient with heart disease: benefits, risks, and controversies. Anesth Analg 1997;85:517–528.
12. Pavlin DJ, Chen C, Penaloza DA, et al. Pain as a factor complicating recovery and discharge after ambulatory surgery. Anesth Analg 2002;95:627–634.
13. Williams BA, Kentor ML, Vogt MT, et al. Economics of nerve block pain management after anterior cruciate ligament reconstruction: potential hospital cost savings via associated postanaesthesia care unit bypass and same-day discharge. Anesthesiology 2004;100:697–706.
14. Liu SS, Block BM, Wu CL. Effects of perioperative central neuraxial analgesia on outcome after coronary artery bypass surgery: a meta-analysis. Anesthesiology 2004;101:153–161.
15. Rigg JR, Jamrozik K, Myles PS, et al. Epidural anaesthesia and analgesia and outcome of major surgery: a randomised trial. Lancet 2002;359:1276–1282.
16. Liu SS, Wu CL. Effect of postoperative analgesia on major postoperative complications: a systematic update of the evidence. Anesth Analg 2007;104:689–702.
17. Nygard E, Kofoed KF, Freiberg J, et al. Effects of high thoracic epidural analgesia on myocardial blood flow in patients with ischemic heart disease. Circulation 2005;111:2165–2170.
18. Procedure Specific Postoperative Pain Management Working Group. Available at: http://www.postoppain.org/frameset.htm. Accessed May 19, 2008.
19. Myles PS, Leslie K, Chan MT. Avoidance of nitrous oxide for patients undergoing major surgery: a randomized controlled trial. Anesthesiology 2007;107:221–231.
20. Horlocker TT, Wedel DJ, Benzon H, et al. Regional anesthesia in the anticoagulated patient: defining the risks (the second ASRA Consensus Conference in Neuraxial Anesthesia and Anticoagulation). Reg Anesth Pain Med 2003;28:172–197.

CHAPTER 38

Ultrasound Guidance for Peripheral Nerve Blockade

Brian D. O'Donnell

CASE FORMAT: REFLECTION

A 95-year-old, 63-kg woman fell down a flight of stairs. She sustained a comminuted midhumeral fracture to her right arm and a Lisfranc fracture-dislocation of her right foot. Both fractures required operative management. Other than mild ecchymosis around her right eye and some tenderness in her right flank, she had suffered no other injuries.

The patient had a history of falls and sustained a hip fracture 3 years earlier, which required a hemiarthroplasty, performed under general anesthesia. At that time, she was discovered to have aortic stenosis with a gradient of 85 mm Hg across the aortic valve. No cardiothoracic surgical intervention was planned. Before her fall, she was independently mobile and self-caring, living in sheltered accommodation. Her medication consisted of aspirin 75 mg daily and metoprolol 10 mg daily. She had no known drug allergies.

On examination, the patient's vital signs were as follows: temperature, 36.5 °C; blood pressure, 155/75 mm Hg; heart rate, 52 beats per minute; and respiratory rate, 16 breaths per minute. The patient's breath sounds were vesicular. Auscultation of her precordium revealed a loud pansystolic murmur loudest at the left sternal border, radiating to the carotids. There was a palpable thrill on the anterior chest wall. Her physical examination was otherwise unremarkable.

The patient's electrocardiograph reading revealed sinus rhythm with left axis deviation and left ventricular hypertrophy (Fig. 38.1). A transthoracic echocardiogram was performed and showed concentric left ventricular hypertrophy, severe aortic stenosis, and mild mitral regurgitation. The gradient across the aortic valve was estimated to be 105 mm Hg with an estimated valve surface area of less than 0.5 cm^2.

Following discussion with the patient, it was decided to proceed with both surgeries consecutively under regional anesthesia. An 18-gauge intravenous cannula was placed on the dorsum of the patient's left hand, and 1 L of Hartmann's solution was slowly administered. Routine electrocardiograph, pulse oximetry (SaO$_2$), and noninvasive blood pressure were attached and used for hemodynamic monitoring throughout the case. A 35% oxygen mask was used to deliver supplemental oxygen.

A SonoSite Titan unit (SonoSite, Titan, Bothwell, WA) with a 7- to 10-MHz Linear 38 mm probe was used to fa-

cilitate nerve localization. A sterile transparent cover was placed over the transducer, and sterile ultrasound gel was used as an acoustic couplant. The nerve block solution consisted of equal parts 2% (20 mg/mL) lidocaine with 1:200,000 adrenaline mixed with 0.5% (5 mg/mL) bupivacaine. Clonidine was added to this solution. The final block solution contained 10 mg/mL lidocaine, 2.5 mg/mL bupivacaine, and 7.5 μg/mL clonidine. In total, 20 mL of block solution was used (200 mg lidocaine, 50 mg bupivacaine, and 150 μg clonidine).

Anesthesia for the open reduction internal fixation of the foot fracture was performed using combined sciatic and femoral blocks. With the patient in a supine position, the right groin was prepared aseptically and was scanned to reveal the femoral vessels and femoral nerve. Once the femoral nerve was identified and centered in the scanning field, a Stimuplex A50 needle (B. Braun Medical, Melsungen, Germany) was introduced at the lateral edge of the scanning probe. The needle was advanced under direct vision, in long axis, toward the femoral nerve. On reaching the nerve, a test dose of 0.5 mL of block solution was injected and observed to surround the nerve, and an additional 4.5 mL of block solution was injected (Fig. 38.2).

Next, the patient's sciatic nerve was blocked at a level just proximal to the popliteal fossa. With the patient still in the supine position, the lateral thigh was prepared aseptically. Flexing the knee slightly, the ultrasound transducer was placed transversely in the popliteal fossa. The popliteal vessels, tibial, and peroneal nerves were identified. The tibial nerve was centered in the scanning field and traced proximally to visualize the site at which the sciatic nerve bifurcated. At this level, a Stimuplex A100 needle (B. Braun Medical) was inserted in the lateral thigh at the level of the scanning probe. The needle was advanced under direct vision, in long axis toward the sciatic nerve. On reaching the nerve, a test dose of 0.5 mL of block solution was injected and observed to surround the nerve. An additional 7.5 mL of block solution was injected, which facilitated complete bathing of the nerve in local anesthetic solution (Fig. 38.3).

Finally, the brachial plexus on the patient's right side was blocked using a supraclavicular approach. With the patient in a supine position, the right supraclavicular fossa was prepared aseptically. The ultrasound probe was placed in an anteroposterior orientation, and the area was scanned to reveal the supraclavicular artery, the first rib, the pleura, and the brachial plexus. Once the brachial plexus was identified and centered in the scanning field, a Stimuplex A50 needle was introduced at the anterior edge of the scanning probe. It was then advanced under direct vision, in long axis, toward the brachial plexus. On reaching the plexus, a test dose of 0.5 mL of block solution was injected and observed to fill the brachial plexus sheath. An additional 6.5 mL of block solution was injected (Fig. 38.4).

Motor and sensory block was tested in the distribution of the brachial plexus, femoral, and sciatic nerves. Once satisfactory anesthesia had been achieved, sedation was provided using 2 mg midazolam. Surgery proceeded uneventfully, taking 4.5 hours in total. During the surgery, the patient received 2 L of Hartmann's solution, 1.5 g cefuroxime, and 2 g intravenous paracetamol. At the end of surgery, she fulfilled the recovery room bypass criteria and was discharged pain free from the operating room to the ward. Postoperative pain was managed with a combination of oral oxycodone and paracetamol. The patient made an uneventful recovery from anesthesia and surgery and was discharged to convalescent care on the fifth postoperative day.

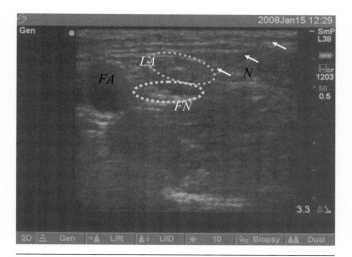

Figure 38.2 • Ultrasound-Guided Femoral Nerve Block. The image shows the performance of a femoral nerve block with needle visible in the long axis of the ultrasound beam. FN, femoral nerve; FA, femoral artery; N, needle; LA, local anesthetic (test dose, 0.5 mL).

Why choose a peripheral nerve block?

Improved Outcome? Outcome studies have not shown improved morbidity and mortality rates with the use of peripheral nerve blocks. Studies to date have been underpowered to detect such rare occurrences as perioperative death. Outcomes such as pain, nausea and vomiting, ambulation, and time to hospital discharge, however, have all been improved with the use of peripheral nerve block in many clinical contexts.[1–3] Brachial plexus blocks have been associated with improved pain outcomes following upper limb surgery.[4–6] A combination of

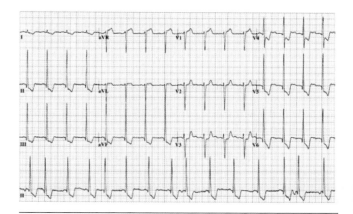

Figure 38.1 • Twelve-lead electrocardiograph showing features of left ventricular hypertrophy. Voltage criteria for LVH include:

Limb leads

- R wave in lead 1 plus S wave in lead III >25 mm
- R wave in lead aVL >11 mm
- R wave in lead aVF >20 mm
- S wave in lead aVR >14 mm

Precordial leads

- R wave in leads V4, V5, or V6 >26 mm
- R wave in leads V5 or 6 plus S wave in lead V1 >35 mm
- Largest R wave plus largest S wave in precordial leads >45 mm

(Reproduced with permission from Edhouse J, Thakur RK, Khalil JM. ABC of clinical electrocardiography conditions affecting the left side of the heart. BMJ 2002;324:1264–1267.)

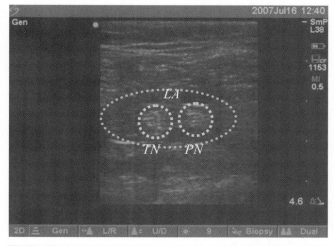

Figure 38.3 • Ultrasound-Guided Sciatic Nerve Block. Image showing the two parts (tibial and common peroneal) of the sciatic nerve in the proximal popliteal fossa surrounded by local anesthetic. TN, tibial nerve; PN, common peroneal nerve; LA, local anesthetic.

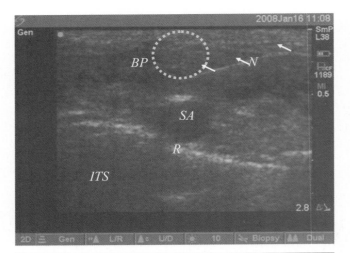

Figure 38.4 • Ultrasound-Guided Supraclavicular Brachial Plexus Block. Image showing the performance of a supraclavicular brachial plexus block, with needle visible in the long axis of the ultrasound beam. SA, subclavian artery; R, first rib; BP, brachial plexus (resembles a bunch of grapes); N, needle; ITS, intra-thoracic space.

TABLE 38.1 Physicochemical Properties of Local Anesthetics

	pKa	Protein Binding (%)	Lipid Solubility
Lidocaine	7.8	65	366
Bupivacaine	8.1	96	3460

peripheral nerve blocks facilitated excellent anesthesia and postoperative analgesia in this case.

Reduced Physiologic Insult? General anesthesia agents cause significant cardiac depression, vasodilatation, and hemodynamic derangement.[7] Although these physiologic changes are normally well tolerated in health, this patient had severe aortic stenosis, which predisposes to anesthesia-related cardiovascular morbidity and mortality.

General anesthesia also alters respiratory mechanics, resulting in lung atelectasis and intrapulmonary shunt, thereby predisposing the patient to postoperative complications such as hypoxemia and pneumonia.[8] Regional anesthesia permits targeted anesthesia of surgical site and facilitates surgery in awake or lightly sedated, cooperative patients. The unwanted aforementioned physiologic derangements were avoided in this case.

Lower Level Monitoring Required? Monitoring for this surgery under general anesthesia would have necessitated the placement of invasive arterial and central venous cannulae.[9] Vasopressor support, to correct predictable hemodynamic derangement accompanying general anesthesia, may have been required. Effective peripheral nerve block obviated the need to use general anesthesia in this case.

Why use a mixture of lidocaine, bupivacaine and clonidine?

The physicochemical properties of lidocaine and bupivacaine are summarized in Table 38.1.[10] Lidocaine with a pKa of 7.7 has a rapid onset of action. Bupivacaine, with 98% protein binding, will provide an extended block well into the postoperative period. Clonidine has been shown to prolong brachial plexus blocks when administered into the perineural space.[11,12]

Why ultrasound guidance?

Block Success Rates? Poor success rates have hampered the use and development of peripheral nerve block techniques. Blind techniques rely on imprecise end points such as paraesthesia or motor response to nerve stimulation. Ultrasound guidance facilitates placing the block needle directly adjacent to the target nerve, allowing visualization of needle, nerve, and injectate. Needle reposition is facilitated, ensuring circumferential spread of injectate around the nerve. Ultrasound guidance has been shown to increase the likelihood of a successful block (from 80% to 95%) when compared with nerve stimulation for three-in-one blocks.[13,14] The only study evaluating brachial plexus block techniques suggests equivalence between ultrasound and nerve stimulation.[15] Currently, comparative studies have not been performed with sciatic nerve block.

Onset Time? Not only have poor success rates hampered peripheral nerve block development, slow block onset times similarly make peripheral nerve blocks a less attractive anesthetic option. When compared with general anesthesia, peripheral nerve blocks have been shown to take on average 11 minutes longer to provide effective anesthesia.[16] Ultrasound guidance permits deposition of a local anesthetic agent directly adjacent to the nerve structure. The physicochemical properties of local anesthetic agents (pKa, lipid solubility) and the relative concentration of the drug (2% vs. 0.25%) largely determine block onset times. Also, the closer the solution is deposited to the nerve, the faster the agent will work. Therefore, greater precision in injectate placement as seen with ultrasound guidance, has resulted in a reduction in block onset time.[15,17]

Reduction in Dose? The dose of the local anesthetic agent used to perform peripheral nerve blocks has been greatly reduced when compared with traditional techniques. Marhofer et al[14] demonstrated a reduction in dose when ultrasound was compared with nerve stimulation for three-in-one block. Casati et al[18] estimated the ED-50 of 0.5% ropivacaine for femoral nerve block to be 15 mL under ultrasound guidance and 26 mL for nerve stimulation. Willschke et al[19] used as little as 0.075 mL/kg for ilioinguinal/iliohypogastric blocks in children. Clinical experience, as illustrated in this case, suggests the potential to dramatically reduce the dose of the agent required to produce successful peripheral nerve block. However, the optimal dose of local anesthetic agent for brachial plexus and sciatic blocks has not yet been defined.

In summary, ultrasound guidance permitted the safe and effective conduct of regional anesthesia in a patient with upper and lower limb fractures, for whom general anesthesia carried significant risks. Improved block success rates and reduced onset times as seen with ultrasound guidance provided the confidence to proceed using regional anesthesia alone. In this case, ultrasound guidance permitted same-day treatment of both upper and lower limb fractures, which may not have been possible with other nerve localization techniques because of dose limitations.

KEY MESSAGES

In experienced hands, ultrasound guidance

1. Permits precise nerve localization and perineural local anesthetic deposition.

2. Facilitates a reduction in local anesthetic dose.

3. Improves the success rates of nerve block techniques.

4. Speeds the onset time of peripheral nerve block.

QUESTIONS

1. Does ultrasound guidance facilitate reducing the dose of local anesthetic agent needed to perform successful neural blockade.

   Answer: Yes. Ultrasound guidance permits precise perineural needle and injectate placement. Visualization of circumferential perineural spread is accepted as the end point for ultrasound-guided peripheral nerve block. This permits neural blockade with very small volumes of local anesthetic agent (Riazi S, Carmichael N, Awad I, et al. Effect of local anaesthetic volume (20 vs 5 ml) on the efficacy and respiratory consequences of ultrasound-guided interscalene brachial plexus block. Br J Anaesth 2008;101:549–556).

2. Does ultrasound guidance make the practice of regional anesthesia under deep sedation or general anesthesia safe?

   Answer: No, occult intraneural injection or intraneural catheter placement resulting in nerve injury is still possible. Conscious patients may report pain or dysesthesia should this occur. Deep sedation and general anesthesia will abolish this feedback. Real-time ultrasound guidance may detect needle tip position, but it may not prevent an operator-dependent phenomenon such as intraneural injection. It is best practice to perform regional anesthesia in conscious patients.

3. Does ultrasound guidance improve the safety of regional anesthetic techniques?

   Answer: The term safety implies clinical efficacy without adverse event or harm. There is no conclusive evidence demonstrating an improvement in patient safety with the use of ultrasound guidance for regional anesthesia. In expert hands, ultrasound guidance reduces local anesthetic dose, speeds block onset and facilitates avoidance of important related structures (arteries and veins). It may appear logical that these conditions confer a greater level of safety than blind techniques. This has not been borne out by prospective data as of yet.

References

1. Liu SS Wu C. Effect of postoperative analgesia on major postoperative complications: a systematic update of the evidence. Anesth Analg 2007;104:689–702.
2. Richman JM, Liu SS, Courpas G, et al. Does continuous peripheral nerve block provide superior pain control to opioids? A meta-analysis. Anesth Analg 2006;102:248–257.
3. Liu SS, Strodtbeck WM, Richman JM, Wu CL. A comparison of regional versus general anesthesia for ambulatory anesthesia: a meta-analysis of randomized controlled trials. Anesth Analg 2005;101:1634–1642.
4. Hadzic A, Williams BA, Karaca PE, et al. For outpatient rotator cuff surgery, nerve block anesthesia provides superior same-day recovery over general anesthesia. Anesthesiology. 2005;102:1001–1007.
5. Singelyn FJ, Lhotel L, Fabre B. Pain relief after arthroscopic shoulder surgery: a comparison of intraarticular analgesia, suprascapular nerve block, and interscalene brachial plexus block. Anesth Analg 2004;99:589–592.
6. Hadzic A, Arliss J, Kerimoglu B, et al. A comparison of infraclavicular nerve block versus general anesthesia for hand and wrist day-case surgeries. Anesthesiology 2004;101:127–132.
7. Akata T. General anesthetics and vascular smooth muscle: direct actions of general anesthetics on cellular mechanisms regulating vascular tone. Anesthesiology 2007;106:365–391.
8. Magnusson L, Spahn DR. New concepts of atelectasis during general anaesthesia Br J Anaesth 2003;91:61–72.
9. The Association of Anaesthetists of Great Britain & Ireland. Recommendations for Standards of Monitoring During Anaesthesia and Recovery, 4th Ed. http://www.aagbi.org/publications/guidelines/docs/standardsofmonitoring07.pdf. Accessed March 6, 2009.
10. Strichartz GR, Sanchez V, Arthur GR, et al. Fundamental properties of local anesthetics. II. Measured octanol:buffer partition coefficients and pKa values of clinically used drugs. Anesth Analg 1990;71:158–170.
11. Iohom G, Machmachi A, Diarra DP, et al. The effects of clonidine added to mepivacaine for paronychia surgery under axillary brachial plexus block. Anesth Analg 2005;100:1179–1183.
12. Hutschala D, Mascher H, Schmetterer L, et al. Clonidine added to bupivacaine enhances and prolongs analgesia after brachial plexus block via a local mechanism in healthy volunteers. Eur J Anaesthesiol 2004;21:198–204.
13. Marhofer P, Schrogendorfer K, Koinig H, et al. Ultrasonographic guidance improves sensory block and onset time of three-in-one blocks. Anesth Analg 1997;85:854–857.
14. Marhofer P, Schrogendorfer K, Wallner T, et al. Ultrasonographic guidance reduces the amount of local anesthetic for 3-in-1 blocks. Reg Anesth Pain Med 1998;23:584–588.
15. Casati A, Danelli G, Baciarello M, et al. A prospective, randomized comparison between ultrasound and nerve stimulation guidance for multiple injection axillary brachial plexus block. Anesthesiology. 2007;106:992–996.

16. Liu SS, Strodtbeck WM, Richman JM, Wu CL. A comparison of regional versus general anesthesia for ambulatory anesthesia: a meta-analysis of randomized controlled trials. Anesth Analg. 2005;101:1634–1642.

17. Williams SR, Chouinard P, Arcand G, et al. Ultrasound guidance speeds execution and improves the quality of supraclavicular block. Anesth Analg 2003;97:1518–1523.

18. Casati A, Baciarello M, Di Cianni S, et al. Effects of ultrasound guidance on the minimum effective anaesthetic volume required to block the femoral nerve. Br J Anaesth 2007;98:823–827.

19. Willschke H, Bösenberg A, Marhofer P, et al. Ultrasonographic-guided ilioinguinal/iliohypogastric nerve block in pediatric anesthesia: what is the optimal volume? Anesth Analg. 2006;102: 1680–1684.

CHAPTER 39

Continuous Ambulatory Regional Anesthesia

Jason Van der Velde

FORMAT: REFLECTION

A 56-year-old woman was scheduled for an elective arthroscopic shoulder rotater cuff repair and subacranial decompression. She was a well-controlled asthmatic, on regular budesonide 200 μg through a metered dose inhaler who had never required hospital admission for her asthma.

In the preoperative assessment clinic, a continuous ambulatory regional anesthetic technique was recommended to the patient for optimal pain management. Specific informed consent was obtained for perineural interscalene catheter placement prior to general anaesthesia after discussing the risks, benefits, alternatives, and management of potential complications. Motor and sensory examination of her shoulder was performed at this clinic appointment.

On the day of surgery, the catheter was placed in the anesthetic room with standard monitoring and intravenous (IV) access. Real-time ultrasound was used for guidance throughout the procedure, which was conducted under standard aseptic conditions consisting of sterile skin preparation and draping of both patient and equipment.

After infiltration of skin and subcutaneous tissue with a local anesthetic, an 18-gauge thin-walled needle was inserted into the interscalene space between the anterior and the middle scalene muscle. Preservative-free bupivacaine (0.5% 20 mL) with 1:200,000 epinephrine was injected. A 20-gauge polyamide catheter was inserted through the needle to a depth of 3 cm beyond the needle tip. The catheter was secured with a clear adhesive dressing. The patient was noted to have both a dense motor and sensory block 30 minutes later.

General anesthesia was then induced with fentanyl 100 μg and propofol 150 mg. Anesthesia maintenance was achieved with sevoflurane and a 50:50 oxygen:air mix through a laryngeal mask airway. An uneventful 2-hour procedure followed under general anesthesia without catheter infusion. Paracetamol 1g was administered intravenously during the procedure.

The patient was pain free in the postanesthesia recovery area. Having confirmed the correct position of the perineural catheter with a thoracic inlet radiograph, a disposable elastomeric infusion pump was attached and set to infuse plain preservative-free 0.25% bupivacaine at 5 mL per hour.

On conclusion of the day's operating list, the anesthetist visited the patient on the ward. Instructions initially given during the preoperative clinic were reiterated to both the patient and her husband. These instructions were reinforced with a patient information leaflet. The leaflet explained how to use the catheter, cautioned the patient to care for the insensate arm, and described the possible drainage that could occur. In addition, the sheet mentioned side effects including a sagging eyelid, smaller pupil, slight redness of the eye, and a possible decrease in deep breathing especially while lying down. The day and time when the catheter should be removed were written on the sheet. The patient was discharged home that evening, in care of her husband, with the contact numbers of the orthopaedic admissions ward, the district nurse team, and a letter for her general practitioner.

The patient awoke at home at 3:00 AM with pain in the lateral deltoid only. Her husband telephoned the ward, and an immediate admission was initiated. On arrival, the patient's pain scores were found to be 7/10, and rescue pain relief (intramuscular morphine) was prescribed as required. The perineural infusion was maintained for an additional 48 hours, as it continued to provide excellent pain relief to all other aspects of her shoulder. The patient was discharged home on minor analgesics thereafter, and her outpatient rehabilitation and recovery continued uneventfully.

CASE DISCUSSION

Although greatly improving patients' long-term quality of life, shoulder procedures can be extremely painful. Immediate postoperative pain is costly, particularly in terms of length of hospital stay and rehabilitation time. With the number of procedures predicted to increase as the population ages, novel approaches to pain management are constantly being sought.

Anesthetic and Analgesic Options

Pain is greatly exacerbated in the rehabilitation phase of treatment, particularly during physiotherapy. This pain has been shown to have a direct bearing on the functional outcome of the procedure.[1] Current postoperative analgesic regimens should ideally include a multimodal prescription of oral minor analgesics combined with rescue opioids.

In this particular patient, it is unclear whether this avenue has been fully explored prior to her initial discharge home. It appears that she had a single dose of IV paracetamol intraoperatively, and no nonsteroidal anti-inflammatory drugs

TABLE 39.1 Comparison of Local Anesthetics

		Lidocaine	Bupivacaine	Levobupivacaine	Ropivacaine
Block duration (min)	Plain	60–120	180–360	180–360	140–200
	With epinephrine	90–180	300–480		160–220
Onset		Rapid	Slow	Slow	Moderate
Sensory block		Dense	Dense	Dense	Dense
Motor block		Moderate	Dense	Dense	Moderate
Safety		Moderately cardiotoxic	Highly cardiotoxic	Improved safety over bupivacaine	Favorable safety profile compared to bupivacaines, with less diaphragmatic impairment

(NSAIDs) were given, possibly because of exaggerated anxiety that this may worsen her asthma. Aspirin and NSAIDs may cause bronchoconstriction in approximately 10% of asthmatic patients, although they also relieve it in approximately 0.3% of patients.[10] As the primary mechanism is believed to be inhibition of the cyclooxygenase 1 (COX-1) enzyme, patients with aspirin sensitivity often display cross-reactions to nonselective NSAIDs that inhibit the COX-1 enzyme.[11] Because acetaminophen is a weak inhibitor of the COX-1 enzyme, patients with aspirin-induced asthma should not take more than 1000 mg in a single dose, but COX-2 selective NSAIDs appear to be safe in this patient population.[11]

Regional anesthesia is the cornerstone of multimodal analgesic regimens. Single-shot plexus blocks were first used to reduce the amount of systemic opioids administered perioperatively. The interscalene brachial plexus block provides analgesia that is superior to morphine in shoulder arthroplasty.[2] The advantages of a single-shot nerve block may be extended using perineural local anesthetic infusions. They have the additional benefit of expediting and improving functional recovery. The safety and efficacy of various continuous regional anesthesia techniques using portable infusions or patient-controlled boluses of local anesthetic agents through indwelling perineural catheters has been demonstrated.[3]

Interscalene brachial plexus blockade may be combined with a general anesthetic or used as the primary anesthetic technique for shoulder arthroscopy. Regional anesthesia for shoulder arthroscopy has been shown to require significantly less nonsurgical intraoperative time (53 ± 12 vs. 62 ± 13 minutes, $p = .0001$) and also decreased post-anesthesia care unit stay (72 ± 24 vs. 102 ± 40 minutes, $p = .0001$) compared with general anesthesia.[4] Administration of regional anesthesia resulted in significantly fewer unplanned admissions for severe pain management, sedation, or nausea/vomiting than general anesthesia and was accompanied by a failure rate of 8.7%. The increasing use of ultrasound to guide perineural catheter placement may lead to improved success rates.

Pain management during the transition from a dense surgical block to an analgesic block is a challenge. This may occur when using a dilute local anesthetic solution. If a long-acting local anesthetic agent is used to establish the block, as in the case presented (Table 39.1), at about 16 hours postinsertion, gaps may become evident as patchy pain. These gaps may occur in the early hours of the morning, when staffing levels are low or when an ambulatory patient is at home. It is therefore preferable to establish blocks with a short-to-medium acting agent such as 1% prilocaine, lidocaine, or mepivacaine. If there is an area not covered by the infusion, this will become evident a few hours post procedure, thus facilitating an early alternative analgesic strategy.[9]

Patient Selection Weighed Against Potential Complications

Shoulder arthroscopy and arthroplasty are performed in many centers as ambulatory procedures using continuous ambulatory regional anesthesia techniques to control postoperative pain.[5] Patient satisfaction is high,[6] the technique has reduced oral opioid requirements and sleep disturbances while improving range of motion.

Although regional anesthetic techniques provide site-specific analgesia with minor, if any, systemic side effects,[7] it is important to remember that whereas the technique itself does not always require inpatient supervision, the patients' premorbid condition may. Patients must be able to manage at home with the risks posed by an insensate limb. Appropriate patient selection weighed against potential complication risks, education, and follow-up are crucial when prescribing outpatient infusions.

Regional anesthesia is not associated with a greater incidence of neurologic complications than general anesthesia. The American Society of Anesthesiologists closed-claims studies suggest that the majority of reported neurological complications are actually associated with general anesthesia and incorrect patient positioning.

Complications such as hematoma formation, hoarseness, and Horner's syndrome have been reported. These issues are attributed to needle misplacement or local anesthetic either spreading to upper cervical nerve roots (C_3, C_4) or anteriorly to block the phrenic nerve in front of the anterior scalene muscle.

All patients should be counseled regarding the high incidence of varying degrees of ipsilateral diaphragm paralysis. This occurs subclinically in most patients and is rarely an issue unless there is a significant cardiac or respiratory comorbidity. Moderate or severe functional limitation or a baseline room-air oxygen saturation of less than 96% is not necessarily a contraindication for regional anesthesia, but inpatient supervision should be mandated to manage any potential pulmonary complications.

More serious side effects of regional anesthesia include vasovagal attacks, pneumothoraces, total spinal anesthesia, high epidural block, and inadvertent intravascular injection. The latter are very rare and will usually present perioperatively, allowing immediate management.

If ambulatory catheter dislocation or pump malfunction occurs, particularly early on during ambulatory regional anesthesia, patients are at high risk of experiencing severe surgical pain and are usually unresponsive to oral opioids and require hospital re-admission. Patients should therefore not be discharged home if they will be alone and need to be counseled to take prompt actions if block failure occurs. Patients should also be made aware of early signs of systemic local anesthetic toxicity and should be able to demonstrate clearly how to disconnect the infusion pump and access urgent medical help if this occurs.

Infusion Considerations

Three interscalene catheter infusion strategies have been compared:[8] continuous infusion alone, basal infusion with patient-administered boluses, and patient-controlled boluses alone. A basal infusion of 5 mL/h of bupivacaine 0.125% combined with patient-controlled analgesia boluses (2.5 mL/30 min) proved to be the most appropriate technique.

Electronic pumps, although costly, are useful for accurate quantification of the agent infused. They are an ideal delivery option for in-hospital use. On the other hand, elastomeric disposable pumps appear to be more reliable because of simplicity.[9] They are essentially high-flow resistance devices and therefore are inherently safer in preventing inadvertent boluses of large amounts of local anesthetic. They are ideal for ambulatory home use because they are less bulky than electronic pumps.

There are logistical and financial advantages to undertaking shoulder surgery in an ambulatory setting; however, the approach is limited by postoperative pain being inadequately controlled by oral medication alone. Additional continuous ambulatory regional anesthesia appears to meet the challenge of providing a reliable extension of postoperative analgesia following painful surgery.

KEY MESSAGES

1. Regional anesthesia is the cornerstone of multimodal analgesia following painful surgery. Its benefits could be extended beyond hospital stay by continuous ambulatory perineural infusions.

2. Continuous ambulatory regional anesthesia decreases length of hospital stay by providing analgesia that permits greater passive limb mobility and the avoidance of IV opioids. Patient selection and counseling is paramount.

QUESTIONS

1. Is a long-acting local anesthetic agent ideal for establishing the initial block before starting a continuous ambulatory infusion?

   Answer: No. It is preferable to establish blocks with a short-to-medium acting agent to diagnose and manage inadequate or patchy analgesia before a patient's discharge.

2. What steps can be taken to avoid inadvertent intravascular injection of local anesthetic?

   Answer: Inadvertent intravascular injection of local anesthetic is best avoided by maintaining verbal contact with the patient, frequent aspirations, looking for disappearance of motor twitch after injection of the first mL of local anesthetic solution (or tissue expansion with visualization of the needle tip with ultrasound guidance), and using an adrenalin-containing test solution to evaluate and re-evaluate a perineural catheter.

3. What is the management of inadvertent intravascular injection of bupivacaine resulting in systemic toxicity?

   Answer: The cornerstone of bupivacaine systemic toxicity is a 1.5mL/kg bolus of intralipid 20% over 1 minute followed by an infusion at 0.25mL/kg/min over 20 minutes whilst continuing all necessary cardiopulmonary resuscitative efforts. Repeating boluses at 5 minute intervals thereafter or increasing the rate of infusion to 0.5mL/kg/min until a stable circulation is restored may be considered.

References

1. Cameron B. Factors affecting the outcome of total shoulder arthroplasty. Am J Orthop 2001;30:613–623.
2. Richman JM, Liu SS, Wu C, et al. Does continuous peripheral nerve block provide superior pain control to opioids? A meta-analysis. Anesth Analg 2006;102:248–257.
3. Capdevila X, Dadure C, Bringuier S, et. Al. Effect of patient-controlled perineural analgesia on rehabilitation and pain after ambulatory orthopedic surgery. Anesthesiology 2006;105:566–573.
4. D'Alessio J, Rosenblum M, Shea K, et al. A retrospective comparison of interscalene block and general anesthesia for ambulatory surgery shoulder arthroscopy. Regional Anesthesia 1995;20:62–68.
5. Ilfeld B, Wright T, Enneking K, et al. Shoulder arthroplasty as an outpatient procedure using ambulatory perineural local anesthetic infusion: a pilot feasibility study. Anesth Analg 2005;101:1319–1322.
6. Fredrickson MJ, Ball CM, Dalgleish AJ. Successful continuous interscalene analgesia for ambulatory shoulder surgery in a private practice setting. Reg Anesth Pain Med 2008;33:122–128.
7. Bryan N, Swenson J, Greis E, et al. Indwelling interscalene catheter use in an outpatient setting for shoulder surgery: Technique, efficacy, and complications. J Shoulder Elbow Surg 2007;16:388–395.

8. Singelyn F, Seguy S, Gouverneur J. Interscalene brachial plexus analgesia after open shoulder surgery: continuous versus patient-controlled infusion. Anesth Analg 1999;89:1216–1220.

9. Russon K, Sardesai A, Ridgway S, et al. Postoperative shoulder surgery initiative (POSSI): an interim report of major shoulder surgery as a day case procedure. BJA 2006;97:869–873.

10. Babu KS, Salvi SS. Aspirin and asthma. Chest 2000; 118: 1470–1476.

11. Knowles SR, Drucker AM, Weber EA, Shear NH. Management options for patients with aspirin and nonsteroidal anti-inflammatory drug sensitivity. Ann of Pharmacother 2007; 41:1191–1200.

CHAPTER 40

Postoperative Analgesia in a Trauma Patient With Opioid Addiction

Brian D. O'Donnell

FORMAT: STEP BY STEP

A 19-year-old male was brought to the emergency department by ambulance following a motor vehicle accident. He was a restrained rear seat passenger who suffered an open fracture to his right femur after retropulsion of the driver's seat onto his knee. He had no other injuries.

On examination, the patient's vital signs were as follows: heart rate, 110 beats per minute; blood pressure, 105/65 mm Hg; respiratory rate, 24 breaths per minute; temperature, 35.5°C; and SaO_2, 98% on room air. Primary and secondary trauma surveys revealed an open midshaft of femur fracture with bone protruding through a wound on the anterior thigh. The wound was soiled with particulate matter from the crash site. The patient's Glasgow Coma Scale score was 15, there were no external signs of head injury, and he had no memory loss. He was extremely agitated and complaining of severe pain. Trauma radiology included a lateral cervical spine, chest, and pelvic radiographs (all of which showed normal results). His hemoglobin level was 11.4 g/dL, and coagulation as well as biochemistry parameters were normal.

Of note, this young man was a heroin user. He had smoked heroin for 3 years and had recently begun injecting because of diminished drug effect. The absolute quantity of heroin use could not be determined. The patient had never been on a treatment program, and his last "fix" was 4 hours before the accident.

In the emergency room, a 14-gauge intravenous (IV) cannula was placed, and the patient received 2 liters of Hartmann's solution. Pain was managed with 25 mg IV morphine sulphate with little effect. The patient received 1.5 g cefuroxime, 500 mg metronidazole, and a tetanus inoculation. He was scheduled for emergency surgery, and the operating room was alerted and made ready for his arrival.

On initial preoperative assessment in the emergency room, the patient was very agitated and complaining of severe pain.

How might the patient's pain and agitation be managed before surgery?

Acute pain after trauma originates from nociceptors at the site of injury.[1] Nociceptor activation results in a pain signal being conveyed along sensory fibers in peripheral nerves to the spinal cord and via a variety of pathways to several areas within the brain. The femoral nerve is the peripheral nerve that supplies sensation to the femur.[2] This patient had received 25 mg IV morphine without analgesic benefit. His recent conversion from smoked to IV heroin use suggests tolerance to opiates. Tolerance to opiates is defined as a right-shift in the dose response curve, resulting in higher drug doses needed to produce the desired effect.[3] In patients taking long-term opiates, adequate analgesia is difficult to achieve.[4] Agitation in this setting may be as a result of pain. Keep in mind that agitation may be caused by injuries such as head trauma, hypoxia from pneumothorax, or hypovolemic shock resulting from blood loss. Agitation may also be caused by opiate withdrawal. Because this patient had a recent "fix," and primary and secondary surveys had outruled head, chest injury, and hemorrhagic injury, it was assumed that pain was the primary cause of agitation. The presence of an occult injury causing agitation was considered at all times. Peripheral nerve block is one appropriate analgesic option in these circumstances.

Following a thorough preoperative assessment, the attending anesthesiologist decided to manage pain in the emergency room using a femoral nerve block.

The procedural aspects of the femoral nerve block were explained to the patient, who provided verbal consent for the block. He agreed to cooperate and remain still during the block. Electrocardiogram, noninvasive blood pressure, and SaO_2 monitors were attached. The open fracture was covered with a sterile surgical drape, and the patient's groin was prepared aseptically. A Sonosite Titan unit (SonoSite, Titan, Bothwell, WA) with a linear 38-mm 7-to 10-MHz probe was used to guide block placement. A sterile transparent cover was placed over the ultrasound probe, and sterile ultrasound jelly was used as an acoustic couplant. The patient's groin was scanned to reveal the femoral vessels and femoral nerve. A Stimuplex A50 needle (B. Braun Medical, Melsungen, Germany) was advanced under direct vision in long axis toward the femoral nerve (Fig. 40.1). Once the needle reached the desired perineural space, 0.5 mL of 2% lidocaine with 1:200,000 adrenaline was injected after careful aspiration. The solution was observed to surround the nerve. An additional 9.5 mL of 2% lidocaine with 1:200,000 adrenaline was then slowly injected (Fig. 40.2). Over the next 10 minutes, the patient's pain improved, and his level of agitation lessened.

Approximately 90 minutes later, the patient was moved to the operating room where surgical toilet of the wound and intramedullary nailing of the femur fracture was planned. Although lucid and cooperative, the patient was anxious and requested general anesthesia, as he did not want to be awake during surgery.

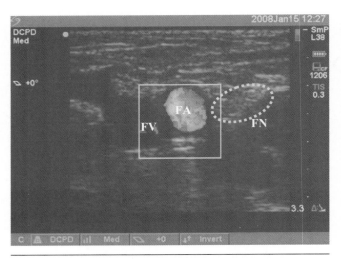

Figure 40.1 • Image Showing the Femoral Artery, Vein, and Nerve with the Use of Directional Color-flow Doppler. FA, femoral artery; FN, femoral nerve; FV, femoral vein.

How should anesthesia be provided for this man?

Both general and spinal anesthesia were considered. Spinal anesthesia would facilitate rapid and effective anesthesia. However, the combination of vasodilation associated with spinal anesthesia and relative hypovolemia from the femur fracture may have precipitated dramatic hemodynamic instability. Spinal anesthesia would necessitate turning the patient into the lateral position to gain access to the central neuraxis. This maneuver would have been technically difficult because of the patient's open femur fracture. In view of the patient's

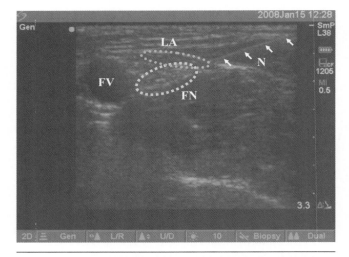

Figure 40.2 • Image Showing a Femoral Nerve Block being Performed with the Block Needle Visualized along the Long Axis of the Ultrasound Beam. FA, femoral artery; FN, femoral nerve; LA, 0.5-mL test dose local anesthetic; N, needle with arrows depicting needle path.

preference and these factors, the anesthesiologist decided to proceed with general anesthesia.

The patient was considered to have a full stomach, as he had suffered a painful traumatic injury and had received opiate analgesics, both known to predispose to impaired gastric emptying.[5] Routine monitoring (electrocardiogram, noninvasive blood pressure, SaO_2) was attached to the patient, and a second 16-gauge IV line was placed. General anesthesia was induced using a rapid sequence technique with propofol, suxamethonium, and the Sellick maneuver. The patient's airway was managed with an 8.5-mm cuffed endotracheal tube secured at 23 cm at the incisors. Anesthesia was maintained with 50% oxygen in air and 3% sevoflurane. Intraoperative analgesia consisted of 2 g IV paracetamol and 75 mg IV diclofenac sodium. The surgery took 3 hours to complete. During this time, an additional 4 liters of Hartmann's solution was administered. No blood products were administered, and the patient remained hemodynamically stable throughout the procedure. His hemoglobin level was 9.1 g/dL at the end of surgery.

On emergence in the recovery room, the patient complained of mild pain in his leg and could demonstrate return of femoral nerve motor function by flexing his quadriceps muscles. Over the next 30 minutes, his pain increased.

How might pain be managed in the postoperative setting?

Multimodal analgesia involves the administration of two or more analgesic agents that have a different mechanism of action.[6] The American Society of Anesthesiologists Task Force on Acute Pain Management advocates the use of multimodal analgesia for the management of acute pain.[7] Multimodal analgesic regimens have been shown to provide superior analgesia compared with single agents.[8,9] Nonsteroidal anti-inflammatory drugs (NSAIDs) and paracetamol are standard components to multimodal analgesia. Opiates administered enterally or parenterally are used in combination with paracetamol and NSAIDs for the treatment of severe pain. Because of this patient's tolerance to opioid medications, effective analgesia would be difficult to achieve with an opiate-based analgesia regimen.

A continuous femoral nerve block would provide excellent analgesia in this setting. Femoral catheters have been used successfully to provide analgesia following femur fracture in non–opioid-dependent patients.[10,11] As the initial femoral nerve block had worn off, it was safe to proceed with inserting a femoral catheter. Placing a catheter under anesthesia (general or regional) is a controversial matter. It might be argued that the advent of ultrasound guidance minimizes the risk of inadvertent intraneural needle or catheter placement. However, it is accepted that an awake patient, reporting dysesthesia or pain during a nerve block procedure, is an early warning of intra-neural injection. Therefore, peripheral nerve blocks are probably best placed in patients who can report symptoms of intraneural injection.[12] Pain on intraneural injection has been disputed as a reliable indicator of intraneural injection.[13] In this case, however, it was judged prudent to allow the initial rescue block to wear off before placing the perineural catheter.

The patient's right groin was fully prepared aseptically under sterile conditions. A hernia towel covered the groin and facilitated access to the expected puncture site. The ultrasound probe was covered with a sterile sheath, and sterile ultrasound jelly was used both inside and outside the sheath as an acoustic couplant. An 18-gauge Tuohy needle and epidural catheter set were used (Fig. 40.3). The groin was scanned to reveal the femoral vessels. The Tuohy needle was inserted in long axis toward the femoral nerve. On contact with the nerve, 0.5 mL 2% lidocaine with 1:200,000 adrenaline was injected and observed to be just outside the perineural space. Minor adjustments were made to the needle tip position, and another 0.5 mL injectate confirmed satisfactory needle tip placement. An additional 9 mL of 2% lidocaine with 1:200,000 adrenaline was injected to dilate the space to accommodate the perineural catheter. The catheter was placed through the needle approximately 2 cm beyond the needle tip. Correct catheter placement was confirmed by observing the location of injectate administered through the catheter. Next, the catheter was tunneled to a site lateral and distal to the insertion site and secured with Steri-Strips (3M, St. Paul, Minnesota, USA) and a transparent dressing. An infusion of 0.25% bupivacaine at a rate of 5 mL per hour was commenced and continued for 3 days post-operatively. The catheter was removed on the third postoperative day.

The patient made an uneventful recovery from anesthesia and surgery and had excellent analgesia provided by a combination of femoral nerve catheter, diclofenac sodium 75 mg twice daily, and 1g paracetamol four times per day. On the first postoperative day, the patient received counseling on heroin cessation and agreed to be placed in a methadone treatment program.

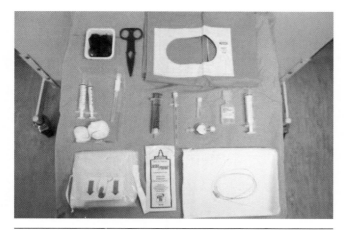

Figure 40.3 • Image Showing the Equipment used to Place an Ultrasound-Guided Perineural Catheter. Note the standard aseptic preparation pack with sterile fenestrated drape, an 18-gauge Tuohy needle, catheter, and attachments (standard epidural kit from B. Braun Medical, Melsungen, Germany). Also note sterile ultrasound gel and a sterile sheath with which to cover the ultrasound probe, providing a sterile interface between patient and ultrasound probe.

KEY MESSAGES

1. Heroin use and subsequent opioid tolerance reduce the efficacy of opioid analgesics necessitating an alternate approach to acute pain management.

2. A mechanistic approach to pain management identified femoral nerve block as an appropriate component of an analgesic regimen for femur fracture.

3. Femoral nerve block formed a component of the multimodal analgesic regimen used in this case, which also consisted of NSAIDs and paracetamol.

4. Ultrasound guidance facilitated the precise placement of needle, injectate, and catheter adjacent to the femoral nerve.

5. Regional anesthesia should ideally be performed only when patients are able to report symptoms of neural injury.

QUESTIONS

1. What is meant by the terms opiate tolerance and addiction?

   Answer:
   • Opioid tolerance is a predictable pharmacological adaptation to continued opioid exposure resulting in a rightward shift in the dose-response curve. Patients require increasing amounts of the drug to maintain the same pharmacological effects.
   • Addiction:
     ○ Psychological dependence: Need for a specific psychoactive substance either for its positive effects or to avoid negative effects associated with its withdrawal.
     ○ Physical dependence: State of adaptation to a substance characterized by the emergence of a withdrawal syndrome during abstinence

2. Why was the femoral nerve catheter placed only when the initial block had worn off?

   Answer: Inadvertent intraneural injection or catheter placement may result in serious nerve injury. Patients will usually report pain or dysesthesia should these occur during catheter placement (patient feedback). A nerve, which has already been blocked with local anesthetic solution, loses patient feedback and therefore, the potential exists to inflict serious nerve injury. It is best practice to allow the initial block to wear off before placing the perineural catheter.

3. Does ultrasound guidance make the practice of regional anesthesia under deep sedation or general anesthesia safe?

   Answer: No, occult intraneural injection or intraneural catheter placement resulting in nerve injury is still possible. Conscious patients may report pain or dysesthesia should this occur. Deep sedation and general anesthesia will abolish this feedback. Real-time ultrasound guidance may detect needle tip position, but it may not prevent an operator-dependent phenomenon such as intraneural injection. It is best practice to perform regional anesthesia in conscious patients.

References

1. Fink WA. The pathophysiology of acute pain. Emerg Med Clin N Am 2005;23:277–284.
2. Enneking FK, Chan VW, Greger J, et al. Lower-extremity peripheral nerve blockade: essentials of our current understanding. Reg Anesth Pain Med 2005;30:4–35.
3. Mitra S, Sinatra RS. Perioperative management of acute pain in the opioid-dependent patient. Anesthesiology 2004;101: 212–227.
4. Carroll IR, Angst MS, Clark JD. Management of perioperative pain in patients chronically consuming opioids. Reg Anesth Pain Med 2004;29:576–591.
5. Murphy DB, Sutton JA, Prescott LF, et al. Opioid-induced delay in gastric emptying: a peripheral mechanism in humans. Anesthesiology 1997;87:765–770.
6. Kehlet H, Dahl JB. The value of "multimodal" or "balanced analgesia" in postoperative pain treatment. Anesth Analg 1993;77:1048–1056.
7. Ashburn MA, Caplan RA, Carr DB, et al. Practice guidelines for acute pain management in the perioperative setting: an updated report by the American Society of Anesthesiologists Task Force on Acute Pain Management. Anesthesiology 2004;100: 1573–1581.
8. Elia N, Lysakowski C, Trame' r MR, et al. Does multimodal analgesia with acetaminophen, nonsteroidal anti-inflammatory drugs, or selective cyclooxygenase-2 inhibitors and patient-controlled analgesia morphine offer advantages over morphine alone? Anesthesiology 2005;103:1296–1304.
9. Cepeda MS, Carr DB, Miranda N, et al. Comparison of morphine, ketorolac, and their combination for postoperative pain: results from a large, randomized, double-blind trial. Anesthesiology. 2005;103:1225–1232.
10. Mutty CE, Jensen EJ, Manka MA, et al. Femoral nerve block for diaphyseal and distal femoral fractures in the emergency department. J Bone Joint Surg Am 2007;89:2599–2603.
11. Stewart B, Tudur Smith C, Teebay L, et al. Emergency department use of a continuous femoral nerve block for pain relief for fractured femur in children. Emerg Med J. 2007;24:113–114.
12. Hu P, Harmon D, Frizelle H. Patient comfort during regional anesthesia. J Clin Anesth 2007;19:67–74.
13. Bigeleisen P. Nerve puncture and apparent intraneural injection during ultrasound-guided axillary block does not invariably result in neurologic injury. Anesthesiology 2006;105: 779–783.

CHAPTER 41

Alzheimer's Disease and Anesthesia

Owen O'Sullivan

CASE FORMAT: REFLECTION

An 81-year-old, 50-kg woman presented to the emergency department following a fall at home. She was accompanied by her daughter, who witnessed her mother tripping and falling awkwardly on her right side. The patient was in obvious distress when her right hip was moved and appeared to have a swollen and bruised right thigh. She was agitated, and staff had difficulty obtaining a relevant history from her. The patient's vital signs were as follows: blood pressure, 170/80 mm Hg; heart rate, 104 beats per minute; temperature, 36.2°C; and respiratory rate, 20 breaths per minute.

A collateral history from the patient's daughter reveals a recent diagnosis of Alzheimer's disease (AD) following a steady decline in cognitive function over the last 3 years. The patient was also being treated for hypothyroidism and depression. She had an uneventful cholecystectomy 5 years ago. The patient was taking the following medications once daily: donepezil 5 mg, thyroxine 50 μg, and omeprazole 40 mg.

Clinical examination of respiratory and cardiovascular systems was noncontributory, and on neurological assessment, no sensory-motor deficits were found. Intravenous access was established, and samples were taken for full blood count, coagulation profile, urea and electrolytes, thyroid function, and glucose. IV morphine sulphate 5 mg was administered before transferring the patient to the radiology department. Radiology revealed a fractured neck of the femur on the right. A computed tomography brain scan was also performed, which showed no acute changes. The results of the laboratory investigations are summarized in Table 41.1. The patient consented for a bipolar hemiarthroplasty.

At the preoperative assessment, the anesthetist felt that the risks of performing a regional block outweighed the benefits, particularly as it appeared that the patient would be very uncooperative and was unlikely to reliably report symptoms (e.g., paraesthesia). The anesthetist elected to perform the procedure under general anesthetic, supplemented with regional anesthesia. Standard monitoring was applied preoperatively, consisting of pulse oximetry, electrocardiogram, and noninvasive blood pressure monitoring. Anesthesia was induced with fentanyl 50 μg, propofol 80 mg, and vecuronium 6 mg and was maintained with sevoflurane in a mixture of oxygen and air. An orotracheal tube was inserted. After induction, an episode of bradycar-

dia (32 beats per minute) was effectively treated with glycopyrrolate 200 mg, and six boluses of phenylephrine 50 μg were required to maintain a mean arterial pressure of ≥65 mm Hg. Oropharyngeal temperature was monitored, and a warming blanket as well as warmed intravenous fluids were used.

After the patient's blood pressure was stabilized, a right-sided femoral nerve block was performed, aseptically, under ultrasound guidance. A total of 20 mL of 0.25% levobupivicaine with 100 mg of clonidine was administered. The surgical procedure was well tolerated. Intraoperatively, proparacetamol 1g was administered intravenously.

On completion of the procedure, residual neuromuscular block was reversed with neostigmine (plus glycopyrronium). The patient was extubated at an appropriate point and transferred to the recovery room. The recovery staff felt she was grimacing and bringing her hand to her right thigh. She remained drowsy and disorientated when engaged, not responding to direct questioning about pain. Morphine 2 mg was given intravenously, and after about 50 minutes in recovery, the patient appeared settled and was transferred to the surgical ward. Postoperative analgesia was prescribed as paracetamol 1 g orally/rectally every 6 hours and morphine 5 mg (0.1 mg/kg) intramuscularly as required.

Over the next few days, the patient was more agitated than normal, and the nursing staff found it difficult to assess the patient's pain intensity. After 5 days, the agitation had settled, and the patient was transferred to a rehabilitation unit. She made a good recovery, however, her daughter felt she was more confused and less independent 3 weeks after surgery.

CASE DISCUSSION

AD is the most common form of dementia, affecting an estimated 5.1 million Americans. In the United States, an estimated $148 million is spent annually on AD and other dementias; 1 in 8 individuals over 65 years of age has this neurodegenerative disease, rising to almost half aged 85 or older.[1] With life expectancy ever increasing and no cure at hand, the impact of AD in day-to-day medical practice increases each year. The German physician Alois Alzheimer first described the disease in 1906. He noted microscopic changes at autopsy in the brain of a

TABLE 41.1 Results of Laboratory Investigations

Hb	10.3g/dL (↓)	Na$^+$	144 mmol/L
WCC	10.4×10^9/L	K$^+$	4.5 mmol/L
Plt	289×10^9/L	Urea	8.2 mmol/L (↑)
INR	1.1	Creatinine	122 μmol/L (↑)
APTT	38 seconds	TSH	3.3 mIU/L
Glucose	6.9 mmol/L	Thyroxine	145 nmol/L (↑)

APTT, activated partial thromboplastin time; Hb, hemoglobin; INR, international normalized ratio; K$^+$ potassium; Na$^+$, sodium; Plt, platelets; TSH, thyroid-stimulating hormone; WCC, white cell count.

51-year-old woman who died after 4 years of progressive dementia. His findings included abnormal clumps (amyloid plaques) and tangled bundles of fibers (neurofibrillary tangles), now considered the hallmarks of the disease that bears his name.

AD is a gradually progressive condition. Problems with memory are the first symptoms, with other aspects of cognition and behavior (difficulty performing everyday tasks, understanding, and speaking) developing later in the disease's course. Late-stage symptoms of AD such as anxiety, aggression, and wandering herald the inevitable requirement for total care.

The definitive diagnosis of AD can only be made on postmortem examination of the patient's brain. The *Diagnostic and Statistical Manual*, 4th edition[2] provides one example of many criteria used to diagnose probable AD (Table 41.2).

The exact pathogenesis of the disease remains unknown, however, it is thought that the loss of cholinergic neurons in the forebrain basal nuclei plays a central role in the characteristic memory and learning deficits.[3] The etiology of AD is also unknown, however, several risk factors have been identified. The most important of these is advancing age and family history (particularly in early-onset AD). A number of specific genes have been implicated in the development of early-onset AD, in which the onset of AD is before 65 years of age. Genetic mutations on chromosomes 1, 14, and 21 have been identified in many of these cases, inherited in an autosomal dominant fashion, which make up less than 5% of all AD cases. Polymorphisms of the apolipoprotein E gene on chromosome 19 have also been identified as altering susceptibility for AD.[4]

In recent years, there has been increasing interest regarding an Alzheimer's-anesthesia link. In vitro studies have shown halothane and isoflurane to promote amyloid oligomerization.[5,6] This process has been replicated in vivo in transgenic mice, however, it did not result in additional cognitive decline in cognitively impaired mice.[7] To date, human studies have shown no conclusive link between exposure and risk of developing AD.[8,9] Such a link, if one did exist, would be very difficult to demonstrate, largely because anesthesia is administered to facilitate surgery (often emergency), and isolating its effect from other elements such as the surgical stress response can be difficult. Although the patient described herein showed subjective evidence of deterioration postoperatively, keep in mind that AD is a progressive disorder, and deterioration is inevitable.

TABLE 41.2 Diagnostic Criteria for Alzheimer's Type Dementia

Multiple Cognitive Deficits Involving

A. Memory impairment and one or more of the following:
   - Aphasia
   - Apraxia
   - Agnosia
   - Disturbance of executive functioning

B. With impairment and a significant decline in social or occupational functioning as a result of these deficits

C. A gradual onset and continuing cognitive decline

D. Not caused by
   - Other central nervous system conditions that cause progressive deficits in memory and cognition (e.g., cerebrovascular disease, Parkinson's disease)
   - Systemic conditions known to cause dementia (e.g., hypercalcemia, hypothyroidism)
   - Substance-induced conditions

E. Not occurring exclusively during the course of a delirium

F. Not better explained by another psychiatric disorder (e.g., a major depressive disorder, schizophrenia)

Adapted from American Psychiatric Association. Diagnostic and Statistical Manual of Mental Disorders, 4th ed. Arlington, VA: American Psychiatric Association, 1994.

TABLE 41.3 General Considerations Regarding Anesthesia for the Elderly

Pharmacological Considerations	Other General Considerations
Reduced minimum alveolar concentration	Increased likelihood of ischemic heart disease and cerebrovascular insufficiency
Reduced intravenous anesthetic dose requirements	Decreased lung volumes
Increased proportion of body fat	Decreased response to hypercapnia and hypoxemia
Reduction in skeletal muscle	Increased closing capacity
Reduced renal clearance	Increased incidence of atelectasis and postoperative respiratory tract infections
Reduced hepatic metabolism and albumin production	Deep vein thrombosis is more common
Increased α-glycoprotein production	Increased incidence of diabetes mellitus
Of particular importance in positioning:	Impaired hearing
Limited joint movement	Increased intraoperative heat loss
Weak bones	
Thin skin	

There is no cure yet for AD. The mainstay of symptomatic treatment at present is the use of cholinesterase inhibitors (donepezil in this case), which increase the amount of acetylcholine available in the depleted cholinergic nerves. In terms of anesthetic considerations, these drugs have systemic cholinergic features. This can translate into reduced heart rate variability and increased susceptibility for bradycardia, as we saw in this patient. Extreme bradycardia should be treated with an anticholinergic drug, which does not cross the blood-brain barrier (e.g., glycopyrrolate). Cholinesterase inhibitors also appear to antagonize the effects of neuromuscular blocking agents.[11]

Preoperative assessment should involve the patient's family or caregivers, as the patient's ability to understand, communicate, and cooperate may be significantly impaired. Explanations and questions should be simple and stated in a clear fashion. Multiple comorbidities are common in this age group, and time may be required to establish these as well as to ascertain the patient's regular medications. In a trauma patient with poor communication, efforts should be made to rule out concealed injury (e.g., rib fractures, intracranial trauma). If agitation is a major feature, small amounts of judiciously administered benzodiazepine may be required.

Acquiring consent for patients with AD can prove difficult. It is up to the doctor to establish the patient's capacity to understand information and make an informed decision or seek consent from a relevant other. There is no clear standard or formal guideline available at present. Wishes of relatives and any advance directives should be taken into consideration. Legal aspects relating to consent also vary in different jurisdictions. A diagnosis of dementia does not automatically assume incompetence. AD is progressive; therefore, in early stages, patients will retain enough cognitive capacity to consent themselves. The difficult task is to establish at what point a patient be protected from making a "bad decision." It is not clear whether the patient in this case retained sufficient cognitive function to make an informed decision or whether an effort to establish competence was made. This was certainly a deficiency in her management. It would seem unlikely that the otherwise uncooperative, agitated patient was able to give a meaningful consent.

In preparing for anesthesia, each patient should be evaluated on an individual basis taking into consideration comorbid conditions and the procedure itself. Regional techniques can be challenging because of poor cooperation and agitation, however, they allow minimal disturbance of mental capacities. Sedative premedications may worsen confusion and agitation. Monitoring should take into account potential of poor functional reserve. General considerations of anesthesia in the elderly should be taken into account (Table 41.3).

Pain management may be challenging and is often undertreated in elderly patients with cognitive impairment. One study of elderly patients posthip fracture showed that cognitively impaired patients received only one-third the amount of opioid analgesia compared with cognitively intact individuals.[12] Possible reasons for this include poor pain assessment in patients with communication difficulties and concern for using analgesics, which may deteriorate cognitive function or other comorbidities. This is despite the fact that inadequate analgesia can lead to poorer clinical outcomes, cognitive dysfunction, depression, longer hospital stays, and compromised pulmonary function.[13]

Appropriate pain assessment tools should be utilized, using self-reporting (preferable) or nonverbal cues as appropriate to patient's degree of understanding and communication. Facial expression may be affected in late dementia adding further complication to assessment. Once an appropriate tool has been selected, it should be used consistently with regular reassessment. Assessment should include duration of pain relief, ability to ambulate and adequately cough, side effects, and patient satisfaction. Analgesia using an epidural route, local anesthetic infiltration, or peripheral nerve blockade can reduce opioid requirement. If opioids are required, an appropriate route of administration should be chosen. Patient-controlled analgesia may be beyond the cognitive or physical ability of the patient. Intramuscular injection results in slower absorption and possible toxicity with repeated dosing and should therefore be avoided. The use of nonsteroidal anti-inflammatory drugs is often restricted in the elderly population because of altered metabolism and excretion leading to drug accumulation.

Although regional anesthesia techniques were welcome in this case scenario, performing them in an uncooperative patient or under general anaesthesia is questionable. Ultrasound guidance does not protect from intraneural (or intravascular) injection. A better option in this patient would have been an iliacus block. Spread of local anesthetic beneath the iliacus fascia produces a high success rate of anesthesia of both the femoral and lateral cutaneous nerve of the thigh (which innervates the anterolateral thigh, the incision area).[14] As this is a compartment block, it can be performed safely in anesthetized patients. The needle insertion point is high at the patient's thigh in the gutter between the sartorius and quadriceps muscle. A blunt needle is inserted perpendicular to the skin. An initial loss of resistance is identified on penetrating the fascia lata. A second loss of resistance indicates penetration of the fascia iliaca. Performed preoperatively in this case, it would have avoided the need for systemic opioids with associated side effects. To extend the duration of the block, a continuous iliacus block could have been subsequently administered under general anesthesia, leaving an epidural catheter in place and using a standard infusion of local anesthetic solution (e.g., levobupivacaine 0.2% titrated to effect).

KEY MESSAGES

1. AD is increasing in prevalence with increasing life expectancy.

2. Cholinesterase inhibitors, the mainstay of treatment, have anesthetic implications.

3. Anesthesia should be tailored on an individual basis taking into consideration the degree of patient cooperation as well as comorbid conditions. Patient consent and pain management may be particularly challenging.

QUESTIONS

1. Has anesthesia been shown to cause AD?

   Answer: Despite significant interest into the possibility of anesthesia causing AD, to date, there is no evidence of such a link in humans. However, even if there were a link between the two, this would be very hard to demonstrate because it is difficult to isolate anesthetic factors from other factors surrounding surgery (e.g., pain, surgical stress responses). In vitro studies using halothane and isoflurane have resulted in cellular processes (amyloid oligomerization) that are similar to those thought to cause AD.

2. Can patients with AD consent to surgical procedures?

   Answer: Keep in mind that a diagnosis of dementia does not automatically assume incompetence. AD is progressive, and early in the disease, patients may retain enough cognitive capacity to consent themselves. It is the responsibility of the treating doctor to establish whether this capacity has been retained or if consent should be sought from a relevant other. There are no guidelines available at present to aid this process, and importantly, legal aspects of consent vary across different jurisdictions. The wishes of family members and advance directives should also be considered.

3. What elements are important in the postoperative pain management of a patient with AD?

Answer: Appropriate and consistent pain assessment tools should be employed in managing analgesia in patients with AD. Self-reporting is still preferable, however, nonverbal cues may need to be utilized as the disease and communicative abilities deteriorate. Keep in mind that the commonly used nonverbal cue of facial expression will also be affected later in the disease. When an appropriate tool is established, it should be applied regularly, especially during movement and coughing. Side effects attributable to analgesics should also be noted. Opioid-sparing measures such as the use of epidural or peripheral nerve blocks should decrease the likelihood of such side effects. If opioids are required, the most appropriate means of administering them should be chosen. Patient-controlled analgesia devices require an adequate level of cognitive function and physical dexterity to operate. Pharmacologic alterations that occur in the elderly should also be considered.

References

1. Alzheimer's Association. Every 72 seconds someone in America develops Alzheimer's. Alzheimer's Disease Facts and Figures 2007. Available at www.alz.org. Accessed May 17, 2008.
2. American Psychiatric Association. Diagnostic and Statistical Manual of Mental Disorders, 4th ed. Arlington, VA: American Psychiatric Association, 1994.
3. Coyle JT, Price DL, DeLong MR. Alzheimer's disease: a disorder of cortical cholinergic innervation. Science 1983;219:1184–1190.
4. Farrer LA, Cupples LA, Haines JL, et al. Effects of age, sex, and ethnicity on the association between apolipoprotein E genotype and Alzheimer disease. A meta-analysis. APOE and Alzheimer disease meta-analysis consortium. JAMA 1997;278:1349–1356.
5. Eckenhoff RG, Johansson JS, Wei H, et al. Inhaled anesthetic enhancement of amyloid-beta oligomerization and cytotoxicity. Anesthesiology 2004;101:703–709.
6. Xie Z, Dong Y, Maeda U, et al. The inhalation anesthetic isoflurane induces a vicious cycle of apoptosis and amyloid beta-protein accumulation. J Neurosci 2007;27:1247–1254.
7. Bianchi SL, Tran T, Liu C, et al. Brain and behavior changes in 12-month-old Tg2576 and nontransgenic mice exposed to anesthetics. Neurobiol Aging 2008;29:1002–1010.
8. Gasparini M, Vanacore N, Schiaffini C, et al. A case-control study on Alzheimer's disease and exposure to anesthesia. Neurol Sci 2002;23:11–14.
9. Bohnen NI, Warner M, Kokmen E, et al. Alzheimer's disease and cumulative exposure to anesthesia: a case-control study. J Am Geriatr Soc 1994;42:198–201.
10. Livingston G, Katona C. How useful are cholinesterase inhibitors in the treatment of Alzheimer's disease? A number needed to treat analysis. Int J Geriatr Psychiatry 2000;15:203–207.
11. Sánchez Morillo J, Demartini Ferrari A, Roca de Togores López A. Interaction of donepezil and muscular blockers in Alzheimer's disease. Rev Esp Anestesiol Reanim 2003;50:97–100.
12. Morrison RS, Siu AL. A comparison of pain and its treatment in advanced dementia and cognitively intact patients with hip fracture. J Pain Symptom Manage 2000;19:240–248.
13. Karani R, Meier DE. Systemic pharmacologic postoperative pain management in the geriatric orthopaedic patient. Clin Orthop Relat Res 2004;:26–34.
14. Barrett J, Harmon D, Loughnane F, et al. Peripheral nerve blocks and peri-operative pain relief. 1st ed. Philadelphia: Saunders; 2004.

Sickle Cell Disease

Siun Burke

FORMAT: REFLECTION

A 4-year-old boy was scheduled on the emergency trauma list for a right hand nerve and tendon repair. The boy was of West African origin and had only recently arrived in the country. He sustained a right hand laceration 6 hours previously when he ran into a glass door. On preoperative assessment, the child was pale and irritable; he was complaining of thirst, as he had been kept fasting since arrival to the hospital in preparation for surgery. At 15 kg, he was in the 40th percentile for weight. His mother said he lost about "a cup full" of blood earlier.

There were multiple venipuncture marks on the child's left arm; the pediatrician had difficulty with venipuncture and decided that as the child's operation was imminent, he should have a cannula inserted and blood taken under general anesthesia instead.

Finally, the anesthetist asked the child's mother if there was any family history of blood diseases or problems with general anesthesia. She had limited English and was anxiously trying to calm her son. The child's mother said he was from a healthy family, although he seemed to get coughs and colds more frequently than her other children. He never had a general anesthetic, but other family members had undergone uneventful anesthesia.

Two hours later, after 8 hours of fasting, the operating room finally became available. With routine monitors in place, the child had an uneventful inhalational induction, and a 20-gauge cannula was inserted in his left forearm. A laryngeal mask airway was placed, and the child resumed spontaneous respiration of an oxygen, nitrous oxide, and sevoflurane mixture. The fraction of inspired oxygen was 0.3. Maintenance fluids were commenced at 50 mL per hour. A tourniquet was inflated to 100 mm Hg above the patient's systolic blood pressure, and the surgeon proceeded to repair the tendons and nerves. On closer inspection, the surgeon discovered more extensive injuries than expected and informed the anesthetist that he would require at least 2 more hours of operating time.

An hour later, the child started to become hypotensive. His blood pressure was 70/34 mm Hg and he was tachycardic with a heart rate of 139 beats per minute. His oxygen saturation read 92%, and his temperature was 33.2°C. Information for the patient's arterial blood analysis is shown in Table 42.1.

The patient's inspired oxygen concentration was increased to 70%, he was volume resuscitated with crystalloid and red cell concentrate, actively rewarmed, and the surgery was expedited.

In the recovery room, the child complained of severe pain and continued to have a low oxygen saturation of 91% and PO_2 was 65 mm Hg.

Hemoglobin analysis confirmed that the child had sickle cell disease (SCD). He was transferred to the high-dependency unit, managed with supplemental oxygen, fluid and blood resuscitation, and judicious opioid analgesia.

Two days later, the patient developed shortness of breath, a wheeze, and a high temperature of 39.4°C. His chest radiograph showed a new right upper lobe pulmonary infiltrate (Fig. 42.1). This finding was diagnosed as acute chest syndrome (ACS), and the child was started on ceftriaxone, clarithromycin, and regular paracetamol.

On postoperative day 5, the patient was discharged to the general ward. His family was counseled regarding his sickle cell status, its implications for other family members, and for any future illnesses and general anesthetics the child may have.

CASE DISCUSSION

Discussion points:

1. Pathophysiology of SCD
2. Preoperative screening for sickle cell status
3. Optimal perioperative management SCD
4. Acute chest syndrome

PATHOPHYSIOLOGY OF SCD

SCD is an autosomal recessive disease that results from the substitution of valine for glutamic acid at position 6 of the β-globin gene, leading to production of a defective form of hemoglobin, hemoglobin S (HbS). Patients who are homozygous for the HbS gene have sickle cell disease. Patients who are heterozygous for the HbS gene are carriers of the condition (sickle cell trait). Under stressful conditions, carriers may display some clinical manifestations. If both members of a couple are carriers, they have a 25% risk of producing a child who is homozygous for the HbS gene.

TABLE 42.1 Arterial Blood Analysis

		Normal Values
PO_2	9.2 kPa	11–14 kPa
PCO_2	8.5 kPa	4–6.5 kPa
Ph	7.19	7.35–7.45
Bicarbonate	19 mEq/L	22–26 mEq/L
Lactate	4 mmol/L	<2 mmol/L
Hemoglobin	6.4 g/dL	10–12 g/dL

The hallmark of SCD is a group of devastating symptoms known collectively as a *sickle cell crisis*. Sickle cell crises are episodes of pain that occur with varying frequency and are usually followed by remission.[1]

In the case history presented herein, the fact that the patient's siblings were well and underwent uneventful general anesthesia in the past does not preclude this child from having a sickle cell crisis, as the risk of heterozygous parents producing a homozygous child is 25%.

Deoxygenated HbS is 50 times less soluble in blood than deoxygenated adult hemoglobin. Deoxygenation of HbS leads to hydrophobic interactions between HbS molecules causing the classic sickle shape. The sickle-shaped red blood cells have reduced deformability, thereby obstructing the microvasculature. This results in vicious cycle of tissue hypoxia and acidosis, which promotes further sickling.[2] Also the impaired stability of HbS leads to increased breakdown of the molecule resulting in the release of large amounts of toxic iron and heme compounds into the cell. This produces oxidant damage to the cell membrane, disruption of the phospholipid bilayer, protein distribution, and normal membrane function. This results in increased adhesion to the vascular endothelium inducing endothelial damage and dysfunction. The endothelial regulatory balance between vasoconstriction and vasodilatation and pro- and anti-coagulation is disturbed, leading to ischemia, vaso-occlusion, and pain.[2]

Preoperative Screening for Sickle Cell Status

Sickle cell disease is a genetic disorder affecting diverse populations. Those at risk include African, Hispanic Mediterranean, Middle Eastern, and Asian Indian. The perioperative period is a well-recognized and predictable time of disease exacerbations.[3] Preoperative screening of at-risk populations is recommended as a method to decrease perioperative morbidity. A solubility test is used to screen for SCD, a deoxygenating agent is added to the blood, and if 25% or more of the hemoglobin is HbS, the cells will sickle and form a turbid suspension. For confirmation, abnormal samples undergo further testing, either hemoglobin electrophoresis or high-pressure liquid chromatography.[4]

The National Institute for Clinical Excellence guideline on preoperative testing, June 2003, states that all patients of ethnic origin considered to be at risk, whose sickle cell status is unknown, should be offered screening with genetic counseling before anesthesia and surgery.[5] The advantages and disadvantages of preoperative screening for sickle cell status are summarized in Table 42.2. A preoperative screening test for the child in the case history presented herein would have detected his sickle cell status and allowed the anesthetist to tailor an anesthetic that would have avoided any factors that precipitate sickling.

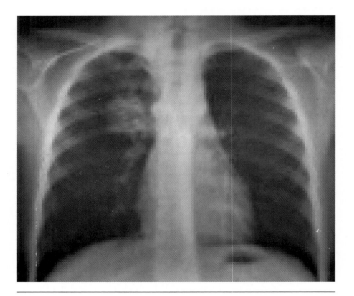

Figure 42.1 • Chest Radiograph Showing a Right Upper Lobe Infiltrate.

TABLE 42.2 Preoperative Screening for Sickle Cell Status

Advantages of Preoperative Screening

- Avoids the potential disaster of a perioperative sickle cell crisis in a patient with undiagnosed sickle cell disease.

- As heterozygous parents and siblings may be asymptomatic, there may not be a family history in patients with sickle cell disease.

Disadvantages of Preoperative Screening

- Low yield of positive test results.

- Low risk of a crisis if every patient considered at risk for sickle cell disease receives a well-conducted general anesthetic avoiding factors that precipitate sickling.

- Risks of indiscriminate preoperative screening resulting in unnecessary surgical cancellations, surgical delays, duplication of screening, and misdiagnosis.

- Children often consider venipuncture to be the worst part of the hospital experience.

- Lack of appropriate medical follow-up and parental counseling in the busy perioperative period.

- Increased diversity of mixed-race populations with low accuracy of self-reported ethnicity.

- Cost of screening.

The patient had been fasting for several hours preoperatively without intravenous fluids, and intraoperative maintenance fluids were minimal without adjustment for fasting time or blood loss. A tourniquet was used for more than 2 hours, which contributed to hypoxia and acidosis. The operating room was cold, there was no warming apparatus, and the child's temperature dropped significantly. His hemoglobin level was not checked preoperatively.

Optimal Perioperative Management of Patients With SCD

AVOID HYPOXIA

As many patients with SCD have impaired oxygen delivery secondary to pulmonary damage, widespread vasculopathy, increased blood viscosity, anemia, impaired vascular regulation, and disturbed nitrous oxide signaling. Controlled ventilation with a high-inspired oxygen concentration would have improved oxygenation in this patient's case.

Although in vitro evidence of increased sickling in the presence of acidosis exists, no benefit has been detected from alkalinization. Tourniquet use may increase hypoxia and acidosis, but there are reports of uneventful use in SCD, and each case should be considered independently.[6] Judicious use of a tourniquet at minimal inflation pressures and for the minimum time possible may have reduced the degree of acidosis evident in the child presented in this case.

HEMOGLOBIN DILUTION

Intravascular dehydration increases hemoglobin concentration and consequently the rate of sickling. All patients should be adequately hydrated preoperatively, and careful attention must be paid to intraoperative fluid balance. However, there is no evidence to support aggressive fluid hydration of patients with SCD.[6] In the case described herein, the child should have been commenced on intravenous fluids preoperatively with careful calculation of pre- and intraoperative fluid deficits.

DILUTION OF SICKLE CELLS

Perioperative red cell transfusion remains a controversial topic. A large prospective randomized trial published in 1995 found no benefit to aggressive transfusion (HbS <30) compared with a conservative transfusion strategy, but there was a higher incidence of transfusion-related complications[7] (Table 42.3).

AVOID HYPOTHERMIA

Hypothermia has been suggested as a perioperative trigger for SCD complications, however, there is no publication to demonstrate a link. As normothermia is a basic standard of anesthetic care for the general surgical population, it should also be a goal for patients with SCD.

A preoperative diagnosis of SCD in the case presented herein would have ensured a careful approach to fluid management, accounting for preoperative blood loss and duration of fasting, minimum use of a tourniquet, and strict maintenance of the child's temperature throughout the procedure.

ACS

ACS is defined as a new lobar infiltration on a chest radiograph accompanied by fever greater than 38.5°C, respiratory

TABLE 42.3 Perioperative Transfusion in Sickle Cell Disease[8]

Group 1	Children who are currently well and undergoing minor surgery (myringotomy)	No transfusion
Group 2	Children who are currently well and undergoing intermediate surgery (tonsillectomy)	May require top-up transfusion to Hb 8–10 g/dL, HbS level will remain elevated
Group 3	Children with a history of major SCD complications (stroke, ACS) or a history of hospital admissions for painful crises or children undergoing major surgery (intra-abdominal or thoracic procedures)	Exchange transfusion to achieve HbS level <30% Total Hb should not exceed 12 g/dL

ACS, acute chest syndrome; Hb, hemoglobin; Hbs, hemoglobin S; SCD indicates sickle cell disease.
Adapted from Sickle Cell Disease Transfusion; Clinical Guideline Great Ormond Street Hospital for Children, NHS Trust.[8]

distress, or chest pain.[9] It is a frequent cause of hospital admission and the leading cause of mortality in young adult SCD patients. Repeated episodes predispose individuals to chronic pulmonary disease including pulmonary hypertension. The incidence following invasive surgical procedures such as intra-abdominal procedures or joint replacement is approximately 10% to 15%.[10] Risk factors include HbSS genotype, low fetal haemoglobin (HbF) concentrations, and high steady-state leukocyte and hemoglobin concentrations. Nearly half of the patients are in the hospital for a diagnosis other than ACS, with superimposition of the disorder during hospital care. Specific causes can be identified in approximately 38% of patients, infections in 29%, and fat embolism in 9%. Infections are equally divided between bacterial viral mycoplasma and chlamydial infections suggesting a macrolide antibiotic as an important treatment adjunct.[10]

The pathophysiology of ACS is linked to hypoxic pulmonary vasoconstriction. The combination of regional hypoxia and vasoconstriction will not only increase HbS polymerization and sickling but will also increase capillary transit time causing exacerbation of endothelial dysfunction via mediators such as hypoxia, cytokines, and free radical species.

ACS is typically detected 48 hours postoperatively. Prevention requires early mobilization, good control of surgical pain, incentive spirometry, physiotherapy, and attention to pulmonary function. Rates of complications and mortality figures are age dependent, increasing in individuals over 20 years of age.

TABLE 42.4 Causes of Acute Chest Syndrome

Infectious Causes	Noninfectious Causes
Bacteria	
• Pneumococcus	• Pulmonary infarction
• Gram-negative bacteria	• Hypoventilation secondary to rib infarction or opioid administration
• Chlamydia pneumonia	
• Mycoplasma pneumonia	
	• Fat embolism
	• Pulmonary edema
Viruses	
• Respiratory syncytial virus	
• Parainfluenza	
• Influenza	

Adapted from Credit Valley Hospital Clinical Practice Guideline. Management of Sickle Cell Disease in Children, 2004.[9]

Treatment involves supplemental oxygenation and ventilatory support as required; bronchodilators should be used to treat bronchospasm and antibiotics if pneumonia supervenes. Inhaled nitric oxide may improve alveolar-arterial oxygen gradients and reduce pulmonary artery pressure (Table 42.4).

KEY MESSAGES

1. Sickle cell disease is an autosomal recessive disease that results in production of a defective form of hemoglobin, hemoglobin S (HbS). Deoxygenation of HbS causes the classic sickle shape with reduced deformability that obstructs the microvasculature.

2. According to the National Institute for Clinical Excellence guidelines, all patients of ethnic origin considered to be at risk, whose sickle cell status is unknown, should be offered screening with genetic counseling before anesthesia and surgery.

3. Optimal perioperative management of patients with SCD requires avoiding factors that may precipitate a sickle cell crisis (e.g., hypoxia, acidosis, intravascular dehydration, hypothermia, and venous stasis).

4. ACS is the leading cause of mortality in young adults with SCD. It is defined as a new lobar infiltration on chest radiograph accompanied by fever greater than 38.5°C, respiratory distress, or chest pain.

QUESTIONS

1. Which organs are affected by sickle cell disease?

Answer: Sickle cell disease is a multisystemic disease which impacts many major organs. The kidneys may undergo hypertrophy, develop tubular acidosis, tubular deficiencies, proteinuria, nephritic syndrome, and end stage renal disease. The lungs develop pulmonary hypertension in 5% to 30% of patients. The spleen may undergo autoinfarction and hyposplenism. Skin manifestations include chronic leg ulcers and there may be osteonecrosis of the femoral and humeral heads. The eye may develop retinitis proliferans.

2. By what mechanism does HbS arise?

Answer: HbS arises when a single nucleotide substitution CTG for GAG in the sixth codon of the beta globin gene results in the substitution of phenylalanine for glutamic acid. One in 14 people of African heritage are asymptomatic carriers of sickle cell anaemia. One in 700 newborns of African heritage is affected by sickle cell anaemia.

3. What are the benefits of hydroxyurea treatment in sickle cell disease?

Answer: Hydroxyurea is a cytotoxic drug that reduces the production of red cells containing a high level of sickle haemoglobin which tend to arise from rapidly dividing precursors and favours the production of fetal haemoglobin.[11] The number of white blood cells and platelets are also reduced. The metabolism of hydroxyurea results in the release of nitric oxide which also stimulates HbF production. Increased concentration of HbF results in decreased red cell sludging and vaso-occlusion with subsequent decreased ischaemia and necrosis. An increased production of nitric oxide results in more normal vascular tone and decreased pulmonary artery hypertension. In a study of 299 patients by Charache et al.,[11] the incidence of painful crises reduced from 4.5 to 2.5 per year; the rates of acute chest syndrome and blood transfusion also reduced considerably. After 9 years, there was a 40% reduction in mortality in those who received hydroxyurea. Recommendations for hydroxyurea therapy include patients with frequent pain episodes, history of acute chest syndrome, other severe vaso-occlusive events, or severe symptomatic anaemia.

References

1. Koshy M, Weiner SJ, Miller ST, et al. Surgery and anesthesia in sickle cell disease. Cooperative study of sickle cell diseases. Blood 1995;86:3676–3684.
2. Firth PG. Anaesthesia for peculiar cells—a century of sickle cell disease. BJA advance access published on September 1, 2005. Br J Anaesth 2005;95:287–299.
3. Buck J, Davies SC. Surgery in sickle cell disease. Hematol Oncol Clin North Am 2005;19:897802.
4. Crawford MW, Galton S, Abdelhaleem M. Preoperative screening for sickle cell disease in children: clinical implications. Can J Anesth 2005;52:1058–1063.
5. The use of routine preoperative tests for elective surgery. NICE Guidelines, June 2003.

6. Tobin JR, Butterworth J. Sickle cell disease: dogma, science, and clinical care. Anesth Analg 2004;98:283–284.

7. Buck J, Casbard A, Llewelyn C, et al. Preoperative transfusion in sickle cell disease: a survey of practice in England. Eur J Haematol 2005;75:14–21(8).

8. Transfusion guidelines for neonates and older children. Br J Haema 2004;124(4):433–453.

9. Credit Valley Hospital, Clinical practice guideline: Management of Sickle Cell Disease in Children. 2004.

10. Stuart MJ, Nagel RL. Sickle cell disease. Lancet 2004;364:1343–1360.

11. Charache S, Barton FB, Moore RD, et al. Hydroxyurea and sickle cell anemia. Clinical utility of a myelosuppressive "switching" agent. The Multicenter Study of Hydroxyurea in Sickle Cell Anemia. *Medicine (Baltimore)* 1996;75:300–326.

CHAPTER 43

Anaphylaxis

Mansoor A. Siddiqui

CASE FORMAT: STEP BY STEP

A 27-year-old man was admitted to the accident and emergency department, feeling febrile, with a 1-day history of abdominal pain, nausea, and vomiting for the last 12 hours. He had been fit and healthy in the past and was not taking any medication. The patient smoked 10 cigarettes per day, and drank alcohol occasionally. He had not been eating or drinking for 8 hours before admission and had vomited twice during the preceding 3 hours. He had not undergone surgery in the past and had no known drug allergies.

The patient's examination revealed the following: temperature, 37.8°C; dehydration, mild; heart rate, 110 beats per minute; blood pressure, 90/50 mm Hg; respiratory rate, 20 breaths per minute on auscultation; and normal vesicular breathing. On abdominal palpation, there was tenderness in the right iliac fossa. The patient's airway was evaluated as Mallampati grade I with normal dentition. Investigations showed the following: hemoglobin, 16.8 g/dL; hematocrit, 0.41; white blood cell count, 13.5×10^9; and platelets, 198×10.

The patient was diagnosed as having acute appendicitis and was scheduled for emergency open appendicectomy by the surgical team. An 18-gauge intravenous (IV) cannula was inserted and fluid resuscitation commenced. After receiving 500 mL of Hartmann's solution, the patient's heart rate decreased to 90 beats per minute, and his blood pressure increased to 110/60 mm Hg. A dose of prophylactic antibiotic (co-amoxiclav, 1.2 g) was administered at the surgeon's request and the patient was transferred to the operating room.

After preoxygenation for 3 minutes, anesthesia was achieved using fentanyl 100 μg, propofol 250 mg, and suxamethonium 100 mg as part of a rapid sequence induction. A cuffed oroendotracheal tube (inner diameter, 8.5 mm) was inserted without difficulty and fixed at 23 cm after auscultating for bilateral air entry. Atracurium 40 mg was administered 5 minutes later.

Two minutes after atracurium administration, the patient's airway pressure was noted to increase rendering his lungs progressively more difficult to ventilate. On examination, his face was flushed, and urticarial rashes were observed on his skin. His heart rate was 120 beats per minute, and his blood pressure was 80/40 mm Hg. On auscultation, the patient's chest was wheezy, and air entry decreased bilaterally. Marked facial swelling occurred in 2 to 3 minutes.

What is the differential diagnosis?

Clinically, it is neither possible nor necessary to differentiate between anaphylaxis and anaphylactic reactions at the time of presentation, as both respond to the same treatment. Symptoms of anaphylaxis have their onset within minutes but occasionally can occur late following exposure to the causative agent. Symptoms can be masked under general anesthesia (Table 43.1).

Individuals with a history of atopy, asthma, or food allergies appear to be at increased risk of latex allergy but possibly not anaphylaxis to neuromuscular-blocking drugs.[5,6] There is evidence that patients receiving β-blockers (showing unopposed α-adrenergic effects and therefore being more resistant to adrenaline) and those with asthma suffer more severe reactions.[13,14]

Additional differential diagnoses to consider include vasovagal reactions. They can mimic anaphylaxis and are characterized by hypotension, bradycardia, pallor, weakness, nausea, vomiting, and diaphoresis. Urticaria, pruritus, angioedema, tachycardia, and bronchospasm, however, are not vasovagal responses.

Acute respiratory decompensation from severe asthma attacks, foreign body aspiration, and pulmonary embolism can mimic respiratory symptoms suggestive of anaphylaxis, but other characteristics such as pruritus, urticaria, and angioedema are lacking.

Seizure disorders, myocardial infarction, and arrhythmias can be readily distinguished clinically. Patients with hereditary angioedema do not exhibit pruritus and urticaria; a family history is usually present.

It is likely that this patient has had an allergic reaction or anaphylaxis to one of the substances he received in the perioperative period.

What is the pathophysiology of anaphylaxis?

Any drug administered in the perioperative period can cause a severe immune-mediated hypersensitivity reaction after exposure to a foreign protein (antigen) that stimulates immunoglobulin E (IgE) production. Non–immune-mediated reactions account for 30% to 40% of hypersensitivity reactions.[4] They neither involve IgE nor prior exposure to this antigen.

It is not possible to clinically differentiate between immune and non–immune-mediated reactions. Anaphylactoid reactions are more likely to involve skin features (94% vs. 72%),[5,6] and anaphylactic reactions are more severe.[5]

The time course of anaphylaxis can be classified as uniphasic, protracted, or biphasic. Reactions typically follow a

TABLE 43.1 Clinical Manifestations of Suspected Anaphylactic Reactions

Organ System	Symptom	Sign	Specific Sign During Anesthesia
Cutaneous	Itching	Rash, erythema, flushing, urticaria, angioedema	
Respiratory	Lump in the throat Hoarseness Dysphonia Dyspnea	Stridor Wheezing Pulmonary edema Cyanosis	Difficult to ventilate ↑Peak airway pressure SpO_2 ↑$EtCO_2$
Cardiovascular	Angina Light-headedness Faintness	Tachycardia Arrhythmias Hypotension Cardiac arrest	↓ $EtCO_2$ ↑Hematocrit ST segment, T-wave changes
Gastrointestinal	Nausea Abdominal pain	Vomiting Diarrhea	

Adapted from Soetens FM, Vercauteren MP. Allergic reactions during anaesthesia: diagnosis and treatment. Jurnalul Roman de Anestezie Terapie Intensiva 2008;15:43–50.

uniphasic course, that is, they respond rapidly to treatment and do not recur. In some patients, symptoms may fail to improve or may worsen as the effect of adrenaline wears off (protracted anaphylaxis); however, 20% will be biphasic in nature.[7] The second phase usually occurs after an asymptomatic period of 1 to 8 hours, but there may be a delay of up to 24 hours. Prolonged observation in these cases is needed.[8]

How would this case be managed intraoperatively?

Anaphylaxis is a medical emergency that requires immediate treatment. Even a severe anaphylactic reaction is associated with a prompt and successful response to appropriate treatment in most patients. This patient should be managed aggressively according to the existing Association of Anaesthetists of Great Britain and Ireland guidelines:[3]

1. Stop administration of all agents likely to have caused anaphylaxis.
2. Call for help.
3. Maintain airway, give 100% oxygen, and lay patient flat with legs elevated.
4. Give epinephrine (adrenaline). This may be given intramuscularly in a dose of 0.5 mg to 1.0 mg (0.5 to 1 mL of 1:1,000) and may be repeated every 10 minutes according to the arterial pressure and pulse until improvement occurs. Alternatively, 50 to 100 μg intravenously (0.5 to 1 mL of 1:10,000) over 1 minute has been recommended for hypotension with titration of further doses as required.
5. Start rapid IV infusion with colloids or crystalloids. Adult patients may require 2 to 4 liters of crystalloids.

Secondary therapy consists of:

1. Antihistamines (chlorpheniramine 10 to 20 mg by slow IV infusion)

2. Corticosteroids (100 to 500 mg hydrocortisone IV slowly)
3. Bronchodilators may be required for persistent bronchospasm

The patient was immediately commenced on 100% oxygen. With help on the way, the adrenaline ([1:10,000], 50–100 μg over 1 minute) was administered, followed by two additional increments. A rapid infusion of 0.9% sodium chloride was started. The patient was positioned supine with the legs slightly elevated. At this point, his blood pressure increased to 100/50 mm Hg. His airway pressure normalized, and ventilation of his lungs was once again easy. The surgery was restarted, and the patient was stabilized, chlorpheniramine 10 mg was administered by slow IV infusion. Hydrocortisone 100 mg was administered intravenously. At this point, the patient was hemodynamically stable with a heart rate of 90 beats per minute, blood pressure of 110/70 mm Hg, and clear chest on auscultation. His skin looked normal. Surgery proceeded to laparotomy because of peritonitis. The surgeon requested muscle relaxation.

What would be the additional management of choice?

In terms of anaphylactic risk, neuromuscular blocking agents (NMBAs) could be classified into three groups: high risk (succinylcholine and rocuronium), intermediate risk (vecuronium, pancuronium), and low risk (mivacurium, atracurium, cisatracurium).[2]

As cross-reactivity between NMBAs occurs in up to 60% of patients, no other agent should be used without prior testing.[2] Thus, the best additional prophylactic strategy would be to avoid using NMBAs, which implies an attempt to deepen anesthesia, taking advantage of muscle relaxation produced by inhalational agents. If this step fails to provide adequate relaxation, and bearing in mind that succinylcholine is the most likely culprit in this scenario, a short-acting low-anaphylactic-risk NMBA such as mivacurium may be used. This drug may have the extra advantage of not requiring reversal, thus minimizing further histamine release. Pretreatment with antihistamines and corticosteroids in this case may limit the severity of potential reactions, although there is currently little evidence to support their routine use for this sole purpose.

Following administration of mivacurium 8 mg, surgery was finished quickly, and the patient's trachea was extubated uneventfully.

A blood sample (5–10 mL) was taken in three plain bottles for mast cell tryptase measurement. The first sample was taken about 15 minutes after the event, the second after 1 hour, and the third after 6 hours. The samples were spun, separated, and refrigerated at 4°C for testing within 48 hours (can be stored at −20°C for longer).

How would this patient be managed postoperatively?

Posttreatment observation of these patients is required, because of the potential for the second phase of reactivity. The anesthetist should take responsibility in investigating the patient for the cause of anaphylaxis.

This patient was admitted to the high-dependency unit overnight. The serum concentration of mast cell tryptase taken 1 hour after the reaction was 27 ng/mL (normal <1 ng/mL).

This abnormal result confirms that the patient had an anaphylactic reaction, but it does not identify the cause. Serum mast cell tryptase measurement has a positive predictive value for the diagnosis of anaphylaxis of 95.3% and a negative predictive value of 49%.[6] Thus, a negative test does not rule out anaphylaxis completely. Also, tryptase levels are unlikely to be elevated in mild systemic reactions.

The patient should be advised about the importance of further testing before discharge. For these tests, the patient is sent to an allergologist in a regional allergy center. The radioallergosorbent test is a technique for measuring antigen-specific antibodies in serum. If a fast result is needed, this is the test of choice based on the fact that the concentration of specific IgE antibodies is the same during the reaction as after 4 to 6 weeks.[16]

Skin tests (which may take the form of skin prick or intradermal tests) should be done 6 weeks after the reaction. Before 4 weeks, the intracellular stocks of histamine and other mediators are still lower than normal, therefore increasing the probability of a false-negative result. For the same reason, drugs that could modify the skin's response have to be avoided (e.g., antihistamines, angiotensin-converting enzyme inhibitors, nonsteroidal anti-inflammatory drugs, vasoconstrictors, neuroleptics). Because of the risk of life-threatening reactions, challenge tests are not done except for local anesthetics.[15]

A copy of the entire patient's records (i.e., copies of anesthetic chart, drug charts, full details of reaction, and reports of tests done) is sent to both the allergologist and the general practitioner. In addition:

- Patients and their family members are to be informed about the incident. A full account of the events, a written record of the reaction, and advice regarding future anesthetics should be given. The patient is encouraged to carry an anesthetic card or medic alert bracelet.

- The primary and attending team, if different, are also informed about the incident and are given a copy of case notes.
- The National Medicines Board or appropriate body should be informed regarding the incident. A national database may allow physicians to determine the precise incidence of allergic reactions to various substances relative to their market share, thus making comparisons between countries possible.
- The case is discussed at a departmental mortality and morbidity meeting. Ideally, a departmental policy regarding follow-up and a standard checklist of actions should be designed and implemented.

KEY MESSAGES

1. Anaphylaxis is a severe, potentially fatal systemic allergic reaction with a variable clinical picture. There is no valid predictor of anaphylaxis, and previous exposure is not necessary.

2. Epinephrine in incremental doses is the mainstay of early treatment.

3. Further evaluation, diagnostics, and reporting are highly desirable in the interest of the patient and the anesthetist when faced with subsequent surgery. Diagnosis is made with intraoperative tests (mast cell tryptase) and postoperative tests (radioallergosorbent tests for specific IgE antibodies and skin tests).

QUESTIONS

1. What is anaphylaxis and what is its incidence during anesthesia?

   Answer: Anaphylaxis is a severe allergic reaction to any stimulus, usually having sudden onset and usually lasting less than 24 hours, involving one or more body systems and producing one or more symptoms such as hives, flushing, itching, angioedema, stridor, wheezing, shortness of breath, vomiting, diarrhea, and shock. The incidence of anaphylaxis is estimated to be between 1 in 10,000 and 1 in 20,000 anesthesia cases.

2. Which substance is most often associated with anaphylactic reactions during anesthesia?

   Answer: Any substance or drug administered in the perioperative period can potentially produce life-threatening immune-mediated hypersensitivity reactions. Neuromuscular blocking agents (55%), latex (22.3%), and antibiotics (14.7%) are the substances most frequently associated with anaphylactic reactions.

3. What are the principles of intra- and postoperative management of anaphylaxis?

   Answer: Anaphylactic reactions cannot be clinically distinguished from non–immune-mediated reactions (which account for 30%–40% of hypersensitivity reactions). Therefore, any suspected anaphylactic reaction must be extensively investigated using combined peri- and postoperative testing to confirm the nature of the reaction, to identify the causative substance, and to provide recommendations for future anesthetics.

Guidelines have been issued by the Association of Anaesthetists of Great Britain and Ireland to standardize the emergency treatment of anaphylaxis.[3] These are:

a. Stop administration of all agents likely to have caused anaphylaxis.
b. Call for help.
c. Maintain airway, give 100% oxygen and lay patient flat with legs elevated.
d. Give adrenaline. This may be given intramuscularly in a dose of 0.5 mg to 1 mg (0.5 to 1 mL of 1:1000) and may be repeated every 10 minutes according to the arterial pressure and pulse until improvement occurs.

     Alternatively, 50 to 100 μg intravenously (0.5 to 1 mL of 1:10,000) over 1 minute has been recommended for hypotension with titration of further doses as required.
e. Start rapid IV infusion with colloids or crystalloids.

Secondary therapy consists of:

1. Give antihistamines (chlorpheniramine 10—20 mg by slow IV infusion)
2. Give corticosteroids (100—500 mg hydrocortisone IV slowly)
3. Bronchodilators may be required for persistent bronchospasm.

References

1. Mertes PM, Lexenaire MC, Alla F. Anaphylactic and anaphylactoid reactions occurring during anaesthesia in France 1999–2000. Anaesthesiology 2003;99:536–545.
2. Laxenaire MC, Mertes PM. Anaphylaxis during anaesthesia. Br J Anaesthesia 2001; 87:549–558.
3. Lang DM, Alpern MB, Visitainer PF, et al. Increased risk for anaphylactic reactions from contrast media in patients in B-adrenergic blockers or with asthma. Ann Inter Med 1991; 115:270–276.
4. Lang DM. Anaphylactoid and anaphylactic reactions. Hazards of B blockers. Drugs Saf 1995;12:299–304.
5. Mertes PM, Laxenaire MC. Allergy and anaphylaxis in anaesthesia. Minerva Anestesiol 2004;70:285–291.
6. Stark BJ, Sullivan TJ. Biphasic and protracted anaphylaxis. J Allergy Clin Immunol 1986;78:76–83.
7. Sampson HA, Munoz-Furlong A, Campbell RL, et al. Second symposium on the definition and management of anaphylaxis: summary report—second National Institute of allergy and infectious disease/food allergy and anaphylaxis network symposium. J Allergy Clin Immunol 2006;117:391–397.
8. Association of Anaesthetists of Great Britain and Ireland: Suspected anaphylactic reactions associated with anaesthesia. London 2003. http://www.aagbi.org. Accessed May 2008.
9. Mertes PM, Laxenaire MC. Adverse reactions to neuromuscular blocking agents. Curr Allergy Asthma Rep 2004;4:7–16.
10. Laroche D, Lefrancois C, Gerard J, et al. Early diagnosis of anaphylactic reactions to neuromuscular blocking drugs. Br J Anaesth 1992;69:611–614.
11. Soetens FM, Vercauteren MP. Allergic reactions during anaesthesia: diagnosis and treatment. Jurnalul Roman de Anestezie Terapie Intensiva 2008;15:43–50.

Persistent Postsurgical Pain

Peter John Lee

FORMAT: REFLECTION

A 64-year-old woman presented to her general practitioner with a lump in the left upper quadrant of her left breast. On examination, a hard nodule was detected, and she was referred to a general surgeon for further investigation. Mammography and breast biopsy confirmed the presence of a 3-cm invasive adenocarcinoma. Computed axial tomography showed no evidence of metastatic disease. The patient was scheduled for a left mastectomy and axillary node clearance.

The patient had previously undergone a total abdominal hysterectomy under general anesthesia. She was taking pravastatin 20 mg daily for dyslipidemia but was otherwise fit and healthy. She was anxious at the postoperative interview and was particularly apprehensive about pain after her operation, as she had experienced considerable pain following her hysterectomy.

Physical examination of the patient was unremarkable apart from the lump in her left breast, and the results of a full blood picture, urea, and electrolytes were all normal. Her electrocardiogram and chest radiograph were unremarkable.

Before surgery, and with standard monitoring in progress, a paravertebral block was performed on the patient. The third thoracic vertebral body was identified with the patient in a sitting position, and, under aseptic conditions, following local infiltration, a 22-gauge Tuohy needle was inserted 3 cm lateral to the most cephalad aspect of the spinous process. The needle was advanced to 3.5 cm to make contact with the transverse process. The needle was then "walked" above the transverse process until a loss of resistance to air confirmed the correct location. A catheter was inserted into the paravertebral space, and following a test dose, bupivacaine 0.5% 20 mL was administered.

Anesthesia was induced using propofol 180 mg, and muscle relaxation was achieved with atracurium 35 mg. Following tracheal intubation, anesthesia was maintained with inhaled sevoflurane in an air/oxygen mixture.

Paracetamol 1000 mg and diclofenac 75 mg were administered intravenously during surgery. Surgery was completed within 1 hour, and the patient's trachea was extubated following reversal with glycopyrrolate and neostigmine.

In the postanesthesia care unit, the patient reported a pain score of 4, in which a score of 0 represented no pain, and 10 represented the worst possible pain. The patient was prescribed paracetamol 1000 mg and diclofenac sodium 75 mg as required. The paravertebral block catheter was removed before she was transferred to the ward.

On the first postoperative day, the patient complained of mild pain while at rest and moderate-to-severe pain during physiotherapy and while mobilizing. The paracetamol was discontinued, and the patient commenced on co-codamol (codeine phosphate 15 mg/paracetamol 500 mg). The patient reported some relief from pain at rest and was discharged on the fourth postoperative day.

Three months later, after an outpatient consultation, the surgical team reported that the patient complained of moderate pain in the left axilla for which she took paracetamol and ibuprofen. She was referred to a pain specialist for further treatment.

CASE DISCUSSION

Persistent postsurgical pain (PPSP) is defined as pain that developed after a surgical procedure, is of at least 3 months' duration in which other causes for the pain have been excluded, and whereby the possibility that the pain is continuing from a preexisting problem has been explored and excluded.[1] Women who undergo breast surgery experience chest wall, breast, or scar pain (11%–57%), phantom breast pain (13%–24%), and arm and shoulder pain (12%–51%). The incidence of pain in one or more of these sites is close to 50% 1 year after breast surgery for cancer.[2]

Risk Factors for PPSP

There are several risk factors for PPSP[3] (Table 44.1).

Demographic and Psychosocial Factors Age is a risk factor for the development of PPSP. The incidence of PPSP after mastectomy is 26% in patients older than 70 years, 40% in those 50 to 69 years, and 65% in those 30 to 49 years.[4] Preoperative anxiety, although a predictor of clinically meaningful acute pain,[5] is not an independent contributor to the prediction of either the presence or the intensity of PPSP after breast surgery.[6] Prescribing an anxiolytic in this case could have relieved the patient's anxiety and decreased acute postoperative pain.

TABLE 44.1 Risk Factors for Persistent Postsurgical Pain

1. Demographic and psychosocial factors
2. Preoperative pain
3. Type of surgery
4. Concomitant treatments
5. Genetic factors
6. Postoperative pain

Preoperative Pain　The evidence on preoperative pain as a risk factor for PPSP is conflicting. A retrospective study showed a significant correlation between preoperative breast pain and phantom breast syndrome.[7] A prospective trial found no correlation between preoperative breast pain and the risk of developing PPSP.[6]

Type of Surgery　PPSP is more common after breast-conserving surgery than after radical surgery.[8]

Concomitant Treatments　There is a higher incidence of PPSP in patients who undergo chemotherapy[9] or radiotherapy.[6] The patient in this scenario would certainly undergo chemotherapy or radiotherapy following surgery.

Genetic Factors　A genetic influence on the development of PPSP has been shown in animals.[10] Three genetic variants of the gene encoding catechol-O-methyltransferase have been identified, and five combinations of these variants are strongly associated with variation in the sensitivity to experimental pain and with the development of a long-term pain disorder.[11]

Postoperative Pain　Severe acute pain after breast surgery is a risk factor for the development of PPSP,[6] and adequacy of postoperative analgesia is an important determinant of PPSP.[12].

Decreasing the Incidence of PPSP

Peripheral and central sensitization of the nervous system is implicated in the development of PPSP. Nociception-induced hyperalgesia observable in the postoperative period is a consequence of surgical tissue and nerve trauma.[13] Nociceptive inputs alter subsequent sensory nervous system processing, both peripheral and central.[14] This neuroplasticity is initially excitatory (termed *sensitization*) and develops from activation (acute, transient, and activity-dependent) via modulation (subacute, slower, still reversible functional changes) through to modification (chronic structural and architectural changes).[13] Nociceptive excitatory neuroplasticity is expressed clinically as increased sensitivity to pain. Peripheral nervous system excitation increases sensitivity to painful stimulus in the area of damaged tissue.

Changes Underlying the Development of PPSP

Providing adequate postoperative analgesia after breast surgery decreases the incidence and intensity of PPSP. Because it has

been theorized that PPSP results from sensitization, the blockade of sensitization by regional technique may help with prevention. Paravertebral block for breast surgery decreases the incidence of pain symptoms, the intensity of motion-related pain, and the intensity of pain at rest at 12 months.[15] Multimodal analgesia with gabapentin and topical application of a eutectic mixture of local anesthetic decreases the postoperative analgesic requirements and the incidence and intensity of PPSP 3 months after breast surgery.[16] Multimodal analgesia using a continuous paravertebral block and regular acetaminophen and parecoxib decreased the incidence of PPSP at 10 weeks.[12]

Although satisfactory analgesia at rest was achieved in this case, movement-evoked pain was described as moderate to severe and was not treated adequately. The paravertebral catheter could have been left in situ, and an infusion of local anesthetic could have been administered postoperatively or a combination of nonsteroidal anti-inflammatory drugs and paracetamol with opioids administered regularly. The use of multimodal analgesia techniques, which has been shown to provide optimal dynamic pain relief with minimal side effects, may prevent PPSP.

The perioperative use of tricyclic antidepressants and anticonvulsants may also benefit in the prevention of PPSP. The antiepileptic drugs gabapentin and pregabalin are efficacious in the treatment of neuropathic pain associated with diabetic peripheral neuropathy and postherpetic neuralgia.[17] Pregabalin binds to the alpha$_2$delta subunit of calcium channels, reducing depolarization-induced calcium influx and thereby decreasing the release of excitatory neurotransmitters, including glutamate, noradrenaline and substance P.[17] A single dose of gabapentin administered to patients before mastectomy decreases postoperative morphine consumption and pain during movement.[18] Gabapentin, as part of a multimodal analgesic regimen, decreased the incidence of PPSP at 10 weeks after breast surgery.[19] Gabapentin could certainly have been used in this case.

Excitatory neurotransmitters, acting through N-methyl-D-aspartate receptors, are implicated in the process of sensitization and development of PPSP. Ketamine, an N-methyl-D-aspartate receptor antagonist, is an antihyperalgesic drug that modulates excitatory neurotransmission, decreasing both mechanical hyperalgesia around the wound and incidence of residual pain in patients undergoing bowel surgery.[20] As part of a multimodal analgesic technique along with intraoperative epidural anesthesia, ketamine reduces the incidence of PPSP 1 year after major digestive surgery.[21]

There are no specific recommendations regarding the use of ketamine in this scenario.

Perioperative administration of the N-methyl-D-aspartate receptor antagonist amantadine did not prevent the development of postmastectomy pain syndrome in patients who underwent breast surgery with axillary lymph node dissection.[22]

KEY MESSAGES

1. The incidence of PPSP following breast surgery is 48%.

2. Severe acute postoperative pain is the most significant risk factor for PPSP after breast surgery.

3. Multimodal analgesic techniques, including conduction blockade by regional technique, reduce the incidence and severity of PPSP.

4. The gabapentinoid antiepileptic drugs (gabapentin and pregabalin), and the N-methyl-D-aspartate receptor antagonist ketamine show promise in perioperative prevention of PPSP.

QUESTIONS

1. What is the definition of PPSP?

Answer: PPSP is defined as pain that developed after a surgical procedure, is of at least 3 months' duration in which other causes for the pain have been excluded, and whereby the possibility that the pain is continuing from a preexisting problem has been explored and excluded.

2. What techniques have been successfully used to reduce the incidence of PPSP after breast surgery?

Answer: Providing adequate postoperative analgesia after breast surgery decreases the incidence and intensity of PPSP. Multimodal analgesia using continuous paravertebral block and regular acetaminophen and parecoxib, or a eutectic mixture of local anesthetic and gabapentin has decreased the incidence of PPSP after breast surgery.

3. In what way might pregabalin prevent sensitization of the pain system?

Answer: Pregabalin binds to the alpha$_2$delta subunit of calcium channels in neurons, reducing depolarization-induced calcium influx and thereby decreasing the release of excitatory neurotransmitters, including glutamate, noradrenaline, and substance P at the level of the dorsal horn.

References

1. Macrae WA. Chronic pain after surgery. Br J Anaesth 2001;87: 88–98.
2. Perkins FM, Kehlet MD. Chronic pain as an outcome of surgery. Anesthesiology 2000;93:1123–1133.
3. Macrae WA. Can we prevent chronic pain after surgery? In: Shorten GD, Carr D, Harmon D, et al, eds. Postoperative Pain Management. Philadelphia: Saunders Elsevier, 2006:259–264.
4. Smith WCS, Bourne D, Squair J, et al. A retrospective cohort study of post-mastectomy pain syndrome. Pain 1999;83:91–95.
5. Katz J, Poleshuck E, Andrus CH, et al. Risk factors for acute pain and its persistence following breast cancer surgery. Pain 2005;119:16–25.
6. Poleshuck EL. Risk factors for chronic pain following breast cancer surgery: a prospective study. J Pain 2006;7:626–634.
7. Kroner K, Krebs B, Skov J, et al. Immediate and long-term phantom breast syndrome after mastectomy: incidence, clinical characteristics and relationship to pre-mastectomy breast pain. Pain 1989;36:327–334.
8. Tasmuth T, Kataja M, Blomqvist C, et al. Pain and other symptoms after different treatment modalities of breast cancer. Ann Oncol 1995;6:453–459.
9. Tasmuth T, Kataja M, Blomqvist C, et al. Treatment-related factors predisposing to chronic pain in patients with breast cancer—a multivariate approach. Acta Oncol 1997;36:625–630.
10. Seltzer Z, Wu T, Max MB, et al. Mapping a gene for neuropathic pain-related behaviour following peripheral neurectomy in the mouse. Pain 2001;93:101—106.
11. Diatchenko L, Slade GD, Nackley AG, et al. Genetic basis for individual variations in pain perception and the development of a chronic pain condition. Human Mol Genet 2005;14:135–143.
12. Iohom G, Abdalla H, O'Brien J, et al. The associations between severity of early postoperative pain, chronic postsurgical pain and plasma concentration of stable nitric oxide products after breast surgery. Anesth Analg 2006;103:995–1000.
13. Wilder-Smith OH, Tassonyi E, Crul BJP, et al. Quantitative sensory testing and human surgery: effects of analgesic management on postoperative neuroplasticity. Anesthesiology 2003;98: 1214–1222.
14. Woolf CJ, Salter MW. Neuronal plasticity: increasing the gain in pain. Science 2000;288:1765–1769.
15. Kairaluoma PM, Bachmann MS, Rosenberg PH, et al. Preincisional paravertebral block reduces the prevalence of chronic pan after breast surgery. Anesth Analg 2006; 103: 703–708.
16. Fassoulaki A, Triga A, Melemeni A, et al. Multimodal analgesia with gabapentin and local anaesthetics prevents acute and chronic pain after breast surgery for cancer. Anesth Analg 2005; 101:1427–1432.
17. Ben-Menacern E. Pregabalin pharmacology and its relevance to clinical practice. Epilepsia 2004;45:13–18.
18. Dirks J, Fredensborg BB, Christensen D, et al. A randomized study of the effects of single-dose gabapentin versus placebo on postoperative pain and morphine consumption after mastectomy. Anesthesiology 2002;97:560–564.
19. Gilron I. Is gabapentin a broad-spectrum analgesic? Anesthesiology 2002;97:537—539.
20. De Kock M, Lavand'homme P, Waterloos H, et al. 'Balanced analgesia' in the perioperative period: is there a place for ketamine? Pain 2001;92:373–380.
21. Lavand'homme P, De Kock M, Waterloos H, et al. Intraoperative epidural analgesia combined with ketamine provides effective preventive analgesia in patients undergoing major digestive surgery. Anesthesiology 2005;103:813–820.
22. Eisenberg E, Pud D, Koltun L, et al. Effect of early administration of the N-methyl-D-aspartate receptor antagonist amantadine on the development of postmastectomy pain syndrome: a prospective pilot study. J Pain 2007;8:223–229.

CHAPTER 45

Opioid-Induced Hyperalgesia

James O'Driscoll

FORMAT: REFLECTION

A 29-year-old, ASA II (American Society of Anesthesiologists), 80-kg male admitted to the plastic surgery department sustained significant injuries to his right hand while as a passenger in a car involved in a road traffic accident. He had extensive lacerations to both the palmar and dorsal aspects of his right, dominant hand and had clinical evidence of tendon and nerve damage. He also had fractures of the first and second phalanges of his third finger. It was therefore proposed to explore and repair the wound under anesthesia.

The patient had a history of intravenous (IV) drug abuse (heroin) but was not currently using and had been abstinent for 2 months. He also had a history of long-term, well-controlled asthma and was using salbutamol and beclamethasone metered-dose inhalers. His examination was unremarkable.

The various options for anesthesia including general, regional, and combined techniques were discussed with the patient. He requested a general anesthetic and refused all offers of regional/nerve blockade despite explanation of these techniques and reassurance regarding efficacy and safety.

On arrival in the operating room, appropriate monitoring was established, and after preoxygenation with 100% oxygen, anesthesia was induced with 2 μg midazolam, 250 mcg fentanyl, and 300 mg propofol. A size 4 laryngeal mask airway was placed, and the position was confirmed by auscultation and capnography. Anesthesia was maintained uneventfully with sevoflurane in an oxygen/air mixture and assisted ventilation in a pressure support mode until return of spontaneous ventilation. Analgesia administered consisted of 2 g paracetamol IV, 75 mg diclofenac IV, 15 mg morphine IV, and wound infiltration by a surgeon at end of the procedure with 10 mL 0.25% bupivacaine. The total anesthesia time was 3 hours, and the patient's vital signs were stable throughout.

After the procedure, the patient was transferred to the postanesthesia care unit (PACU), and 10 minutes later, he began to complain of pain. His Verbal Rating Scale score was 8 out of 10 (scale, 0–10), his pulse was 110 beats per minute, and noninvasive blood pressure was 140/88 mm Hg. Further bolus doses of morphine were administered to a total of 10 mg in accordance with PACU protocol. Twenty minutes later the patient complained again of pain and was reviewed by the anesthetist. He gave the patient two further

boluses of 5 mg morphine and noted that the pain seemed out of proportion for the procedure given the multimodal approach taken, particularly the local infiltration. The patient's Verbal Rating Score at this stage remained at 8, his heart rate was 100 beats per minute, and noninvasive blood pressure was 140/94 mm Hg. As soon as the patient had settled, he was discharged from the PACU to the general ward on oral paracetamol and diclofenac around the clock as well as oxycodone as required for breakthrough pain.

Two hours later, the anesthetist was called to review the patient's pain on the ward. The patient reported increased pain scores (Verbal Rating Score, 7) and had not responded to oral analgesia in the form of oxycodone. His heart rate was 110 beats per minute and noninvasive blood pressure was 150/88 mm Hg. Morphine-based patient-controlled analgesia was prescribed in addition to regular paracetamol as well as nonsteroidal anti-inflammatory drugs, and the patient seemed to have improved when reviewed 1 hour later.

In the morning, the acute pain team reviewed the patient, and he reported moderate pain control. Examination of the patient-controlled analgesia delivery system showed a total consumption of 120 mg of morphine over 16 hours and a bolus demand/delivery ratio of 4:1. It was felt that his pain control was suboptimal despite all the appropriate measures.

The patient subsequently made a full recovery and never demonstrated any evidence of a return to IV drug abuse. In the weeks following surgery, the patient reported that pain control was excellent.

CASE DISCUSSION

The finding of increased postoperative pain and postoperative opioid consumption in a patient receiving a high rather than a low intraoperative opioid dose indicates the possibility of opioid-induced hyperalgesia (OIH) in this patient. Alternatively, this patient may have experienced acute tolerance to analgesic opioid effects. No firm conclusions can be drawn. Differentiation between OIH and tolerance requires a method directly assessing pain sensitivity, and implementing such a method into clinical practice is difficult.

OIH

OIH is a phenomenon whereby opioid drugs prescribed to alleviate pain may paradoxically make the patient more sensitive to painful stimuli. There is strong animal evidence for the phenomenon particularly with long-term opioid administration.[1] There is, however, a growing body of evidence for its occurrence in humans. OIH is most commonly described in the setting of long-term use or withdrawal from long-term use as is the case of the patient described herein.[2] Increased pain sensation after opioids for acute pain has also been reported, particularly with remifentanil.[3]

Various potential mechanisms have been proposed, but none appears to be definitive. There may be sensitization of peripheral nociceptors, enhanced production and release, or decreased reuptake of nociceptive neurotransmitters, or sensitization of second-order neurons. We do know that c-fos expression is increased and that blockade of N-methyl-D-aspartic acid or excitatory amino acid receptors prevent hyperalgesia associated with opioid use.[4]

Management of OIH

The first step is to have a high index of suspicion and to identify patients who may be at risk of developing OIH. Currently, this group would mainly be those on long-term opioid therapy. Any opioid has the potential to cause OIH. A multimodal approach to analgesia is essential, as the use of adjuvants (regional anesthesia, clonidine, ketamine) attenuates/blocks the development of OIH.[4]

There was potential for improvement in the management of our patient. It would be important to discover the exact reasons for patient refusal of regional anesthesia (even just as adjuvant) and to address his concerns in an attempt to change his mind. It is very likely that a brachial plexus block would have provided optimal intra- and postoperative analgesia in his case. Perhaps the addition of other drugs such as clonidine or ketamine may have helped once pain control was found to be unsatisfactory in the PACU. Gabapentin has been shown to prevent OIH in rats, explained by the fact that neuropathic pain and OIH share common pathophysiologic mechanisms.[5] Another important observation is that OIH is often related to a particular drug in a particular patient. Therefore, rotating drugs both in the acute and long-term pain setting can help to reduce this phenomenon.[4] As soon as a high-dose, opioid-induced hyperalgesic effect is suspected, dose reduction of the causative agent and/or switching to another opioid agonist (in this case fentanyl or sufentanil) is a logical next step.

KEY MESSAGES

1. OIH is a pronociceptive phenomenon that can occur with acute or long-term opioid administration.

2. Disappearance of opioid treatment effects coupled with unexplained pain expansion may indicate OIH.

3. The cornerstone of managing OIH is dose reduction of the culprit opioid and the use of multimodal analgesia.

QUESTIONS

1. What is OIH, and in what clinical settings is it likely to occur?

   Answer: OIH is a clinical condition whereby opioid drugs such as morphine or any opioid drug prescribed to relieve pain may paradoxically increase the patient's perception of pain. The exact mechanism by which this occurs is unknown, but there is strong evidence for the involvement of several nociceptive pathways and regulatory mechanisms such as the excitatory amino acids and N-methyl-D-aspartic acid receptor. OIH has most often been described in the setting of long-term pain, in patients with prolonged exposure to opioid medication. It has also been described following acute exposure to opioids such as remifentanil.

2. Can OIH be prevented?

   Answer: Little is known about the exact mechanism, thereby making strategies for prevention difficult. It is known that a multimodal approach to analgesia in both the acute and chronic settings is essential. This also limits exposure to opioid medications and all their undesirable effects.

3. What is the treatment for OIH?

   Answer: Treatment of OIH can be difficult when it does occur. Keep in mind that reducing the dose or changing to a different opioid can help alleviate the problem. Drug rotation is becoming a common strategy in the long-term use of opioids for pain management to maintain efficacy and reduce side effects. In addition, clonidine and ketamine may be added to the armamentarium of pain management in these cases.

References

1. Zissen MH, Zhang G, McKelvy A, et al. Tolerance, opioid-induced allodynia and withdrawal associated allodynia in infant and young rats. Neuroscience 2007;144:247–262.
2. Meyer M, Wagner K, Benvenuto A, et al. Intrapartum and postpartum analgesia for women maintained on methadone during pregnancy. Obstet Gynecol 2007;110:261–266.
3. Schmidt S, Bethge G, Forster MH, et al. Enhanced postoperative sensitivity to painful pressure stimuli after intraoperative high dose remifentanil in patients without significant surgical site pain. Clin J Pain 2007;23:605–611.
4. Koppert W, Schulz M. The impact of opioid-induced hyperalgesia for postoperative pain. Best Pract Res Clin Anaesthesiol 2007;21:65–83.
5. Van Elstraete AC, Sitbon P, Mazoit JX, Benhamou D. Gabapentin prevents delayed and long-lasting hyperalgesia induced by fentanyl in rats. Anesthesiology 2008;108:484–494.

CHAPTER 46

Transurethral Resection of Prostate Syndrome

John Dowling

A 74-year-old, 92-kg man (American Society of Anesthesiologists II with long-standing, well-controlled hypertension) was admitted for transurethral resection of prostate (TURP) for benign prostatic hypertrophy. He had an uneventful inguinal hernia repair under general anesthesia 8 years previously. His medications included a β-adrenergic antagonist (bisoprolol) and an HMG Co-A reductase inhibitor (pravastatin).

The patient underwent a full preoperative evaluation including a past medical and anesthetic history and relevant physical examination. Table 46.1 summarizes his preoperative blood results. The patient's preoperative electrocardiogram (ECG) reading was normal.

What are the main anesthetic considerations for this patient?

TURP is performed by passing a loop through a special cystoscope (resectoscope). Using direct visualization and continuous irrigation, prostatic tissue is resected by applying a cutting current to the loop. This procedure is performed on a predominantly elderly population, therefore, anesthesia carries a mortality risk of 0.2% to 6%, which correlates best with the American Society of Anesthesiologists' physical status scale. Although this patient is on statins, because he is 74 years old, he has a high chance of cerebrovascular and cardiovascular atherosclerotic disease. In addition, being hypertensive increases his risk of perioperative myocardial events because of possible left ventricular hypertrophy. His ECG reading, however, was normal. Despite the fact that β-blockers reduce the patient's ability to compensate for hypotension, they should be continued in the perioperative period, as they have proven benefit in terms of perioperative morbidity/mortality in patients with ischemic heart disease.

A neuraxial block is considered the most suitable technique for TURP, although general anesthesia has a similar morbidity and mortality profile. A subarachnoid block to T10 is desirable, as it provides excellent anesthesia without important hypotension for the patient and adequate perineal and pelvic floor relaxation for the surgeon. Compared with general anesthesia, regional anesthesia appears to reduce the incidence of postoperative deep venous thrombosis, and it is less likely to mask signs of bladder perforation symptoms or TURP syndrome.

As there were no contraindications to a neuraxial anesthetic technique, a spinal anesthetic was planned for the procedure and discussed with the patient.

Upon arrival at the operating room, a wide-bore (16-gauge) cannula was inserted in the patient's left wrist, and 500 mL of Hartmann's solution was administered. Standard monitoring was instituted (ECG, oxygen (O_2) saturation, and noninvasive blood pressure monitoring). Forty percent O_2 was administered via a Venturi fixed performance mask. A spinal anesthetic was performed at the level of L3 to L4 with the patient in the sitting position under strict aseptic conditions. Three mL of 0.5% hyperbaric bupivacaine was injected into clear, free-flowing cerebrospinal fluid. After 10 minutes, a motor and sensory block to the level of T10 was noted and deemed adequate for starting the procedure. The attending anesthetist kept in regular verbal contact with the patient. A senior surgical trainee began the procedure with his consultant surgeon supervising at chair side. Baseline monitoring (immediately post-spinal blockade) showed a heart rate of 66 beats per minute, blood pressure of 114/74 mm Hg, O_2 saturation of 99%, and the patient's ECG trace showed normal sinus rhythm.

Fifty minutes into the procedure, the patient complained of a headache and dizziness and was noted to be somewhat confused and restless. His heart rate was found to have fallen to 52 beats per minute, and he was noted to be hypertensive (blood pressure, 162/106 mm Hg). The patient became progressively more anxious and in addition was now dyspneic. He then complained of feeling cold, and a subsequent temperature measurement showed him to be markedly hypothermic (33.8°C).

What differential diagnosis should be considered at this stage?

- TURP syndrome
- Hypoxia
- Hemorrhage
- Myocardial infarction
- Cerebrovascular event
- Hypothermia
- Bladder perforation
- Septicemia (gram-negative)

What is the most likely diagnosis, and how could this be rapidly ascertained?

The most likely diagnosis is TURP syndrome and could be confirmed via a stat sodium (showing hyponatremia).

TABLE 46.1 Preoperative Blood Results

Measured Variable	Preoperative Value	Normal Range
Na^+	136	135–146 mEq/L
K^+	4.1	3.5–5.0 mEq/L
Creatinine	0.087	0.06–0.12 mmol/L
Urea	4.4	2.5–6.7 mmol/L
Hemoglobin	14.7	14–17 g/dL
White blood cells	5.7	$4.3–10.8 \times 10^9$/L

The classic triad of features that constitute the TURP syndrome are (a) dilutional hyponatremia, (b) fluid overload with consequent pulmonary and cerebral edema, and (c) glycine toxicity.[1]

In the TURP procedure, resecting prostatic tissue opens up the large and extensive network of prostatic venous plexuses. Continuous irrigation is used to distend the bladder and remove blood and tissue from the operative view. A hypo-osmotic glycine solution is most commonly utilized for this purpose because of its favorable optical and electrical properties in transurethral surgery. A variable amount of this irrigating solution will be absorbed intravascularly over the course of the procedure. Absorption of large amounts of this fluid (>2 L) results in a constellation of symptoms commonly described as TURP syndrome.

The critical physiologic derangement of central nervous system function is not only hyponatremia, but also acute hypoosmolality because the blood-brain barrier is largely impermeable to sodium but freely permeable to water. The cerebral edema caused by acute hypo-osmolality can increase intracranial pressure with consequent bradycardia, hypertension, and neurologic symptoms.[1]

What factors influence the volume of solution absorbed intravascularly?

1. Hydrostatic pressure, which is determined by the height of the irrigating fluid above the patient. The irrigating bag must be kept as low as possible to achieve adequate flow of irrigant (usually 60–70 cm).
2. Number and size of opened venous sinuses
3. Procedure duration and experience of the operating surgeon. The most important preventive measure during surgery is preserving the prostatic capsule. Violation of the capsule aids entry of irrigation fluid into the periprostatic and retroperitoneal space.
4. Venous pressure: More fluid is absorbed if the patient is hypovolemic or hypotensive.[2] Of note, smoking is the only patient factor known to be associated with large-scale fluid absorption during TURP.[9]

What are the origins and manifestations of the classic triad of symptoms?

1. Dilutional hyponatremia found in TURP syndrome is a hypervolemic hyponatremia representing excess total body water with normal total body sodium. In general, if the serum sodium concentration falls to 120 mEq/L, signs and symptoms of dilutional hyponatremia may ensue.
2. Fluid overload may give rise to pulmonary edema and cardiac failure especially in individuals with preexisting cardiovascular compromise, as well as cerebral edema.
3. Glycine toxicity results in impairment of consciousness and transient blindness. This is thought to be related to glycine acting as an inhibitory neurotransmitter at both central nervous system and retinal sites.[1]

What other signs and symptoms may indicate the presence of or an evolving TURP syndrome?

1. Cardiovascular system: The presence of hypertension and bradycardia may reflect a hypervolemic state; hypotension may then ensue representing emerging cardiac failure. In addition, glycine is known to be directly cardiotoxic to the myocardium.
2. Central nervous system: Confusion and agitation progressing to unconsciousness reflects hyponatremia, cerebral edema, and glycine toxicity.
3. Pulmonary system: Fluid overload may result in pulmonary edema and hypoxemia.
4. Hematologic system: Dilutional anemia may ensue.
5. Nausea and vomiting may result from hyperammonemia—in severe cases progressing to encephalopathy (ammonia is a major by-product of glycine metabolism).
6. Hypothermia may occur as a result of using a cold irrigant solution.[3]

An arterial blood gas analysis was quickly performed, and the results are shown in Table 46.2.

How could the most obvious abnormalities be explained?

The patient's Na^+ measurement of 111 mEq/L reflects a decrease in serum Na of 25 mEq/L. A diagnosis of TURP syndrome can be made on the basis of the arterial blood gas findings. Typically, if the serum Na^+ levels drop to below 120 mEq/L, signs and symptoms of water intoxication will be seen.[1] In addition, the blood gas shows that the patient was

TABLE 46.2 Intraoperative Arterial Blood Gas

Measured Value	Result	Normal Range
pH	7.38	7.35–7.45
pO_2	9	11–14.5 kPa
pCO_2	4.8	4.5–6.0 kPa
Na^+	111	135–146 mEq/L
K^+	4.7	3.5–5 mEq/L
Cl^-	102	100–106 mEq/L
Base excess	1.2	−2–+2
Hemoglobin	12.6	14–17 g/dL

hypoxemic (PO_2 of 9), indicating respiratory compromise and probable pulmonary edema. A dilutional anemia is also seen (hemoglobin level of 12.6), reflecting the large intravascular fluid load.

What would be the emergency management in this case?

Treating TURP syndrome depends on early recognition, and therefore, the anesthetist should maintain a high degree of clinical vigilance. Initial management should follow the airway breathing and circulation guidelines (ABC). The operating surgeon should be informed, and the procedure should be discontinued as soon as sites of bleeding have been controlled.[5] Cardiovascular compromise including bradycardia and hypotension may require treatment with anticholinergic and/or adrenergic agents, particularly in this case, in which the patient has been on β-blocker therapy.

Subsequently, the surgery was rapidly terminated, and the patient was monitored in the recovery room. His SpO_2 was between 92% and 95% on a Venturi face mask delivering 60% O_2. A 12-lead ECG was performed, which showed widening of the QRS complex on the ECG trace (Fig. 46.1).

What arrhythmias and other cardiac manifestations may be seen in a patient with TURP syndrome?

When serum sodium levels fall to less than 120 mEq/L, signs of cardiovascular depression can occur; less than 115 mEq/L may cause bradycardia, widening of the QRS complex, ST-segment elevation, ventricular ectopic beats, and T-wave inversion.[3] A serum sodium level of less than 110 mEq/L may cause respiratory and cardiac arrest.

The patient subsequently developed severe respiratory distress and was unable to maintain adequate O_2 saturations on high-flow O_2.

A diagnosis of pulmonary edema was made on the basis of clinical and radiology findings (Fig. 46.2). The patient was intubated, and transfer to the intensive care unit was arranged. He was ventilated using a synchronized intermittent mandatory ventilatory mode. He was also started on a hypertonic saline infusion to slowly correct his hyponatremia (at a rate of approximately 1 mmol/L per hour). When hemodynamically stable, the patient was started on a bolus of intravenous frusemide to treat his fluid overload and consequent pulmonary edema. Twenty-four hours later, the pulmonary edema and hyponatremia had resolved, the patient was extubated, and he made an uneventful recovery.

What are the current controversies regarding treatment of TURP syndrome?

In the past, fluid restriction was suggested as a potential therapy to improve hyponatremia, yet this method did not address the hypovolemia and low cardiac output that frequently followed the discontinuation of irrigating solution. Several studies support the use of hypertonic saline in the correction of the existing hyponatremia.[2,3] Treatment is recommended when measured serum sodium is below 120 mEq/L or when there are obvious signs and symptoms of hyponatremia. In addition, studies have shown a higher frequency of neurological disability and death among individuals who either did not receive or when there was a delay in instituting hypertonic saline therapy.[6] As a general rule, a correction of serum sodium by 1 mmol/L per hour may be considered as a safe rate but should be guided by improvements in the patient's neurological status. Hypertonic saline 3% is suggested as an initial fluid therapy, which can be adjusted in relation to serial serum sodium measurements and clinical improvement of the patient. Hypertonic saline has been shown to counteract

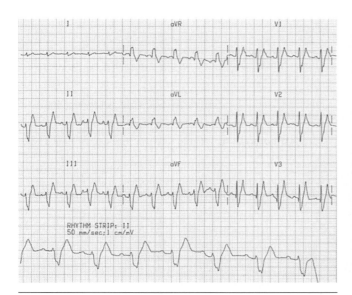

Figure 46.1 • QRS Widening on Electrocardiogram.

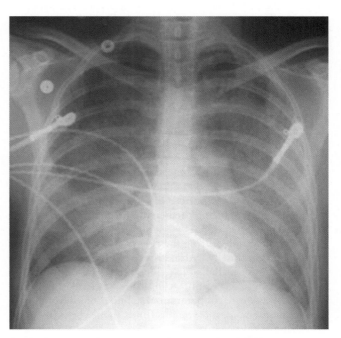

Figure 46.2 • Pulmonary Edema.

cerebral edema and expand plasma volume; the theoretical risk of causing pulmonary edema has not been seen in clinical usage.[7]

Although the risk of pontine myelinolysis is more immediate in the setting of chronic hyponatremia, the literature still advocates a gradual sodium correction even in the acute phase.[6]

Intravenous frusemide may be used to counteract the acute pulmonary edema and promote diuresis. No studies advocate its routine use in the treatment of fluid absorption, and in fact, it may exacerbate a preexisting hyponatremic hypovolemic picture. In situations when pulmonary edema is not established, the best practice is probably to withhold frusemide until the patient is hemodynamically stable and a hypertonic saline infusion has been started.[8]

Preventive measures, such as low-pressure irrigation, might reduce the extent of fluid absorption but do not eliminate this complication. Alternative surgical techniques, such as the use of bipolar resectoscopes and prostate vaporization may influence fluid absorption and its consequences.

KEY MESSAGES

1. Absorption of small amounts of fluid occurs in 5% to 10% of patients undergoing TURP and results in an easily overlooked mild TURP syndrome.
2. Most symptoms appear 30 to 45 minutes after surgery is completed, at which time hyponatremia is explained by natriuresis and not by dilution. However, symptoms related to fluid absorption develop in 3% to 5% of patients.
3. Furosemide should be used cautiously. In the absence of pulmonary edema, its use should be best delayed until the patient is hemodynamically stable and hypertonic fluid therapy has been instituted.
   Judicious correction of hyponatremia with hypertonic saline has been shown to improve patient outcome.

QUESTIONS

1. **What key precautions can surgeons and anesthetists take to prevent the occurrence of TURP syndrome?**

   Answer: The likelihood of developing TURP syndrome can be lessened by limiting the surgical procedure's duration, by reducing the height and thus pressure of the irrigating solution, by attempting to preserve the prostatic capsule during the resection, by ensuring the patient is optimally hydrated preoperatively, and compensating for intraoperative blood loss (often difficult to appreciate). As continuous absorption of irrigating fluid may be assumed, only minimal volumes of Na containing maintenance intravenous fluids should be infused during the procedure.

2. **What is the main advantage of performing the procedure under neuraxial blockade rather than general anesthesia?**

   Answer: With the patient awake, it is possible to keep in constant verbal contact with him and thus detect any early signs of confusion or restlessness, which may indicate an evolving TURP syndrome. This aspect of patient monitoring is lost with general anesthesia.

3. **What are the attributes of an ideal irrigation fluid for TURP? How are these similar to those that are currently available?**

   Answer: The ideal irrigation fluid should be optically clear, nonelectrolytic (and therefore nonconductive of the electrosurgical current) and isotonic. Numerous nonconductive fluids are available, such as glycine 1.5%, sorbitol 3%, mannitol 5%, and sterile water. The most commonly used irrigation fluid, glycine 1.5% solution is optically clear and non-electrolytic but hypo-osmolar (200 mOsm/L); therefore, large amounts may be absorbed systemically through the vascular prostate bed. Direct toxicity and metabolism of glycine can account for some of the neurologic symptoms of TURP syndrome. The 6-carbon alcohols, mannitol and sorbitol, both act as osmotic diuretics, in slightly varying concentrations. Solutions approximating 3% of either of the 6-carbon alcohols are most often used. These solutions are purposely prepared moderately hypotonic to maintain their transparency. Sterile water offers a very clear view of the operating field (and is therefore often used for cystoscopy), but it is highly hypotonic and may result in hemolysis of erythrocytes and possible renal failure when absorbed in large amounts through vascular openings.

References

1. Gravenstein D. Transurethral resection of the prostate syndrome: a review of the pathophysiology and management. Anesth Analg 1997;84:438–446.
2. Hahn RG. Fluid absorption in endoscopic surgery. Br J Anaesth 2006; 96:8–20.
3. Porter M, McCormick B. Anaesthesia for transurethral resection of the prostate. Update in Anaesthesia 2003;16.Article 8.
4. Scheingraber S, Heitmann L, Werner W, et al. Are there acid base changes during transurethral resection of the prostate? Anesth Analg 2000;90:946–950.
5. Ghanem AN, Ward JP. Osmotic and metabolic sequelae of volumetric overload in relation to the TURP syndrome. Br J Urol 1990;66:71–78.
6. Ayus JC, Krothapalli RK, Arieff AI. Treatment of symptomatic hyponatremia and its relation to brain damage. N Engl J Med 1987;317:1190–1195.
7. Beal JL, Freysz M, Berthelon G, et al. Consequences of fluid absorption during transurethral resection of the prostate using distilled water or glycine 1.5 per cent. Can J Anaesth 1989;36: 278–282.
8. Crowley K, Clarkson K, Hannon V, et al. Diuretics after transurethral prostatectomy: a double-blind controlled trial comparing frusemide and mannitol. Br J Anaesth 1990;65:337–341.
9. Hahn RG. Smoking increases the risk of large-scale fluid absorption during transurethral prostatic resection. J Urol 2001; 166:162–165.

CHAPTER 47

Anesthesia and Sleep-Disordered Breathing

Leon Serfontein

CASE FORMAT: STEP BY STEP

A 47-year-old, 5′ 7″, 85-kg (body mass index, 29.4 kg/m^2) male was scheduled for a semiurgent posterior cervical discectomy following acute C7–8 disc herniation with radicular symptoms to his right hand.

The patient had a history of chronic "neck problems" requiring intermittent use of nonsteroidal anti-inflammatory drugs for analgesia. He had no other medical problems of note. He had smoked 10 to 15 cigarettes a day for 20 years. Ten years previously, he had undergone general anesthesia for an inguinal hernia repair, after which he had awoken with a very sore, hoarse throat. He was told subsequently that it had been "very difficult to insert the breathing tube." No notes or further details of the event were available. The patient was taking an herbal throat spray at night, which he believed helped reduce snoring.

On examination, the patient was of stocky build and slightly overweight with a potentially difficult airway on assessment (Mallampati grade III, thyromental distance 6 cm, a short neck with a large circumference and limited mobility especially on extension). His blood pressure was 150/90 mm Hg, and his pulse rate was 85 beats per minute. All other clinical observations were normal.

The laboratory investigations were as follows: full blood count, hemoglobin, 16.8 g/dL; hematocrit, 0.51; platelets, 218 × 10^9/L; electrolytes, normal. The electrocardiogram reading showed no abnormalities.

What conclusions derived from the assessment could have important implications for this patient's perioperative management?

- The likelihood of difficulty in airway management and/or intubation.
- High suspicion of previously undiagnosed obstructive sleep apnea (OSA). The presence of polycythemia may indicate severe OSA (Table 47.1).

What is the relationship between difficult intubation and OSA?

Patients with difficult airways are at substantially increased risk of OSA.[3] Conversely, the possibility of difficulty with airway management and intubation should be considered in patients with known or suspected OSA.[4]

OSA is a syndrome characterized by periodic, partial, or complete obstruction of the upper airway during sleep. There are practice guidelines for the perioperative management of patients with OSA.[16] A good starting point is to stratify the patients using the terms mild, moderate, and severe as defined by the laboratory where the study was done.[16]

Which important details in the patient's history need to be investigated to support the diagnosis of OSA?

Symptoms and signs of OSA are listed in Table 47.1. The strongest of these associations are snoring, witnessed apneas, and obesity. Other risk factors include male gender,[12] aging,[13] menopausal status,[14] black race,[15] alcohol, and smoking.

Given the fact that no formal diagnosis of OSA can be made at this time, how should this patient be managed?

This patient should be managed as if he has OSA. Up to 20% of adults have at least mild OSA.[6] In a substantial number of these patients, the condition remains undiagnosed and untreated.[5]

Ideally, the severity of OSA may be determined by sleep studies. If a sleep study is not available, such patients should be treated as if they have moderate sleep apnea unless one or more of the signs or symptoms is severely abnormal (e.g., markedly increased body mass index or neck circumference, respiratory pauses that are frightening to the observer), in which case they should be treated as if they have severe sleep apnea.[16] In addition, polycythemia in this patient's case may indicate severe OSA.

If a sleep study had been done, the results should be used to determine the perioperative anesthetic management of a patient. Because procedures differ among laboratories, the American Society of Anesthesiologists' Task Force on Perioperative Management of Patients with OSA recommends that stratification of OSA should be done using the terms none, mild, moderate, or severe as defined by the laboratory where the study was done rather than the actual apnea-hypopnea index (the number of episodes of sleep-disordered breathing per hour). If this is not indicated, it may be approximated as shown in Table 47.2.

An anesthetic plan was discussed with the patient. He was told that an awake fiberoptics-assisted intubation would be

TABLE 47.1 Symptoms[7,9] and Signs[10] Associated With Increased Risk of Obstructive Sleep Apnea[11]

Snoring (prominent, habitual)	Obesity
Witnessed apneas (gasping/choking)	Increased neck circumference
Excessive/persistent daytime sleepiness	Hypertension
Family history	Presence of difficult airway predictors
	Right heart failure*
	Polycythemia*

*Severe obstructive sleep apnea.

TABLE 47.2 Statification of Patients with Obsructive Sleep Apnea[9]

Severity of OSA	Adult AHI	Pediatric AHI
None	0–5	0
Mild OSA	6–20	1–5
Moderate OSA	21–40	6–10
Severe OSA	>40	>10

AHI, apnea-hypopnea index; OSA, obstructive sleep apnea.
Reproduced with permission from Gross JB, Bachenberg KL, Benumof JL, et al. Practice guidelines for the perioperative management of patients with obstructive sleep apnea: a report by the American Society of Anesthesiologists Task Force on Perioperative Management of patients with obstructive sleep apnea. Anesthesiology 2006;104:1081–1093.

performed. The patient was very anxious and requested premedication. Diazepam 10 mg was prescribed orally.

Assuming that the patient is likely to suffer from OSA, what would be the advantages of using an asleep technique for instrumenting the airway?

Provided that spontaneous ventilation is maintained, or the ability to ventilate the patient is confirmed before a long-acting muscle relaxant is given, advantages include: (a) eliminating the need for sedation (awake technique) and (b) the ability to better gauge the potential for or the degree of obstruction and the likelihood of requiring devices to improve airway patency postoperatively (e.g., nasal airway, continuous positive airway pressure machine).

What are the main considerations regarding the choice of drugs used for anesthesia and analgesia in this patient in the perioperative period?

- Premedication with sedatives or opioids should ideally be avoided.
- Drugs used during general anesthesia should be chosen and dosed in such a way to minimize the extent and duration of any inhibitory effect on this patient's ability to maintain normal airway patency and ventilation postoperatively.
- The provision of adequate postoperative analgesia should be accomplished in a multimodal fashion to reduce the need for opioids. This includes the use of paracetamol, nonsteroidal anti-inflammatory drugs, and local anesthetics for incision infiltration. This patient would have conceivably benefited from wound infiltration with a long-acting local anesthetic.

In the anesthetic induction room on the morning of surgery, a 14-g cannula was inserted. Midazolam 4 mg and fentanyl 100 mg were given intravenously in incremental doses, as well as glycopyrrolate 200 μg. Following topicalization of

the airway, an orotracheal tube 8.5 was inserted with fiberoptic assistance. Anesthesia was induced with propofol and maintained with sevoflurane delivered in a mixture of 50:50 oxygen:nitrous oxide. Vecuronium 8 mg was given for muscle relaxation. Following prone positioning, the surgery proceeded uneventfully and was finished 2 hours later. Throughout the course of the surgery, the patient received paracetamol 2 g, diclofenac sodium 75 mg, and morphine 8 mg intravenously.

What are the important safety considerations when extubating this patient's trachea?

- Full reversal of neuromuscular blockade should be ensured and neuromuscular recovery should be ascertained (preferably with a nerve stimulator) before extubation.
- Extubation should occur with an oral or nasopharyngeal airway in place and only after spontaneous ventilation is established and the patient is conscious (rousable).
- The preferred recovery position for the patient is the lateral posture.[1] Placing his head in the sniffing position and displacing the mandible forward will further reduce the tendency for airway collapse.[2]
- Continuous positive airway pressure therapy should be applied if obstruction occurs despite the simple measures mentioned in this list (and in all cases of diagnosed OSA whereby the therapy has been prescribed or used preoperatively).

After reversal of neuromuscular blockade, the patient was extubated awake in the supine position. In the recovery area, he complained of pain and was given a further 4 mg of morphine in incremental doses. He desaturated a number of times to as low as 92%, and the anesthesiologist decided that supplemental oxygen should be continued on the ward. After a stable period of around 45 minutes, the patient was sent back to the ward. Approximately 6 hours after admission to the ward, the patient was found by a nurse to be unarousable, with minimal breathing efforts and a SpO_2 of 70%. His radial pulse was palpable, and his blood pressure was 85/55 mm Hg.

After an unsuccessful attempt at intubation by the anesthetic trainee on call, a laryngeal mask airway was inserted, and a total of 800 mcg naloxone was given in increments intravenously. The patient responded well to these measures over the course of the next 20 minutes. He subsequently removed the laryngeal mask airway himself. The patient was taken to the intensive care unit fully conscious with a SpO_2 of 96% on a 35% oxygen mask and recovered from the event with no permanent sequelae.

What simple measures could have minimized/prevented this complication?

- Although supplemental oxygen is mandatory in the postoperative period, to the inexperienced observer, this may mask the presence of obstructive episodes by reducing recurrent desaturation. This may have been the case in this patient.
- Patient positioning: The literature supports an improvement in apnea-hypopnea index scores when adult patients with OSA sleep in the lateral, prone, or sitting positions rather than the supine position in the nonperioperative setting. This would suggest that positional measures may be of use to prevent airway collapse even in the postoperative setting, although the literature does not provide specific guidance in this regard. It is unclear if this patient was encouraged to maintain a sitting or lateral posture postoperatively.
- An appropriate postoperative nursing environment is crucial. This patient should have ideally spent his recovery period in a high-dependency area. Airway patency was likely to deteriorate postoperatively because of residual levels of anesthetic agents, opioid analgesics, or drugs used for sedation.
- Monitoring: The literature is insufficient to offer guidance regarding the appropriate duration of postoperative respiratory monitoring in patients with OSA. However, hospitalized patients who are at increased risk of respiratory compromise from OSA should have continuous pulse oximetry monitoring after discharge from the recovery room. If frequent or severe airway obstruction or hypoxemia occurs during postoperative monitoring, initiating nasal continuous positive airway pressure or nasal intermittent positive pressure ventilation should be considered.[16]

Would there be an alternative to benzodiazepines in this case?

Gabapentin, as a potential multimodal perioperative drug, would have been a more suitable drug choice. Since its introduction in 1993 as an adjunctive anticonvulsant, its use has extended into more acute situations, particularly in the perioperative period.

Gabapentin is known to decrease preoperative anxiety; significantly lower Visual Analog Scale anxiety scores have been shown in patients given gabapentin as opposed to placebo before knee surgery.[17] Gabapentin has been proven to blunt hemodynamic response to laryngoscopy and intubation. Patients receiving 800 mg of gabapentin 1 hour before surgery had significantly decreased mean arterial pressure and heart rate during the first 10 minutes after endotracheal intubation compared with either 400 mg gabapentin or placebo.[17]

A meta-analysis of gabapentin administration for acute postoperative pain showed that a single preoperative dose of

KEY MESSAGES

1. OSA is a syndrome characterized by periodic, partial, or complete obstruction of the upper airway during sleep.
2. Patients with difficult airways are at substantially increased risk of OSA.[3] Conversely, the possibility of difficulty with airway management and intubation should be considered in patients with known or suspected OSA.[4]
3. Practice guidelines exist for the perioperative management of patients with OSA.[16] They target the preoperative assessment (risk stratification) and preparation, intraoperative (choice of anesthesia technique), and postoperative management (analgesia, oxygenation, patient positioning and monitoring).

gabapentin 1200 mg or less decreased pain intensity at 6 and 24 hours postoperatively. Twenty-four-hour cumulative opioid consumption was also significantly reduced.[17]

It is likely that this patient would have benefited from gabapentin 900 mg administered 1 to 2 hours before surgery, and the advantages include anxiolysis, decreased pressor response to intubation, and less acute postoperative pain. Repeated doses, however, carry the risk of increased sedation and withdrawal phenomenon.

Another option for this patient would have been a remifentanil infusion used for sedation during fiberoptic intubation.

QUESTIONS

1. How is OSA defined?

   Answer: OSA is defined as cessation of airflow for >10 seconds despite continuing ventilatory effort, 5 or more times per hour of sleep, and usually associated with a decrease in SaO_2 of >4%.

2. What symptoms and signs are associated with an increased risk of OSA?

3. Which predictors for difficult mask ventilation are commonly associated with OSA?

   Answer: History of snoring, obesity, and advanced age are commonly associated with OSA.

Snoring (prominent, habitual)	**Obesity**
Witnessed apneas (gasping/choking)	Increased neck circumference
Excessive/persistent daytime sleepiness	Hypertension
Family history	Presence of difficult airway predictors
	Clinical features of right heart failure*
	Clinical features of polycythemia*

*Severe OSA.

References

1. Isono S, Tanaka A, Nishino T. Lateral position decreases collapsibility of the passive pharynx in patients with obstructive sleep apnea. Anesthesiology 2002;97:780–785.

2. Connolly LA. Anesthetic management of obstructive sleep apnea patients. J Clin Anesth 1991;3:461–469.

3. Hiremath AS, Hillman DR, James AL, et al. Relationship between difficult tracheal intubation and obstructive sleep apnoea. Br J Anaesth 1998;80:606–611.

4. Siyam MA, Benhamou D. Difficult endotracheal intubation in patients with sleep apnea syndrome. Anesth Analg 2002;95:1098–1102.

5. Phillips B. Sleep apnoea: underdiagnosed and undertreated. Hospital Practice 1996;31: 193–194.

6. Young T, Peppard PE, Gottlieb DJ. Epidemiology of obstructive sleep apnea: a population health perspective. Am J Respir Crit Care Med 2002;165:1217–1239.

7. Grunstein RR, Wilcox I. Sleep-disordered breathing and obesity. Ballieres Clin Endocrinol Metab 1994;8:601–628.

8. Davies RJ, Stradling JR. The relationship between neck circumference, radiographic pharyngeal anatomy, and the obstructive sleep apnoea syndrome. Eur Respir J 1990;3: 509–514.

9. Hillman DR, Platt PR, Eastwood PR. The upper airway during anaesthesia. Br J Anaesth 2003;91:31–39.

10. Ballieres Clin Endocrinol Metab 1994; 8: 601–28. Flemons WW. Clinical practice. Obstructive sleep apnea. New Engl J Med 2002; 347:498–504.

11. Davies RJ, Ali NJ, Stradling JR. Neck circumference and other clinical features in the diagnosis of obstructive sleep apnoea syndrome. Thorax 1992;47;101–105.

12. Pillar G, Malhotra A, Fogel R, et al. Airway mechanisms and ventilation in response to resistive loading during REM sleep: the influence of gender. Am J Respir Crit Care Med 2000;162: 1627–1632.

13. Bixler EO, Vgontzas AN, Ten Have T, et al. Effects of age on sleep apnoea in men: prevalence and severity. Am J Crit Care Med 1998;157:144–148.

14. Young T. Menopause, hormone replacement therapy, and sleep-disordered breathing: are we ready for the heat? Am J Respir Crit Care Med 2001;163:597–598.

15. Redline S, Tisher PV, Hans MG, et al. Racial differences in sleep-disordered breathing in African-Americans. Am J Respir Crit Care Med 1997;155:186–192.

16. Gross JB, Bachenberg KL, Benumof JL, et al. Practice guidelines for the perioperative management of patients with obstructive sleep apnea: a report by the American Society of Anesthesiologists Task Force on Perioperative Management of patients with obstructive sleep apnea. Anesthesiology 2006;104:1081–1093.

17. Kong VKF, Irwin MG. Gabapentin: a multimodal perioperative drug? Br J Anaesth. 2007;99:775–786.

CHAPTER 48

Herbal Medicine and Anesthesia

Ashit Bardhan and Craig Dunlop

CASE FORMAT: REFLECTION

A 33-year-old woman presented at term in spontaneous labor, requesting analgesia. She had previously had a normal vaginal delivery, during which she had received effective epidural analgesia. She had no significant medical problems, had experienced an uneventful pregnancy, had no allergies, and denied taking any medications. Epidural analgesia was offered and informed consent was obtained.

After establishing intravenous access, an epidural catheter was inserted aseptically on the first attempt in the L3–4 interspace. Effective analgesia was obtained. The patient had an uneventful labor and gave birth about 6 hours later to a live male infant by normal vaginal delivery. Before discharge from the labor ward, the epidural catheter was removed. She remained an inpatient for another day before being discharged home.

The following day at home, the patient began to develop central back pain and an associated headache. Both were relieved with simple analgesia including paracetamol and diclofenac. She did not seek medical attention at this point. The headache did not recur, but the back pain returned and gradually increased in severity over the subsequent 48 hours. By this stage, she was in severe pain with restricted mobility and presented to the emergency department for review. She was afebrile and generally well, reported no altered sensation or weakness of the lower limbs, and no symptoms of bladder or bowel disturbance. Examination revealed tenderness over the epidural insertion site with no neurologic signs in the lower limbs. She required opiate analgesia to provide effective pain relief.

The patient's blood test results were as follows: hemoglobin, 12.6 g/dL; white blood cell count, 13.5 × 10⁹/L elevated; neutrophils, 10.22 × 10⁹/L (elevated); platelets, 220 × 10⁹/L; erythrocyte sedimentation rate, 83 mm/hr elevated; international normalized ratio, 1.0; activated partial thromboplastin time, 30 seconds; sodium, 133 mmol/L; potassium, 3.9 mmol/L; urea, 4.8 mmol/L; and serum creatinine, 64 mmol/L.

A differential diagnosis of epidural abscess or epidural hematoma was considered, and the patient was admitted for further investigation and analgesia. An urgent neurosurgical consultation was requested, and a magnetic resonance imaging scan of the lumbar spine was performed (Fig. 48.1).

The magnetic resonance imaging scan revealed an epidural hematoma located at L3–4 with significant thecal

sac compression. In the absence of objective neurologic signs, the patient was managed conservatively, with analgesia as required and mobilization as tolerated.

The patient's history was reviewed for possible risk factors for epidural hematoma. At this stage, she admitted to taking oral Arnica when labor began to "reduce perineal bruising and aid healing following delivery." She had omitted to mention this at the time, as she felt that herbal remedies were safe and were not classified as medicines. By the time of the epidural insertion, she had taken three doses of two tablets. Examination of the packaging revealed no information as to active constituents. An Internet search suggested that Arnica montana contained "coumarin derivatives" and may potentiate anticoagulant effects. More formal evidence was limited to a journal letter stating that ingestion may result in an anticoagulant effect from coumarin constituents.[1]

The patient's symptoms improved over the course of 4 days, and she was discharged home. She was reviewed 3 weeks later and had complete pain resolution.

DISCUSSION

Complementary and alternative medicine is increasing in popularity, encompassing herbal and dietary supplements as well as alternative medical theories such as homeopathy and traditional Chinese medicine. Estimates of usage in patients vary from 4.8% to 42%.[2–6] Of these percentages, approximately 70% of patients are thought to not routinely disclose their usage to medical staff,[4] as in the patient described in this case. The danger lies with the assumption that the term *natural* is synonymous with *safe*. A survey of herbal medicine use in parturients showed that only 14.6% of those using herbal remedies considered them to be medications.[2]

Although the therapeutic profile of Arnica provides a possible explanation as to the occurrence of epidural hematoma in the patient in this case, a causal relationship could not be retrospectively ascertained. Also, she would have been likely to be offered an epidural even if the information regarding Arnica usage had been provided. A coagulation screen before insertion may have been prudent.

Under United States law, herbal and homeopathic medications are classified as dietary supplements, thus exempting them from regulations applicable to the introduction of prescription medicines.[7] The effect of this classification is to reinforce the belief that they are not drugs and additionally has

179

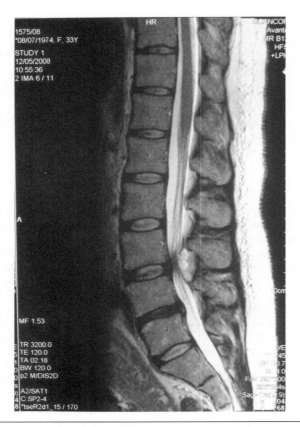

Figure 48.1 • Magnetic Resonance Image of the Spine, Lateral View.

removed the incentive to generate evidence for therapeutic or adverse effects. The presence and concentration of active constituents is often extremely difficult to assess and may vary among brands.[8] Licensing requirements in the United Kingdom are somewhat more rigorous but still fall short of preclinical animal and controlled clinical trials considered standard in the pharmaceutical industry.[9]

Of the more well-known supplements, the effects of most concern in the perioperative period are those of cardiovascular instability, drug interactions, altered coagulation, and altered sedation. Ephedra (ma-huang) may precipitate hypertension and has been associated with cerebrovascular accidents, arrhythmias, myocardial infarction, and sudden cardiac death.[10–12] Garlic and ginkgo may alter platelet aggregation and prolong bleeding times,[13] while ginseng may have a procoagulant effect.[14] Kava, St. John's Wort, and Valerian root may all increase sedative effects and prolong emergence.[13] Diet may also provoke serious adverse effects. Grapefruit juice is known to inhibit cytochrome CYP3A4, which plays a role in metabolism of statins and in this setting, may precipitate rhabdomyolysis.

Traditional Chinese herbal medicine may be even more challenging in that patients may be prescribed complex combinations of ingredients, leading to difficulty in assessment of what they are actually taking. Additionally, these herbal medicines commonly contain significant contaminants, such as heavy metals.[15] One of the few prospective studies investigating outcomes followed a cohort of 601 patients in Hong Kong

and examined the incidence of adverse events in the perioperative period.[16] In their population, 80% of patients took self-prescribed traditional Chinese herbal medicine, and they found an increased risk of adverse effects in the preoperative period including hypokalemia and prolonged activated partial thromboplastin time. No significant association was found between the use of any type of traditional Chinese herbal medicine and the occurrence of either intraoperative or postoperative events.

There is little information regarding guidelines for managing patients taking herbal medications in the perioperative period. The American Society of Anesthesiologists has published a leaflet for doctors containing information about more commonly encountered substances,[7] as well as an information leaflet for patients.[17] Awareness of the risks and direct questioning, along with patient education, remain the cornerstone of management.

KEY MESSAGES

1. The use of herbal medicine is often not reported to medical staff.
2. Although often assumed to be "natural" and thus innocuous, herbal medicines may potentially have significant adverse effects.
3. Manufacture of herbal medicines is not governed by the same strict criteria as that of conventional pharmaceuticals.
4. Good quality evidence of therapeutic or adverse effects of herbal medications is lacking, leading to reliance on anecdotal incidents and case reports.

QUESTIONS

1. What are the readily available herbal preparations that may increase bleeding tendency?

   Answer:
   • Garlic: Has antiplatelet effects and may potentiate warfarin resulting in an increase in international normalized ratio.
   • Ginger: Inhibits thromboxane synthetase, increasing bleeding time.
   • Ginkgo: May increase bleeding in patients taking anticoagulant or antithrombotic therapy.
   • Ginseng: Variable. May have antiplatelet properties, but may also reduce effectiveness of warfarin.
   • Also: Arnica, feverfew, vitamin E.[7]

2. Which herbal products should be discontinued before surgery?

   Answer: Garlic, ginseng, and Valerian root should be discontinued at least 1 week before surgery. St. John's Wort should be discontinued at least 5 days before surgery. Ephedra, ginkgo, Kava, and licorice should be discontinued at least 1 day beforehand.[18]

3. **Does St. John's Wort decrease the efficacy of digoxin?**

Answer: Yes. St. John's Wort is a potent inducer of the hepatic cytochrome P450 microsomal enzymes, thus increasing the metabolism of digoxin. This additionally affects levels of warfarin, theophylline, cyclosporine, anticonvulsants, and antiretrovirals.[10]

References

1. Shiffman MA. Warning about herbals in plastic and cosmetic surgery (letter). Plast and Reconstr Surg 2001;108:2180–2181.
2. Skinner CM, Rangasami J. Preoperative use of herbal medicines: a patient survey. B J Anaesth 2002;89:792–795.
3. Tsen LC, Segal S, Pothier M, et al. Alternative medicine use in presurgical patients. Anesthesiology 2000;93:148–151.
4. Kaye AD, Clarke RC, Sabar R, et al. Herbal medications: current trends in anesthesiology practice—a hospital survey. J Clin Anesth 2000;12:468–471.
5. Hepner DL, Harnett, M, Segal S, et al. Herbal medicine use in parturients. Anesth Analg 2002;94:690–693.
6. Eisenberg DM, Davis RB, Ettner SL, et al. Trends in alternative medicine use in the United States, 1990–1997: results of a follow-up study. JAMA 1998;280:1569–1575.
7. American Society of Anesthesiologists. Considerations for anesthesiologists: what you should know about your patients' use of herbal medicines and other dietary supplements. 2003. Available at www.asahq.com. Accessed: May 2008.
8. Harkey MR, Henderson GL, Gershwin ME, et al. Variability in commercial ginseng products: an analysis of 25 preparations. Am J Clin Nutr 2001;73:1101–1106.
9. Medicines and Healthcare Products Regulatory Agency. Safety of herbal medicinal products. 2002. Available at www.mhra.gov.uk. Accessed: May 2008.
10. Hodges PJ, Kam PC. The peri-operative implications of herbal medicines. Anaesthesia 2002;57:889–899.
11. Drew A. Herbal medicines: ma huang. Current Therapeutics July 2000;82–83.
12. Haller C, Benowitz N. Adverse cardiovascular and central nervous system events associated with dietary supplements containing ephedra alkaloids. N Engl J Med 2000;343:1833–1838.
13. Ang-Lee MK, Moss J, Yuan CS. Herbal medicines and perioperative care. JAMA 2001; 286:208–216.
14. Yuan CS, Wei G, Dey L, et al. American ginseng reduces warfarin's effect in healthy patients: a randomized, controlled trial. Ann Intern Med 2004;141:23–27.
15. Kam PCA, Liew S. Traditional Chinese herbal medicine and anaesthesia. Anaesthesia 2002;57:1083–1089.
16. Lee A, Chui PT, Aun CST, et al. Incidence and risk of adverse perioperative events among surgical patients taking traditional chinese herbal medicines. Anesthesiology 2006;105:454–461.
17. American Society of Anesthesiologists. What you should know about herbal and dietary supplement use and anesthesia. 2003. Available at www.asahq.com. Accessed: May 2008.
18. Heyneman CA. Preoperative considerations: which herbal products should be discontinued before surgery? Crit Care Nurse 2003;23:116–124.

CHAPTER 49

Levosimendan and Acute Heart Failure

Dorothy Breen

CASE FORMAT: REFLECTION

A 47-year-old female presented to the emergency department with increasing shortness of breath. In the preceding week, she had woken several times during the night unable to breathe or lie flat. The patient had no history of chest pain or palpitations, was well known to the cardiology service, and had a history of ischemic cardiomyopathy. Six years previously, she had undergone coronary artery bypass graft surgery; she also had a pacemaker in situ. Her medications were frusemide 20 mg twice per day, bisoprolol 10 mg once per day, and enalapril 5 mg once per day. On examination, the patient was alert but cyanosed and in marked respiratory distress. Her respiratory rate was 35 beats per minute; pulse,105 beats per minute, regular; and blood pressure, 130/75 mm Hg. On auscultation, crepitations were audible at both lung bases. Examination of the cardiovascular system revealed an elevated jugular venous pressure, displaced apex, and a third heart sound. The emergency physician administered 60% oxygen by face mask and 60 mg of frusemide intravenously. The following tests were ordered: arterial blood gases (Table 49.1), full blood count, urea, electrolytes, glucose, creatinine, liver function tests, troponin level (Table 49.2), and an electrocardiogram. The patient's chest radiograph is shown in Figure 49.1. There was some clinical improvement, but oxygen saturation measured by pulse oximetry was 89%. It was decided to notify the intensive care team. Continuous positive airway pressure (CPAP) via face mask (positive end-expiratory pressure, 10 cm water; 60% oxygen) and an intravenous infusion of glyceryl trinitrate were commenced. In the intensive care unit, an echocardiograph was performed, and left ventricular ejection-fraction was estimated at 20%. This was a notable reduction from previous estimates. Troponin levels were not elevated, and there were no new changes on the electrocardiogram. Six hours after admission, the patient was found to be tolerating CPAP well but desaturated rapidly if the mask was removed even for brief periods. In addition, her renal function had started to deteriorate. The intensivist reviewed her and commenced dobutamine 5 µg/kg per minute. The following day, the patient still required face mask CPAP, glyceryl trinitrate, and regular intravenous frusemide 60 mg three times daily. A different intensivist was now on duty and found the situation unchanged except that the patient's renal parameters had continued to deteriorate (Table 49.2). He decided to administer levosimendan in place of dobutamine. A bolus dose of 6 mcg/kg followed by an infusion of 0.2 µg/kg per minute was administered. Six hours later, the patient developed rapid atrial fibrillation at 130 beats per minute. Her blood pressure remained stable, and she was treated with amiodarone. She also received potassium supplementation, as her plasma potassium concentration had decreased to 3.0 mmol/L. Over the next 24 hours, the patient's dyspnea improved significantly, but her renal function continued to deteriorate (Table 49.2).

REVIEW

This patient presented with an episode of severe acute on chronic heart failure. Despite the frequency with which this clinical situation occurs, therapeutic options are limited, and as many as 25% of patients die within 6 months of presentation.[1] This patient was initially treated with oxygen, diuretics, and a peripheral vasodilator. Current guidelines emphasize these treatments as the cornerstones of therapy.[2,3] Loop diuretics are by far the most common agents used in this setting despite the lack of data from large clinical trials on their use.[4] The absence of hypotension in this case facilitated the use of a vasodilator (glyceryl trinitrate). CPAP was well tolerated and alleviated the patient's initial hypoxemia (Table 49.1).

The onset of renal dysfunction is of concern. Inadequate renal blood flow caused by poor cardiac output and hypovolemia resulting from aggressive diuresis contributed in this instance (Table 49.2). Short-term inotropic support is said to be indicated when there is evidence of hypoperfusion (i.e., the onset of renal dysfunction in this case). Dobutamine was the initial agent chosen for this purpose. However, the evidence to support the use of inotropes in this setting is not clear.[5,6] β-Agonists (e.g., dobutamine) and phosphodiesterase inhibitors (e.g., milrinone) are typically chosen for their ability to inodilate. More recently, levosimendan has received attention as a novel inotrope for this purpose. Levosimendan enhances myocardial sensitivity to calcium by binding to cardiac troponin C and does so in a calcium-dependent manner. Thus, the effect is greatest at times of high intracellular calcium concentration (i.e., during systole) and least at times of low intracellular calcium concentration (i.e., during diastole). Unlike other agents, levosimendan is capable of improving contractility without increasing myocardial oxygen demand. In addition, it activates adenosine triphosphate-dependent potassium channels in vascular smooth muscle producing peripheral and coronary vasodilation. In theory, these properties make levosimendan an ideal agent for use in

TABLE 49.1 Arterial Blood Gases Taken in the Emergency Room

	FiO$_2$ 0.6 via Venturi Face Mask	FiO$_2$, 0.6; PEEP,10 cm Water via CPAP
pH (7.35–7.45)	7.64	7.62
PaCO$_2$ (7.35–7.45)	31 mm Hg	33 mm Hg
PaO$_2$ (85–100 mm Hg)	55 mm Hg	85 mm Hg
Bicarbonate (22–26 mEq/L)	33 mmol/L	32 mmol/L

CPAP, continuous positive airway pressure; PEEP, positive end-expiratory pressure.

The most striking finding is hypoxemia, which corrects with the application of CPAP via face mask. Note also that alkalemia is present. The elevated bicarbonate level indicates metabolic alkalosis, but there is no evidence of respiratory compensation; in fact, the PaCO$_2$ is low. There are two acid-base processes here: metabolic alkalosis and respiratory alkalosis. The metabolic alkalosis is most likely caused by diuretic therapy, and the respiratory alkalosis is caused by tachypnea resulting from pulmonary edema.

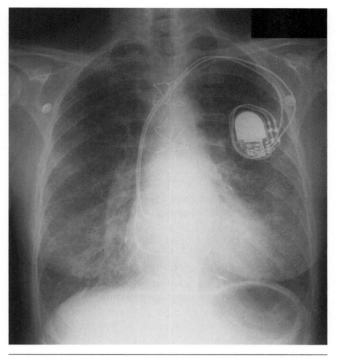

Figure 49.1 • The Patient's Chest Radiograph on Admission. A pacemaker and evidence of previous sternotomy are clearly seen. The heart is enlarged. There is a diffuse bilateral infiltrate with Kerley B lines (predominantly at the right base). The appearances are consistent with pulmonary edema.

TABLE 49.2 Biochemical Results Obtained at 0, 12, and 24 Hours After Admission

Values	Initial	12 Hours	24 Hours
Sodium (135–145 mmol/L)	130	131	133
Potassium (3.5–5.5 mmol/L)	3.1	3.5	3.0
Urea (3.0–8.0 mmol/L)	10	16	26
Creatinine (0.07–0.1 mmol/L)	0.10	0.14	0.16
Magnesium (0.7–1.0 mmol/L)	0.61	0.92	1.0
Bilirubin (μmol/L)	6		11
GGT (0–50 U/L)	15		21
ALP (32–110 U/L)	44		32
LDH (110–250 U/L)	122		118
AST (0–40 U/L)	22		23
ALT (0–40 U/L)	26		34
Glucose (4.0–7.5 mmol/L)	6.3	14.6	8.2
Troponin (0.0–0.2 ng/mL)	0.03	0.05	
BNP pg/mL	752	705	575

ALP, alkaline phosphatase; ALT, alanine aminotransferase; AST, aspartate aminotransferase; BNP, B-type natriuretic peptide; GGT, γ-glutamyl transferase; LDH, lactate dehydrogenase.

The initial presence of hyponatremia, hypokalemia, and hypomagnesemia indicate chronic loop diuretic use. At 12 hours, the electrolyte abnormalities have been corrected, but the patient's renal function has started to deteriorate. The result at 24 hours shows a disproportionate elevation in the urea: creatinine ratio (normally, 50–100:1); this most likely represents dehydration as a result of high-dose diuretic use. Hypokalemia recurs after levosimendan administration. Plasma BNP levels are elevated to those seen in congestive cardiac failure, although there is some decline with therapy.

this patient. The deteriorating renal function prompted the second intensivist to change from dobutamine to levosimendan in the patient discussed in this case.

In the setting of acute heart failure, levosimendan is the most widely studied inotrope to date. Encouraging results from initial studies have fueled enthusiasm for the drug. The RUSSLAN investigators explored the safety and efficacy of levosimendan versus placebo in patients with left ventricular failure following myocardial infarction. Five hundred patients were randomized to receive either placebo or levosimendan in one of four different dosing regimens.[7] Levosimendan administered at 0.1 to 0.2 μg/kg per minute had equivalent incidences of hypotension and ischemia when compared with placebo. Although not a primary end point, mortality was lower in the levosimendan group at 14 days (11.7% vs. 19.6%) and 180 days (22.6% vs. 31.4%).

The LIDO trial examined 203 patients similar to the present case (low output heart failure and documented left ventricular ejection fraction <0.35).[8] Patients were randomly assigned to receive either levosimendan (24 μg/kg bolus followed by an infusion of 0.1 μg/kg per minute) or dobutamine (5–10 μg/kg per minute) each for 24 hours. The primary end point of the trial was the proportion of patients showing hemodynamic improvement as measured by ≥30% increase in cardiac output and a ≤ 25% reduction in pulmonary capillary wedge pressure. A significantly greater proportion of patients in the levosimendan group compared with the dobutamine group (28% vs. 15%) reached this endpoint. Analysis of mortality data revealed a significantly greater mortality rate in the dobutamine group at both 31 days (8% vs. 17%) and 180 days (26% vs. 38%).

Subgroup analysis in the LIDO trial showed that the use of β-blockers, as in the case described, enhanced the hemodynamic effects of levosimendan but diminished those of dobutamine. Furthermore, decreases in mean potassium levels were observed in the levosimendan group over the 24 hours of the study. Despite initial supplementation, the patient's potassium levels fell with the administration of levosimendan in this case (Table 49.2).

This study and others led to the inclusion of levosimendan for use in patients with symptomatic low-output cardiac failure without hypotension in the 2004 European heart failure guidelines.[2] The durations of action of levosimendan and dobutamine differ. Levosimendan has an active metabolite OR-1896 that has a long half-life. The clinical hemodynamic effects of levosimendan can persist for up to 7 to 9 days after discontinuation of the drug. In this respect, the validity of comparing a 24-hour infusion of levosimendan with a 24-hour infusion of dobutamine has been questioned.[9]

The CASINO study was designed to enroll 600 patients with acute decompensated heart failure. Patients were randomized to receive a 24-hour infusion of levosimendan, dobutamine, or placebo.[5,10,11] The trial was terminated after 299 patients were enrolled because of improved outcome in the levosimendan group. Mortality at 6 months was 18% for the levosimendan group, 28.3% for the placebo group, and a remarkable 42% in the dobutamine group.

Two larger clinical trials have been designed to confirm these initial positive findings regarding the use of levosimendan. REVIVE-11 compared levosimendan with placebo in 600 patients with acute decompensated heart failure and left ventricular impairment similar to this case (ejection fraction ≤ 35%). Patients in the levosimendan group had better symptomatic improvement, greater decreases in plasma B-type natriuretic peptide (BNP) levels, and shorter duration of hospital stay when compared with those who received placebo.[12] Patients taking levosimendan showed a trend toward a greater mortality at 90 days (35 deaths in the placebo group vs. 45 in the levosimendan group). Mortality was not a primary end point of REVIVE-11, but the outcome data seem at odds with earlier smaller studies. Atrial fibrillation developed in the patient described in this case following levosimendan administration. In REVIVE 11, atrial fibrillation, hypotension, and ventricular tachycardia occurred more frequently with levosimendan than with placebo.

This patient had symptomatic improvement and a decrease in BNP levels when switched to levosimendan. To determine if this result translates into improved survival, the evidence from larger outcome studies is needed.

SURVIVE represents the largest outcome study to date of levosimendan use in patients with acute decompensated heart failure.[13] In this recently published randomized, double-blind, international trial, 1327 patients were assigned to receive a 24-hour infusion of either dobutamine (5–40 μg/kg per minute) or levosimendan (bolus, 12 μg/kg followed by an infusion 0.1–0.2 μg/kg per minute). Despite a decrease in plasma BNP levels, there was no difference in mortality at 31 days (12% in the levosimendan group vs. 14% in the dobutamine group) or at 180 days (26% in the levosimendan group vs. 28% in the dobutamine group). It has been observed that the failure to demonstrate survival benefit in the SURVIVE study could in part be attributed to the fact that some patients had low systolic pressure and may have been in cardiogenic shock, rendering them unsuitable for treatment with levosimendan.[10] The patient described in this case presented with severe acute on chronic heart failure. Subgroup analysis of the SURVIVE data has shown that a trend toward a lower 31-day mortality rate was observed in those with a prior history of heart failure.

Is levosimendan a better choice than dobutamine for the patient described here? Given the available evidence to date, no clear case can be made for a better outcome with the use of one agent over another. Proponents of levosimendan can be reassured by the amount of data that exists when compared with other agents currently in use for acute heart failure.[2,10] Future trials should focus on subgroups that may benefit most from levosimendan. Patients such as the woman described in this case (on β-blocker therapy, with acute on chronic heart failure, and normotensive) represent a potential target population for such further study.

KEY MESSAGES

1. Levosimendan is a novel inodilator, and its mode of action is mediated via myocardial sensitization to calcium.

2. Smaller studies point to the safety and efficacy of levosimendan in relieving symptoms, reducing BNP levels, and improving hemodynamic profile.

3. The largest clinical trial to date failed to show a long-term mortality benefit when compared with dobutamine.

QUESTIONS

1. What is the mechanism of action of levosimendan?

   Answer: Levosimendan is a positive isotrope which enhances myocardial sensitivity to calcium by binding troporin C in a calcium sensitive manner.

2. In patients with acute decompensated heart failure, does levosimendan confer a survival advantage compared to dobutamine?

   Answer: Probably not. The best evidence (SURVIVE TRIAL) indicates similar mortality for patients who received on or other of these drugs at 31 and 180 days.

3. What is the duration of action of levosimendan?

   Answer: Although usually administered by continuous infusion, clinical hemodynamic effects can persist for 7 to 9 days after discontinuation of the infusion due to an active metabolite with a long elimination half life.

References

1. Mebazza A, Nieminen M, Packer M, et al. Levosimendan vs. dobutamine for patients with acute decompensated heart failure. The SURVIVE randomized trial. JAMA 2007;297:1883–1891.
2. Nieminen MS, Bohm M, Cowie MR, et al. ESC Committee for Practice Guidelines (CPG). Executive summary of the guidelines on the diagnosis and treatment of acute heart failure: the task force on acute heart failure of the European society of cardiology. Eur Heart J 2005;26:384–416.
3. Heart failure society of America: HFSA 2006 comprehensive heart failure practice guidelines. Evaluation and management of patients with acute decompensated heart failure. J Card Fail 2006;12:86–103.
4. Allen LA, O'Connor CM. Management of acute decompensated heart failure. Can Med Assoc J 2007;176:787–805.
5. De Luca L, Colucci WS, Nieminen MS, et al. Evidence-based use of levosimendan in different clinical settings. Eur Heart J 2006;27:1908–1920.
6. Thackray S, Eastaugh J, Freemantle N, et al. The effectiveness and relative effectiveness of intravenous inotropic drugs acting through the adrenergic pathway in patients with heart failure: a meta-regression analysis. Eur J Heart Fail 2002;4:515–529.
7. Moiseyev VS, Poder P, Andrejevs N, et al. Safety and efficacy of a novel calcium sensitizer, levosimendan, in patients with left ventricular failure due to an acute myocardial infarction. A randomized, placebo-controlled, double-blind study (RUSSLAN). Eur Heart J 2002;23:1422–1432.
8. Follath F, Cleland JG, Just H, et al. Efficacy and safety of intravenous levosimendan compared with dobutamine in severe low-output heart failure (the LIDO study): a randomised double-blind trial. Lancet 2002;360:196–202.
9. Delaney A, Bradford C, McCaffrey J, et al. Is there a place for levosimendan in the intensive care unit? Crit Care Resusc 2007;9: 290–292.
10. Cleland JG, Ghosh J, Freemantle N, et al. Clinical trials update from and cumulative meta-analyses from the American college of cardiology: WATCH, SCD-HeFT, DINAMIT, CASINO, INSPIRE, STRATUS-US, RIO-Lipids and cardiac resynchronisation therapy in heart failure. Eur J Heart Fail 2004;6: 501–508.
11. Zairis MN, Apostolatos C, Anastasiadis P. The effect of a calcium sensitizer or an inotrope or none in chronic low output decompensated heart failure: results from the calcium sensitizer or an inotrope or none in low output decompensated heart failure (CASINO). J Am Coll Cardiol 2004;43: 206A–207A.
12. Teerlink JR, Packer M, Colucci WS, et al. Levosimendan provides rapid and sustained relief in patient global assessment of acutely decompensated heart failure: the REVIVE 11 study. J Card Fail 2006;12:S86.

CHAPTER 50

Antiplatelet Agents, Low-Molecular-Weight Heparin, and Neuraxial Blockade

Leon Serfontein

CASE FORMAT: REFLECTION

A 67-year-old, 83-kg man diagnosed with a rectal carcinoma was scheduled for an abdominoperineal resection. On initial screening, there was no evidence of metastatic disease. The patient had dyslipidemia, long-standing well-controlled hypertension, and coronary artery disease. Six months previously, he had presented to the emergency department with chest pain and was diagnosed with unstable angina for which he had undergone coronary angioplasty with stenting of two vessels. Since then, he had been angina-free and had good exercise tolerance (able to walk briskly for 20 to 30 minutes and to climb two flights of stairs without rest or shortness of breath). He had stopped smoking after his cardiac event but admitted to smoking 10 to 15 cigarettes a day for nearly 35 years prior to that.

The patient was currently taking the following medications once per day: aspirin 150 mg, atorvastatin 20 mg, diltiazem 360 mg, and esomeprozole 20 mg. He had discontinued clopidogrel 7 days previously as per the surgeon's instruction.

The patient's cardiorespiratory examination was unremarkable. His vital signs were as follows: temperature, 36.7°C; pulse rate, 76 beats per minute; blood pressure, 145/80 mm Hg; and respiratory rate, 18 breaths per minute.

The patient's electrocardiogram reading revealed sinus rhythm with no evidence of ischemia or previous infarction, and his chest radiograph was normal. An echocardiogram performed after his stenting showed mild concentric left ventricular hypertrophy, left ventricular ejection fraction of 60%, and normal valves.

The results of the patient's blood work were as follows: full blood count, normal (hemoglobin, 13.4 g/dl; platelets, 190×10^9/L); electrolytes, normal; coagulation screen, normal (international normalized ratio, 0.9; activated partial thromboplastin time, 25 seconds); and cholesterol, 6.5 mmol/L.

An anesthetic plan was discussed with the patient on the evening before surgery. It was decided to place a thoracic epidural catheter for perioperative pain management before inducing general anesthesia. As the patient was anxious, diazepam 10 mg was prescribed. It was noted that enoxaparin 40 mg had been administered subcutaneously at 6:00 PM.

The patient arrived to the operating room at 8:30 on the following morning, and standard monitoring was applied. An intravenous 16-gauge cannula was inserted in his left hand, followed by insertion of an epidural at the T9–10 interspace with the patient in the sitting position. Blood was aspirated through the epidural catheter and failed to clear on flushing or on incremental withdrawal of the catheter. The epidural catheter was reinserted at T8–9 without complications. After administration of a negative test dose (lidocaine 2% with adrenaline 1:200,000 U/mL), preoxygenation (100% oxygen tidal breathing for 3 minutes) was performed, and general anesthesia was induced. The patient received fentanyl 100 μg, propofol 160 mg, and vecuronium 8 mg intravenously. Anesthesia was maintained with sevoflurane in air:oxygen (50:50). Another 16-gauge cannula was inserted in the patient's right external jugular vein. A bolus of bupivacaine 0.25% 10 mL was administered via the epidural catheter in divided doses followed by an infusion of bupivacaine 0.125% with fentanyl 2 mcg/mL at 10 mL.hr^{-1}. The surgical registrar inserted a urinary catheter. After infusion of the first liter of Hartmann's solution, paracetamol 2 g and diclofenac 75 mg were administered intravenously.

As surgery proceeded, "generalized ooze" was noted in the operative field. The patient's hemodynamic stability was maintained with intravenous fluids and intermittent boluses of phenylephrine (total, 400 mcg). Hartmann's solution (2500 mL), hydroxy-ethyl 6% (130:4) (500 mL), and two units of packed red blood cells were administered intraoperatively. The patient's measured total blood loss was 1400 mL.

At 12:00, the patient's trachea was extubated, and he was taken to the high-dependency unit. During the next 24 hours, he complained of abdominal pain intermittently, and bolus doses of bupivacaine 0.25% (6 mL each) were administered per epidural with good effect. The patient also complained of weakness in his legs but was reassured by the nurses that it was a normal effect of the epidural. Upon instruction from the surgical team, enoxaparin 40 mg subcutaneously was administered at 6:00 on the evening of the operative day.

At 3:00 PM on the first postoperative day, the patient complained of back pain and was unable to move his lower limbs. A magnetic resonance imaging scan was performed, which identified a large epidural hematoma extending from T7 to T11. An emergency decompressive laminectomy was performed to evacuate the hematoma. The patient recovered with a degree of residual lower body muscle weakness and sensory loss, which improved partially over the course of the subsequent 6 months.

DISCUSSION

Antiplatelet Agents and Neuraxial Blocks

Antiplatelet agents are commonly prescribed for primary and secondary prevention of cardiovascular disease and to decrease the incidence of acute cerebrovascular and cardiovascular events. Long-term dual therapy with aspirin and clopidogrel in this patient was indicated to maintain patency of his coronary stents.[1,2]

In the case described, the anesthetist and the surgical team were confronted with the need to balance the risk of increased blood loss if the antiplatelet agents were continued during the perioperative period, with that of coronary thrombosis if the drugs were stopped abruptly. In a meta-analysis of 41 studies evaluating aspirin-related bleeding risks in a wide range of surgical procedures, aspirin was found to increase the rate of bleeding complications (ranging from mild to severe) by a factor of 1.5 without an increase in surgical mortality or morbidity (with the exception of intracranial surgery and possibly transurethral prostatectomy).[3]

The well-established benefits of epidural anesthesia had to be weighed against the rare but potentially devastating complication of epidural hematoma.[4,5] This decision should be made on an individual basis, but any attempt to make an evidence-based decision is limited by the rarity of epidural hematomata. The American (American Society of Regional Anesthesia and Pain Medicine) and European guidelines summarize other evidence-based reviews and represent the collective experience of recognized experts in the field.

The elimination half-life of clopidogrel is short (4 hours), but recovery from the drug is long (7 days) because of irreversible platelet inhibition.[8] Neuraxial blockade is therefore contraindicated in a patient who has taken clopidogrel within seven days.[7] In the case of the patient described herein, neuraxial block was appropriately performed 7 days after clopidogrel had been discontinued. This interval should be extended to 14 days for ticlopidine, another thienopyridine derivative.[6]

Nonsteroidal anti-inflammatory drugs do not appear to add to the risks of neuraxial blockade, except when used in combination with other drugs that affect clotting mechanisms.[6] This patient received a low-molecular-weight heparin (LMWH) preoperatively as well as aspirin. If a nonsteroidal anti-inflammatory drug were to be administered, a cyclooxygenase-2 selective inhibitor would have been a better choice in this case because of its minimal effect on platelet function.[6]

Timing of Needle Placement and Catheter Removal

It is necessary to time epidural needle placement and catheter removal relative to the timing of anticoagulant drug administration. This patient was at moderate-to-high risk for developing venous thromboembolism, making LMWH an important part of his management.[9]

Epidural needle insertion should be performed at least 10 to 12 hours after the preceding dose of LMWH. The same interval should be allowed to elapse from the last dose of LMWH until the epidural catheter is removed. As will be highlighted later, this step may have to be altered in patients at

greater risk of epidural hematoma. In the case of therapeutic anticoagulation with LMWH, this time period should be further extended to 24 hours.[7] After the removal of an epidural catheter, a minimum of 2 hours should elapse before subsequent LMWH administration.[7]

The previously mentioned guidelines apply to once-daily dosing of LMWH, which was applied in the patient described herein and which approximates European practice. Although the biochemistry and pharmacology of LMWHs vary, there is a lack of comparative studies. Experience in Europe indicates that the incidence of epidural hematoma associated with different LMWHs is similar.[7]

Managing High-Risk Patients

The incidence of epidural hematoma is less than 1 in 150,000 epidurals and less than 1 in 220,000 spinal anesthetics.[10] In patients receiving a LMWH, the incidence of epidural hematoma is approximately 1 in 3000 patients undergoing continuous epidural anesthesia and 1 in 40,000 patients undergoing spinal anesthesia.[11] Several patient characteristics have been associated with an increased risk of developing spinal hematoma after neuraxial anesthesia (Table 50.1).[12] Based on these, the patient in this case was at greater risk of this particular complication. He had received nonsteroidal anti-inflammatory drugs (aspirin and diclofenac) in conjunction with other anticoagulants and a vessel puncture on catheter insertion. Ideally, the subsequent dose of LMWH should be delayed for 24 hours after the traumatic puncture.[6,7]

TABLE 50.1 Risk Factors for Developing Spinal Hematoma

Patient Factors
Female gender
Increased age
Impaired hemostasis
Anatomic anomalies of spinal cord/vertebral column
Anesthetic Factors
Repeated, difficult needle/catheter placement
Traumatic (bloody) punctures
Epidural (cf. spinal) technique
Thromboprophylaxis Management Factors
LMWH with concomitant antiplatelet or anticoagulant administration
LMWH administration in the presence of an indwelling epidural catheter
Immediate pre-, intra-, or early postoperative LMWH administration
Twice-daily LMWH dosing

LMWH, low-molecular-weight heparin.
Modified from Horlocker TT, Wedel DJ, Benson H. Regional anesthesia in anticoagulated patients: defining the risks. Reg Anesth Pain Med 2003;28:172–198.

The provision of safe neuraxial anesthesia/analgesia concurrent with anticoagulation requires education of the entire patient care team. Patients at increased risk should be identified by and to the responsible clinicians and nurses. One option in this case would have been to avoid greater concentrations (>1.25%) of bupivacaine for "top-ups," thus allowing better assessment and earlier detection of neurologic dysfunction. Magnetic resonance imaging is the diagnostic tool of choice for detecting epidural hematoma. Emergency decompressive laminectomy is the treatment of choice.[13,14] Overall, a less severe preoperative neurological deficit and early hematoma evacuation (within 6 hours) are associated with better neurological recovery.[15,16]

Newer and more effective anticoagulants are continuously being developed. Examples include the new synthetic pentasaccharide fondaparinux, and razaxaban, each of which has potent antifactor Xa activity and is intended for thromboprophylactic use. Because of their efficacy and longer elimination half-lives, these drugs pose additional problems for the anesthetist. Alternative anesthetic and analgesic techniques should be considered for patients considered to be at unacceptably high risk of epidural hematoma. Safer neuraxial alternatives such as spinal (cf. epidural) anesthesia or peripheral nerve blockade are among these options. In general, superficial limb blocks, the anatomical landmarks for which are well defined or easily visualized with ultrasound imaging and performed where a developing hematoma can be easily accessed and compressed, are not contraindicated in patients receiving anticoagulation.[7]

KEY MESSAGES

1. Neuraxial blockade is contraindicated in a patient who has taken clopidogrel within 7 days.

2. Epidural needle insertion as well as epidural catheter removal should be performed at least 10 to 12 hours after the preceding dose (prophylactic regimen) of LMWH.

3. Magnetic resonance imaging is the diagnostic tool of choice for detecting epidural hematoma, and emergency decompressive laminectomy is the treatment of choice.

4. A less severe preoperative neurological deficit and early hematoma evacuation (within 6 hours) are associated with better neurological recovery.

QUESTIONS

1. How could the risk of epidural hematoma associated with neuraxial anesthesia be minimized?

   Answer:
   • Identifying patients at unacceptably high risk and considering alternative anesthetic/analgesic techniques such as peripheral nerve blocks when feasible.
   • Performing spinal anesthesia in preference to epidural anesthesia when possible.
   • Timing needle insertion and epidural catheter removal appropriately in the presence of perioperative anticoagulation (to occur at the nadir of anticoagulant activity).

   An indwelling epidural catheter should not be removed while the patient is therapeutically anticoagulated.
   • Avoiding combinations of drugs (perioperatively) that independently alter coagulation.

2. What are the symptoms of cord compression from an epidural hematoma?

   Answer: Symptoms include severe back pain, new-onset, or persisting sensory or motor deficit outlasting the expected duration of the neuraxial block and bowel or bladder dysfunction within the postoperative period.

3. Following removal of an indwelling epidural catheter, how long is the wait before the next dose of prophylactic heparin could be safely administered?

   Answer: A minimum of 2 hours.

References

1. Burger W, Chemnitius JM, Kneissl GD, Rücker G. Low-dose aspirin for secondary cardiovascular prevention—cardiovascular risks after its preoperative withdrawal versus bleeding risks with its continuation—review and meta-analysis. J Int Med 2005;257:399–414.

2. Bergqvist D, Wu CL, Neal JM. Anticoagulation and neuraxial regional anesthesia: perspectives. Reg Anesth Pain Med 2003;28:163.

3. Rodgers A, Walker N, Schug S, et al. Reduction of postoperative mortality and morbidity with epidural or spinal anaesthesia: results from overview of randomised trials. Br Med J 2000;321:1.

4. ACC/AHA/SCAI Guideline update for percutaneous coronary intervention. Executive summary. J Am Coll Cardiol 2006;47:216–235.

5. AHA/ACC Guidelines for secondary prevention for patients with coronary and other atherosclerotic vascular disease: 2006 update. Circulation 2006;113:2363–2372.

6. Second Consensus Conference on Neuraxial Anesthesia and Anticoagulation. April 25–28, 2002.

7. Horlocker TT, Wedel DJ, Benson H. Regional anesthesia in anticoagulated patients: defining the risks. Reg Anesth Pain Med 2003;28:172–198.

8. Weber AA, Braun M, Hohlfeld T, et al. Recovery of platelet function after discontinuation of clopidogrel treatment in healthy volunteers. Br J Clin Pharmacol 2001; 52:333–336.

9. Anonymous. Practice parameters for the prevention of venous thromboembolism. The Standards Task Force of The American Society of Colon and Rectal Surgeons. Dis Colon Rectum 2000; 43:1037–1047.

10. Horlocker TT, Wedel DJ, Schroeder DR, et al. Preoperative antiplatelet therapy does not increase the risk of spinal hematoma with regional anesthesia. Anesth Analg 1995;80:303–309.

11. Horlocker TT, Wedel DJ. Neuraxial block and low molecular-weight heparin: balancing perioperative analgesia and thromboprophylaxis. Reg Anesth Pain Med 1998;23:164.

12. Horlocker TT, Wedel DJ. Anticoagulation and neuraxial block: historical perspective, anesthetic implications, and risk management. Reg Anesth Pain Med 1998;23:129–134.

13. Binder DK, Sonne DC, Lawton MT. Spinal epidural hematoma. Neurosurg Q 2004;14:51–59.

14. Vandermeulen EP, Van Aken H, Vermylen J. Anticoagulants and spinal–epidural anesthesia Anesth Analg 1994;79:1165–1177.

15. Kreppel D, Antoniadis G, Seeling W. Spinal hematoma: a literature survey with meta- analysis of 613 patients. Neurosurg Rev 2003;26:1–49.

16. Lawton MT, Porter RW, Heiserman JE, et al. Surgical management of spinal epidural hematoma: relationship between surgical timing and neurological outcome. J Neurosurg 1995;83:1–7.

CHAPTER 51

Neuroprotection During Cerebral Aneurysm Surgery

Peter John Lee

CASE FORMAT: REFLECTION

A 54-year-old, 65-kg woman presented to the emergency department with sudden-onset severe headache, vomiting, and drowsiness. Her Glasgow Coma Scale score was 13. Computed axial tomography showed diffuse subarachnoid hemorrhage (SAH) from an aneurysm. Four-vessel cerebral angiography was performed and revealed a ruptured aneurysm on the anterior communicating artery. Nimodipine 60 mg was administered to the patient orally, and phenytoin 975 mg was administered intravenously over 20 minutes. The patient was scheduled to undergo aneurysm clipping on the following morning.

The patient had a 10-year history of hypertension for which she took indapamide 2.5 mg and atenolol 25 mg each morning. She denied symptoms of cardiac disease but admitted to smoking 20 cigarettes each day for 20 years. The patient denied cocaine use.

On arrival to the operating room, the patient's GCS score had deteriorated to 11. Her blood pressure was 140/90 mm Hg, and her heart rate was 85 beats per minute. She had no focal neurological deficit.

The results of a full blood picture, urea, electrolytes, and blood glucose performed in the emergency department were all normal. Electrocardiograph and chest radiograph readings were unremarkable. Two units of cross-matched blood were made available.

Standard monitoring was commenced in the operating room, and a 16-gauge intravenous (IV) cannula was inserted (an 18-gauge IV cannula was already in situ). A cannula was placed in the patient's left radial artery for arterial pressure monitoring. Fentanyl 150 µg IV was administered. Anesthesia was induced with propofol 150 mg, and muscle relaxation was achieved with vecuronium 8 mg. Following tracheal intubation, anesthesia was maintained with inhaled sevoflurane at one minimum alveolar concentration in an air/oxygen mixture. A nasopharyngeal temperature probe was inserted, and a forced-air cooling blanket was placed on the patient, with the temperature set to 32°C. Immediately before pinning the patient's head in a Mayfield surgical frame, fentanyl 200 µg was administered IV, and her scalp was infiltrated with bupivacaine 0.5% 5 mL.

After incision of the dura and when optimal exposure was obtained, the surgeon announced his intention to place a temporary clip on the A1 segment of the anterior communicating artery.

Shortly after administration of thiopentone 250 mg IV, the patient's blood pressure decreased to 80/45 mm Hg. The nasopharyngeal temperature was 35.1° C. Arterial blood gas, electrolyte, and glucose analysis were performed as shown here:

pH	7.37	Na^+	140 mmol/L^{-1}
pCO_2	6.3 kPa	K^+	5.1 mmol/L^{-1}
pO_2	11.3 kPa	Cl^-	100 mmol/L^{-1}
HCO_3^-	25 mmol/L	Glucose	12 mmol/L^{-1}
BE	0 mmol/L		
SaO_2	96%		

After placement of the temporary clip, IV phenylephrine boluses of 50 µg were administered as required to maintain the patient's blood pressure within a mean arterial pressure of 70 to 80 mm Hg. Ninety minutes later, after placing the permanent clip on the aneurysm, the surgeon removed the temporary clip. The total surgical blood loss was approximately 200 mL and was replaced with 250 mL colloid. Normal saline 2000 mL was administered over the course of the operation. The surgery lasted for 150 minutes.

During surgical closure, the cooling blanket temperature setting was increased to 38°C. Fentanyl 200 µg was administered at this time. The inspired concentration of inhalational agent was decreased, and reversal of neuromuscular block was achieved using glycopyrrolate 500 µg and neostigmine 2.5 mg. The patient's trachea was extubated when she demonstrated a satisfactory spontaneous ventilatory pattern and nasopharyngeal temperature was 37°C. Twenty minutes after discontinuing the inhalational agent, the patient had emerged sufficiently to obey commands. She did not cough with extubation, and her blood pressure was 135/92 mm Hg at the time.

The patient was transferred to the postanesthesia care unit where she was noted to be drowsy but rousable with a Glasgow Coma Scale score of 14. She had no focal neurological deficit. Morphine was administered intravenously to a total of 8 mg, titrated to patient request, and she was transferred to the high-dependency unit for continued monitoring.

Cerebral angiography 2 weeks after surgery showed obliteration of the aneurysm and no additional aneurysms. The patient was maintained on nimodipine for 21 days after surgery and was discharged home having made a full neurological recovery.

CASE DISCUSSION

Cerebral aneurysms have a prevalence of 0.2% to 9.9% in the general population.[1] The incidence of SAH resulting from ruptured cerebral aneurysms ranges from 6 to 16 per 100,000, depending on the population under study.[2,3] In the United States, this figure accounts for 25,000 to 30,000 cases of SAH per year.[4]

The application of temporary clips to a cerebral artery during surgical exploration and repair of an intracranial aneurysm is performed when the risk of rupture is high. Temporary clipping causes a period of focal cerebral ischemia and the anesthetist should institute measures for neuroprotection in this situation.

Neuroprotection

Neuroprotective strategies are intended to modify intra-ischemic cellular and vascular biological responses to deprivation of the cellular energy supply to increase tissue tolerance to ischemia and/or reperfusion resulting in improved outcome.[5] Uncontrolled release of glutamate during ischemia and the consequent excessive stimulation of postsynaptic receptors are implicated in the initiation of neuronal injury, a process known as *excitotoxicity*. Neuronal apoptosis occurs early during ischemia and is responsible for some of the continued neuronal loss that is seen following the insult.

Blood Pressure

Maintaining a high normal cerebral perfusion pressure (CPP) can augment collateral blood flow to the ischemic penumbra, minimize secondary injury, and result in improved neurological outcome. This is particularly germane when a temporary clip has been applied, and collateral perfusion to affected areas can occur through Willisian channels, pial-to-pial collaterals, or leptomeningeal pathways. CPP should be maintained at a greater level in patients who are chronically hypertensive and whose autoregulatory curves are shifted to the right. It may be best to maintain the blood pressure of such individuals close to their pre-SAH measurements. In this case, the anesthetist maintained the mean arterial pressure between 70 to 80 mm Hg; in the absence of accurate data on the patient's baseline blood pressure, this is acceptable management.

Partial Pressure of Carbon Dioxide

During periods of focal cerebral ischemia, ventilation should be altered to ensure normocapnia. Hypercapnia can cause intracerebral "steal" by preferentially vasodilating vessels in the noninjured area and decreasing intracellular pH. Hypocapnia does not cause the putative inverse-steal phenomenon and can increase the size of the region at risk of ischemic damage. The hypercapnia seen in the arterial blood gas analysis in this case (pCO_2, 6.3 kPa) should have been corrected promptly.

Blood Glucose

Hyperglycemia increases damage in focal ischemia and is an independent predictor of poor outcome in patients who have focal ischemic injury. During incomplete ischemia, glucose is metabolized anaerobically by glycolysis, with a resultant accumulation of lactic acid and decrease in pH. The buffering capacity of the brain is exceeded, and reactive oxygen species are generated leading to cell membrane rupture and neuronal necrosis. The hyperglycemia noted in this patient should have been corrected.

In clinical practice, it is advisable to avoid glucose-containing solutions and to correct hyperglycemia aggressively (target concentration, 5–9 mmol/L^{-1}) in patients with focal cerebral ischemia.

Temperature

Hypothermia can offer some degree of neuroprotection in focal and global ischemia. Early studies have shown that hypothermia decreases cerebral metabolic rate (CMR) in a temperature-dependent fashion, with the greatest effect at very low temperatures (18°C–22°C) achievable only with cardiopulmonary bypass. The effects of mild hypothermia (cooling to 32°C–35°C) were found to be negligible. Reduction in brain temperature by 2°C to 4°C has been shown to be neuroprotective in rats. The protective effects of hypothermia are more likely to be dependent on changes at several steps in the ischemic cascade than on change in CMR alone. Possible mechanisms include suppression of glutamate release and decrease in nitric oxide production leading to a reduction in free radical-triggered lipid peroxidation. Disappointingly, a prospective trial has shown that short-duration intraoperative hypothermia (33°C) did not improve 3-month neurologic outcome after craniotomy for good-grade patients with aneurysmal subarachnoid hemorrhage.[6]

Hypothermia causes shivering with increased oxygen demand, is associated with arrhythmias and cardiac ischemia, decreased platelet activity, disordered coagulation, and increased infection rate.

The conflicting nature of such study results as well as the paucity of prospective trials in the area leave many anesthetists unsure of hypothermia's role in neuroprotection. The mild hypothermia achieved in the patient discussed in this case would have provided little neuroprotection and may have contributed to the delay in emergence. A timely emergence is important so that prompt neurologic examination can be performed.

Without doubt, hyperthermia has adverse effects on the postischemic brain. Spontaneous hyperthermia, common in the postischemic brain, is associated with poor outcome in humans and should be treated aggressively.[7]

IV Anesthetic Agents

The protective effect of barbiturates in focal cerebral ischemia has been shown in one human trial and in numerous animal trials.

This effect is thought to be caused by suppression of the CMR, which produces a progressive decrease in electroencephalographic activity and a reduction in the rate of adenosine 5-triphosphate depletion. It may also result from cerebral blood flow (CBF) redistribution to peri-ischemic areas, free radical scavenging, and potentiation of γ-aminobutyric acid activity.

The potential for barbiturates to confer long-term neuroprotection has not been investigated.

Propofol may have beneficial effects on cerebral physiology. It decreases CMR and CBF. It can also protect the brain against ischemic injury in rats. Neuroprotection by propofol might result from a direct scavenging effect on reactive oxygen species generated during ischemia and reperfusion.[8] Propofol, compared with nitrous oxide and fentanyl, decreases neuronal injury and favorably modulates apoptosis-regulating proteins for at least 28 days. This suggests that propofol could be neuroprotective over a long postischemic period, particularly if the insult is mild.[9] Because propofol has negative inotropic and vasodilatory properties, it may decrease CPP if a large dose is administered rapidly.

Ketamine increases intracranial pressure, CMR, and CBF. However, it also inhibits glutamatergic neurotransmission at the N-methyl-D-aspartate receptor, which is highly activated by the excitatory transmitter release that occurs during ischemia. There are no human data supporting the use of ketamine in brain protection.

Lidocaine blocks apoptotic cell death in vitro, and, in antiarrhythmic doses, it decreases infarct size and improves neurologic outcome in a rat model of transient ischemia.[10] Opioids (such as fentanyl, used in this case) are useful adjuncts as they limit the need for higher-dose volatile anesthetics with attendant cerebral vasodilation and increased CBF. Evidence as to whether opioids produce neuroprotection is lacking. The short half-life of fentanyl in moderate doses allows timely postsurgical neurological evaluation.

The use of thiopentone in this patient was appropriate. Propofol can also be used as a neuroprotective agent and can circumvent the delayed emergence seen with large doses of barbiturates.

Inhalational Anesthetic Agents

Inhalational anesthetic agents can decrease ischemic cerebral injury. Both halothane and sevoflurane reduce the volume of infarction after focal ischemia.[11] This occurs because these agents attenuate excitotoxicity by inhibiting glutamate release and postsynaptic glutamate receptor-mediated responses. The neuroprotection offered by isoflurane, and possibly other inhalational agents, appears to be short-lived; a reduction in neurologic injury is seen when evaluated at 2 days but not 14 days after ischemic injury.[12]

Like the barbiturates, most inhalational anesthetic agents produce progressive electroencephalographic depression in a dose-dependent manner, with a similar reduction in CMR.

Halothane is a potent cerebral vasodilator that can produce a marked increase in intracranial pressure. Hyperventilation can be used to prevent this increase but must be instituted before introducing the halothane, as the vasodilatory effects occur faster than the onset of metabolic suppression. Enflurane is a less potent cerebral vasodilator and more potent depressant of CMR. Greater doses of enflurane produce cerebral seizure activity when combined with hypocarbia. Isoflurane is the least potent cerebral vasodilator and most effectively decreases CMR. Greater intracranial pressure increases with its use, hyperventilation minimizes the effect and can be safely instituted after introduction of the agent. Desflurane and sevoflurane have similar properties to isoflurane. The lower blood-gas solubility of desflurane and sevoflurane allow more prompt awakening.

Interestingly, sevoflurane has been shown to provide longer-term protection in an experimental model of focal cerebral ischemia. The use of sevoflurane in the patient presented in this case was appropriate.

"Triple-H" Therapy

Vasospasm after surgery is a major cause of morbidity and mortality following SAH. Constriction of the cerebral arterial vasculature occurs as free subarachnoid blood under high pressure comes into contact with the surfaces of vessels, particularly in the basal cisterns. The mainstay of medical treatment of cerebral vasospasm, in addition to calcium channel blockade with nimodipine, is "triple-H" therapy: hypervolemia (an increase in the volume of circulating plasma), induced arterial hypertension, and hemodilution. Postoperative "triple-H" therapy has been used in many centers, on the basis that it augments CBF, prevents delayed ischemia, and improves clinical outcome. However, the efficacy of "triple-H" therapy has not been proven by prospective study.[13] Although induced hypertension results in a significant increase in regional CBF and brain tissue oxygenation, hypervolemia/ hemodilution induce only a slight increase in regional CBF, while brain tissue oxygenation does not improve[14] (Table 51.1).

KEY MESSAGES

1. Maintaining a high normal CPP can augment collateral blood flow to the ischemic penumbra, minimize secondary injury, and result in improved neurological outcome.
2. Hyperglycemia increases damage in focal neurologic ischemia and is an independent predictor of poor outcome in patients who have focal ischemic injury.
3. Hyperthermia has adverse effects on the postischemic brain.
4. The efficacy of "triple-H" therapy (hypervolemia −[an increase in the volume of circulating plasma], induced arterial hypertension, and hemodilution) has not been proven by prospective study.

QUESTIONS

1. What is neuroprotection?

   Answer: Neuroprotection is modification of intraischemic cellular and vascular biological responses to deprivation of the cellular energy supply to increase tissue tolerance to ischemia and/or reperfusion resulting in improved outcome.

2. What is the best ventilatory strategy to use during general anesthesia for cerebral aneurysm repair?

   Answer: Ventilation should be carried out to achieve normocapnia. Hypercapnia can cause intracerebral "steal" by preferentially vasodilating vessels in the noninjured area and decrease intracellular pH. Hypocapnia can increase the size of the region at risk of ischemic damage.

3. What inhalational agents are suitable for use in a case in which neuroprotection is desirable?

   Answer: Desflurane and sevoflurane are suitable for use in a case in which neuroprotection is desirable. Both of these agents offer some neuroprotection with easy control

TABLE 51.1 Evidence-Based Status of Plausible Interventions to Reduce Perioperative Ischemic Brain Injury

Intervention	Pre-ischemic Efficacy in Experimental Animals	Post-ischemic Efficacy in Experimental Animals	Pre-ischemic Efficacy in Humans	Post-ischemic Efficacy in Humans	Sustained protection in experimental animals	Sustained protection in humans
Moderate hypothermia	+ +	+ +	−/+	+ +*	+ +	+ +
Mild hyperthermia	− − −	− − −	− −	− −	− −	− −
Hyperventilation	− −	− −	− −	− −	− −	− −
Normoglycemia	+ +	− −	+	+	+ +	− −
Hyperbaric oxygen	+ +	− −	− −	−/+	− −	− −
Barbiturates	+ +	−	+	−	− −	− −
Propofol	+ +	+	−	−	− −	− −
Etomidate	− − −	− −	− −	− −	− −	− −
Nitrous oxide	−	− −	− −	− −	− −	− −
Isoflurane	+ +	− −	− −	− −	+ +	− −
Sevoflurane		− −	− −	− −	+ +	− −
Desflurane	+ +	− −	− −	− −	− −	− −
Lidocaine	+ +	− −	+	− −	− −	− −
Ketamine	+ +	− −	− −	− −	− −	− −
Glucocorticoids	− − −	− −	− −	− −	− −	− −

+ +, repeated physiologically controlled studies in animals/randomized, prospective, adequately powered clinical trials; +, consistent suggestion by case series/retrospective or prospective small sample size trials, or data extrapolated from other paradigms; −/+, inconsistent findings in clinical trials; may be dependent on characteristics of insult; −, well-defined absence of benefit; − −, absence of evidence in physiologically controlled studies in animals/randomized, prospective, adequately powered clinical trials; − − −, evidence of potential harm; *, out-of-hospital ventricular fibrillation cardiac arrest. Reproduced with permission from Fukuda S, Warner DS. Cerebral protection. Br J Anaesth 2007; 99:10–17.

of vasodilation. The low blood-gas solubility of these agents allows prompt awakening.

References

1. Rinkel GJ, Djibuti M, Algra A, et al. Prevalence and risk of rupture of intracranial aneurysms: a systematic review. Stroke 1998; 29:251–256.
2. Linn FH, Rinkel GJ, van Gijn J. Incidence of subarachnoid hemorrhage: role of region, year, and rate of computed tomography: a meta-analysis. Stroke 1996;27:625–629
3. Broderick JP, Brott T, Tomsick T, et al. The risk of subarachnoid hemorrhage in blacks as compared to whites. N Engl J Med 1992;326:733–736.
4. van Gijn J, Rinkel GJE. Subarachnoid hemorrhage: diagnosis, causes and management. Brain 2001;124:249–278.
5. Fukuda S, Warner DS. Cerebral protection. Br J Anaesth 2007; 99:10–17.
6. Todd MM, Hindman BJ, Clarke WR, et al. Mild intraoperative hypothermia during surgery for intracranial aneurysm. N Engl J Med 2005;352:135–145.
7. Kammersgaard LP, Jorgensen HS, Rungby JA, et al. Admission body temperature predicts long-term mortality after acute stroke: the Copenhagen Stroke Study. Stroke 2002; 33:1759–1762.
8. Sitar SM, Hanifi-Moghaddam P, Gelb A, et al. Propofol prevents peroxide-induced inhibition of glutamate transport in cultured astrocytes. Anesthesiology 1999;90:1446–1453.
9. Engelhard K, Werner C, Eberspacher E, et al. Influence of propofol on neuronal damage and apoptotic factors after incomplete cerebral ischaemia and reperfusion in rats: a long-term observation. Anesthesiology 2004;101:912–917.
10. Lei B, Cottrell JE, Kass IS. Neuroprotective effect of low-dose lidocaine in a rat model of transient focal cerebral ischemia. Anesthesiology 2001;95:445–451.
11. Warner DS, McFarlane C, Todd M, et al. Sevoflurane and halothane reduce focal ischaemic brain damage in the rat. Possible influences on thermoregulation. Anesthesiology 1993; 79:985–992.
12. Kawaguchi M, Kimbro JR, Drummond JC, et al. Effects of isoflurane on neuronal apoptosis in rats subjected to focal ischaemia. J Neurosurg Anesthesiol 2000;12:385.
13. Treggiari MM, Walder B, Suter PM, et al. Systematic review of the prevention of delayed ischemic neurological deficits with hypertension, hypervolemia, and hemodilution therapy following subarachnoid hemorrhage. J Neurosurg 2003;98:978.
14. Muench E, Horn P, Bauhuf C, et al. Effects of hypervolaemia and hypertension on regional cerebral blood flow, intracranial pressure, and brain tissue oxygenation after subarachnoid haemorrhage. Critical Care Med 2007;35:1844–1851.

CHAPTER 52

Anesthesia for Cerebral Aneurysm Coiling

Ashit Bardhan

A 65-year-old, 75-kg male was admitted to the emergency department with a severe headache and decreased level of consciousness. His Glasgow Coma Scale score was 14. A computed tomographic scan showed subarachnoid hemorrhage (SAH). An angiogram demonstrated (Fig. 52.1) that the source of the SAH was an 8-mm posterior communicating artery aneurysm.

The patient had smoked 3 to 5 cigarettes per day for the previous 30 years. He walked 2 kilometers each day on level ground and denied chest pain or dyspnea on exertion. He had undergone an appendectomy at 16 years of age for which the anesthetic had been uneventful.

The patient's neurologic examination revealed a Glasgow Coma scale of 14 (Table 52.1); he opened his eyes in response to voice (3), was oriented and conversing (5), and obeyed commands (6). He was judged to be Hunt and Hess grade II (Table 52.2) and also grade II by World Federation of Neurological Surgeons Grading (Table 52.3). His pupils were 6 to 7 mm in diameter, were equal, and reacted normally to light. He had no neurologic deficit. Electrocardiogram (ECG) and chest radiograph readings were unremarkable. The patient's serum urea was 6.5 mmol/L; creatinine, 85 mmol/L; sodium, 130 mmol/L; and glucose, 8.5 mmol/L. His hemoglobin concentration was 14.6 g/dL, and his white blood cell count was 12×10^9/L.

The patient had been fasting for 6 hours and had received 60 mg of oral nimodipine (additional doses had been prescribed every 4 hours thereafter). A prophylactic dose of phenytoin 1.125 g (15 mg/kg) had been administered intravenously on admission over 30 minutes in the emergency department.

In view of the hyponatremia, the patient's estimated fluid losses were replaced with 0.9% sodium chloride. As part of the multidisciplinary approach to managing a cerebral aneurysm, the neurosurgeon and neuroradiologist discussed definitive treatment options such as clipping and coiling of the aneurysm. On the basis of findings of the International Subarachnoid Aneurysm Trial (ISAT)[1] trial, they decided to proceed to coiling of the aneurysm on the following day.

On the next morning, the patient received the prescribed dose of nimodipine. He received no premedicant, as he volunteered that it was not necessary. In the neuroradiology suite, standard monitors (ECG, SpO$_2$, and noninvasive

blood pressure) were applied. One 16-gauge cannula was inserted on the dorsum of the patient's left hand after 1% lignocaine infiltration at the site. A 20-gauge arterial cannula was inserted in the left radial artery for invasive monitoring of blood pressure also after local infiltration with 1% lignocaine. After 3 minutes of preoxygenation with 100% oxygen, anesthesia was induced using intravenous propofol 200 mg and fentanyl 150. Muscle relaxation was achieved with intravenous atracurium 40 mg. Anesthesia was maintained using an infusion of propofol (target control infusion targeted plasma concentration was 4 ng/L) and remifentanil (target control infusion, 6–9 ng/L). Bispectral index monitoring was commenced and maintained <60 by titrating the propofol infusion. Convected warm air was circulated on the patient's body (Bair Hugger; Arizant Inc, Eden Prairie, MN), for which the temperature was set at 38°C. Once the right femoral artery was successfully cannulated, 100 IU/kg of heparin was administered. Three minutes later, the activated clotting time was 345 seconds. Using a microcatheter, the neuroradiologist catheterized the aneurysm and then successfully deposited platinum coils within the aneurysm sac until it was occluded. Propofol and remifentanil infusion were discontinued. Reversal of neuromuscular block was achieved by administering 2.5 mg neostigmine and 500 µg glycopyrrolate. During the procedure, 1 L of 0.9% sodium chloride had been administered. Within 12 minutes of discontinuing the anesthetic agents, the patient was able to obey commands, and his trachea was extubated without coughing. He was transferred to the postanesthesia care unit, and after 30 minutes, he was oriented, alert, awake, and comfortable. His vital signs were normal and he was discharged to the neurosurgical observation ward. Regular nimodipine and phenytoin were prescribed for 3 weeks, and the patient was scheduled for a repeat cerebral angiogram in 6 months.

CASE DISCUSSION

ISAT

The ISAT is the only large-scale, multicenter, prospective, randomized control trial that has compared endovascular coiling and neurosurgical clipping for ruptured intra-cerebral aneurysm. A total of 2143 patients were randomly allocated, 1073 to the endovascular and 1070 to the neurosurgical arms. The trial included patients with ruptured aneurysms that

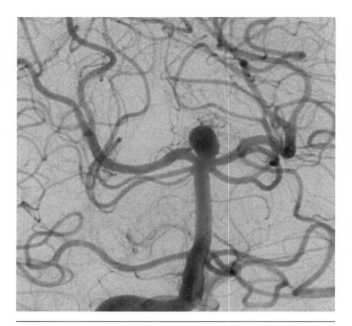

Figure 52.1 • Precoiling Angiogram.

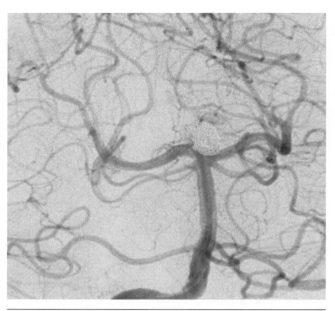

Figure 52.2 • Postcoiling Angiogram.

TABLE 52.1 Glasgow Coma Scale

Score	6	5	4	3	2	1
Eyes	N/A	N/A	Opens eyes spontaneously	Opens eyes in response to voice	Opens eyes in response to painful stimuli	Does not open eyes
Verbal	N/A	Oriented, converses normally	Confused, disoriented	Utters inappropriate words	Incomprehensible sounds	Makes no sounds
Motor	Obeys commands	Localizes painful stimuli	Flexion / withdrawal to painful stimuli	Abnormal flexion to painful stimuli	Extension to painful stimuli	Makes no movements

N/A, not applicable.

TABLE 52.2 Hunt and Hess Grading Scale for Subarachnoid Hemorrhage

Grade	Clinical Description
I	Asymptomatic or minimal headache and slight nuchal rigidity
II	Moderate- to- severe headache, nuchal rigidity, no neurological deficit other than cranial nerve palsy
III	Drowsiness, confusion, or mild focal deficit
IV	Stupor, moderate- to- severe hemiparesis, and possibly early decerebrate rigidity and vegetative disturbance
V	Deep coma, decerebrate rigidity, and moribund appearance

TABLE 52.3 World Federation of Neurological Surgeons Grading Scheme for Subarachnoid Hemorrhage

Grade	Glasgow Coma Scale	Motor Deficit
I	15	Absent
II	13 or 14	Absent
III	13 or 14	Present
IV	7–12	–
V	3–6	–

were amenable to treatment with clipping or coiling. Patients randomly allocated to coiling experienced a 23.7% incidence of neurological dependency or death compared with a 30.6% incidence in patients randomized to clipping. These results showed that the absolute benefit of coiling over clipping was 7.4%. This figure equates to a number needed to treat of 14 patients, for one to avoid death or dependency at 1 year after rupture.

Several aspects of this study need to be emphasized to place the findings into proper clinical perspective. Only 22.4% of the initially screened 9559 patients with ruptured aneurysms underwent randomization; <10% of the patients were at high clinical risk, and approximately 95% of them had aneurysms in the anterior cerebral circulation with a size of <10 mm. Complete occlusion of the aneurysm was achieved more often in the surgically treated group compared with the endovascularly treated group (82 vs. 66%). Late aneurysm rebleeding was more common in the coiled group (0.2% per year) than in the open surgical group (0.06% per year); however, rebleeding was uncommon in both treatment groups and did not reverse the benefit of endovascular treatment at 7-year follow-up.[2]

What is coiling of a cerebral aneurysm?

Coiling is a procedure in which a microcatheter is inserted through the femoral artery, navigated into the aneurysm sac allowing detachable coils to be advanced into the sac until the aneurysm is occluded. The original coils are named Guglielmi Detachable Coils after Dr. Guido Guglielmi, the developer of the technique.

What are the advantages of coiling?

Coiling is a minimally invasive procedure. It also avoids the complications associated with craniotomy. Recovery time is shorter than after clipping. Within the setting described of the ISAT trial, coiling was associated with a better outcome (in terms of neurologic dependency or death) than surgical clipping.

How is the decision made to coil a cerebral aneurysm?

Several factors are important in deciding if an aneurysm is suitable for coiling. The following factors favor coiling: small aneurysm sac size (but not too small, >3 mm), favorable neck size (not wide), no branches coming out of the dome of the aneurysm, certain locations where surgical access is difficult (basilar artery, parophthalmic artery), advanced age, and severe systemic disease. Approximately 7 out of 10 ruptured aneurysms are suitable for coiling. In many cases, aneurysms can be secured using either technique.

What is the optimal timing for intervention?

Cerebral vasospasm usually develops 3 to 12 days after SAH, lasts on average 2 weeks, and affects 60% to 70% of patients with SAH. It frequently results in cerebral ischaemia, and is the major cause of morbidity and mortality in these patients. After SAH has been diagnosed, it should be repaired at the earliest possible time before cerebral vasospasm develops.

What is the role of nimodipine?

Nimodipine, a calcium channel blocker, improves outcome after SAH.[3] Nimodipine therapy (60 mg orally or by nasogastric tube every 4 hours; maximal daily dose 360 mg) should be started in all patients at admission and continued for 21 days. Nimodipine administered as a continuous infusion is no more effective than when administered orally, but it is associated with a greater incidence of hypotension. Intravenous nimodipine should be administered via a central venous catheter. In addition, the infusion system must be protected from light. If an adequate and stable blood pressure (systolic blood pressure 130–150 mm Hg) cannot be maintained, hemodynamic management takes priority over nimodipine administration. In general, nimodipine renders patients prone to hypotension, especially when they are intravascularly depleted and during anesthesia induction. As nimodipine does not reliably relieve angiographically documented vasospasm, its beneficial effect may be caused by a general brain protective mechanism.[2]

How is grading and neurologic assessment used?

Clinical grading scales such as that of Hunt and Hess [4] or the World Federation of Neurological Surgeons [3] are used to standardize clinical assessment and to estimate patients' prognosis. Focal neurologic deficits and change in mental status are the basis of the Hunt and Hess grading scale, which has been used as a predictor of outcome. A frequently overlooked part in this classification is that, if patients have medical comorbidities, such as hypertension, severe atherosclerotic disease, chronic pulmonary disease, diabetes mellitus, and severe vasospasm, the grade should be the next less favorable one. The World Federation of Neurosurgical Societies has introduced a new grading system that has more accurate prognostic value and is partially based on the Glasgow Coma Scale of patients on arrival.[5] Knowledge and understanding of the grading scales are required for effective communication among physicians, assessment of the severity of the patient's underlying pathophysiologic abnormalities, and rational planning of the perioperative anesthetic management.[2]

What type of electrolyte abnormalities may occur?

Common electrolyte abnormalities include hyponatremia, hypokalemia, hypomagnesemia, and hypocalcemia. Hypomagnesemia occurs in more than 50% of patients with SAH and is associated with delayed cerebral ischemia and poor outcome.[6,7] If hyponatremia is caused by the syndrome of inappropriate anti-diuretic hormone secretion, normovolemia should be maintained with isotonic saline.[8]

Which type of anesthetic technique is generally used to facilitate coiling?

Conscious sedation, "neurolept" anesthesia, and general anesthesia have been described. Anesthetists in most hospitals use general anesthesia with tracheal intubation.[7] Airway management using a laryngeal mask airway has also been advocated.

What types of premedication are used?

If the patient is alert and very anxious, an anxiolytic can be prescribed.[8] A small dose of benzodiazepine is usually sufficient. On the other hand, in cases of altered consciousness, sedative premedication should be avoided. Opiates are best avoided, as they can cause respiratory depression. The patient might already be taking a calcium channel antagonist such as nimodipine as a neuroprotective agent or for decreasing the incidence of vasospasm. Anticonvulsants, corticosteroids, and antibiotics might be used as premedicants depending on the patient's status and requirements. In patients with obesity or gastroesophageal reflux, H_2- receptor antagonists such as ranitidine or metoclopramide are used to decrease the risk of pulmonary aspiration of gastric contents.[9]

What type of electrocardiographic changes take place?

SAH can be associated with marked systemic and pulmonary hypertension, cardiac arrhythmias, myocardial dysfunction and injury, and neurogenic pulmonary edema. ECG abnormalities (e.g., QT_c prolongation, repolarization abnormalities) have been reported in 25% to 100% of cases, along with an increase in serum concentration of cardiac troponin in 17% to 28%, of creatine kinase- MB isoenzyme in 37%, and of left ventricular dysfunction in 8% to 30% of cases. In most cases, myocardial dysfunction seems to correlate more with the degree of neurologic deficit than with the severity of ECG abnormalities.[2] Cardiac injury and dysfunction usually resolve over time and do not seem to directly affect morbidity and mortality.[10]

What type of monitoring is used?

Monitoring standards in a neuroradiology interventional suite should be equivalent to those available in the operating room. Invasive blood pressure monitoring and urine output measurement are required. A central venous catheter is not regularly inserted, as large fluid shifts are not expected. Neurophysiologic monitoring is used in some hospitals but is not a common practice.

What are the principles of anesthetic management?

The goal during anesthesia induction for repair of cerebral aneurysms is to minimize the risk of aneurysm rupture. The incidence of aneurysm rupture during induction is approximately 2%.[11] As there is no skull decompression during the procedure, the risk of aneurysm rupture is present until it is coiled successfully. Anesthesia is maintained by total intravenous anesthesia or a combination of low-dose propofol and remifentanil in conjunction with small dose of a volatile agent. Cannulation of the femoral artery is associated with greatest stimulation. Overall, the anesthetic requirement is not great. Systemic hypotension should be avoided, and "low-normocapnia" should be maintained. During emergence, if the aneurysm is secured, a systolic blood pressure of 160 mm Hg has been reported to result in a favorable outcome. The safe upper limit for an unsecured aneurysm is not clear.[7]

What type of complications are possible?

Non-central nervous system complications include contrast allergic reactions, contrast nephropathy, and groin or retroperitoneal hematomata. Central nervous system complications can be categorized based on the timing of the procedure: intraprocedural, early, and late postprocedural. Intraprocedural complications include rebleed from aneurysm rupture or ischemic stroke caused by vessel occlusion (from thrombosis, embolization, branch occlusion, or dissection). Early postprocedural complications include rebleeding and delayed thromboembolism. The main late postprocedural complication is aneurysm regrowth (from coil compaction or aneurysm growth).

CONCLUSION

Anesthesia for coiling of cerebral aneurysms requires a thorough understanding of the pathophysiology of SAH. Anesthesia is provided in a setting with which the anesthetist may not be familiar; often, trained assistance is not readily available, and there is the potential for catastrophic complications such as re-bleeding or perforation.

KEY MESSAGES

With respect to the anesthetic care of patients undergoing coiling of cerebral aneurysms:

1. It is necessary for the anesthetist to familiarize him/herself with the neuroradiology suite before undertaking care of such patients.

2. Thorough neurologic assessment of the patient is required pre- and postoperatively.

3. Maintaining hemodynamic stability throughout the procedure is important to avoid the risk of secondary injury caused by hypoperfusion or aneurysm rupture.

4. Communication between the anesthetist and the interventional team is important.

QUESTIONS

1. What is the principal finding of the ISAT trial?

   Answer: The principal finding of the ISAT trial is that patients randomly allocated to coiling experienced a 23.7% incidence of neurologic dependency or death compared with a 30.6% incidence in patients randomized to clipping.

2. What nimodipine regimen is indicated in patients with SAH?

   Answer: Nimodipine (60 mg orally or by nasogastric tube every 4 hours; maximal daily dose, 360 mg) should be administered to all SAH patients at admission and continued for 21 days.

3. What electrolyte abnormalities are most commonly associated with SAH?

Answer: Common electrolyte abnormalities associated with SAH include hyponatremia, hypokalemia, hypomagnesemia, and hypocalcemia.

References

1. Molyneux A, Kerr R, Yu L, et al. International Subarachnoid Aneurysm Trial (ISAT) of neurosurgical clipping and endovascular coiling in 2413 patients with intracranial aneurysm: a randomised comparison of effects on survival, dependency, seizures, rebleeding, subgroups and aneurysm occlusion. Lancet 2005;366: 809–817.

2. Priebe HJ. Aneurysmal subarachnoid haemorrhage and the anaesthetist. Br J Anaesth 2007;99:102–118.

3. Drake CG, Hunt WE, Sano K, et al. Report of World Federation of Neurological Surgeons Committee on a universal subarachnoid haemorrhage grading scale. J Neurosurg 1988;68:985–986.

4. Hunt WE, Hess RM. Surgical risk as related to time of intervention in the repair of intracranial aneurysms. J Neurosurg 1968;28:14–20.

5. Avitsian R, Schubert A. Anaesthetic considerations for intraoperative management of cerebrovascular disease in neurovascular surgical procedures. Anesthesiol Clin 2007;25:Issue 3.

6. Van den Bergh WM, Algra A., van der sprenkel JW, et al. Hypomagnesemia after SAH. Neurosurgery 2003;52:276–282.

7. Lakhani S, Guha A, Nahser SC. Anaesthesia for endovascular management of cerebral aneurysm. Eur J Anaesthesiol 2006;23: 902–913.

8. Rosas AL. Anaesthesia for INR: part II: preoperative assessment, premedication. Internet J Anesthesiol 1997;1. Available at: www.ispub.com/ostia/index.php?xmlFilepath=journals/ija/vol1n2/neuroan2.xml. Accessed February 27, 2009.

9. Ahmed A. Anaesthesia for interventional neuroradiology. J Ayub Med Coll Abbottabad 2007;19:80–84.

10. Diebert E, Barzilai B, Braverman A, et al. The clinical significance of elevated troponin I in patients with non traumatic subarachnoid haemorrhage. J Neurosurg 2003;98:741–746.

11. Tsementzis SA, Hitchcock ER. Outcome from 'rescue clipping' of ruptured intracranial aneurysm during induction of anaesthesia and endotracheal intubation. J Neurol Neurosurg Psychiat 1985;48:160–163.

CHAPTER 53

Emergency Reversal of Rocuronium-Induced Neuromuscular Blockade Using Sugammadex

Mohan Mugawar

CASE FORMAT: REFLECTION

A 38-year-old female (American Society of Anesthesiologists physical status I) presented with radicular low back pain of 3 months' duration. After appropriate investigations and discussion of the treatment options with her, she was scheduled for elective lumbar laminectomy. The patient's medical history was unremarkable. She had undergone uneventful general endotracheal anesthesia for a tonsillectomy at 5 years of age and spinal anesthesia for an elective caesarean section 2 years previously.

The preoperative evaluation revealed a moderately obese woman who was 165 cm in height and weighed 85 kg. Cardiorespiratory assessment was normal. Preoperative laboratory data were within the normal ranges. The airway assessment revealed prominent upper incisors, interincisor gap >3 cm, thyromental distance 8 cm, and Mallampati grade II. The patient's neck appeared short; the cervical spine mobility was normal. In the operating room, an intravenous (IV) cannula was inserted, and an infusion of compound sodium lactate commenced. Routine standard monitoring was applied including neuromuscular monitoring using train-of-four stimulation (TOF watch).

After 3 minutes of preoxygenation, anesthesia was induced by an experienced anesthesiologist with fentanyl 100 µg and propofol 200 mg. With some difficulty, positive pressure was applied via face mask, and some chest expansion was noted; rocuronium IV 1.2 mg/kg was administered. Mask ventilation became progressively more difficult after the administration of rocuronium despite vigorous jaw thrust and placement of an appropriately sized oral airway. Three attempts at rigid laryngoscopy were made—the first two by the initial anesthetist and the third by another senior colleague who was called to assist. Having optimized head and neck position, Macintosh 3, 4 and McCoy blades were used without acquiring a view even of the arytenoids. Between laryngoscopy attempts, manual ventilation was attempted using a two- operator technique; these attempts, however, were unsuccessful. Insertion of a laryngeal mask airway did not enable effective manual ventilation. These attempts at securing a patent airway had taken approximately 4 minutes. The patient became profoundly hypoxic with SpO$_2$ <80%. While urgent preparation was made for cricothyrotomy, sugammadex 16 mg/kg was administered by rapid IV bolus (the drug was available because trials of sugammadex were underway at the institution). Ninety seconds later, it became possible to deliver a breath (100% oxygen) to the patient's lungs via face mask and Guedel airway. Shortly afterward, the patient resumed spontaneous ventilation and regained consciousness. SpO$_2$ rapidly returned to 97% to 99%. Reassessment of the patient revealed a TOF ratio of 0.9, 115 seconds after sugammadex administration (Fig. 53.1).

The patient was fully conscious, alert, well oriented, neurologically intact, hemodynamically stable, and thereafter maintained oxygen saturation of 100% on room air. She was observed for 2 hours in a postanesthetic care unit and was stable without any signs of recurarization. After complete recovery from anesthesia, a full explanation of the events was made to the patient, and the events were recorded in detail in her medical record. The patient was provided with written information regarding her airway management and was asked to relay this to any future anesthetist and to her primary care physician. She was also advised about the option of obtaining a Medic Alert bracelet. Her surgery was rescheduled, and awake fiberoptic intubation was planned.

CASE DISCUSSION

Sugammadex (Org 25969) is the first selective muscle relaxant binding agent, designed to reverse the steroidal neuromuscular blocking agents (NMBAs), particularly rocuronium.[1] It is a modified γ-cyclodextrin, forms inactive tight 1:1 complexes with, and functions as an irreversible chelating agent for aminosteroidal NMBAs. The administration of sugammadex results in a rapid decrease in the concentration of free rocuronium in the plasma and subsequently in the synaptic cleft at the neuromuscular junction, resulting in rapid normalization of neuromuscular function. Sugammadex has no effect on acetylcholinesterase or any receptor system in the body. Therefore, the need for administering anticholinesterases and anticholinergic (-muscarinic) agents and the associated adverse effects are avoided. Sugammadex-rocuronium complexes are highly hydrophilic and are therefore excreted rapidly and in a dose-dependent manner. Sugammadex is biologically inactive and appears to be safe and well tolerated by patients.[2] Sugammadex reverses profound NMB induced by aminosteroidal nondepolarizing NMB agents rapidly and effectively in a dose-dependent manner.[3–5] The optimal dose required to reverse profound blockade has not yet been fully elucidated. However, sugammadex administration in doses of 4, 8, 12, and 16 mg/kg resulted in reversal of profound rocuronium-induced

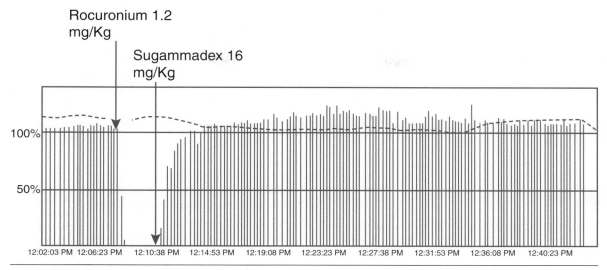

Figure 53.1 • TOF-Watch SX trace (Bluestar Enterprises, Inc, Chanhassen, MN) of the twitch height and T4/T1 ratio after IV administration of rocuronium and sugammadex. Recovery of twitch height (T1) of 90% and TOF ratio of 0.9 returned approximately 115 seconds after sugammadex administration.

NMB to a TOF ratio of 0.9 in (mean values) of 15.8, 2.8, 1.4 and 1.9 minutes, respectively.[3] (The TOF ratio taken to indicate adequate reversal of/recovery from NMB is 0.9, as this level is required for normal function of vital muscle groups, including those of the pharynx, to avoid postoperative respiratory complications.[6,7])

Administering sugammadex in clinical practice could decrease the incidence of postoperative residual curarization. Use of sugammadex could also facilitate the use of rocuronium for rapid sequence induction by providing a faster onset/offset of NMB profile compared with succinylcholine. As in the patient described in this case, sugammadex offers the potential to rapidly terminate profound NMB if the anesthetist is confronted with a "cannot intubate, cannot ventilate" situation.

KEY MESSAGES

1. Sugammadex is a selective, novel reversal agent of NMB induced by aminosteroid nondepolarizing NMB agents.
2. Administration of sugammadex 8 mg/kg can reverse profound rocuronium-induced NMB in approximately 90 seconds.
3. A TOF ratio of 0.9 or greater is the threshold that corresponds to adequacy of reversal of/recovery from NMB.

QUESTIONS

1. What is the mechanism of action of sugammadex?

   Answer: Sugammadex is a modified γ-cyclodextrin, forms inactive tight 1:1 complexes with, and functions as an irreversible chelating agent for aminosteroidal NMBAs.

2. What is the TOF ratio normally accepted to indicate adequate reversal of /recovery from NMB?

   Answer: 0.9

3. What hemodynamic adverse effects are associated with sugammadex administration?

   Answer: None of clinical importance. Sugammadex is biologically inactive and appears to be safe and well tolerated by patients.[2]

References

1. Bom A, Bradley M, Cameron K, et al. A novel concept of reversing neuromuscular block: chemical encapsulation of rocuronium bromide by a cyclodextrin-based synthetic host. Angew Chem Int Ed Engl 2002;41:266–270.
2. Naguib M. Sugammadex: another milestone in clinical neuromuscular pharmacology. Anesth Analg 2007;104: 575–581.
3. de Boer HD, Driessen JJ, Marcus MAE, et al. Reversal of rocuronium-induced (1.2 mg/kg) profound neuromuscular block by sugammadex. Anesthesiology 2007;107:239–244.
4. Sparr HJ, Vermeyaen KM, Beaufort AM, Rietbergen H, et al. Early reversal of profound rocuronium induced neuromuscular blockade by sugammadex in a randomised multicenter study. Anesthesiology 2007;106:935–943.
5. Suy K, Morias K, Cammu G, et al. Effective reversal of moderate rocuronium-or vecuronium-induced neuromuscular block with sugammadex, a selective relaxant binding agent. Anesthesiology 2007;106:283–288.
6. Eriksson LI, Sundman E, Olsson R, Nilsson L, et al. Functional assessment of the pharynx at rest and during swallowing in partially paralysed humans: simultaneous videomanometry and mechanomyography of awake human volunteers. Anesthesiology 1997;87:1035–1043.
7. Kopman AF. Surrogate endpoints and neuromuscular recovery (editorial). Anesthesiology 1997;87:1029–1031.

CHAPTER 54

Awareness During Anesthesia

Justin Lane

CASE FORMAT: STEP BY STEP

A 36-year-old primigravida presented for emergency ovarian cystectomy. At 30 weeks' gestation, she had been in the hospital for 2 days with severe abdominal pain, nausea, and vomiting. Intramuscular pethidine (meper-idine) 50 mg and prochlorperazine 12.5 mg were administered to control the symptoms. The patient, a nurse, had no history of anesthesia-related problems.

On assessment the patient, was found to be normotensive (blood pressure, 115/75 mm Hg), with a pulse rate of 92 beats per minute. Her blood glucose was normal, and in her laboratory workup, it was noted that she had an increased white blood cell count 17 × 10 9/L and serum urea 11 mg/dL. An ultrasound of the patient's abdomen and pelvis confirmed the diagnosis of ovarian cyst torsion. Assessment of her upper airway revealed Mallampati grade II and thyromental distance of 7 cm. Her incisor separation and mandibular mobility were normal. In view of her history and abnormal serum urea, she was commenced on Hartmann's solution at 200 mL per hour to improve her hydration status before surgery. The anesthetic plan was discussed with the patient. A general anesthetic was described, using a "rapid sequence induction" technique, and a transversus abdominis plane block[1] was to be performed intraoperatively for analgesia.

Following application of standard monitors, a rapid sequence induction of anesthesia and tracheal intubation were performed using sodium thiopentone (5 mg/kg) and suxamethonium (1.5 mg/kg) after denitrogenation[2] (preoxygenation with 100% oxygen for 5 minutes). A wedge was placed under the patient's right buttock to decrease the likelihood of supine hypotension. Sevoflurane End tidel (ET) 0.5% to 0.8% in nitrous oxide/oxygen (50:50 mixture), vecuronium, and fentanyl were administered according to the anesthetist's clinical judgment. Although BIS monitoring[3] (Aspect Medical Systems, Norwood, MA) was applied (and BIS was <60 throughout the surgery), the anesthetist titrated sevoflurane administration according to the patient's heart rate and blood pressure rather than to the BIS value. The difficult airway cart was kept in the operating room. A fetal monitor was applied before induction and was monitored by the attending obstetrician.

What factors relevant to this case influence the risk of intraoperative awareness?

Pregnancy is associated with as great as 30% decrease in minimum alveolar concentration value.[2] Analysis of the American Society of Anesthesiologists closed claims database[4] has identified five factors that increase the risk of recall under general anesthesia: (a) female gender, (b) gynecological/obstetrical procedures, (c) use of opioids, (d) use of muscle relaxants, (e) and lack of use of a volatile anesthetic agent. At least four of these factors apply to the patient in this case. It is likely that the emergency nature of the procedure also increases the risk.

Following an uneventful surgical procedure, the patient's trachea was extubated, and she was transferred to the postanesthesia care unit. Routine postanesthesia monitoring was carried out in the postanesthesia care unit. A combination of regular intravenous paracetamol every 6 hours and intramuscular pethidine (meper-idine) 50 mg every 4 hours was prescribed as were antiemetics and supplemental oxygen. The transverse abdominis plane (TA) block performed intraoperatively appeared to be effective, as no analgesics were administered in the postanesthesia care unit. Hartmann's solution 125 mL per hour was administered until the patient could tolerate fluids orally.

On the second postoperative day, the patient informed the surgeon that she thought she recalled hearing alarms and people discussing her case while the operation was in progress.

What is awareness under anesthesia?

Awareness is a rare complication of general anesthesia, which can have serious psychological sequelae for the patient and serious financial implications for the hospital in which it occurs. It can be classified as: (a) awareness with explicit memory—the patient has conscious recollection of intraoperative events or (b) awareness with implicit memory—the patient has no recollection of intraoperative events.[5]

One to two people per thousand may describe some degree of awareness during their anesthetic; of these, 33% describe pain as part of their experience.[6] More than 50% of "aware" patients describe hearing conversations and sounds within the operating room. About 25% of such patients have experiences relating to endotracheal tube insertion.

Any suggestion of a case of awareness under anesthesia must be followed up (Table 54.1). A review of the anesthetic

TABLE 54.1 Protocol for Managing Possible Case of Awareness Under Anesthesia[6,10,11]

Visit the patient as soon as possible after the event.
Take a full history and document the patient's exact memory of events, conversations, names, events, and sounds.
Check with other staff who would have been present in theatre during the event.
Review the anaesthesia case notes for evidence of a possible cause, e.g., tachycardia, hypertension in the case of "light anaesthesia."
Give a full explanation of events to the patient.
Plan for patient follow up, including psychological support.
Reassure the patient that further safe general anaesthesia is possible.
Try to determine the cause, review the notes, and check the machine and circuit.
Notify the patient's GP.
Make a detailed record of the event for future reference.

TABLE 54.2 Anesthetic Factors Contributing to Awareness

- Equipment problems: empty vaporizer, circuit leak
- Drug errors: mislabeled syringes, inadequate drug doses
- Technique: opioid use, light anesthesia in emergency situations
- Airway problems: laryngospasm, difficult intubation

Reproduced with permission from Osborne G, Bacon A, Runciman K, et al. Crisis management during anaesthesia: awareness and anaesthesia. Quality and Safety in Health Care 2005;14;16–25.

record for the procedure is the first step. The drugs and doses administered should be verified if possible. The levels of volatile agents used alone or in combination with nitrous oxide should be noted. It may be necessary to check the service date on the anesthetic machine, especially the vaporizer. The anesthetist involved in the case should visit the patient, and a witness should be present. The purpose of the visit is to elicit a full history of what the patient experienced and in particular, what he or she heard. It is certainly not to deny the possibility that awareness under anesthesia may have occurred. The patient should be reassured that the claims are taken seriously, and that if she wishes to discuss the issue further, it will be facilitated. Detailed notes regarding the claim should be made at the time of the initial interview. A full range of support services should be made available including psychologists and counselors. If an explanation is possible, it should be provided. The patient will also require reassurance that further anesthesia can be given safely. The patient's general practitioner (primary care doctor) needs to be informed of the incident. The relevant medical indemnity organization and the hospital management should also be informed (Table 54.1).

The responsible anesthetist arranged to meet with the patient in the presence of a hospital representative on the day after she described her experience to the surgeon. The meeting took place in a quiet consulting room, and as she described her recollections, the patient became tearful. She described great difficulty in sleeping and feeling anxious since her operation. She asked what her anesthetist had done that allowed her to be aware of her surroundings during the operation.

In general, what factors contribute to the occurrence of awareness in modern anesthetic practice?

Patients undergoing specific types of surgical procedures are at greater risk of awareness:[6]

- Cardiac surgery: up to 1 in 100
- Trauma and emergency surgery: up to 1 in 20
- Emergency caesarean section under general anesthesia: 4 in 1000.

The patient's question (regarding the anesthetist's role) is understandable and legitimate, as anesthetic factors can predispose a patient to awareness (Table 54.2).

KEY MESSAGES

1. Intraoperative awareness occurs more commonly in females and in patients undergoing obstetric-related surgery, cardiac surgery, or emergency procedures.
2. BIS monitoring does not decrease the incidence of intraoperative recall/awareness.[7,8] Intraoperative awareness can occur even when BIS values are within target ranges.[8]
3. Anesthetic departments should have a readily available protocol in place to deal with possible cases of awareness, should they arise.

QUESTIONS

1. Which patients are at greatest risk of experiencing intraoperative awareness?

   Answer: Females and patients undergoing obstetric-related or cardiac surgery or emergency procedures are at greatest risk of experiencing intraoperative awareness.

2. What is the initial appropriate step in responding to a patient's account of awareness?

   Answer: The responsible anesthetist should visit the patient as soon as possible after the event.

3. What proportion of patients who describe an awareness experience report pain as a dominant element of their recollection?

   Answer: Only 33% of patients who describe an awareness experience report pain as a dominant element of their recollection.

References

1. McDonnell JG, O'Donnell B, Curley G, et al. The analgesic efficacy of transversus abdominis plane block after abdominal surgery: a prospective randomised controlled trial. Anesth Analg 2007;104:193–197.

2. Ni Mhuireachtaigh R, O'Gorman DA. Anesthesia in pregnant patients for nonobstetric surgery. J Clin Anesth 2006;18:60–66.

3. Punjasawadong Y, Boonjeungmonkol N, Phongchiewboon A. Bispectral index for improving anaesthetic delivery and post-operative recovery. Cochrane Database of Systematic Reviews 2007. Issue 4. Art No. CD003843. DOI: 10.1002/14651858. CD003843.pub2

4. The ASA Closed Claims Project. Available at: www.asa closedclaims.org. Accessed October 31, 2007.

5. Anaesthesia UK. Available at: www.anaesthesiauk.com. Accessed October 31, 2007.

6. The Royal College of Anaesthetists. Information for patients. Section 8: Awareness " risks associated with your anaesthetic." Available at: http://www.rcoa.ac.uk/docs/awareness.pdf. Accessed November 23, 2008.

7. Osborne GA, Bacon AK, Runciman WB, et al. Crisis management during anaesthesia: awareness and anaesthesia. Quality and Safety in Health Care 2005;14;16–25.

8. Avidan MS, Zhang L, Burnside BA, et al. Anesthesia awareness and the bispectral index. N Engl J Med 2008;358: 1097–1108.

CHAPTER 55

Mitochondrial Disease and Anesthesia

Dorothy Breen

CASE FORMAT: STEP BY STEP

A 16-year-old, 4'7", 50-kg girl with mitochondrial disease was scheduled for a cochlear implant. The anesthesiologist in charge decided to consult his standard textbooks before reviewing the patient. Unfortunately, he found very little information relevant to mitochondrial disease and anaesthesia.

What is mitochondrial disease, and how does it manifest?

Mitochondrial disease comprises a heterogeneous group of disorders in which the primary abnormalities are errors in the synthesis of mitochondrial proteins caused by defects in nuclear DNA, mitochondrial DNA, or mitochondrial transfer RNA.[1] The mitochondrion is traditionally viewed as the "powerhouse" of the cell, as it contains all the machinery necessary for the Krebs cycle, fatty acid oxidation, and oxidative phosphorylation. The mitochondrion is also unique in that it is the only cellular organelle with its own DNA (mitochondrial DNA). Mitochondrial DNA encodes some of the components of the respiratory chain enzyme complexes. Five enzyme protein complexes are involved in oxidative phosphorylation. Adenosine triphosphate synthesis takes place at complex V. During division of a fertilized ovum, defective mitochondria can become more or less concentrated in one organ or another. Tissues that are postmitotic at birth and have high-energy requirements tend to be most affected (muscle, brain, nerves, retinas, liver, and kidneys), but theoretically, any organ can be involved. Clinical manifestations can range from mild to severe and are progressive over time. All modes of inheritance have been observed, but acquired defects also exist. All these factors contribute to the difficulty in diagnosing patients with mitochondrial disease. These disorders were initially termed the *mitochondrial myopathies*, given that muscle was most often identified as the predominant tissue affected. More recently it is recognized that any organ can be affected at any age; as such, the term *mitochondrial cytopathies* is more appropriate.[2]

Both the girl and her mother were present at the preoperative assessment. The patient's mitochondrial disease had been confirmed as Kearns-Sayre syndrome (KSS). At 9 years of age, she had undergone a muscle biopsy under general anesthesia at a pediatric facility. Her main presenting features were progressive ptosis, skeletal muscle fatigability, and deafness. More recently, she had developed difficulty swallowing and repeated chest infections. Antibiotics were prescribed 2 days previously for a lower respiratory tract infection. The patient's heart rate was 60 beats per minute, blood pressure was 105/60 mm Hg, and her temperature was 37.9°C. The cardiovascular examination was normal, and her lung fields were clear. There was bilateral ptosis and evidence of skeletal muscle wasting.

What factors are important in assessing this patient preoperatively?

Preoperative assessment should take account of the potential for multisystem involvement and the varying degrees of severity. Surgery and anesthesia pose a considerable stress to a patient with an already deranged bioenergy metabolism. Infection in this setting places even further demands. Given the presence of pyrexia and the history of a recent respiratory tract infection, it is wise to postpone the surgery. Furthermore, anesthesia in this patient requires much more detailed assessment and planning. KSS, although rare, is one of the better-described entities in the spectrum of mitochondrial cytopathies that exist (Table 55.1). Cardiac involvement is a feature of KSS, and conduction defects are common. Thorough nervous system and neuromuscular assessment should also be performed to determine the extent of skeletal muscle involvement, neurologic deficit, and presence of seizure disorders. Respiratory function is often impaired in patients with mitochondrial disease. It is important to assess the presence of bulbar symptoms, recurrent aspiration, and respiratory muscle weakness.[3,4]

What tests should be ordered preoperatively?

The results of preoperative spirometry are given in Table 55.2. Full blood count, blood glucose, arterial blood gases, renal, and liver function are presented in Table 55.3. An electrocardiogram, chest radiograph, and echocardiogram were requested and the patient's previous anesthetic record was obtained.

Elevated lactate and blood gas disturbances tend to occur in times of crisis in these disorders. It is important to establish preoperative values, as some patients will have a raised lactate at baseline. The presence of hepatic dysfunction in this patient underscores the multiorgan nature of mitochondrial disease. The finding of left bundle branch block on the electrocardiogram is indicative of the cardiac conduction defects that frequently occur in patients with KSS. Cardiomyopathy has also been described,[5] necessitating an echocardiogram, which was normal in this case. The patient's chest radiograph showed clear lung fields and a normal heart size.

TABLE 55.1 Some of the Described Clinical Syndromes in Mitochondrial Disease

Acronym/Name	Features
KSS (Kearns-Sayre syndrome)	Ophthalmoplegia, cardiac conduction block, deafness, retinitis pigmentosa, and skeletal muscle weakness
MELAS	Mitochondrial encephalomyopathy, lactic acidosis, and stroke-like episodes
MERRF	Myoclonic epilepsy and ragged red fibers on muscle biopsy
NARP	Neuropathy, ataxia, retinitis pigmentosa, and ptosis
MNGIE	Mitochondrial neurogastrointestinal encephalopathy
LHON	Leber hereditary optic neuropathy. Also Wolff-Parkinson-White syndrome and neuropathy
Leigh's syndrome	Subacute sclerosing encephalopathy

What type of premedication should be given?

Any form of sedative as a premedication was omitted in this case. Patients with mitochondrial disease are extraordinarily sensitive to sedatives and hypnotics. Respiratory failure and alterations in conscious level can occur even at low doses.

Fasting can precipitate hypoglycemia and a metabolic crisis. The fasting period should be kept as short as possible. If necessary, dextrose infusions can be used to supplement this period. Lactate-containing intravenous fluids should be avoided.

The previous anesthetic record in this instance showed that the patient had previously safely undergone a nontriggering anesthetic. The patient's mother accompanied her to the operating room. Intravenous access was obtained and standard monitoring instituted.

Anesthesia was induced using 10-mg increments of propofol. Once it was established that the patient's airway could be maintained by manual ventilation, 25 mg of atracurium was administered to facilitate tracheal intubation. Analgesia was achieved using paracetamol 1 g and fentanyl 20 μg. Anesthesia was maintained thereafter via propofol infusion and an air/oxygen mixture.

TABLE 55.2 Spirometry Results

	Predicted	Measured	Predicted (%)
FVC (L)	2.16	1.60	74%
FEV1 (L)	2.14	1.56	73%
FEV1/FVC (%)	99%	98%	99%

Both the FEV1 and FVC are reduced, but the ratio of FEV1/FVC is preserved. These findings are typical of a restrictive lung disease. In this case, it is caused by a respiratory muscle dysfunction. A reduction of FEV1 and FVC in the range 65% to 85% of predicted values signifies that the impairment is mild.

Was this the most suitable anesthetic technique in this case?

In reality, the safest anesthetic technique for patients with mitochondrial disease is not known. Although many patients have undergone anesthesia safely, there have been case reports describing worsening of underlying neurologic deficit, respiratory failure, high-degree atrioventricular block conduction block, malignant hyperthermia, and death following anesthesia.[6–8]

Because of the limited information available in relation to mitochondrial disease and anesthesia, there are no absolute recommendations. Each anesthetic has to be tailored to the individual patient. Malignant hyperthermia has been reported in the setting of mitochondrial cytopathy.[6,7] There are conflicting opinions, however, as to whether a nontriggering technique is required in mitochondrial disease. The use of inhaled anesthetic agents has been widely described.[9] As with other anesthetic drugs, there appears to be enhanced sensitivity to these agents.[10] In patients with KSS who are at risk of serious arrhythmia, isoflurane and sevoflurane are the preferred agents. On the basis of the patient's previous anesthetic history, inhaled agents were not used in this case. Obtaining previous anesthetic records is vital, as so little is known about safety of anesthesia in patients with these disorders.

Patients with myopathy as a predominant feature of their disease are at risk of suxamethonium-induced hyperkalemia. Notwithstanding the additional risk of malignant hyperthermia, it therefore seems prudent to avoid using this agent.

Propofol has been used safely in many patients with mitochondrial disease despite the fact that it can directly impair mitochondrial function. Caution is required with dosages of all hypnotic agents because of extreme sensitivity. A case of induction of anesthesia after as little as 75 mg of thiopentone in an adult has been described.[11]

Metabolic homeostasis during anesthesia for these patients is an important consideration. Ensuring that the patient does not experience hypothermia and shivering is imperative. A normal glucose and acid-base status should also be maintained.

The presence of left bundle branch block is of concern because patients with KSS undergoing anesthesia are at risk of sudden high-grade atrioventricular block.[12] An isoprenaline infusion and access to external/temporary pacing should be available during anesthesia.

TABLE 55.3 Full Blood Count, Blood Glucose, Arterial Blood Gases, and Renal and Liver Function

Sodium (135–145 mmol/L)	143	Hemoglobin (11–15 g/dL)	12.5
Potassium (3.5–5.5 mmol/L)	3.7	White blood cells (4–11 × 10^9/L)	11
Urea (3.0–8.0 mmol/L)	6.2	Red blood cells (3.8–5 × 10^{12}/L)	4.6
Creatinine (0.07–0.1 mmol/L)	0.07	Platelet count (150–440 × 10^9/L)	300
Magnesium (0.7–1.0 mmol/L)	0.89	Hematocrit 34%–47%	38
Bilirubin (μmol/L)	6	Glucose (4.0–7.5 mmol/L)	6.2
GGT (0–50 U/L)	79	Lactate (0.3–2.0 mEq/L)	1.0
ALP (32–110 U/L)	109	pH (7.35–7.45)	7.38
LDH (110–250 U/L)	298	$PaCO_2$ (7.35–7.45)	39
AST (0–40 U/L)	256	PaO_2 (85–100 mm Hg)	89
ALT (0–40 U/L)	240	Bicarbonate (22–26 mEq/L)	24

ALP, alkaline phosphatase; ALT, alanine aminotransferase; AST, aspartate aminotransferase; LDH, lactate dehydrogenase. Full blood count, glucose, electrolytes, lactate and renal parameters are all within normal limits. Hepatic dysfunction indicates liver involvement in this case. Reassuringly, there is no evidence of hypercapnic respiratory failure. This finding would be consistent with the spirometry findings of only mild restrictive lung disease.

At the end of the procedure, values obtained for capillary glucose concentration and arterial blood gas estimation were similar to those obtained preoperatively. The patient's temperature was 36.5°C, but there were no twitches evident following train-of-four nerve stimulation. An additional 50 minutes elapsed before four twitches could be elicited. The anesthesiologist then discontinued the propofol and administered 100% oxygen. Following tracheal extubation, the patient was observed in the postanaesthesia care unit for an extended period. Her vital signs were normal, and she appeared comfortable.

Was the delay in recovery of neuromuscular function to be expected?

Administering a standard dose of atracurium (0.5 mg/kg) in this patient most likely contributed to the prolonged action. As with other anesthetic agents, patients with mitochondrial disease are extraordinarily sensitive. When possible, these agents should be avoided, as they contribute to postoperative respiratory muscle weakness.[13,14] They have been used safely, however, at reduced dosage and with careful monitoring of neuromuscular function. Shorter-acting agents are preferable. The likelihood of renal or hepatic dysfunction (present in this case) makes atracurium and cisatracurium the agents of choice.

KEY MESSAGES

1. The anesthetic management plan should be tailored to the individual patient.

2. Surgery should be delayed if there is evidence of concurrent infection.

3. Maintenance of normothermia, normoglycemia, and acid-base status is imperative.

4. Lactate-containing solutions should be avoided.

QUESTIONS

1. Can mitochondrial cytopathies present in adulthood?

   Answer: Yes.

2. Can suxamethonium be safely administered to patients with a mitochondrial cytopathy?

   Answer: No. Opinion is divided on whether such patients are at risk of malignant hyperthermia. Patients with myopathy are at additional risk of suxamethonium induced hyperkalemia.

3. Is Ringer's Lactate a suitable choice as replacement fluid in these patients?

   Answer: No. It contains lactate.

References

1. Muravchick S, Levy RJ. Clinical implications of mitochondrial dysfunction. Anesthesiology 2006;105:819–837.
2. Cohen BH, Gold DR. Mitochondrial cytopathy in adults: what we know so far. Cleve Clin J Med 2001;68:625–642.
3. Gold DR, Cohn BH. Treatment of mitochondrial cytopathies. Semin Neurol 2001;21:309–325.
4. Barohn RJ, Clanton T, Zarife S, et al. Recurrent respiratory insufficiency and depressed ventilatory drive complicating mitochondrial myopathies. Neurology 1990;40:103–106.
5. Tveskov C, Angelo-Nielsen K. Kearns-Sayre and dilated cardiomyopathy. Neurology 1990;40:553–554.
6. Ohtani Y, Miike T, Ishitsu T, et al. A case of malignant hyperthermia with mitochondrial dysfunction (letter). Brain Dev 1985;7:249.
7. Fricker R, Raffelsberger T, Rauch-Shorny S, et al. Positive malignant hyperthermia susceptibility *in vitro* test in a patient with mitochondrial myopathy and myoadenylate deaminase deficiency. Anesthesiology 2002;97:1635–1637.
8. Casta A, Quackenbush EJ, Houck CS, et al. Perioperative white matter degeneration and death in a patient with a defect

in mitochondrial oxidative phosphorylation. Anesthesiology 1997;87:420–425.

9. Shipton EA, Prosser DO. Mitochondrial myopathies and anaesthesia. Eur J Anaesthesiol 2004;21:173–178.

10. Morgan PG, Hoppel CL, Sedensky MM, et al. Mitochondrial defects and anesthetic sensitivity. Anesthesiology 2002;96: 1268–1270.

11. James RH. Thiopentone and opthalmoplegia plus. Anaesthesia 1985;40;88.

12. Kitoh T, Mizuno K, Otagi T, et al. Anesthetic management for a patient with Kearns-Sayre syndrome. Anesth Analg 1995; 80:1240–1242.

13. Wisely NA, Cook PR. General anaesthesia in a man with mitochondrial myopathy undergoing eye surgery. Eur J Anaesthesiol 2001;18:333–335.

14. Edmonds JL. Surgical and anesthetic management of patients with mitochondrial dysfunction. Mitochondrion 2004;4: 543–548.

CHAPTER 56

Emergence Agitation in Pediatric Patients

Mansoor A. Siddiqui

CASE FORMAT: REFLECTION

A 5-year-old boy was scheduled for inpatient surgery for elective bilateral myringotomy and ventilator tube insertion. He had been fit and healthy and was not taking any medication. He had not undergone anesthesia in the past. The boy's mother told him that "he is going to the hospital to have his ears fixed, and he is going to be asleep for that." On examination in the day ward, the boy appeared anxious. He was offered toys but, unlike the other children in the ward at that time, he did not play with them. Both of his parents were present, and they also looked anxious. The boy tended to hold onto to his mother and seemed afraid when the nurses or doctors approached.

The patient's heart rate was 120 beats per minute, his blood pressure was 100/50 mm Hg, and his respiratory rate was 25 breaths per minute. He had not taken food or drink for 6 hours before his early morning admission. His upper airway was evaluated as Mallampati grade I with normal dentition (no loose teeth). Informed consent was obtained from his parents for rectal administration of analgesic suppositories. The boy was premedicated with midazolam 0.5 mg/kg orally 30 minutes before his scheduled procedure.

The child's mother accompanied him into the operating room. With standard monitors (electrocardiogram, noninvasive blood pressure, and SpO_2) in place, anesthesia was induced with oxygen (O_2)/nitrous oxide (N_2O) and sevoflurane as he sat in his mother's lap. He was then gently positioned on the operating table. Intravenous (IV) access was obtained with a 22-gauge IV cannula, and a size 2 laryngeal mask airway was inserted. Anesthesia was maintained with sevoflurane (1%–3% inspired) in O_2/N_2O (1:2). Diclofenac and paracetamol suppositories were administered before the procedure began.

The procedure was carried out uneventfully in approximately 10 minutes. While the patient was breathing spontaneously, sevoflurane and N_2O were discontinued (replaced by 100% O_2), and the laryngeal mask airway was removed while he was still deeply anesthetized. The patient's mouth and oropharynx were gently suctioned. Three minutes later, he started to move his arms and legs and pushed the face mask away. At this stage, he was transferred to the recovery room where he quickly became extremely agitated. He started crying, calling for his "mama." He persistently reached for his ears and vomited once.

During this period of agitation, the patient's heart rate was 140 beats per minute, his blood pressure was 120/70 mm Hg, and his respiratory rate was 35 breaths per minute. He was reassured by the nurse, administered O_2 40% via face mask, and his mother was invited into the recovery room. His mother's presence helped to calm the child to some extent. Fentanyl 0.5 mcg.kg^{-1} was administered intravenously. Over 5 to 10 minutes, his agitated behavior resolved, his heart rate decreased to 95 beats per minute, his blood pressure to 100/50 mm Hg, and his respiratory rate decreased to 25 breaths per minute. The child appeared content and comfortable sitting in his mother's lap.

After the boy was observed and monitored for 30 minutes in the recovery room, he was transferred to the inpatient ward where he remained for another 3 hours until he had eaten, drank, passed urine, and his vitals signs were at preoperative levels. He was reviewed in the inpatient ward by the anesthetist before discharge, whose note in the medical record described him as "comfortable and calm." The patient was discharged home with a prescription for oral analgesics (paracetamol and ibuprofen) "as required" for 5 days.

Two days after discharge, the boy's parents reported to their family doctor that he was reluctant to eat and was sleeping for only 1 to 2 hours at a time. They also noted that, despite receiving the maximum prescribed doses of paracetamol and ibuprofen, he continued to complain of discomfort. They were reassured and advised to continue to administer oral analgesics as required. Three days later, the parents reported that the abnormal eating and sleeping pattern appeared to have resolved.

CASE DISCUSSION

Emergence agitation can manifest as a number of behavioral patterns that children display during recovery from anesthesia. Two scales that have been used to categorize and grade postoperative behavior in children are the Post Anesthetic Behavior Scale (Table 56.1)[1] and the Pediatric Anesthesia Emergence Delirium scale (Table 56.2).[2]

The Pediatric Anesthesia Emergence Delirium scale score demonstrates negative correlation with a child's age and time to awakening and is significantly greater in children who receive sevoflurane than in those who receive halothane.[2]

TABLE 56.1 Postanesthetic Behavior Scale

1. Sleeping
2. Awake, calm
3. Irritable, crying
4. Inconsolable crying
5. Severe restlessness, disorientation, thrashing around

Reproduced with permission from Cole JW, Murray DJ, McAkiter JD, et al. Emergence behaviour in children: defining the incidence of excitement and agitation following anesthesia. Pediatr Anesth 2002:12:442–447.

Emergence agitation is distressing for the child and his or her parents; its incidence will also influence the numbers of nurses needed to staff the recovery room. It can be associated with physical injury and can prolong the patient's stay in the postanesthetic care unit/recovery room[3] (Table 56.3).

STRATEGIES TO DECREASE EMERGENCE AGITATION

It is important to identify patients with risk factors for emergence agitation, so that appropriate measures can be taken.

Anxiety

As many as 65% of children undergoing anesthesia and surgery develop intense anxiety, preoperatively.[4] Preoperative anxiety is a subjective feeling of tension, apprehension, nervousness, and worry. Some of the causes of increased anxiety include separation from parents, uncertainty about anesthesia or surgery and about the outcome of the operation.[5] Preoperative anxiety is an important etiological factor in the development of emergence agitation.

The incidence of postoperative agitation/delirium is greater in anxious (9.7%) compared with nonanxious (1.5%) children.[3] Increased preoperative anxiety is also associated with greater postoperative pain, analgesic consumption, postoperative anxiety, sleep disturbance, and altered eating patterns in 5- to 12-year-old children.[3] Preoperative preparation of children, their parents, and their environment are

TABLE 56.2 Pediatric Anesthesia Emergence Delirium Scale

1. The child makes eye contact with the caregiver.
2. The child's action is purposeful.
3. The child is aware of his or her surrounding.
4. The child is restless.
5. The child is inconsolable.

Reproduced with permission from Sikich N, Lerman J. Development and psychometric evaluation of the pediatric anesthesia emergence delirium scale. Anesthesiology 2004;100:1138–1145.

TABLE 56.3 Possible Etiological Factors Related to Emergence Agitation

Patient Factors
Age[14,15]
Child's temperament[15]
Preoperative anxiety[9]
Parent's anxiety[11]
Hypoxia[36]
Hypercarbia[36]
Hypoglycemia[36]
Hyponatremia[36]
Surgical Factors
Otorhinolaryngologic surgery[14,15]
Pain[16,19]
Anesthetic Factors
Rapid emergence[19]
Choice of inhalational agent (60% with sevoflurane vs. 20% with halothane)[19]
Intrinsic characteristics of anesthetic agents[16,37,38]
Residual drug effects (e.g., ketamine, droperidol, hyoscine, atropine)[36]
Midazolam[1]

important in decreasing preoperative anxiety. Preparing children for surgery can prevent psychological and behavioral manifestations of anxiety.[6] Various distraction techniques have been used to decrease preoperative anxiety in the anesthetic induction room, the including presence of clown doctors[7] and a handheld video game.[8]

Temperament

A child's baseline temperament may be associated with the likelihood of his or her developing emergence agitation. Children with a history of temper tantrums are more likely to develop emergence agitation.[9] Various scales exist to assess a child's baseline temperament. One such scale is EASI (emotionality, activity, sociability, and impulsivity), for which reliability has been demonstrated.[10] Younger, more emotional, more impulsive, and less sociable children are more likely to develop emergence agitation. Parents of children in this group were also significantly more anxious.[11]

Parental Presence During Anesthesia Induction

Parental presence during induction of anesthesia can be used to treat or reduce preanesthetic anxiety. It has been shown to enhance the effect of oral midazolam premedication on emergence behavior of children undergoing general anesthesia.[12] Parental presence has no additive effect on the child's compliance during the anesthetic induction.[12] A combination of written, pictorial, and verbal information would improve the process of informed consent.[13]

Age

Emergence agitation is observed more frequently in preschool children.[14,15] Possible etiologic factors include psychological immaturity, genetic predisposition, and the type of procedure.[1,16–18]

Anesthetic Factors

Emergence agitation occurs in 60% of children after sevoflurane anesthesia.[19] A central nervous system excitatory effect of sevoflurane[20] and epileptiform activity during induction with sevoflurane have been reported.[21] Induction using sevoflurane alone is associated with a greater incidence of emergence agitation compared with when N_2O is coadministered (35% vs. 5%).[22] Whether awakening occurs rapidly or slowly does not appear to influence the incidence of emergence agitation (35.7% vs. 32, 6% respectively)[16] (Table 56.4).

Surgical Factors and Adjunct Medications

Surgical procedures involving otorhinolaryngologic surgery and head and neck surgery are associated with a greater incidence of emergence agitation. It has been speculated that this is caused by a "sense of suffocation."[23]

Postoperative pain has been consistently implicated as an important cause of emergence agitation.[16,19,23,24] In children, emergence agitation and pain behavior may be indistinguishable.[25] The presence of pain as a predisposing factor to postoperative agitation explains the effectiveness of analgesic drugs, either in prophylaxis or treatment of agitation. Opioid administration considerably decreases the incidence of postoperative agitation[26] (Table 56.5).

One or more of these interventions may be selected for managing children at greatest risk for emergence agitation.

Long-Term Consequences

Emergence agitation in the recovery room is usually self-limiting and resolves without pharmacologic intervention.[1,3] However, long-term sequelae can result. New maladaptive behaviors such as nightmare crying, enuresis, separation

TABLE 56.4 Modification of Anesthetic Technique to Minimize Likelihood of Emergence Agitation

- Using nerve blocks to minimize postoperative pain
- Parental presence during induction of anesthesia[12]
- Caudal anesthesia for lower abdominal surgery[38]
- Avoiding inhalational agents especially those with low solubility[19]
- Using total IV anesthesia[37]
- IV bolus of propofol at the end of surgery[39]

TABLE 56.5 Adjunct Medications

- Midazolam 0.2 mg/kg premedication[40–42]
- Clonidine µg/kg orally premedication[43]
- Clonidine 1 to 3 mcg/kg intraoperatively (decreases incidence of emergence agitation from 39% to 0%)[44,45]
- Ketamine 6 mg/kg premedication[46]
- Fentanyl 2 µg/kg intranasally intraoperatively (decreases incidence of emergence agitation from 23% to 2%)[19] or 2.5 µg/kg intravenously[14,26,47]
- Dexmedetomidine 1µg/kg after anesthetic induction[25,41]
- Ketorolac 1 mg/kg intraoperatively[24]

anxiety, and temper tantrums can occur postoperatively in as many as 50% of children.[4] The Post-Hospital Behaviour Questionnaire is designed to evaluate maladaptive behavioral responses in children after surgery. It has shown good test-retest reliability and is a useful standardized tool for assessing postoperative behavior.[27] Using the Post-Hospital Behaviour Questionnaire, it has been shown that children's preoperative anxiety and emergence status were significant predictors of presence or absence of new maladaptive behavior.[11] The odds ratio for one or more new-onset maladaptive behaviors is 1.43 for children with marked emergence agitation.[11]

KEY MESSAGES

1. Emergence delirium in children is defined as "a disturbance in a child's awareness of and attention to his or her environment with disorientation and perceptual alterations including hypersensitivity to stimuli and hyperactive motor behavior in the immediate postoperative period."[2]

2. It is usually a self-limiting condition, appearing in the immediate postoperative period and resolving spontaneously in 5 to 15 minutes[28,29] but can last longer in 2% to 3% of patients.[1,30]

3. Emergence agitation is defined as "a state of mild restlessness and mental distress that, unlike delirium, is not always accompanied by a significant change in behavior."[31]

4. Emergence agitation can result from pain, physiological compromise, or anxiety.[32]

5. As many as 10% to 50% of children (compared with 5% of adults) demonstrate alerted behavior during emergence.[33–35] Age, history of temper tantrums, type of surgery, and the anesthetic technique are important predisposing factors.

QUESTIONS

1. **What is emergence delirium and emergence agitation?**

   Answer: Emergence delirium can be defined as "a disturbance in a child's awareness of and attention to his or her environment with disorientation and perceptual alterations including hypersensitivity to stimuli and hyperactive motor behavior in the immediate postoperative period." Emergence agitation can be defined as "a state of mild restlessness and mental distress that does not always suggest a significant change in behavior."

2. **What are the possible etiological factors contributing to the development of emergence agitation in children?**

   Answer: In children, preoperative anxiety, age, temperament, parents' anxiety, type of surgery, type of anesthetic, and adjunct medications all influence the likelihood of emergence agitation occurring. It is more commonly seen in preschool children, with a history of temper tantrums and those with separation anxiety undergoing ear, nose, and throat surgery under inhalation anesthetic (sevoflurane, in particular). Pain is an important etiological factor.

3. **How can emergence agitation be prevented?**

   Answer: In children, methods to decrease preoperative anxiety include careful explanation (written, verbal, pictorial) to the child of what to expect, psychological preparation, parental presence during anesthesia induction, use of distraction techniques such as clowns or handheld video games, premedication (e.g., clonidine), and effective perioperative analgesia. Other methods include avoidance of inhalational anesthetic agents, administering an IV bolus of propofol before waking the child, the use of regional anesthetic techniques such as caudal block, and perioperative administration of fentanyl, clonidine, dexmedetomidine, or ketorolac.

References

1. Cole JW, Murray DJ, McAlister JD, et al. Emergence behaviour in children: defining the incidence of excitement and agitation following anaesthesia. Pediatr Anesth 2002;12:442–447.
2. Sikich N, Lerman J. Development and psychometric evaluation of the pediatric anesthesia emergence delirium scale. Anesthesiology 2004;100:1138–1145.
3. Voepel-Lewis T, Malviya S, Tait AR. A prospective cohort study of emergence agitation in the pediatric post anesthesia care unit. Anesth Analg 2003;96:1625–1630.
4. Kain ZN, Mayes LC, O'Connor TZ, et al. Preoperative anxiety in children, predictors and outcomes. Arch Pediatr Med 1996; 150:1238–1245.
5. Kain ZN, Caldwell-Andrews AA, Wang SM. Psychological preparation of the parent and pediatric surgical patient. Anesthesiol Clin North Am 2002;20:69–88.
6. Kain ZN, Caldwell-Andrews AA. Preoperative psychological preparation of the child for surgery: an update. Anesthesiol Clin North Am 2005;23:597–614.
7. Laura V, Simona C, Arianna R, et al. Clown doctors as a treatment for preoperative anxiety in children. Pediatrics 2005;116:563–567.
8. Patel A, Schiebe T, Davidson M, et al. Distraction with a handheld video game reduces pediatric preoperative anxiety. Pediatr Anesth, 2006;16:1019–1027.
9. Paul AT, Tonya MP, Susan T, et al. Assessment of risk factors for emergence distress and postoperative behavioural changes in children following general anaesthesia. Pediatric Anesth 2004;14: 235–240.
10. Buss AH, Plomin R. Theory and measurement of EAS temperament: early developing personality traits. Hillsdale, NJ: L. Erlbaum Associates, 1984:98–130.
11. Kain N, Caldwell-Andrews, Mayes LC, et al. Preoperative anxiety and emergence delirium and postoperative maladaptive behaviours. Anesth Analg 2004;99:1648–1654.
12. Arai YC, Ito H, Kandatsu N, et al. Parental presence during induction enhances the effect of oral midazolam on emergence behaviour of children undergoing general anesthesia. Acta Anaesth Scand 2007;51:858–861.
13. Astuto M, Rosano G, Rizzo G, et al. Preoperative parental information and parents' presence at induction of anaesthesia. Minerva Anestesiol 2006;72:461–465.
14. Finkel JC, Cohen IT, Hannallah RS, et al. The effect of intranasal fentanyl on the emergence characteristics after sevoflurane anesthesia in children undergoing surgery for bilateral myringotomy tube placement. Anesth Analg 2001;92:1164–1168.
15. Anono J, Ueda W, Mamiya K, et al. Greater incidence of delirium during recovery from sevoflurane anaesthesia in pre school boys. Anesthesiology 1997:87:1298–1300.
16. Muto R, Miyasaka K, Takata M, et al. Initial experience of complete switch over to sevoflurane in 1550 children. Pediatr Anesth 1993;3:229–233.
17. Welborn LG, Hannallah RS, Norden JM, et al. Comparison of emergence and recovery characteristics of sevoflurane, desflurane, and halothane in pediatric ambulatory patients. Anesth Analg 1996;83:917–920.
18. Wells LT, Rasch DK. Emergence delirium after sevoflurane anaesthesia: a paranoid delusion? Anesth Analg 1999;88: 1308–1310.
19. Naito Y, Tamai S, Shingu K, et al. Comparison between sevoflurane and halothane for paediatric ambulatory anaesthesia. Br J Anaesth 1991;67:387–389.
20. Eger EI. New inhaled anaesthetics. Anesthesiology 1994;80: 906–922.
21. Adachi M, Ikemoto Y, Kubo K, et al. Seizure-like movements during induction of anaesthesia with sevoflurane. Br J Anaesth 1992:68:214–215.
22. Sarner J, Levine M, Davis P, et al. Clinical characteristics of sevoflurane in children Anesthesiology 1995:82:38–46.
23. Eckenhoff JE, Kneale DH, Dripps RD. The incidence and etiology of post anaesthetic excitement. Anesthesiology 1961;22: 667–673.
24. Davis PJ, Greenberg JA, Gendelman M, et al. Recovery characteristics of sevoflurane and halothane in preschool aged children undergoing bilateral myringotomy and pressure equalization tube insertion. Anesth Analg 1999;88:34–38.
25. Berrin I, Mustafa A, Alpern DT, et al. Dexmedetomidine decreases emergence agitation in pediatric patients after sevoflurane anaesthesia without surgery. Pediatr Anesth 2006; 748–753.
26. Cohen IT, Finkel JC, Hannallah RS, et al. The effect of fentanyl on the emergence characteristics after desflurane or sevoflurane anaesthesia in children. Anesth Analg 2002; 94:1178–1181.
27. Vernon DT, Schulman JL, Foley JM. Changes in children's behavior after hospitalization. Am J Dis Child 1966;111:581–593.
28. Olympio MA. Postanesthetic delirium: historical perspectives. J Clin Anesth 1991;3:60–63.
29. Moore JK, Moore EW, Ellion RA, et al. Propofol and halothane versus sevoflurane in paediatric day case surgery: induction and recovery characteristics. Br J Anaesth 2003;90:461–466.
30. Holzki J, Kretz FJ. Changing aspects of sevoflurane in pediatric anesthesia:1975–99 (editorial). Pediatr Anesth 1999;9:283–286.

31. Galford RE. Problems in anesthesiology: approach to diagnosis. Boston, MA: Little, Brown & Company, 1992:341–343.
32. Voepel-Lewis T, Burke C. Differentiating pain and delirium is only part of assessing the agitated child. J Perianesth Nurs 2004; 19:298–299.
33. Lerman J, Davis PJ, Welborn LG, et al. Induction, recovery and safety and characteristics of sevoflurane in children undergoing ambulatory surgery. Anesthesiology 1996;84:1332–1340.
34. Baum VC, Yemen TA, Baum LD. Immediate 8% sevoflurane induction in children: a comparison with incremental sevoflurane and incremental halothane. Anesth Analg 1997;85: 313–316.
35. Lepouse C, Lautner CA, Liu L, et al. Emergence delirium in adults in the post anaesthetic care unit. Br J Anaesth 2006;96: 747–753.
36. Picard V, Dumont L, Pellegrini M. Quality of recovery in children: sevoflurane versus propofol. Acta Anaesthesiol Scand 2000;44:307–310.
37. Cohen IT, Finkel JC, Hannallah RS, et al. Rapid emergence does not explain agitation following sevoflurane anaesthesia in infants and children: a comparison with propofol. Pediatric Anesth 2003; 13:63–67.
38. Aouad MT, Kanazi GE, Siddik-Sayyed SM, et al. Preoperative caudal block prevents emergence agitation in children following sevoflurane anesthesia. Acta Anaesthesiol Scand 2005;49: 300–304.
39. Aouad MT, Yazbeck-Karam VG, Nasr VG, et al. A single dose of propofol at the end of surgery for the prevention of emergence agitation in children undergoing strabismus surgery during sevoflurane anesthesia. Anesthesiology 2007;107:733–738.
40. Ko YP, Huang CJ, Hung YC, et al. Premedication with low dose midazolam reduces the incidence and severity of emergence agitation in pediatric patients following sevoflurane anesthesia. Acta Anesthesiol Sin 2001;39:169–177.
41. Riva J, Lejbussiewicz G, Papa M, et al. Oral premedication with midazolam in paediatric anaesthesia. Effects on sedation and gastric contents. Pediatr Anesth 1997;191–196.
42. Kogan A, Katz J, Erfat R, et al. Premedication with midazolam in young children: a comparison of four routes of administration. Pediatr Anesth 2002;12:685–689.
43. Almenrader N, Pessariello M, Coccetti B, et al. Premedication in children: a comparison of oral midazolam and oral clonidine. Pediatr Anesth 2007;17:1143–1149.
44. Bock M, Kunz P, Schreckenberger R, et al. Comparison of caudal and intravenous clonidine in prevention of agitation after sevoflurane in children. Br J Anaesth 2002;88:790–796.
45. Malviya S, Voepel-Lewis T, Ramamurthi R, et al. Clonidine for the prevention of emergence agitation in young children: efficacy and recovery profile. Pediatr Anesth 2006;16:554–559.
46. Kararmaz A, Kaya S, Turhanoglu S, et al. Oral ketamine premedication can prevent emergence agitation in children after desflurane anaesthesia. Pediatr Anesth 2004; 14:477–482.
47. Galinkin JL, Fazil LM, Cuy RM, et al. Use of intranasal fentanyl in children undergoing myringotomy and tube placement during halothane and sevoflurane anaesthesia. Anesthesiology 2000; 93:1378–1383.

CHAPTER 57

The Acute Pain Team Role in Management of a Patient With Traumatic Upper Limb Amputation

Owen O'Sullivan

CASE FORMAT: STEP BY STEP

A 46-year-old fisherman was taken to the emergency room of a small regional hospital on a Saturday morning. An accident in the harbor area resulted in a traumatic (avulsion) amputation of his forearm proximal to the wrist, and paramedics had attended to him at the site within minutes. The amputated limb had been packed in ice, and bleeding was controlled with direct pressure. On arrival to the emergency department, 2 hours after the accident, he walked in with the aid of coworkers and was immediately brought to the resuscitation room.

An emergency medicine physician promptly carried out a primary survey. The patient's upper airway was patent; vesicular breath sounds were audible on auscultation bilaterally. His heart rate was 120 beats per minute; blood pressure, 190/100 mm Hg; and Glasgow Coma Scale, 15/15. No other injuries were identified. Intravenous access was established, blood was sampled for routine investigations (full blood picture, urea and electrolytes, serum glucose, lactate and arterial blood gas analysis were all normal), an intravenous (IV) morphine bolus was administered (increments of 2 mg IV totalling 12 mg over 80 minutes), and prophylactic antibiotics were administered as the trauma team evaluated the injury. It was decided that, in view of the patient's general good condition and the relatively short injury/decision interval, that replantation should be considered at the regional plastic surgical referral service based in a hospital approximately an hour away. It was decided to transfer the patient urgently. Before transfer, the anesthetic service was contacted, as the patient was still in extreme pain despite cumulative administration of morphine 18 mg IV and paracetamol 2 g IV over approximately 4 hours.

What is the purpose of relieving or managing pain in patients who have suffered traumatic injury?

Apart from humanitarian indications for treating pain after trauma, inadequate analgesia can exacerbate the stress response, which can result in myocardial ischemia and stroke. Untreated pain is also associated with complications such as impaired cough and ileus. However, evidence proving that pain control improves morbidity and mortality in this setting is lacking and (for ethical reasons) difficult to acquire. The more general issue of the association between postoperative pain management and patient outcome has recently been critically reviewed.[1,2]

What are the pain management options for this patient?

The American Society of Anesthesiologists guidelines for the management of acute pain in the perioperative period are summarized in Table 57.1.

At the receiving hospital, the plastic surgeon who decided that the amputated limb was not suitable for replantation assessed the patient. An anesthetist (who had received a medical summary by telephone) arrived to assess the patient. The patient was hemodynamically stable but remained distressed and in pain with a verbal rating scale (VRS) score for pain of 10/10. Having considered the risks and potential benefits (delay in surgery, potential for axillary arterial injury, minimizing operative stress response and anesthetic drug and opioid requirements, and lessening risk of postoperative acute and long-term pain), the anesthetist elected to perform a supraclavicular block and to insert a catheter for continuous titratable analgesia. After explaining the procedure to the patient, full asepsis was observed and the block was performed and catheter inserted under ultrasound guidance using a 21-gauge insulated needle. An initial dose of 25 mL of 0.25% levobupivacaine was administered. The patient was reassessed 20 minutes later, just before transfer and was found to be much more comfortable with a VRS score of 2/10. During this 20-minute interval, the anesthetist provided the acute pain team (APT) (through the on-call pain nurse) with a verbal summary of the case.

Prior to induction of general anesthesia (using a rapid sequence induction technique), the patient reported pain in the limb at rest as VRS of 3/10. Six hours had elapsed since the injury. A further 10 mL of 0.25% bupivacaine was injected through the supraclavicular catheter before surgical incision.

The operation, wound exploration, debridement, and a bone-shortening revision of the stump were uneventful. A continuous infusion of 0.1% bupivacaine (initially 8 mL per hour) was commenced via the supraclavicular catheter at the end of the procedure. Regular paracetamol 1 g IV and diclofenac 75 mg IV were prescribed, as was morphine 10 mg intramuscularly for breakthrough pain. Because the anesthetist was concerned about the risk of the patient developing

TABLE 57.1 Acute Perioperative Pain Management

Institutional policies and procedures for providing perioperative pain management	• Education and training for health care providers • Monitoring of patient outcomes • 24-hour availability of anesthetist providing perioperative pain management • Use of a dedicated acute pain service • Standardized, validated instruments to facilitate the regular evaluation and documentation of pain intensity, the effects of pain therapy, and side effects caused by the therapy
Preoperative evaluation of the patient	• Evaluate patient factors • Type of surgery, expected severity of postoperative pain, underlying medical conditions, the risk-benefit ratio for the available techniques, patient's preferences, or previous experience with pain • A directed pain history, a directed physical examination, and a pain control plan
Preoperative preparation of the patient	• Adjust or continue medications that when suddenly stopped may provoke a withdrawal syndrome • Treatment(s) to reduce preexisting pain and anxiety • Premedication(s) before surgery as part of a multimodal analgesic pain management program • Patient and family education • Include misconceptions that overestimate the risk of adverse effects and addiction
Perioperative techniques for pain management	• Use therapeutic options such as epidural, intrathecal opioids, systemic opioid patient-controlled analgesia, and regional techniques after thoughtfully considering the risks and benefits for the individual patient • Used in preference to intramuscular opioids ordered "as needed" • Special caution should be taken when continuous infusion modalities are used, as drug accumulation may contribute to adverse events • Therapy selected should reflect the individual anesthetist's expertise, as well as the capacity for safe application of the modality in each practice setting (including the ability to recognize and treat adverse effects)
Multimodal techniques for pain management	• Unless contraindicated, all patients should receive an around-the-clock regimen of nonsteroidal anti-inflammatory drugs, COX-2 selective inhibitors, or acetaminophen. • Consider regional blockade with local anesthetics. • Dosing regimens should be administered to optimize efficacy while minimizing the risk of adverse events. The choice of medication, dose, route, and duration of therapy should be individualized.

Adapted from Practice guidelines for acute pain management in the perioperative setting: an updated report by the American Society of Anesthesiologists Task Force on Acute Pain Management. Anesthesiology. 2004;100:1573–1581.

phantom limb pain (PLP), he also prescribed gabapentin 300 mg orally starting on the first postoperative day (300 mg every 12 hours on day 2 and 300 mg every 8 hours on day 3). A written referral was sent to the APT to facilitate follow-up of the patient's pain management.

Can phantom symptoms be prevented after traumatic amputation?

Pain perceived at the site previously occupied by an amputated limb is common and can be very difficult to treat. A Dutch study of upper limb amputees showed that the prevalence of PLP was 51% (95% confidence level, 36%–63%); phantom sensation, 76%; and stump pain, 48.6%.[4] Although most of the patients with PLP reported having "moderate" to "very much" pain, only 4 of 99 respondents received medical treatment for phantom pain. In 77% of cases, the indication for surgery was trauma. The use of N-methyl-D-aspartate receptors has been implicated in the development of PLP, and the use of memantine (an N-methyl-D-aspartate receptor antagonist) in a brachial plexus blockade postoperatively in traumatic upper limb amputations has been shown to decrease the intensity of PLP (but not beyond 6 months.)[5]

Some evidence exists that gabapentin, commonly used in several neuropathic pain syndromes, is useful in treating postamputation PLP.[6] However, a study evaluating its effectiveness when administered for 30 days postoperatively failed to show a reduction in incidence or intensity of postamputation pain.[7] Therefore, its use in the case described is not "evidence based."

Over the following 24 hours, the patient remained relatively comfortable, self-reporting pain as VRS 2 to 4/10. As his first postoperative day was a Sunday, the APT did not review him until his second postoperative day. At this point, the team completed a full pain history (including previous experience of pain and use of pain medications) and examination including the insertion site of the supraclavicular catheter. Gabapentin was discontinued. The APT visited the patient each day, assessing his pain and modifying its management throughout his admission.

What is the role of the APT in the management of such patients?

A variety of organizations have recommended establishing structures to provide dedicated postoperative pain service.[3,8] Rawal identified important components of an acute pain service (APS) in a recent review article[9]:

- Designated personnel for provision of 24-hour APS
- Regular assessment and documentation of pain scores at rest and at movement
- Maintaining scores below a predetermined threshold
- Appropriate assessment tools for children and those with cognitive impairment
- Development of protocols to achieve goals for postoperative mobilization and rehabilitation
- Education of ward nurses
- Patient education
- Regular audit (including cost-effectiveness)

More than 10 years after the relevant recommendations of the Royal College of Anaesthetists,[8] a survey showed that 83% of hospitals in the United Kingdom had an established APS. However, most were open only Monday through Friday with reduced out-of-hours coverage with only 5% covering 24 hours.[10] The establishment of an APS is associated with lesser postoperative pain ratings and can decrease postoperative nausea and vomiting and postoperative urinary retention.[11] A review of 10 economic evaluations of APS programs failed to demonstrate their cost-effectiveness definitively. This review was limited by the poor quality of the evaluations.[12] The establishment of an APS is presently a prerequisite for accreditation for training by the Royal College of Anaesthetists[13] and the Australian and New Zealand College of Anaesthetists. To function optimally, an APT must operate as part of a multidisciplinary acute rehabilitation program.[14] To justify provision of sufficient resources to fully implement the APT "concept," further evidence is required regarding the clinical and economic consequences.

KEY MESSAGES

1. The American Society of Anesthesiologists guidelines for perioperative pain management include the preoperative assessment and preparation of patients and multimodal techniques for pain management.

2. To function optimally, an APT must operate as part of a multidisciplinary acute rehabilitation program.

3. To date, the cost-effectiveness of establishing an APT has not been definitively established.

QUESTIONS

1. What are the important elements of an acute pain team/service?

   Answer: The important elements of an acute pain team/service are (a) designated personnel for provision of 24-hour APS, (b) regular assessment and documentation of pain scores, (c) development of protocols to achieve goals for postoperative mobilization and rehabilitation, (d) education of ward nurses, (e) patient education, and (f) regular audit (including cost-effectiveness).

2. What proportion of upper limb amputees will experience phantom limb symptoms?

   Answer: The majority of upper limb amputees will experience phantom limb symptoms (pain, 51%; phantom sensation, 76%).[4]

3. Is establishment of an APT cost-effective?

   Answer: Although this has not been demonstrated definitively to date, a body of related evidence indicates that establishment of an APT may be cost-effective.

References

1. Lui SS, Wu CL. Effect of postoperative analgesia on major postoperative complications: a systematic update of the evidence. Anesth Analg 2007;104:689–702.
2. White PF, Kehlet H. Postoperative pain management and patient outcome: time to return to work. Anesth Analg 2007;104:487–489.
3. Practice guidelines for acute pain management in the perioperative setting: an updated report by the American Society of Anesthesiologists Task Force on Acute Pain Management. Anesthesiology. 2004;100:1573–1581.
4. Kooijman CM, Dijkstra PU, Geertzen JH, et al. Phantom pain and phantom sensations in upper limb amputees: an epidemiological study. Pain. 2000;87:33–41.
5. Schley M, Topfner S, Wiech K, et al. Continuous brachial plexus blockade in combination with the NMDA receptor antagonist memantine prevents phantom pain in acute traumatic upper limb amputees. Eur J Pain 2007;11:299–308.
6. Bone M, Critchley P, Buggy DJ. Gabapentin in postamputation phantom limb pain: a randomized, double-blind, placebo-controlled, cross-over study. Reg Anesth Pain Med 2002;27:481–486.

7. Nikolajsen L, Finnerup NB, Kramp S, et al. A randomized study of the effects of gabapentin on postamputation pain. Anesthesiology. 2006;105:1008–1015.
8. Working Party of the Commission on the Provision of Surgical Services. Pain after surgery. London: Royal College of Surgeons of England, College of Anaesthetists, 1990.
9. Rawal N. Organization, function, and implementation of acute pain service. Anesthesiol Clin North Am 2005;23:211–225.
10. Powell AE, Davies HT, Bannister J, et al. Rhetoric and reality on acute pain services in the UK: a national postal questionnaire survey. Br J Anaesth 2004;92:689–693.
11. Werner MU, Søholm L, Rotbøll-Nielsen P, et al. Does an acute pain service improve postoperative outcome? Anesth Analg 2002; 95:1361–1372.
12. Lee A, Chan S, Chen PP, et al. Economic evaluations of acute pain service programs: a systematic review. Clin J Pain. 2007;23:726–733.
13. Smith G, Power I, Cousins MJ. Acute pain: is there scientific evidence on which to base treatment [editorial]? Br J Anaesth 1999; 82:817–819.
14. Kehlet H. Acute pain control and accelerated postoperative surgical recovery. Surg Clin North Am 1999;79:431–443.

CHAPTER 58

Occupational Exposure to Anesthetic Agents

Jason Van der Velde

CASE FORMAT: STEP BY STEP

A trainee anesthesiologist lodged a grievance with her hospital attributing the spontaneous abortion of her third pregnancy to exposure to anesthetic gases at work as a causative factor. The hospital's management strenuously denied these allegations citing that its policy of regularly monitoring the operating rooms' air quality showed that her working environment consistently conformed to international occupational health standards. Opinions within the hospital were divided, and considerable tensions mounted over this emotive issue.

Does occupational exposure to anesthetic gases represent a health risk to health care workers?

Most occupational exposure limits (OELs) in force today are loosely based on meta-analysis[1–3] of nine major studies[4–12] carried out between 1971 and 1985 that examined the associations between (a) occupational exposure to nitrous oxide (N_2O) and/or some volatile anesthetic agents and (b) a range of adverse health effects, notably spontaneous abortion. Limitations of these investigations include inadequate power, failure to measure personal exposures, and failure to take account of confounding factors such as the variety or absence of scavenging systems used and any additional environmental pollutants. Several subsequent major studies neither ruled out these concerns, nor demonstrated significant association between exposure and adverse health outcomes.[13–19]

The authors of two large epidemiologic studies have concluded that occupational exposure to volatile agents may be related to immunologic, neurologic, renal, or hepatic toxic effects.[20,21] Observational studies have shown associations between exposure to halogenated agents and a deficit in manual dexterity, headache, depression, anxiety, loss of appetite, memory loss, and change in intellectual function.[22–25] Clearly, it would require substantial collaboration to build a conclusive evidence base.

The adverse health effects associated with N_2O exposure alone are spontaneous abortion (relative risk $\cong$ 1.3 to 1.9) and infertility.[26,27] If the use of N_2O is to fall out of favor, it is conceivable that exposure to other volatile anesthetics will increase. This has been specifically investigated using both environmental and personal monitoring. Fortunately, the occupational exposure to sevoflurane is not greater when it is used alone compared with when sevoflurane and N_2O are administered in combination.[28]

In rodents, long-term exposure to low concentrations of halogenated anesthetic agents impairs curiosity, exploratory behavior, learning and memory function, and increases anxiety.[29] The behavioral changes related to long-term exposure in humans and its associated risk to professional performance have yet to be thoroughly investigated.

A concern raised by pediatric operating room nurses surrounded the interpretation of maximum safe levels of atmospheric sevoflurane. A maximum limit of 2 parts per million (ppm) in the atmosphere was quoted as that set by national health safety legislation. Yet a hospital staff member recalled 18 ppm being monitored during one of the sampling periods. Operating room staff, becoming increasingly concerned for their own safety, were not satisfied by managerial assurances that the manufacturers' recommended safe limit is 20 ppm.

What is an OEL ?

The National Institute of Occupational Safety and Health (NIOSH) in the United States America clearly states that it is unable to identify a safe OEL for waste anesthetic gases.[30] Current recommendations from NIOSH are that potential risks should be minimized by "reducing exposures to the greatest extent possible." Table 58.1 lists the range of advised OELs as set by various international health authorities. Unless indicated, they are expressed as a time-weighted average exposure in an 8-hour working day.[31]

Manufacturers advise a maximum exposure limit to known hazards. In a recent study, formation of micronucleated lymphocytes was compared in two groups of anesthetic personnel exposed to different levels of waste anesthetic agents. The results indicate that the current range of international limits appears to be appropriate (at least in terms of this marker).[32]

Some staff members believed that volatile anesthetic agents were efficiently scavenged in the pediatric operating rooms, whereas others were convinced that, if they could smell the agents, the concentrations present could not be "safe."

What is the difference between personal exposure risk and monitored environmental level?

Operating room anesthetic agent concentrations are usually monitored from a fixed point in the room using photoacoustic infrared spectrometry, "monitored environmental level." Because of air movement and scavenging, anesthetic

TABLE 58.1 Recommended Occupational Exposure Levels for Anesthetic Vapors in Various Countries

	N$_2$O	Halothane	Enflurane	Isoflurane	Sevoflurane	Desflurane
Austria	–	5	–	–	–	–
Denmark	100	5	2	–	–	–
France	–	2	–	–	–	–
Germany	100	5	20	–	–	–
Great Britain	100	10	50	50	–	–
Italy	100	–	–	–	–	–
Norway	100	5	2	2	–	–
Sweden	100	5	10	10	–	–
Switzerland	100	5	10	10	–	–
US-NIOSH	25	2	2	2	2	2
US-ACGIH	50	50	75	–	–	–

US-NIOSH, National Institute of Occupational Safety and Health; US-ACGIH, American Conference of Governmental Industrial Hygienists.

agent levels may not be uniform throughout the room. By placing the sampling device at the shoulder of a staff member, that is, sampling directly from their personal breathing zone, a more accurate "personal exposure level" may be measured. Inhalational induction with sevoflurane and N$_2$O in pediatric practice was found to violate NIOSH-recommended personal exposure levels approximately 50% of the time based on the personal samples but not in the room samples.[33] This personal exposure risk appears to strongly correlate with anesthetic technique and training.

During maintenance of pediatric anesthesia, the use of uncuffed endotracheal tubes and the Ayres T-Piece can lead to greater monitored environmental levels of anesthetic agents.[34] OELs are, however, rarely violated provided efficient pressure/exhaust ventilation, above 12 air exchanges per hour, and efficient active scavenging systems are in place.

Personal exposure risk monitoring reveals that during maintenance of anesthesia with laryngeal mask airways in adults, sevoflurane concentrations frequently exceed 2 ppm and 50 ppm for N$_2$O. Alarmingly, these findings occurred despite the use of low-flow circle circuits, gas scavenging, and correct laryngeal mask airway insertion technique and sizing.[35]

To address increasing staff concerns, the hospital management instituted a thorough review of the areas of the hospital where anesthetic agents were administered or where patients recovering from anesthesia were monitored.

Do areas other than operating rooms pose a risk of occupational exposure to anesthetic agents?

The monitoring for environmental pollutants by direct reading instrumentation such as photoacoustic infrared spectrometry is expensive and restricts normal staff movements, potentially leading to spurious results.

Personal environmental sampling using passive diffusion tubes or by urine collection is cost-effective and a method that staff find both acceptable and convenient. The use of gas chromatography-mass spectrometry for determination of N$_2$O and sevoflurane in urine and environmental samples is accurate and sufficient for this purpose.

The unscavenged use of on-demand N$_2$O:O$_2$ in poorly ventilated labor rooms is widespread. There is a strong positive correlation between environmental concentrations and midwives' biological uptake of N$_2$O. N$_2$O in biological tissues is poorly soluble and therefore should be eliminated rapidly between shifts. Interestingly, 50% of midwives studied had non-zero baseline values of N$_2$O in their urine on arrival to the workplace and these 50% showed very high levels.[36]

It is unlikely that staff working in postanesthesia care units are exposed to important amounts of volatile agents from the low concentrations expired by recovering patients. When compared with their colleagues on surgical wards, biological concentrations of N$_2$O for recovery room personnel were 3.1 ppm versus 1.17 ppm.[37]

Following this risk assessment, a number of simple strategies were investigated to reduce staff exposure.

What means are available to minimize occupational exposure of health care workers to anesthetic agents?

Scavenging When Mapleson D circuits were equipped with an airway pressure-limiting valve allowing direct connection to an anesthetic gas extractor, the ambient levels of sevoflurane and N$_2$O measured in the breathing area around the anesthesiologist decreased from 7 (26) to 1.1 (1) ppm ($p < 0.001$).[38]

Ventilation When surgeons and scrub nurses were asked about symptoms related to occupational exposure, a greater incidence of noticing a "smell of gas" was registered for the group without an extractor (87% vs. 11% in the extractor group, $p = 0.003$). Higher rates were also found for general discomfort (62% vs. 11%, $p = 0.05$), nausea (62% vs. 0%, $p = 0.009$), and headache (62% vs. 0%, $p = 0.009$) in the absence of the extractor.

Anesthetic Practice The practice of anesthesiology is not confined to the operating room. Investigations examining the effects of sevoflurane and N₂O exposure on gene mutation,[39] specifically, the incidence of sister chromatid exchanges in peripheral lymphocytes, concluded that a 2-month rotation out of the operating room environment returned the incidence of gene mutation to that of the general population.

KEY MESSAGES

1. Definitive (level 1) evidence regarding the risk of occupational exposure to anesthetic agents is lacking.

2. Personal environmental monitoring provides the best measure of occupational exposure to anesthetic agents.

3. Exposure can be decreased through training, technical innovation, and optimizing working practices.

QUESTIONS

1. Which adverse health outcomes may be associated with occupational exposure to N₂O?

   Answer: The adverse health effects associated with N₂O exposure alone include spontaneous abortion (relative risk ≅ 1.3 to 1.9) and infertility.

2. What means are available to minimize occupational exposure of health care workers to anesthetic agents?

   Answer: Optimizing scavenging, environmental ventilation, anesthetic practice, and regular personal monitoring can minimize occupational exposure of health care workers to anesthetic agents.

3. What is NIOSH?

   Answer: NIOSH stands for the National Institute of Occupational Safety and Health (in the United States).

References

1. Buring JE, Hennekens CH, Mayrent SL, et al. Health experiences of operating room personnel. Anesthesiology 1985;62: 325–330.
2. Tannenbaum TN, Goldberg RJ. Exposure to anesthetic gases and reproductive outcome: a review of the epidemiologic literature. J Occup Med 1985;27:659–668.
3. Boivin J. Risk of spontaneous abortion in women occupationally exposed to anaesthetic gases: a meta-analysis. Occup Environ Med 1997;54:541–548.
4. Cohen EN, Bellville JW, Brown BW. Anesthesia, pregnancy, and miscarriage: a study of operating room nurses and anesthetists. Anesthesiology 1971;35:343–347.
5. Knill-Jones RP, Rodrigues LV, Moir DD, et al. Anaesthetic practice and pregnancy: controlled survey of women in the United Kingdom. Lancet 1972;1:1326–1328.
6. Rosenberg P, Kirves A. Miscarriages among operating theatre staff. Acta Anaesthesiol Scand 1973;53(Suppl):37–42.

7. Cohen EN, Brown BW, Bruce DL, et al. Occupational disease among operating room personnel: a national study. Anesthesiology 1974;41:321–340.
8. Corbett TH, Cornell RG, Endres JL, et al. Birth defects among children of nurse-anesthetists. Anesthesiology 1974;41:341–344.
9. Knill-Jones RP, Newman BJ, Spence AA. Anaesthetic practice and pregnancy: controlled survey of male anesthetists in the United Kingdom. Lancet 1975;2:807–809.
10. Cohen EN, Brown BW, Bruce DL, et al. A survey of anesthetic health hazards among dentists. J Am Dent Assoc 1975;90: 1291–1296.
11. Cohen EN, Gift HC, Brown BW, et al. Occupational disease in dentistry and chronic exposure to trace anesthetic gases. J Am Dent Assoc 1980;101:21–31.
12. Tomlin PJ. Health problems of anesthetists and their families in the west midlands. Br Med J 1979;1:779–784.
13. Ericson A, Kallen B. Survey of infants born in 1973 or 1975 to Swedish women working in operating rooms during their pregnancies. Anesth Analg 1979;58:302–305.
14. Pharoah POD, Alberman E, Doyle P, et al. Outcome of pregnancy among women in anaesthetic practice. Lancet 1977;1:34–36.
15. Rosenberg PH, Vanttinen H. Occupational hazards to reproduction and health in anesthetists and pediatricians. Acta Anaesthesiol Scand 1978;22:202–207.
16. Axelsson G, Rylander R. Exposure to anaesthetic gases and spontaneous abortion: response bias in a postal questionnaire study. Int J Epidemiol 1982;11:250–256.
17. Heidam LZ. Spontaneous abortions among dental assistants, factory workers, painters, and gardening workers: a follow-up study. J Epidemiol Community Health 1984;38:149–155.
18. Lauwerys R, Siddons H, Misson CB. Anaesthetic health hazards among Belgian nurses and physicians. Int Arch Occup Environ Health 1981;48:195–203.
19. Hemminki K, Kyyronen P, Lindbohm M. Spontaneous abortions and malformations in the offspring of nurses exposed to anaesthetic gases, cytostatic drugs, and other potential hazards in hospitals, based on registered information of outcome. J Epidemiol Community Health 1985;39:141–147.
20. Martínez-Frías ML, Bermejo E, Rodríguez-Pinilla E, Prieto L. Case-control study on occupational exposure to anesthetic gases during pregnancy. Int J Risk Safety Med 1998;11:225–231.
21. Vessey MP, Nunn JF. Occupational hazards of anaesthesia. BMJ 1980;201:696–698.
22. Cook TL, Smith M, Starkweather JA, et al. Behavioral effects of trace and subanesthetic halothane and nitrous oxide in man. Anesthesiology 1978;49:419–424.
23. Levin ED, Bowman RE. Behavioral effects of chronic exposure to low concentrations of halothane during development in rats. Anesth Analg 1986;65:653–659.
24. Zacny JP, Sparacino G, Hoffmann PM, et al. The subjective, behavioral and cognitive effects of subanesthetic concentrations of isoflurane and nitrous oxide in healthy volunteers. Psychopharmacology (Berl). 1994;114:409–416.
25. Zacny JP, Yajnik S, Lichtor JL, et al. The acute and residual effects of subanesthetic concentrations of isoflurane/nitrous oxide combinations on cognitive and psychomotor performance in healthy volunteers. Anesth Analg 1996;82:153–157.
26. Tannenbaum TN, Goldberg RJ. Exposure to anesthetic gases and reproductive outcome: a review of the epidemiologic literature. J Occup Med 1985;27:659–668.
27. Boivin J. Risk of spontaneous abortion in women occupationally exposed to anaesthetic gases: a meta-analysis. Occup Environ Med 1997;54:541–548.
28. Schiewe-Langgartner F. [Exposure of hospital personnel to sevoflurane]. [Article in German]. Anaesthesist. 2005;54:667–672.
29. Ozer M, Baris S, Karakaya D, et al. Behavioural effects of chronic exposure to subanesthetic concentrations of halothane,

sevoflurane and desflurane in rats. Can J Anesth 2006;53: 7653–658.

30. National Institute of Occupational Safety and Health. Criteria for a recommended standard: occupational exposure to anesthetic gases and vapors. Cincinnati: US Dept of Health, Education, and Welfare (DHEW), 1977.

31. Hoerauf KH, Wallner T, Akca O, et al. Exposure To sevoflurane and N$_2$O. Anesth Analg 1999;88:925–929.

32. Wiesner G, Hoerauf K, Schroegendorfer K, et al. High-level, but not low-level, occupational exposure to inhaled anesthetics is associated with genotoxicity in the micronucleus assay. Anesth Analg 2001;92:118–122.

33. Hoerauf K, Wallner T, Akc O, et. al. Exposure to sevoflurane and nitrous oxide during four different methods of anesthetic induction. Anesth Analg 1999;88:925–929.

34. Krajewski W. Occupational exposure to nitrous oxide—the role of scavenging and ventilation systems in reducing the exposure

level in operating rooms. Int J Hyg Environ Health2007;210: 133–138.

35. Hoerauf K, Koller C, Jakob W, et al. Isoflurane waste gas exposure during general anaesthesia: the laryngeal mask compared with tracheal intubation. Br J Anaesth 1996;77:189–193.

36. Henderson KA, Matthews IP, Adisesh A, Hutchings, AD. Occupational exposure of midwives to nitrous oxide on delivery suites. Occup Environ Med 2003;60;958–961.

37. Nayebzadeh A. Exposure to exhaled nitrous oxide in hospitals post-anesthesia care units. Ind Health 2007;45:334–337.

38. Sanabria Carretero P. [Occupational exposure to nitrous oxide and sevoflurane during pediatric anesthesia: evaluation of an anesthetic gas extractor]. [Article in Spanish]. Rev Esp Anestesiol Reanim 2006;53: 618–625.

39. Eroglu A. A comparison of sister chromatid exchanges in lymphocytes of anesthesiologists to non anesthesiologists in the same hospital. Anesth Analg 2006;102:1573–1577.

CHAPTER 59

Fetal Oxygen Saturation and Caesarean Section

Siun Burke

CASE FORMAT: STEP BY STEP

A 28-year-old, 100-kg, term primigravida presented in labor requesting epidural analgesia.

What are the risks associated with epidural analgesia in labor?

See Table 59.1.

The epidural was inserted on the second attempt, and a bolus dose of 10 mL 0.25% bupivacain--e with 50 μg of fentanyl was administered followed by an epidural infusion of levobupivacaine 0.125% at 12 mL per hour. The patient, however, continued to complain of discomfort with each contraction. Four hours later, a vaginal examination revealed minimal progress, and the patient was scheduled for an emergency lower-segment caesarean section.

How should the anesthetist proceed?

A detailed preoperative assessment will enable early identification of a poorly functioning epidural and any potential problems if spinal or general anesthesia is deemed necessary.

On preoperative assessment, the patient's past medical history was unremarkable. However, she had a short stature and was morbidly obese with a body mass index of 46 kg/m^2. Examination revealed a Mallampati grade III airway.

The patient's vital signs were normal; her blood pressure was 120/64 mm Hg, and her heart rate was 92 beats per minute. The epidural block was assessed, and despite augmentation with 20 mL of bupivacaine 0.5%, only extended to T10 and was patchy. The anesthetist explained to the patient that the epidural was ineffective and that the operation would proceed under spinal anesthesia. The patient asked whether any form of anesthesia was superior in terms of neonatal outcome.

How should the anesthetist respond to this query?

A meta-analysis comparing different methods of anesthesia for caesarean section and neonatal acid base status analyzed 27 studies and concluded that spinal anesthesia could not be considered safer than general anesthesia or epidural anesthesia for the fetus.[1]

Adverse maternal circulatory changes associated with spinal anesthesia may result from excessive sympathetic blockade, aortocaval compression, use of vasopressors, and fluid loading.[1] A recent Cochrane review concluded that there was no evidence to show that regional anesthesia was superior to general anesthesia in terms of major maternal or neonatal outcomes.[2] It must be remembered that the absolute risk of maternal mortality associated with general anesthesia for caesarean section is 32 per million, which is 17-fold greater than that with regional anesthesia.[3] The incidence of failed tracheal intubation in the obstetric population, 1 in 250,[4] is as many as 10 times greater than that in the general population. Recognizing the risks to the mother associated with general anesthesia has led to an increased use of regional anesthesia for caesarean deliveries.

The anesthetist reassured the patient that there was no major difference in neonatal outcome between general, spinal, or epidural anesthesia. In view of her elevated body mass index and potentially difficult airway, he felt regional anesthesia was preferable to general anesthesia.

The patient was prescribed antacid prophylaxis, and a 16-gauge intravenous cannula was inserted. In the operating room, with routine monitors in place, the anesthetist proceeded with spinal anesthesia. Following dural puncture with a 25-gauge pencil-point spinal needle and aspiration of clear cerebrospinal fluid, the anesthetist administered 12.5 mg of hyperbaric bupivacaine intrathecally.

What are the risks of administering spinal anesthesia following inadequate epidural for lower-segment caesarean section?

Spinal anesthesia after epidural analgesia may result in an unpredictable final block height. One retrospective review estimated the incidence of high spinal anesthesia to be 11% in patients after prior failed epidural blockade versus fewer than 1% in patients undergoing spinal anesthesia alone.[5] This may be explained by the volume of the dural sac being restricted by fluid in the epidural space. There is controversy regarding the optimal dose of hyperbaric bupivacaine in this setting; some investigators advocate reducing the dose by 20% to 30%,[6] whereas others believe this increases the risk of a second unsatisfactory block.[7]

Whichever approach is used, early recognition of an inadequate epidural block is important to avoid persisting with further doses of epidural local anesthetic. An assessment of the urgency of the situation will help guide further anesthetic management.

Spinal anesthesia should be followed by careful positioning and frequent block assessment. The parturient should be

TABLE 59.1 Complications of Epidural Analgesia

Immediate

Hypotension (systolic blood pressure <100 mm Hg or a decrease of 25% below preblock average)

Urinary retention

Local anesthetic-induced convulsions*

Local anesthetic-induced cardiac arrest*

Delayed

Postdural puncture headache

Transient backache

Epidural abscess or meningitis*

Permanent neurologic deficit*

*Very rare.
Reproduced with permission from Vincent RD Jr, Chestnut DH. Epidural analgesia during labor. American Family Physician 1998;58: 1785–1792.

TABLE 59.2 Determinants of Fetal Oxygenation

Maternal oxygen delivery to the placenta	• Uterine artery blood flow • Oxygen capacity of maternal blood • Oxygen affinity of maternal blood
Oxygen transfer across the placenta	• Oxygen-diffusing capacity
Fetal oxygen-carrying capacity	• Umbilical vein blood flow • Oxygen capacity of fetal blood • Oxygen affinity of fetal blood

assessed regularly for difficulty in phonation, swallowing, breathing, and weakened handgrip. Extra vigilance is required if a bolus has been administered via the epidural in the 30 minutes prior to spinal anesthesia, if the patient weighs more than 120 kg, or if the height is less than 4'8".[6] The use of a combined spinal epidural technique allows a smaller intrathecal dose to be used with the option of "topping up" using the epidural catheter if the block is inadequate.

In this case, the patient was 100 kg, of short stature, and had just received an epidural top-up before spinal anesthesia. After the spinal, the patient's blood pressure decreased to 74/53 mm Hg, and her heart rate dropped to 62 beats per minute. She experienced nausea, removed the wedge, and lay supine. For the first time, late decelerations (fetal heart rate <90 beats per minute) were evident on the cardiotachograph (Fig. 59.1).

What are the determinants of fetal oxygenation?

Oxygen delivery to the fetus (mmol/min) is given by the product of umbilical blood flow and the oxygen content of umbilical venous blood (Table 59.2).

Maternal oxygen delivery to the placenta is affected by uterine artery blood flow, oxygen content of maternal uterine artery blood, hemoglobin concentration, and saturation. Uterine blood flow at term is 10% of cardiac output. Hypotension, uterine contractions, and vasoconstriction can all decrease uterine blood flow.

In the case described, maternal hypotension and desaturation reduced oxygen delivery to the placenta.

The fetus has about 42 mL of oxygen reserves, and its oxygen consumption is 20 mL/min. A fetus deprived of oxygen can survive 10 minutes (rather than 2 minutes one might expect from these values) by shunting blood flow to vital organs and decreasing oxygen consumption.

The fetus has many protective mechanisms to ensure its oxygen extraction capacity. The hemoglobin concentration is higher (15 to 16 g/dL). Fetal hemoglobin is 80% to 90% saturated at a pO_2 of 35mm Hg, whereas adult hemoglobin is only

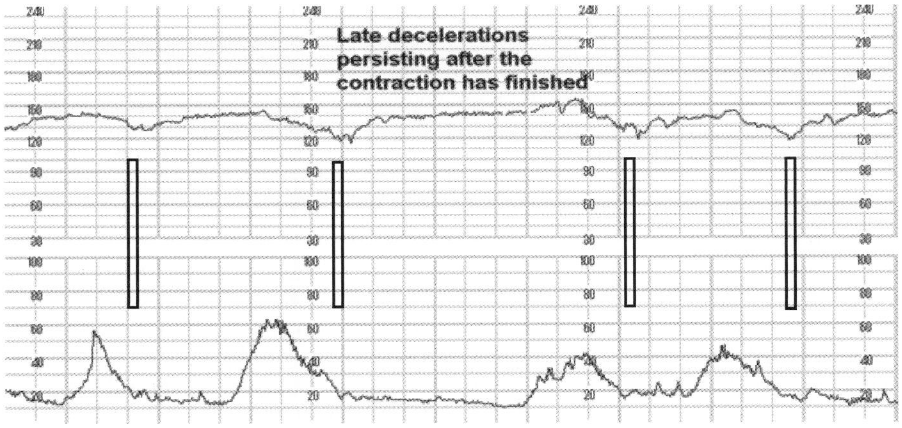

Late decelerations persisting after the contraction has finished

Figure 59.1 • Cardiotachograph Showing Late Decelerations.

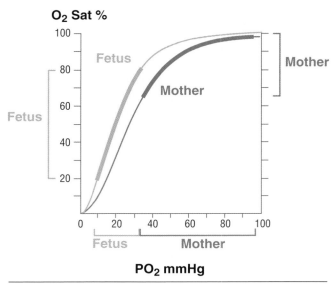

Figure 59.2 • Fetal and Adult Oxyhemoglobin Dissociation Curves.

TABLE 59.3 Umbilical Artery Blood Gas

		Normal Values
pO$_2$	1.8 kPa	2.38 +/−0.9
pCO$_2$	7.2 kPa	7.49 +/−1.13
pH	6.98	7.24 +/−0.07
Base excess	−14	−3.6 +/−2.7
Lactate	6.4	<2

30% saturated at this pO$_2$. This difference is caused by a leftward shift in the fetal oxyhemoglobin dissociation curve.[8] (Fig. 59.2).

Supplemental oxygen (6 L per minute via 40% Ventimask [Flexicare Medical Limited, Mid Glamorgan, United Kingdom]), Hartmann's solution 500 mL, and repeated doses of phenylephrine (100 μg, ×3) were administered rapidly, and the patient was repositioned with a left lateral tilt. Her blood pressure improved to 90/53 mm Hg, and SpO$_2$ increased to 95%.

Is supplemental oxygen beneficial during a caesarean section?

Studies during general anesthesia for caesarean delivery have shown improved pO$_2$ and Apgar scores with increased inhaled fractions of oxygen. A study of hyperoxia versus normoxia in epidural anesthesia showed better umbilical artery base excess in the hyperoxia group.[9] Some investigators believe maternal hyperoxia is necessary to build up a reserve of fetal pO$_2$, as fetal oxygenation ceases after uterine incision after which unexpected delays could cause damage.[10] Patients who undergo spinal anesthesia may be under particular risk because of its restrictive effect on ventilation.

It has been argued that maternal hyperoxia could cause hypoventilation, CO$_2$ retention, and subsequent placental vasoconstriction. Administration of oxygen to the mother at 5 liters per minute has been shown to reduce intervillous blood flow significantly.[11] A maternal FiO$_2$ of 0.6 produces a significant increase in free radical activity in both maternal and fetal blood.[12] Nevertheless, maternal hyperoxia during labor has been shown to increase pO$_2$ in the compromised fetus.[1]

Five minutes later, the patient became distressed, she started to complain of paraesthesia in her arms and difficulty breathing, and then her voice became weak. On examination, there was only minimal chest rise with each inspiration. The oxygen saturation fell to 82%.

How should the anesthetist proceed?

Management of High/Total spinal anesthesia requires early detection and supportive management of airway, breathing, and circulation.

Following preoxygenation, application of cricoid pressure, and induction of general anesthesia, laryngoscopy revealed a Cormack and Lehane grade 3 view.

It was not possible to intubate the trachea, and the oxygen saturation decreased below 70%. The anesthetist managed to manually ventilate the patient via a face mask, and the oxygen saturation increased to 82%.

After several minutes, a baby boy was born. His Apgar scores were 2 and 3 at 1 and 5 minutes, respectively (Table 59.3).

Is umbilical cord blood gas analysis useful in the assessment of the newborn?

Umbilical cord blood gas analysis is now recommended in all high-risk deliveries by both the British and American Colleges of Obstetrics and Gynecology. Umbilical artery pH has a metabolic and a respiratory component, the latter largely determined by maternal respiration. Isolated fetal respiratory acidosis is usually the result of short-lived impairment in the uteroplacental or fetoplacental circulation, and ongoing impairment results in progressive metabolic acidosis caused by anaerobic glycolysis. Consequently, most severe fetal acidosis is mixed. Base excess is independent of respiration and is thus a better index of the metabolic component and key to evaluating the recent prenatal environment.[1] Base excess usually decreases by a total of 3 mmol/L in uncomplicated labor and by 1 mmol/L every 30 minutes under conditions when there are frequent heart rate decelerations. The most profound fetal compromise, uterine rupture, changes pH by 1 mmol/L every 2 to 3 minutes.[13]

Portman et al. developed a validated score for predicting multiorgan impairment following perinatal asphyxia. They found that a score combining a measure of cardiotachograph abnormality, umbilical artery base excess, and low 5-minute Apgar score was strongly associated with morbidity.[14] Lactate measured in umbilical cord blood is almost entirely fetal in origin. Umbilical cord lactate has been shown to correlate with fetal pH and base excess.[15]

The neonate was intubated, stabilized, and transferred to the neonatal intensive care unit. A senior anesthetist arrived, and the mother was intubated with the aid of a gum elastic bougie. The case proceeded uneventfully, and the mother was extubated once fully awake in the recovery room. The neonatologist informed her that the baby had two seizures in the preceding hour and his prognosis was guarded.

KEY MESSAGES

1. Careful preoperative assessment of the parturient will allow early identification of a poorly functioning epidural and of potential problems with spinal or epidural anesthesia. This review will ensure that senior experienced personnel and all necessary equipment are available in case of emergency.

2. Spinal anesthesia following inadequate epidural blockade can result in an unpredictable final block height. Extra vigilance is required if a bolus has been administered via the epidural in the 30 minutes before spinal anesthesia, if the patient weighs greater than 120 kg or if the height is less than 4'8".

3. Early recognition is a key to management of high total spinal anesthesia. Treatment is supportive and begins by addressing airway, breathing, and circulation.

QUESTIONS

1. What population of cardiac output does uterine blood flow constitute at full term?

   Answer: 10%

2. Outline the steps that may resolve peripartum fetal acidosis during caesarean delivery.

   Answer: Oxygen delivery to the fetus (mmol/min) is given by the product of umbilical blood flow and the oxygen content of umbilical venous blood. Maternal oxygen delivery to the placenta is affected by uterine artery blood flow, oxygen content of maternal uterine artery blood, hemoglobin concentration, and saturation. Treating maternal hypotension with a fluid bolus or vasoconstrictors will help to improve fetal oxygenation. A left lateral tilt will reduce the incidence of aortocaval compression, which may compromise fetal blood flow. The oxygen content of maternal blood can be increased by supplying the parturient with supplemental oxygen.

3. What is the clinical presentation of total spinal anesthesia?

   Answer: Total spinal anesthesia may present with increased maternal anxiety, hypotension, bradycardia, paraesthesia and weakness of the arms and hands, difficulty breathing, altered phonation, and loss of consciousness.

References

1. Reynolds F, Seed PT. (2005) Anaesthesia for caesarean section and neonatal acid-base status: a meta-analysis. Anaesthesia 2005; 60:636–653.
2. Afolabi BB, Lesi FEA, Merah NA. Regional versus general anaesthesia for caesarean section. Cochrane Database of Systematic Reviews: Reviews 2006, Issue 4.
3. Hawkins JL. Maternal morbidity and mortality: anesthetic causes. Can J Anesth 2002;49:6R.
4. Hawthorne L, Wilson R, Lyons G, Dresner M. Failed intubation revisited: 17-yr experience in a teaching maternity unit. Br J Anaesth 1996;76:680–684.
5. Furst SR, Reisner LS. Risk of high spinal anesthesia following failed epidural block for cesarean delivery. J Clin Anaesth 1994; Volume 7, Issue 1.
6. Dadarkar P, Philip J, Weidner C, et al. Spinal anesthesia for cesarean section following inadequate labor epidural analgesia: a retrospective audit. Int J Obstet Anesth 2004;13: 239–243.
7. Stocks G. When using spinal anaesthesia for caesarean section after the epidural has failed, the normal dose of spinal anaesthetic should be used. Int J Obst Anesth 14:56–57.
8. Murphy PJ. The fetal circulation. Contin Educ Anaesth Crit Care Pain 2005;5:107–112.
9. Ramanathan S, Gandhi S, Arismendy J, et al. Oxygen transfer from mother to fetus during cesarean section under epidural anesthesia. Anesth Analg 1982;61:576–581.
10. Jordan M. Women undergoing caesarean section under regional anaesthesia should routinely receive supplementary oxygen. Int J Obstet Anesth 2002;11:282–285.
11. Jouppila P, et al. The influence of maternal oxygen inhalation on human placental and umbilical venous blood flow. Eur J Obstet Gynaecol Reproduct Biol 16:151–156.
12. Khaw KS, Wang CC, Ngan Kee WD, et al. Effects of high-inspired oxygen fraction during elective Caesarean section under spinal anaesthesia on maternal and fetal oxygenation and lipid peroxidation. Br J Anaesth. 2002;88:18–23.
13. Ross M. Base excess during cord occlusion. Am J Obstet Gynecol 2003;189:1811–1812.
14. Portman RJ, Carter BS, Gaylord MS, et al. Predicting neonatal morbidity after perinatal asphyxia: a scoring system. Am J Obstet Gynecol 1990;162:174–182.
15. Westgren M, Divon M, Horal M, et al. Routine measurements of umbilical artery lactate levels in the prediction of perinatal outcome. Am J Obstet Gynecol 1995;173:1416–1422.

CHAPTER 60

Vasoconstrictors for Hypotension During Caesarean Section

James O'Driscoll

A fit, healthy 29-year-old primigravida presented for elective lower-segment caesarean section. The indication for surgery was breech presentation of the fetus at 39 weeks' gestation. Preoperative assessment revealed only a history of postoperative nausea and vomiting after a tonsillectomy when the patient was 15 years of age. Hemoglobin concentration was 12.3 g/dL. The options for anesthesia were discussed with the patient, and it was agreed that regional anesthesia in the form of a spinal anesthetic was the most appropriate.

On arrival in the operating room, appropriate monitoring was established (Table 60.1).

What does *appropriate monitoring* mean in this setting?

At this stage, the appropriate monitors are electrocardiogram, noninvasive blood pressure, and SpO_2.

A 16-gauge intravenous cannula was inserted after skin infiltration with 1% lidocaine, and 1500 mL of compound sodium lactate was administered intravenously over 20 minutes.

What is the rationale for fluid preloading before spinal anesthesia?

Fluid preloading before spinal anesthesia is done in an attempt to prevent or decrease the degree of hypotension caused by the regional sympathetic blockade. For patients undergoing lower-segment caesarean section, preloading is no more effective than administering fluid at the time or immediately after performance of the block.[1] Colloid fluids have been shown to be more effective than crystalloids for this purpose.[2]

Bupivacaine (0.5% 2 mL) and fentanyl (25 µg) were injected into the intrathecal space with the patient in the sitting position under aseptic conditions using a 25-gauge pencil-point (Whitacre) spinal needle (BD Medical - Medical Surgical Systems, Franklin Lakes, NJ).

Does the dose of local anesthetic administered influence the likelihood and degree of hypotension?

Lesser doses of local anesthetic, particularly with the addition of opioids, appear to decrease the frequency and degree of hypotension. The most promising preventive strategies are preloading, administering intrathecal opioids (for a local anesthetic-sparing effect), leg compression, or a combination of these methods.[3]

After the spinal anesthetic was administered, the patient was returned to the supine position with left lateral tilt, and ephedrine 6 mg was administered intravenously.

Is prophylactic ephedrine effective in preventing hypotension after spinal block?

Ephedrine has been found to be ineffective in preventing hypotension when used in small doses, and when used in greater doses, it is more likely to cause hypertension.[4]

After 5 minutes, assessment of the patient's perception of cold (ice) revealed a bilateral sensory block to T6 and surgery proceeded. Shortly afterward, the patient complained of nausea, and an additional dose of ephedrine was administered. Her blood pressure remained low at 80/50 mm Hg and did not respond to two additional doses of ephedrine (each 6 mg). At this point, phenylephrine 100 µg was administered intravenously. The patient's systolic blood pressure increased to 110 mm Hg, and her nausea eased. Five minutes later, the patient's blood pressure decreased again (Table 60.1), and she complained of both nausea and discomfort. Again, her blood pressure increased after a bolus of phenylephrine 100 mcg intravenously. Extra doses of phenylephrine were required to maintain her blood pressure at this level, and a live male infant was delivered 25 minutes after the spinal block was administered. His Apgar scores were 9 (at 1 minute) and 10 (at 5 minutes). Umbilical cord pH measurements were arterial, pH 7.2 and venous, pH 7.26. Blood loss during the surgery was approximately 850 mL.

Is phenylephrine more effective than ephedrine in treating systemic hypotension in this setting?

A recent study has shown that phenylephrine is superior to ephedrine when administered by infusion for treatment of hypotension in patients undergoing lower-segment caesarean section under spinal anesthesia. Phenylephrine had less effect on fetal acid-base status, although this finding has not been linked to fetal outcomes in any significant manner.[1,5,6] Although ephedrine and phenylephrine have been the most commonly used and studied agents, other vasoconstrictors such as metaraminol also may be effective.

TABLE 60.1 Vital Signs

	Initial	Block	5 min	10 min	15 min	20 min	25 min	30 min	35 min
Heart Rate	98	110	92	88	76	120	100	98	102
Non-invasive blood pressure (mm Hg)	130/80	138/72	70/42	80/60	110/80	100/72	98/62	116/68	110/62
SpO$_2$ (%)	98	95	96	96	97	94	95	96	96

KEY MESSAGES

1. Early recognition and treatment of hypotension following spinal block for caesarean section is vital for maintaining maternal comfort. Evidence for adverse fetal outcome is lacking.

2. Several strategies for preventing hypotension have been found to be ineffective when used alone but have shown promise in combination.[3]

3. Ephedrine and phenylephrine are the most commonly used vasoconstrictors in this setting; the latter is more effective for treating systemic hypotension and has potentially fewer effects on the fetus.

QUESTIONS

1. Is prophylactic administration of a vasoconstrictor(s) effective in preventing hypotension during a caesarean section?

   Answer: Administering a vasoconstrictor(s) prophylactically can decrease the frequency and magnitude of hypotension after spinal anesthesia for caesarean section but does not reliably do so. No one agent has been shown to be superior to another in terms of prophylaxis.

2. Does fluid preloading decrease the incidence or severity of hypotension during caesarean section under spinal anesthesia?

   Answer: Fluid loading is inconsistent in preventing hypotension in this setting. Preloading seems to be no more effective than what is often called: co- (at the time of block) or post- (immediately after block) loading. Colloids have been shown to be superior to crystalloids for fluid loading but do have the potential to cause adverse effects such as pruritus, allergy, and renal dysfunction.

3. What is the treatment of choice for systemic hypotension following spinal anesthesia for caesarean section?

   Answer: For treatment of hypotension, phenylephrine is more effective than ephedrine, particularly when used by infusion. Phenylephrine also seems to be beneficial in terms of fetal acid base balance with less effect on cord pH measured at delivery, although this does not seem to be related to fetal outcome unless it is abnormal for another reason. Phenylephrine administered by infusion also seems to be superior to phenylephrine administered by bolus dose alone. The optimal strategy seems to be a combination of techniques with anticipation of hypotension, and rapid treatment is a priority.

References

1. Mercier FJ, Bonnet MP, De la Dorie A, et al. Spinal anaesthesia for caesarean section: fluid loading, vasoconstrictors and hypotension. Ann Fr Anesth Reanim 2007;26:688–693.
2. Cyna AM, Andrew M, Emmett RS, et al. Techniques for preventing hypotension during spinal anaesthesia for Caesarean section. Cochrane Database Syst Rev 2006;(4):CD002251.
3. Kaya S, Karaman H, Erdogan H, et al. Combined use of low-dose bupivacaine, colloid preload and wrapping of the legs for preventing hypotension in spinal anaesthesia for caesarean section. J Int Med Res 2007;35:615–625.
4. Lee A, Ngan Kee WD, Gin T. A dose-response meta-analysis of prophylactic intravenous ephedrine for the prevention of hypotension during spinal anaesthesia for elective caesarean delivery. Anesth Analg 2004;98:483–490.
5. Cooper DW, Gibb SC, Meek T, et al. Effect of intravenous vasopressor on spread of spinal anaesthesia and fetal acid-base equilibrium. Br J Anaesth 2007;98:649–656.
6. Ngan Kee WD, Khaw KS. Vasopressors in obstetrics: what should we be using? Curr Opin Anaesthesiol 2006;19:238–243.

INDEX

Page numbers followed by *f* or *t* indicate material in figures or tables, respectively.

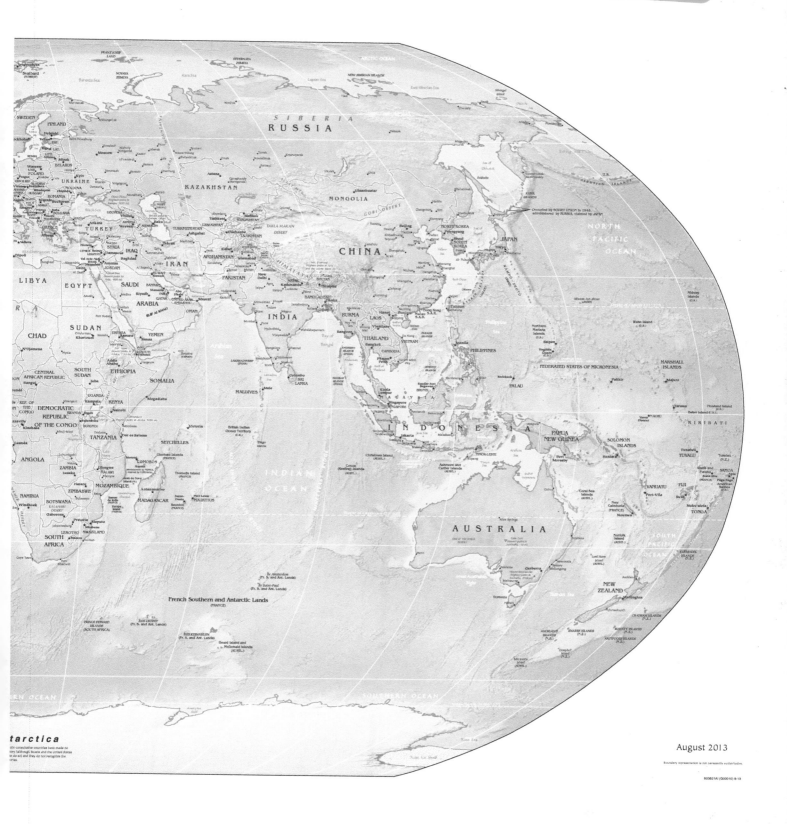

August 2013

AN INTRODUCTION TO
GEOGRAPHY

FROM A CHRISTIAN WORLDVIEW

Second Edition

Robert F. Ritchie IV

Liberty University

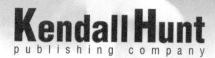

Kendall Hunt
publishing company

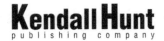

Kendall Hunt
publishing company

www.kendallhunt.com
Send all inquiries to:
4050 Westmark Drive
Dubuque, IA   52004-1840

Copyright © 2011, 2014 by Kendall Hunt Publishing Company

ISBN 978-1-4652-3929-7

Printed in the United States of America
10 9 8 7 6 5 4 3 2 1

Contents

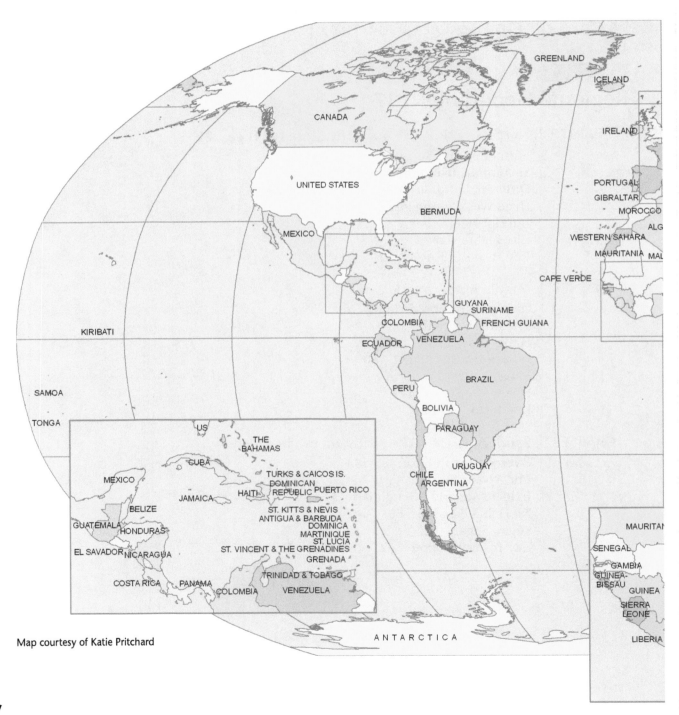

Map courtesy of Katie Pritchard

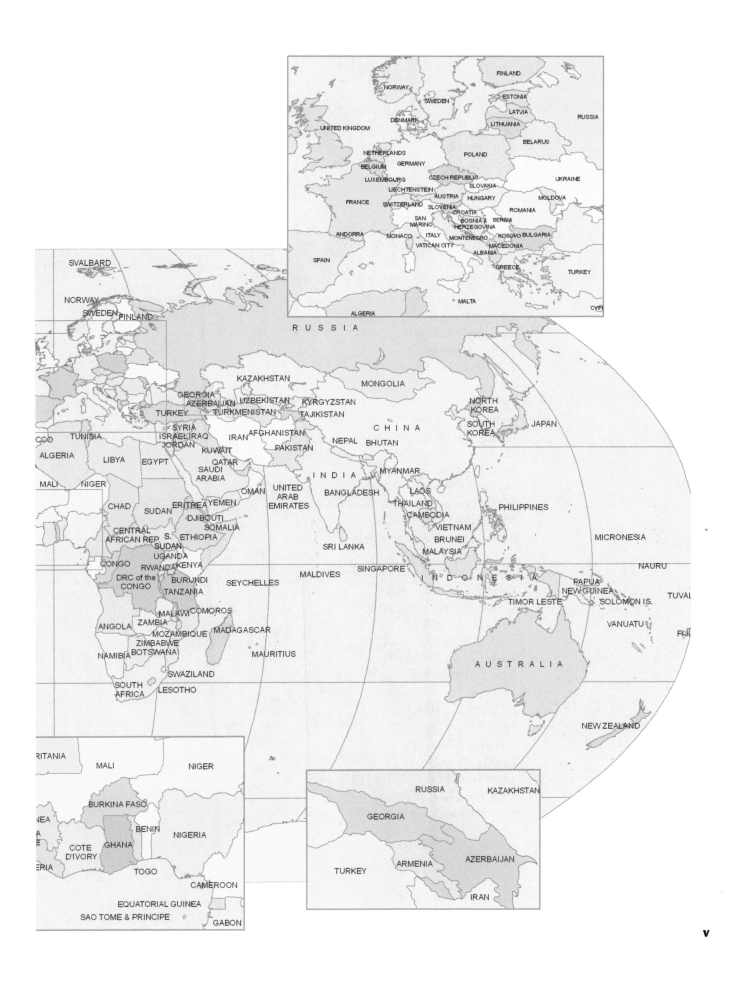

v

UNIT TWO

Human Geography 155

Acknowledgments

This book is written as a compilation of notes from many sources in a somewhat autodidactic endeavor, completed during a tenure of seven years in the classroom at Liberty University. It is a rather humble attempt to inspire students to commit themselves to searching for opportunities to serve others using their talents and spiritual gifts. It is hoped an eclectic approach to this largely unstructured but important and ancient discipline will expose the reader to a plethora of perspectives to current events both contemporary and traditional. In essence, it is argued the culture we experience is ultimately a function of physical geography and we exist at a particular moment in time for the purpose of pursuing opportunities to serve ultimately with an eternal objective in mind. It would, however, not be possible to develop a synthesis with a Christian world view if it were not for the opportunities presented by the ultimate leadership from two powerful Christian scholars: Dr. Roger Schultz, the Dean of the College of Arts and Sciences and the inspirationally brilliant Dr. Emily Heady, the Dean of the College of General Studies.

This book is only possible due to the commitment of very talented and gifted helpers. First the "K" ladies: Katie Hoffmeyer proofed this book and dedicated hours to proofing the manuscript. Katie Wood likewise helped immensely in the later stages of its production as did Kristin Anderson of Kendall-Hunt. Curtis Ross ultimately inspired this effort and demonstrated his consummate talents of motivation as an editor.

I would especially like to thank the Social Studies department of Powhatan High School in Powhatan Virginia for being there at a time in my life when my faith was most tested. Brooks Ann Smith, the department chair, and her team of dedicated historians who showed me what a powerful force for good the public school system truly is and can be. Thank you to my wife and sons for the privilege of serving, albeit rather poorly at times I'm sure.

This book is dedicated to the nearly seven thousand students I have had the joy of teaching and hopefully in some small measure inspired to serve He who Saves us with His pure love.

> 'For to everyone who has, more will be given, and he will have abundance; but from him who does not have, even what he has will be taken away. And cast the unprofitable servant into the outer darkness. There will be weeping and gnashing of teeth.' (Matthew 25: 29–30) NKJV

Introduction to Physical Geography

"And He has made from one blood every nation of men to dwell on all the face of the earth, and has determined their preappointed times and the boundaries of their dwellings, so that they should seek the Lord, in the hope that they might grope for Him and find Him, though He is not far from each one of us." (Acts 17:25–27)

According to the book of Genesis, God created the world. God's creation consists of time and space, and is studied as history and geography, respectively. God's love for this Earth is epitomized by his son Jesus Christ, who gave his life for it. As followers and servants of Jesus, we shall continue to seek opportunities to use our individual talents vocationally. Geography offers an excellent tool for the development of future service strategies. What then is geography? This definition will be discussed in detail later, but for now, geography is basically the study of the Earth's surface and is concerned with spatial concepts. More specifically, the subject of human geography is concerned with various aspects of human activity over space. Any proper study of human geography, however, must begin with an understanding of the planet's physical properties.

This book will survey geography from a regional and human perspective. The regions chosen are somewhat arbitrary and extremely subjective. In the second unit there is an attempt to define general themes and concepts of geography, in Chapter 15, we will observe the globalized world we see today. Mankind has developed various technologies over time by exploiting the resources of a loving Creator through various "revolutions," as we shall discuss in Chapter 16. We proceed to identify culture as changes in human activity in Chapter 17. In Chapter 18, we shall observe how languages and religion changed as people spread over the Earth. Chapter 19 explains the exciting and exponential growth of the human population. By Chapter 20, our interest in the dynamics of human organization will lead us to describe the fundamentals of political geography. Finally, we will observe the growing human imprint on the horizon as we begin to look at the urban landscape in Chapter 21. All of these chapters describe human activity on the surface of planet Earth. We must therefore lay a solid foundation by establishing the properties of this planet that make human activity possible.

The physical properties of planet Earth that we shall focus upon in this introduction to physical geography are shape, spin, tilt, proximity to the Sun's energy, and surface relief. These phenomena work in tandem to create the various climates observed. These climates in turn continue to shape the surface of the Earth, thereby effecting human activities.

Do you think the Earth is round? The Earth is indeed a generally spherically shaped planet. It is actually an oblate ellipsoid, but for the purposes of this course, it will be considered a sphere. A **sphere** is a round, solid form with the surface equally distant from the center. The sphere is an ideal form and varies slightly from the reality of creation. Interestingly, many geologists believe the Earth has actually changed in shape over time, and this change in shape has resulted in both changes to the atmosphere and perhaps even to gravity. Our planet is a sphere suspended in space, it spins on an axis with a 23.5-degree tilt, and it revolves around the Sun. Psalm 74:17 says,

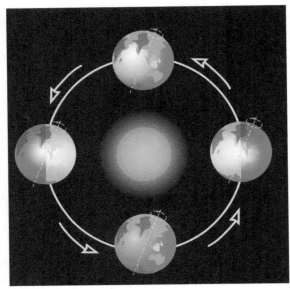

Image © Matthew Cole, 2011. Used under license from Shutterstock, Inc.

"Thou hast set all the borders of the earth; thou hast made summer and winter." Perhaps we can see how the borders of the Earth create the seasons.

The spherical nature of planet Earth is of great importance. The curvature on the surface is approximately 16 feet for every five miles of distance travelled. This curvature is an important consideration in understanding the nature of the Earth and its surrounding atmosphere. Often, students of geography mistakenly see the Earth in a two-dimensional plane, such as that seen on a GPS screen or a map. In fact, it is through the study of geometry we begin to understand the exciting characteristics of the sphere and see how it affects our planet. By looking at a sphere extrinsically (from a distance), we can see that any attempt to divide the sphere results in a lack of symmetry, unless we cut the sphere exactly through the center. The nature of a sphere is such that when it is divided at the center, we explore the concept of the great circle, the circle formed by passing a plane through the exact center of a perfect sphere; this is the largest circle that

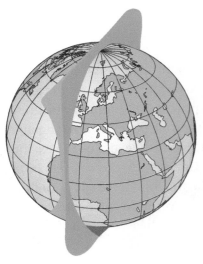

Image © Kendall Hunt Publishing

can be drawn on a sphere's surface. Longitude lines and the equator are examples of **great circles**. A small circle is any place on a sphere where a plane does not go through the center. Latitudes reflect small circles at various angles to the Earth's center, with the angle from the center of the sphere increasing in size when moving from the equator to the poles. The small circle's lack of symmetry offers a way of understanding the circular patterns associated with the atmosphere.

By virtue of its spherical shape, the Earth is witness to a phenomenon called the **Coriolis Effect**. A way of understanding the Coriolis Effect is through a simple illustration. For example, the shortest distance from point A to point B is not necessarily over a mountain, because of its height; but rather, the shortest distance can be around the mountain. Dr. David W. Henderson, in his book, *Experiencing Geometry*, demonstrates the importance of symmetry by illustrating a toy car rolling across a sphere. The toy car would remain on the great circle, but it would fall off a small circle. If you were walking on a small circle, for example, one leg would need to do more work than the other just to stay on a straight line, whereas the symmetry of a great circle would allow you to move your feet at the same speed.

Now consider the Earth's **spin**. Spinning in roughly a 24-hour period, we see a small circle (latitude) is actually moving faster than a great circle as the Earth moves on its axis because the axis of rotation is decreasing in size as one heads towards the poles. This fact may seem counterintuitive, but if one sees the Earth as a circle on a Cartesian coordinate system and the equator is the X line, a Sine function at X (equator) is zero, whereas the Y (poles) would be 1. This illustration numerically reflects the increased angle towards the poles with a decreasing axis of rotation.

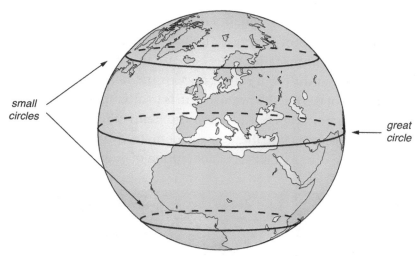

Image © Kendall Hunt Publishing

If this seems a bit confusing, just remember that the Earth is spinning at great speed and, as a sphere, the angle of momentum is perpendicular to the direction of spin. Additionally, the atmosphere is affected by the friction of the surface. Since the shortest distance between two points on a sphere is a great circle, and the angles from the Earth's center (latitude) grow, motion toward the poles picks up speed. To an observer on Earth, these characteristics of sphere and spin appear to create wind and ocean currents moving in a clockwise manner (generally) in the northern hemisphere and counterclockwise (generally) in the southern hemisphere. Imagine a trail of smoke behind a locomotive. Because the train is moving the smoke which in actuality is rising straight up appears to be in a trail behind it. Similarly, our atmosphere is deflected from the earth's surface as the planet is moving under it and appears to be deflecting at an angle. When you think of spin, reflect upon how an ice skater pulls his/her arms in to increase the speed of spin—a function of angular momentum and conservation. The skater is producing a smaller axis of rotation and because the sum total of an objects momentum cannot change the skater's speed increases. Planetary bodies exhibit the same features as they are in a circular path while spinning on an axis. If you can find a globe, look at it from the poles as you spin it. Doing so will help you visualize the aforementioned concepts of great and small circles and axis of rotation; the sum ingredients of the coriollis effect. If you spin the globe, you will find you are hitting it with your hands at an angle because of its tilt.

The **Tilt** of the Earth is about 23.5 degrees. In about 24 hours, a complete **rotation** occurs on this axis. This tilt, also a function of the conservation of angular momentum, holds the Earth in space where its momentum is shared with the moon, as evidenced by the tides. A way of picturing this tilt as a function of the attraction between the Earth and the moon is to think of how your bicycle stays upright when you ride it down the road. The perfect balance of gravitational attraction between the Earth and moon, and to a lesser extent, the other planets in the solar system, help explain the Earth's revolution around the Sun. The combination of tilt and rotation produce differing levels of incoming solar radiation upon the Earth's surface. This alternation between cool night and warm day, combined with the annual revolution, results in the unequal distribution of the Sun's energy. The Earth's **revolution** around the Sun creates the seasons and is of importance to us because this revolution creates a situation where heat is absorbed at different rates between the northern and southern hemispheres. The tendency of the Earth's atmosphere is to attempt to achieve levels of equilibrium. The differing amounts of radiation the hemispheres absorb from the Sun during the different seasons contribute to the climate and weather patterns we see. How does this tilt cause different levels of absorption of energy?

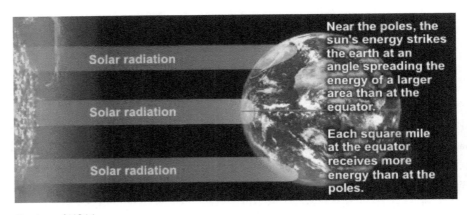

Courtesy of NOAA

Many people think the Earth experiences different extremes of temperature because of the changing proximity to, or distance from, the Sun. Actually, our atmosphere is similar to a microwave oven in that the heat produced is a function of the absorption of solar energy. **Insolation**, or incoming solar radiation, hits the Earth's surface at different **angles of incidence** on the Earth and is then reflected back through the atmosphere at different angles at different levels of latitude called angles of incidence. The differing angles of incidence at different latitudes result in different levels of energy absorbed into the atmosphere as short-wave radiation and then, subsequently, reflected off the Earth's surface into the atmosphere (into outer space) as long-wave radiation. Depending on the **Albedo**—or level of solar radiation reflected from the Earth's surface—of the surface facing the Sun and the amount of moisture in the atmosphere, the resulting reflective long-wave energy will heat up the atmosphere at different rates, depending on altitude. The atmosphere also serves to protect the Earth from certain types of harmful solar radiation through a unique layer of oxygen molecules arranged in threes (triatomic), which is called the **Ozone layer**. We see the different seasons, and even the time of day and latitude determining the different levels of insolation covering the Earth.

The surface of the Earth is a final determining aspect of the different climates we confront. The surface is divided between land and sea. Over 70 percent of the Earth's surface is water, and therefore, varying levels of absorption and reflection of the Sun's radiation occur compared to on land. This varying albedo is also instrumental in accounting for different temperatures and levels of precipitation. Like a giant machine, the Earth is churning and chugging through space, subject to various forces and

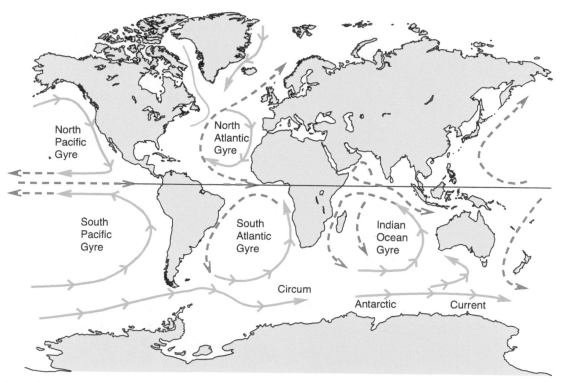

phenomenon, like a spherical battleground attempting to achieve equilibrium. Energy absorbed is cooling in the atmosphere, while the Sun's rays are warming other places. This spinning sphere's surface is releasing and absorbing enormous amounts of energy, and the result are the generally circular patterns of wind and ocean currents we see.

The **ocean currents** of the world are consistent patterns of flow across the Earth's hydrosphere. The currents in large measure are also a function of the moving atmosphere. In the northern hemisphere, we see the winds and ocean currents following a clockwise direction. In the southern hemisphere, these take on the characteristics of a counter-clockwise pattern, in keeping with the Coriolis Effect. In summary, the oceans and seas of the planet tend to absorb and release not retain energy at slower rates than the land and air around them. These currents also tend to distribute the Sun's energy unevenly across the Earth. These currents tend to redistribute energy in a never-ending attempt to redistribute the energy absorbed from the Sun more evenly over the Earth's surface. Hopefully, you are beginning to see how the Earth's shape, its spin, and its topography contribute greatly to the creation of the climates of the world and will see how these climates have affected culture.

The atmosphere, like the oceans themselves, also tends to cool as one goes higher up in elevation. This phenomenon of **orographic lifting** causes air to cool as it rises. As it cools, moisture assumes a lower state of energy, and precipitation may result. After the release of energy, the result is a cooler and dryer air pattern. This sinking phenomenon can occur both locally and globally and is best demonstrated by the global patterns established by **Hadley Cells**. These global cells of varying air pressure account for the general patterns of climate in the world, such as moisture at the equator, dry

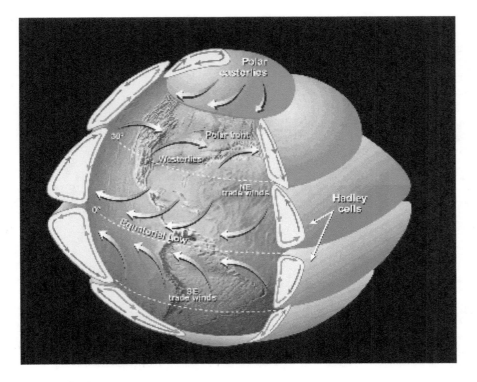

Courtesy of NASA

conditions at 30 degrees north and south, and the global temperate climates where warmer equatorial currents interface with cold, dry, and polar fronts. These colliding cells of varying heat and moisture are turning on the sphere, alternately rising and sinking as they warm and cool. When topography is introduced into the discussion of currents and atmosphere, we begin to be able to define climate and see how the world can be divided into general patterns of weather.

Orographic uplift—the phenomenon of air cooling as it rises—may prevent moisture-laden clouds from rising above mountains with their moisture. As the clouds rise, they cool, and energy is released in the form of winds and heat as precipitation occurs. The result of an ocean-borne current when coming ashore and encountering high terrain can result in a **windward side**, or wet side, of the mountain. Just as we saw with the rise of air in the Hadley cells at 30 degrees north and south, we see the wind absorbing the moisture often creating a dry side, known as the **leeward** side. Here we see how the concepts of latitude, tilt, and spin on a global scale create high-pressure and low-pressure systems rising and falling, and as they come into contact with surface relief, create climates.

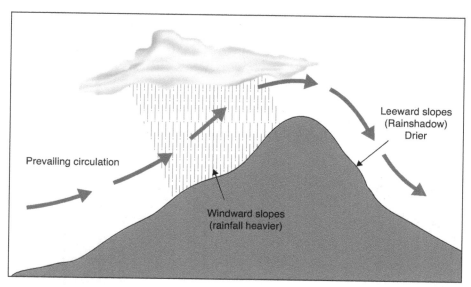

Image © Kendall Hunt Publishing

The different climates of the world therefore describe consistently measured weather patterns and are the result of geostrophic winds blowing ocean currents, resulting in part from the unequal distribution of the Sun's energy on the Earth's surface, combined with the spherical nature of the planet and different latitudes to produce the different climates. **Climates** are defined for the purpose of this class as generalized weather conditions at a given location consistent over long periods of recorded time. For example, the climate in Lynchburg, Virginia, is generally consistent for warmer temperatures and drier conditions in July compared to January. **Weather** is much more variable and can change quickly over time, such as when the Sun comes out at the end of a rainstorm. An easy way to recognize different climates is by their biomes. A **biome** is defined as shared characteristics in animal and plant species

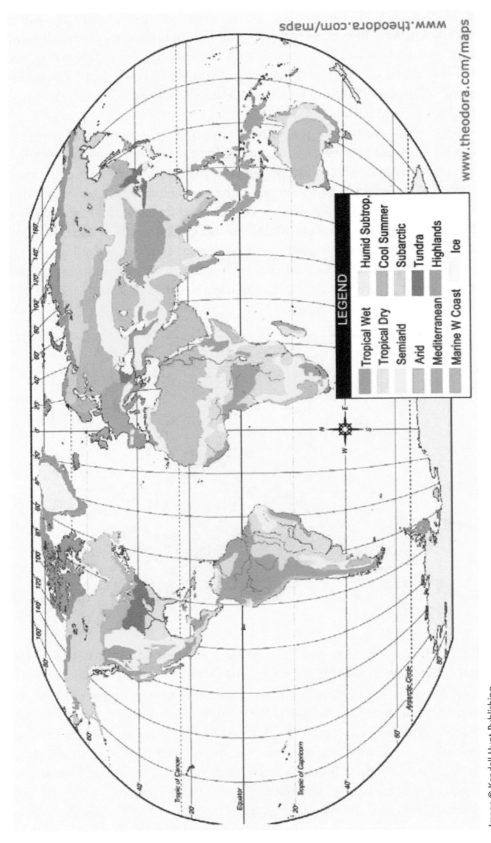

within a particular ecosystem on the Earth's surface and is generally compatible within a particular climate zone.

Brief descriptions of the various world climates and biomes are given as one travels from the equator towards the poles:

Equatorial Climates—these generally occur between the tropics of Cancer and Capricorn located at 23.5 degrees north and south latitude. These tropical climates are characterized by extreme amounts of heat and moisture, in part because they receive the lowest angles of insolation, resulting in a greater release of energy and consequent excitement of atmospheric molecular activity. The moisture may be seasonal in areas, and the result is a high contrast between wet and dry seasons. The biome often associated with this climate is the **rainforest**. Generally, plants within the rainforest are adapted to survive in extremely wet environments by the use of large and thin leaves to enable rapid transpiration and leaf tips to direct moisture from the plant. Plant roots are notoriously shallow and near the surface. Animals are most noted for their extreme diversity. One log, for example, may be home to numerous species.

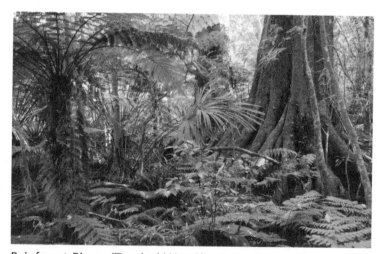

Image © STILLFX, 2011. Used under license from Shutterstock, Inc.

Rainforest Biome/Tropical Wet Climate

The **Dry Climates** vary between semi-arid and arid, depending on amounts of rainfall. The biomes associated with this category generally are marked by **desertification**—an increased degradation or loss of land usage. The deserts of the world are often located between the 15-degree latitude marks north and south, and between rising and falling Hadley Cells, but might also result from colder ocean currents, such as with the Atacama Desert in Chile, or perhaps be the result of relief-blocking moisture through orographic lifting, such as happens in Eastern Australia. We consider the biome here to be that of a **desert**—an area generally recognized by animals able to survive without either much water or physiological adaptations to a dry environment. Plant life generally consists of shrubs and grasses with fewer and smaller leaves and trees becoming noticeably absent. In the New World, we see the predomination of cacti in a similar pattern to Euphorbia in the Old World.

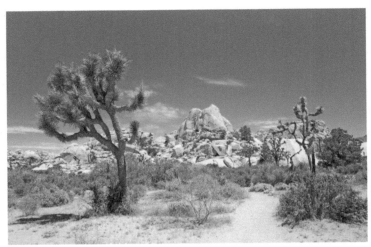

Desert Biome/Arid Climate

The **Temperate Climates**, as the name implies, exist at the higher latitudes from about 30 degrees north and south toward the poles in both the northern and southern hemispheres. These climates reflect the global-scale interaction between the cool, high-pressure air sinking from the poles contacting with the warm air and sea currents turning toward the poles from the equatorial regions. These temperate climates are often cooler and drier as one goes further into the continent where they occur. For example, the proximity of New York to the Canadian land mass results in greater extremes of temperature between summer and winter. Contrasted to this is Virginia, where the proximity of the Atlantic Ocean, with its moderating influence, is felt with the differences between winter and summer much less pronounced. The animals are generally very variable, as are the plants, and the deciduous forest typifies the biomes of this climate zone.

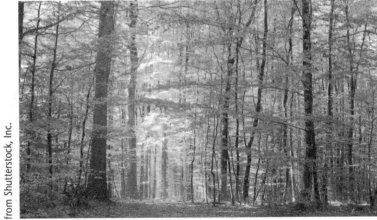

Deciduous Forest/Temperate Climate

The cool, dry air of the high mountainous areas of the Earth is typical of the **highland** climate. The dryness of these intensely cold areas in a sense creates an environment counter-intuitively similar to a desert due to its extremely dry nature. Any moisture in the air is crystallized and may exist for long periods in a solid condition. A highland biome, in particular, is characterized by the plants that have adapted to this climate with needles and a shape generally associated with Christmas trees as the limbs slant down in an imbricated manner resembling the pitch of a roof. This design protects the trees from the harmful effects of ice and wind.

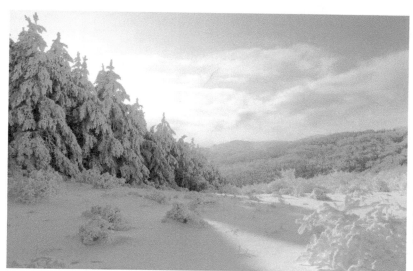

Coniferous Forest/Highland Climate

The **polar** regions of the world are characterized by bitter cold. The polar climates are characterized by extremely dry and cold climatic features and a biome where animals and plants have adapted to these extremes of low temperatures. The most obvious characteristic of the biome, the **tundra**, is the low diversification of the animals. The same amount of animals or biomass may exist in these areas as in other climates and biomes, but generally, the creatures tend to be more homogenous and of the same species.

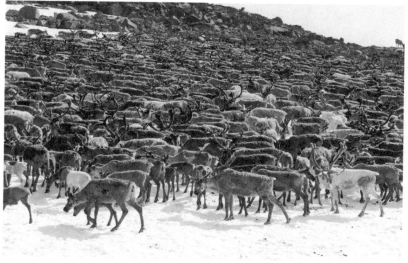

Tundra/Semi Arctic

The final two climates briefly mentioned here are important because they demonstrate the importance of contrasting ocean and land temperatures and air pressure. A cold ocean current next to a warm land mass tends to draw the lower-pressured and warm rising air off the land, and this result is a dry, warm land mass. California and southern Italy are characteristic of this pleasant and somewhat rare **Mediterranean** climate. The opposite phenomenon, however, occurs when the ocean

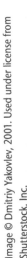
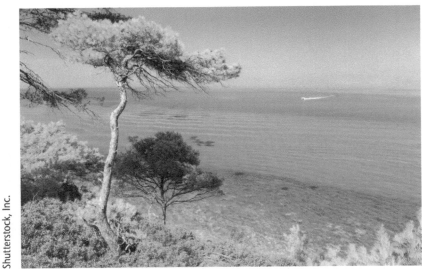

Mediterranean Climate

is warm and the land is cool. This **Maritime** type climate can result in a temperate rainforest biome where ferns and other plants abound; plants in this climate are capable of living in a moist environment. Western Oregon and Washington state are typical of this climate and, along with the Cascade mountain chain, are examples of the windward and leeward effects on climate. Much of Northern Europe epitomizes this type of climate, which is characterized by moderate winters and rainy weather patterns.

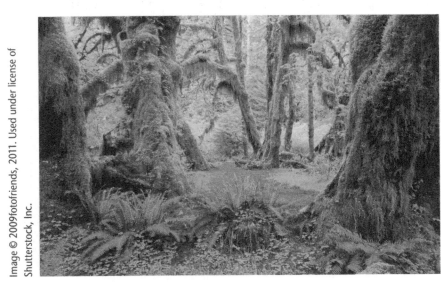

Temperate Rainforest/Maritime Climate

This brief survey is not intended to ignore other forces tend to act upon the Earth's surface. Space here prohibits an in-depth analysis, but the mysterious **Magnetic field** surrounding the Earth also may serve to protect the Earth from harmful effects from outer space. Some experts believe the magnetic fields emanating from other planets in the solar system may serve to further protect the Earth from the harmful effects of space matter. Some scientists also think currents of molten rock or convection currents beneath the Earth's surface may also be responsible for this mysterious phenomenon.[1] Attempting to reconcile tectonic plate activity with the creation of the oceans and seas with the great flood described in Genesis 7:11 offers opportunities for studying the changing surface of the planet. Further exciting opportunities for study exist in the amazing influences of tectonic, hydrospheric, and atmospheric affects upon the Earth's surface. Our planet is truly vibrant and is being shaped and eroded daily under the sovereignty of a Living God.

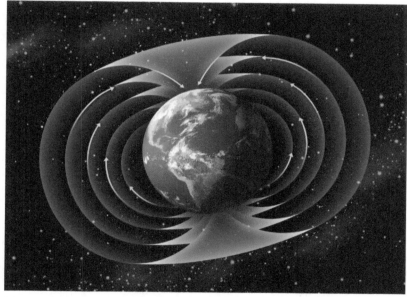

Image © Andrea Danti, 2011. Used under license from Shutterstock, Inc.

Magnetic Field Around the Earth

God has given us a beautiful and enchanted world in which to live. By understanding the various forces and effects that result from the Earth's shape, spin, tilt, and revolution about the Sun, we can determine the reasons for the variations of climate and weather patterns on the Earth as functions of location and topography. Appreciating the physical geography of the Earth is a wonderful starting point for beginning to understand the themes of human geography and the differences in development in the world economy.

---

[1] http://184.154.224.5/~creatio1/index.php?option=com_content&task=view&id=38

KEY TERMS TO KNOW

- Sphere
- Physical geography
- Human geography
- Coriollis Effect
- Great circle
- Currents
- Tilt
- Spin
- Rotation
- Revolution
- Insolation
- Ozone
- Albedo
- Hadley Cells
- Windward
- leeward
- Geostrophic winds
- Orographic uplift
- Adiabatic lapse rate
- Climate
- Weather
- Tropical/Equatorial Wet
- Tropical/Equatorial Wet/Dry
- Dry
- Desertification
- Desert
- Temperate
- Highland
- Polar/Sub-polar
- tundra
- Mediterranean
- Maritime
- Magnetic Field

FURTHER READING

Alex MacGillivray, *Globalization*. (London: Constable & Robinson Ltd., 2006), 288.

Henry Morris, *The Long War Against God*. (Grand Rapids, MI: Baker Books, 1989), 344.

Henderson, *Experiencing Geometry: In Euclidean, Spherical, and Hyperbolic Spaces*. (Upper Saddle River, NJ:Prentice Hall, 2001), 352.

REGIONAL GEOGRAPHY

What is a Regional Approach to Geography?

This book defines geography as a description of the Earth's surface. Anything seen on Earth could technically be described as geographical. A region for the purpose of this book is simply defined as any area studied on the basis of perceived similarities. These similarities can be human in nature as in cultural, physical, climatic, religious, etc. From a physical standpoint, climates and biomes of the world can also contribute to the determination of what constitutes a region. Admittedly very subjective in nature, the discipline of geography with its lack of a formalized structure lends itself to an almost artistic approach to organization that is limited only by the perceived similarities as seen by the observer. The essentially subjective nature of describing geography makes it, therefore, a fascinating discipline and one that can offer a fulfilling lifetime adventure for the student. Everywhere one goes, patterns can be discerned in the various facets of humanity and the environment. Start looking today for opportunities to improve and serve. Make the world even more beautiful!

This book—for the purpose of instruction—describes the following major regions:

1. North America
2. Middle America and the Caribbean
3. South America
4. North Africa and the Middle East
5. Europe
6. Russia
7. Sub-Saharan Africa
8. East Asia
9. South Asia
10. Southeast Asia
11. Central Asia
12. Australia, New Zealand
13. Antarctica and Oceania

The reason for the selection of these areas as regions is generally a function of the physical environment and its obvious effect on culture.

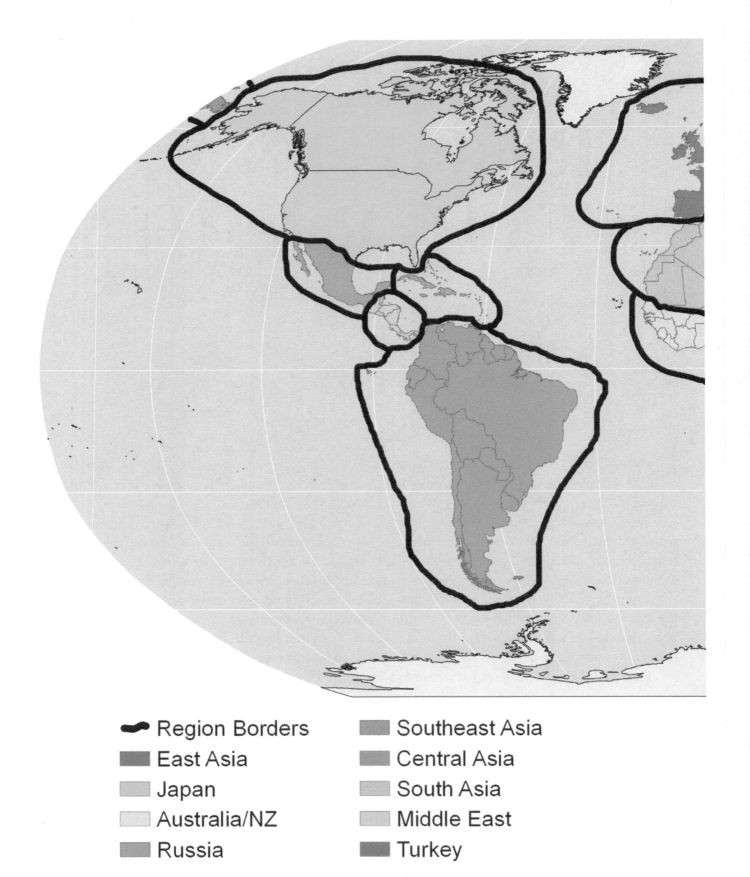

Region Borders

East Asia

Japan

Australia/NZ

Russia

Southeast Asia

Central Asia

South Asia

Middle East

Turkey

Regions generally recognized by geographers. Note: this text diverges slightly from this map.

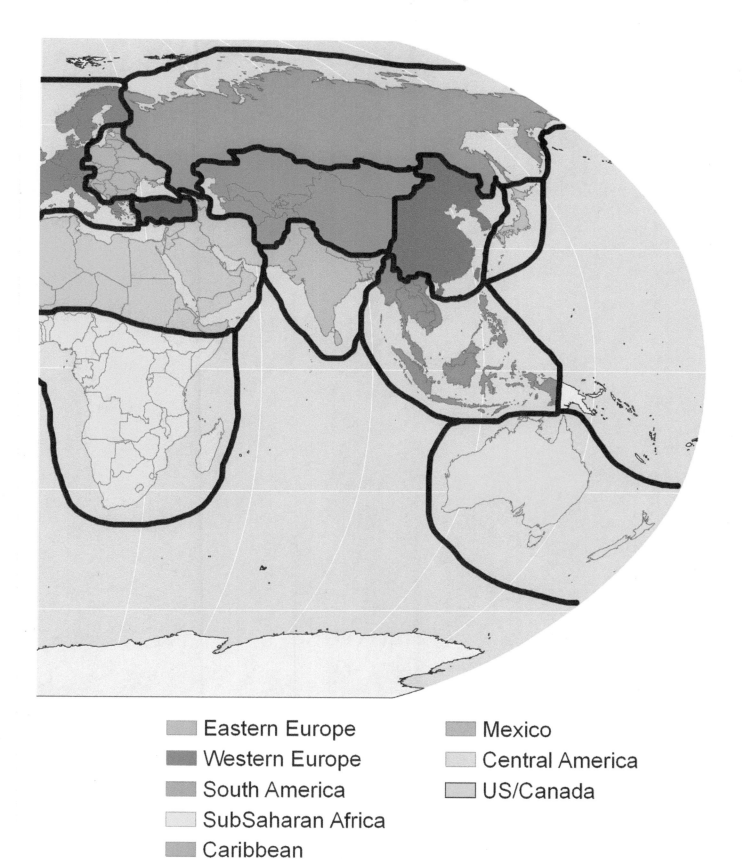

	Eastern Europe		Mexico
	Western Europe		Central America
	South America		US/Canada
	SubSaharan Africa		
	Caribbean		

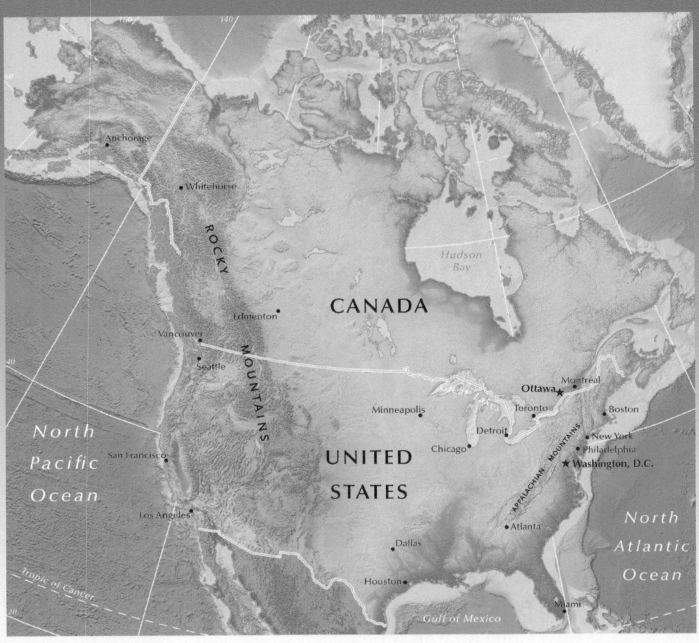

Map courtesy of Katie Pritchard

North America

You are the salt of the earth, but if salt has lost its taste, how shall its saltiness be restored? It is no longer good for anything except to be thrown out and trampled under people's feet. You are the light of the world. A city set on a hill cannot be hidden. Nor do people light a lamp and put it under a basket, but on a stand, and it gives light to all in the house. In the same way, let your light shine before others, so that they may see your good works and give glory to your Father who is in heaven. (Matthew 5:13–16)

A verse commonly heard throughout the university is that from Luke 12:48b. "For everyone to whom much is given, from him much will be required; and to whom much has been committed, of him they will ask the more." To understand how we can help others or to share our hope it is sometimes necessary to honestly assess our strengths and weaknesses. Just as the joy we experience in doing a job well results from diligently reflecting upon both our successes and failures in the past, America's successes are likewise in large measure a function of learning from our past spatially-through geography! Let's see what we can learn about ourselves and how our history has been shaped spatially for the purpose of better serving and providing hope to others!

North America is uniquely placed to fulfill an important role in the world today. From the first footprints left by explorers to the New World, the geography of the continent lent itself to a potentially vibrant culture and one served by the bounties of location and geographic resources. A faithful people clawed an existence out of a few small colonies and set the foundation for a culture destined to be one of the greatest powers on Earth. How God's creation physically intertwined with the creation of a unique culture and history begins with the study of the Earth's surface.

North America is a mid-sized continent in size somewhere between that of Africa and South America. This land area is bordered on two sides by oceans and a gulf.

North America's location and topography have both complemented and facilitated the expansion of European settlement at a time in history when transportation routes demanded harbors and rivers—both of which the continent has in abundance. The placement of North America at middle latitudes ensures it is largely temperate in nature with a unique interaction of topography and climate ideal for agriculture. With oceans bordering both sides of the continent and a gulf to the south, moisture exists in abundance.

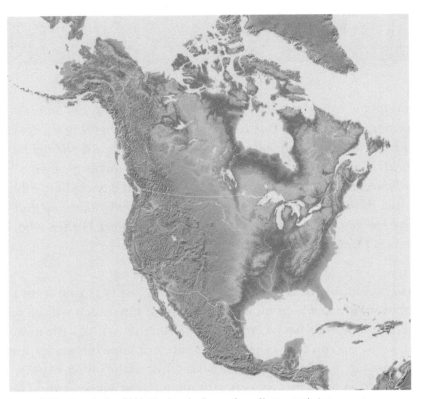

Image © Vitoriano Junior, 2013. Used under license from Shutterstock, Inc.

Funneling and Sunning

The topography of North America interacts with the warm sub-tropical atmosphere to the south by funneling the moisture between the two major mountain chains—the Rockies and the Appalachians; both generally running from north to south. The somewhat funneled and steady rainfall pattern helps to create some of the most productive farmlands in the world. The rivers also follow a pattern of north and south with the major rivers thereby flowing in directions generally advantageous to settlement and transport while uniting the nation **longitudinally**. The mouths of these rivers create some of the world's finest **harbors** and further contribute to the ability to transport goods to international markets. Fine forests of valuable lumber and mature soils in abundance, often watered, have sustained much of the world's population in recent centuries.

The generally latitudinal or east to west movement patterns of settlers from Europe across the North American continent over time seemed to lend itself to what appeared to be a divided culture from the founding of the colonies until the American Civil War. The diffusion of these differing agricultural patterns and their accompanying economies are examples of **Cultural Diffusion**. A southern feudalistic and agrarian society based on servile labor stood in stark contrast to a northern manufacturing center dependent on various transportation outlets or **Nodes**. This ability to connect different networks still is a characteristic of the American economic system and gave the northern or Union views of freedom and the fears of a southern slavocracy an ultimate advantage in movement. Violent war ultimately reconciled different views of freedom and the end of slavery while initiating increased westward expansion in an attempt to spread freedom. Today the cities of the United States still demonstrate patterns of movement often in generally western directions utilizing the latest offerings in various means of transportation.

America's relief affords an excellent opportunity to review some of the aspects of physical geography discussed earlier in this work. The mountains of North America have actually been instrumental in reinforcing from a cultural standpoint the different regions of the North American continent. The rivers likewise have been important in the settlement patterns of North America, and the harbors have served as gateways to the world for the purposes of shipping and the projection of military power. How these factors of relief and the themes of movement have intertwined to create a narrative will be discussed in this section.

The mountains of eastern North America are believed by many scientists to be among the oldest in the world. Possibly some of the finest soils for farming in the United States are in large measure a function of erosion from these mountains. Soils vary and are broken down by the acids from the residue of living organisms (leaves) and tend to chemically break soils down along with physical weathering. Large enough to buffet the extremes of continental climates from the north, the topography nevertheless did not serve as impediments to movement for those self-sufficient settlers seeking to support themselves and their families.

Sectionalism and the City

As the first Americans arrived off of the **easterly** currents at Jamestown, Virginia in 1607, they sought a place of refuge that was near the famed gold of the Spanish but not so near that they could suffer the catastrophic conditions that afflicted Fort Caroline in 1565 (near modern day Jacksonville, Florida). Here the Spanish destroyed a French-speaking colony for venturing too close to their supplies of New World riches. Nevertheless, despite carefully choosing their settlements, the colonists at Jamestown would find themselves geographically challenged. The first English-speaking colonists chose a location relatively near the headquarters of the Indian nation called the Powhatan. Imagine colonists from another culture camping near Washington, D.C., today! To make matters worse, they set up camp in an area that could be compared both to the local dump of the capital city and in a disputed frontier area—a place of contention between two rival nations. Needless to say, the first English-speaking colonists faced spatial challenges, indeed!

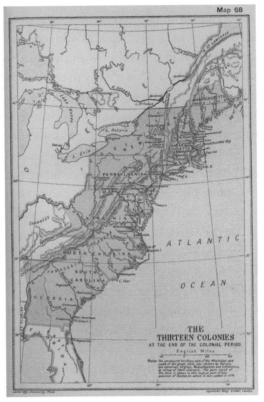

Map source: *The Cambridge Modern History Atlas 1912*, courtesy of the University of Texas Libraries, Perry-Castaneda Library Map Collection.

To the north in Canada and a short time later, the French disembarked their boats at Quebec City in 1608 at what today we would call a **break-bulk point** where the river shallows and prevents further travel by ship. A break-bulk point is where we see one form of transport changed to another such as from a ship to a wagon. Like the patterns of movement to the south, the Canadians followed a generally western pattern and tended to populate the lower regions within 100 miles of what is today the US border. This distribution of population is referred to as an **ecumene** or more habitable region. To the south, the English colonies from New England to Virginia also displayed different cultures reflective of the different climates they experienced and different cultures emerged with fearful implications for freedom.

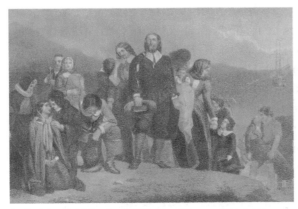

Art by John C. McRae (ca. 1620), from Library of Congress

The movement of the settlers west and the dynamic of a frontier created two different types of agricultural economies. The successful diffusion of these cultures and subsequent population growth would create unique American experiences. As you probably learned in school, the use of tobacco's introduction to the public tended to wear out the soil in the Virginia river lands, and this created a need for more rich soils and the subsequent deforestation of the eastern deciduous forest. As the settlers moved into the interior of the country, the cultural values of private property and the delineation of drawn borders recorded and maintained by the local courthouses reinforced a culture that was both individually competitive and placed a premium on private property rights. Here is where we can see that the intertwining of the topography of North America would ultimately shape a unique and vibrant culture.

While Canadians crossed the windswept prairie, Americans began moving in two different directions and into two different regions, also a function of latitude and moisture. Many of the compromises for union you may have studied in US history also appear to be related to topographic relief and the two different climates seen on map [page 8]. Settlers moved west through the gaps in the Appalachian Mountains into southern states such as Kentucky and Tennessee. Simultaneously to the north, immigrants continued to arrive into coastal harbors and traveled to the Great Lakes through the Erie Canal beginning in the 1820s. This insured the rapid growth of northern cities. The clearing of the northwest bisected the southern culture through the central river valley of the Mississippi and ultimately doomed the southern slave culture.

Different Latitude–Different Attitude

The mighty Mississippi River flowed generally north to south and was fed by the powerful tributaries of the Ohio, Tennessee, Cumberland and Missouri Rivers. This served not only to support inexpensive transport, creating a **gateway city** in New Orleans as American crops and manufacturing spread to the world, but the existence of a river running almost perpendicular to the spread of settlers and culture west seemed to ultimately insure the dominance of a northern culture over a southern one. It also served to inextricably bind the two nations together through trade and transport.

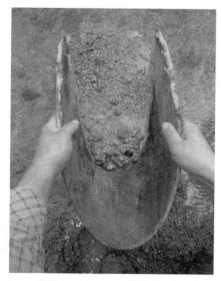

Image © Richard Peterson, 2013. Used under license from Shutterstock, Inc.

The **cultural diffusion** of southern agriculture utilized slaves as a labor source for utilizing cotton as far west as Texas while Americans in the North who were entering into a modern industrialized era experienced a series of religious revivals that embodied a dualistic or **Manichean** perspective and placed a premium on doing good work. This eventually initiated a crusade of sorts to free the slaves in the South. Interestingly, it would be the American West that would bring this issue to full warfare. Northern industry benefited from the physical geography.

Head West, Young People!

When California came into the Union it did so in an expedited manner that upset the national balance. Why the big rush? One word—gold. With an international economy based on **specie** since the age of exploration, the possession of this metal was the fastest ticket to wealth and power of its time. As both the northern and southern cultures eyed each other over this precious resource, the paucity or lack of plantation agriculture in the western region insured California would tend towards a free culture. The subsequent railroad connections and the continued westward movement of a population increasingly marked by immigrants further inflamed passions of freedom. A diffusion of a free and more unionized industrial culture in the north intersected with that of a slave culture based on state's rights in the south. It would seem the American experience was bound to be one of strong unity after the conflagration of war due to the effect of topography and culture.

Interior

The North American continent is blessed with both incredible resources and a culture reflecting a solid and intense Christian work ethic. By the time the American people closed the western frontier by the 1890s, Americans had established important agricultural contributions. A major producer of corn, and marked by an intense work-ethic blended with the faithful legacy of the spiritually minded Puritans and the more capitalistic Jamestown colony, the way was set to lead in manufacturing. Ease of transport connecting resources across the lakes to the emerging cities of New York, Pittsburgh and Chicago kept relative transport rates down. It has been said transportation costs on water range historically from 1:30 to 1:100 relative cost of tonnage to transport on land. This nation of north and south reunited continued to influence the world through the nineteenth and twentieth centuries.

Meanwhile, the continued movement of Americans into the Pacific coast continued unabated as America marched into the global scene as an economic powerhouse. What lured people to California, for example? The answer is jobs and ultimately an opportunity to participate in industries that would change the entire world—such as aviation and Hollywood. World War II presented increased opportunities, in particular, with the proliferation of technologies that enabled people to survive the harsh deserts and to cross them quickly. These technologies included the automobile but also air conditioning. One could argue the southwestern United States and the southeastern part of the deep-south Florida actually presented some of the last frontiers of the continental United States and was finally settled because of the invention of cars and air conditioning!

City Lights

The same world that recognizes McDonald's drive-through food would recognize the automobile culture that poured people west into California where these fast food restaurants would originate. In a sense, the **cultural landscape** of American cities reflects historical movement patterns. In various stages, American westward travel from Jamestown to the Pacific may still be seen when studying America's cities. The first stage of the growth of American cities has generally been from a transportation node such as a river or road. After the arrival of the industrial revolution in the early nineteenth century, people would walk to the factories, often taking the trolley cars to work. Later, the automobile would make the suburbs within reach to the upwardly mobile. Today, fiber optic networks have created corridors in tandem with interstate highways and airports. The vast majorities of these global networks cross or interconnect in North America still. The modern city can demonstrate to the culturally aware the history of the country on its cultural landscape.

We Like Ike! What's the Deal with the Interstate System?

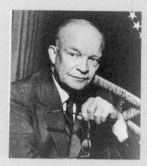

The formal name of the United States interstate system is the "Dwight D. Eisenhower National System of Interstate and Defense Highways." The US interstate system was created by the Federal-Aid Highway Act of 1956, which, as the name suggests, was championed by Eisenhower. The US interstate system was built for both civilian and military purposes. Some of you might be thinking, "Yeah! One in every five miles of road must be straight so that military aircraft can land and take off on them!" Well, maybe. The true military aspects of the interstate system are primarily to facilitate troop movement and to allow for the evacuation of major cities in the event of nuclear war.

The civilian aspects of the Interstate Highway System have helped shape American culture in more ways than we can possibly imagine. Most US interstates pass through the center of cities, which allows people to live outside the city and commute in for work, which has also played a huge role in the creation of suburbs and urban sprawl. The highway system also gives the federal government power over state governments. The US government can withhold interstate highway funds, which are huge amounts of money, from uncooperative state governments. The US government used this tactic to increase the national drinking age to 21 and to lower the blood alcohol level for intoxication to 0.08%. According to the Constitution, both of these issues should be decided by states. However, if they choose to disobey, they don't get their highway money.

(continued)

We Like Ike! What's the Deal with the Interstate System? (continued)

Also, the US highway system allows high speed transportation of consumer products. This makes the prices of everything, from bananas to concrete, cheaper. The result: the US is an automobile culture heavily reliant on fossil fuels for the movement of everything and for virtually all aspects of our lives. Americans are quite unique in this respect. It's also why they are the best stock car racers in the world. Who else has NASCAR? Who is more worried that the price of oil is reaching $150 a barrel?

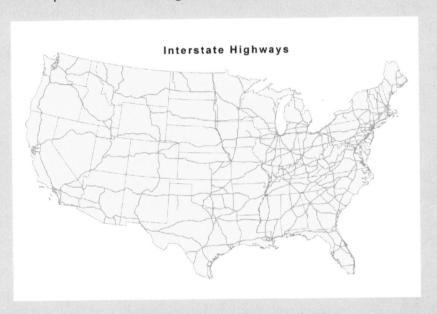

Interstate Highways

From *The Plaid Avenger's World #6 Nuclear Insecurity Edition.* Copyright © 2008, 2009, 2010, 2011, 2012 by John Boyer. Copyright © 2006 by Kendall Hunt Publishing Company. Reprinted by permission.

Resources abound in North America but none would be as valuable as oil. First discovered in Pennsylvania in the 1850's, the United States would begin to actually need imports of oil by the end of the Second World War. Nevertheless, the potential for oil production still exists in various forms and has without question directed America's interest in the world since the fall of the Soviet Union in the 1800's.

California with its terrific harbors and the valuable Puget Sound on the border of the United States and Canada offered priceless gateways to the Pacific—the very same goal of the ancients as they sought the headwaters of the Euphrates River, attempting to circumvent the silk road! But the American story doesn't end on the Pacific coast; rather the western movement patterns of America would transcend regions into the Pacific. In fact, America would expand across the islands of the Pacific and into the Philippines. With two coasts and more good harbors than many continents have, America's role as a military power seemed almost predestined. Many historians in fact

USA GDP =

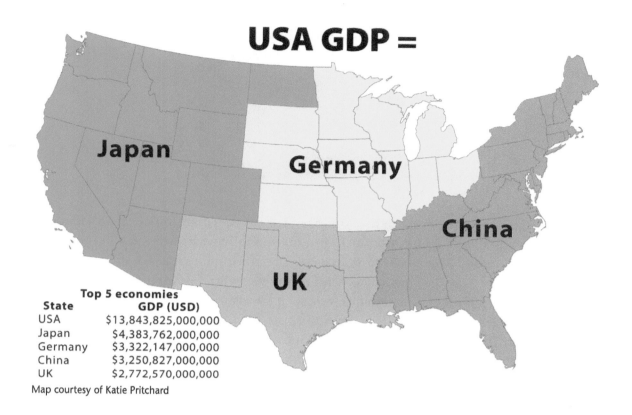

Japan

Germany

China

UK

Top 5 economies	
State	**GDP (USD)**
USA	$13,843,825,000,000
Japan	$4,383,762,000,000
Germany	$3,322,147,000,000
China	$3,250,827,000,000
UK	$2,772,570,000,000

Map courtesy of Katie Pritchard

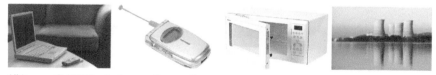

All images © 2007 JupiterImages Corporation

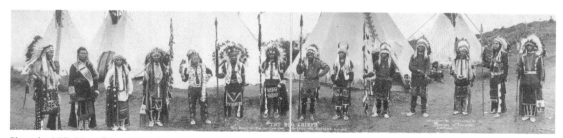

Photo by M.B. Marcell (ca. 1911), from Library of Congress

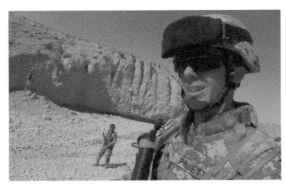

U.S. Air Force photo by SSGT Jacob N. Bailey

believe the high water mark of the American westward expansion or **"manifest destiny"**—or a perception of the rights to occupy spatially westward—would not come until the Vietnam War. Regardless, overseas commitments and treaties would be instrumental in America's growth as a military power with the vast majority of aircraft carriers. America's role as a global power seemed assured by the end of the bipolar world of the 1990's with the fall of communism.

A powerful United States prospered as international networks of fiber optics and space satellites in various levels of Earth orbit maintained an ability to negotiate the globe through GPS and to maintain the security of American interests. Almost like the British Empire, which was based on trade and utilized the waterways to accomplish its business, the United States has overseen an invisible suzerainty over much of the world somewhat unintentionally utilizing the electromagnetic spectrum. With **multinational corporations** or MNC's overseeing an invisible empire of sorts, the American people often stand to benefit both publicly and privately by their profits.

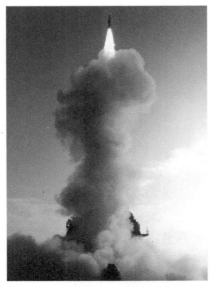

Department of Defense photo by U.S. Navy

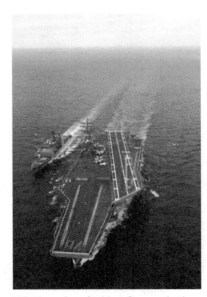

U.S. Navy photo by Mass Communication Specialist 3rd Class Kathleen Gorby

Country	Military Expenditures 2011 (USD)
US	$741,200,000,000
China	$380,000,000,000
India	$92,000,000,000
Russia	$82,500,000,000
Saudi Arabia	$59,090,000,000
France	$54,444,000,000
UK	$50,952,000,000
Turkey	$46,634,700,000
Germany	$42,255,000,000
South Korea	$36,774,000,000
Brazil	$34,170,000,000
Japan	$33,192,000,000
World Total	$2,157,172,000,000

http://www.globalsecurity.org/military/world/spending.htm

From *The Plaid Avenger's World #6 Nuclear Insecurity Edition.* Copyright © 2008, 2009, 2010, 2011, 2012 by John Boyer. Copyright © 2006 by Kendall Hunt Publishing Company.

2011 TOP SALES OF MULTINATIONAL COMPANIES

Company	Home Base	Sales (USD)
Wal-Mart Stores	USA	421.8 billion
Royal Dutch Shell	Netherlands	369.1 billion
ExxonMobil	USA	341.6 billion
BP	UK	297.1 billion
Sinopec-China Petroleum	China	284.8 billion
PetroChina	China	222.3 billion
Toyota Motor	Japan	202.8 billion
Chevron	USA	189.6 billion
Total	France	188.1 billion
ConocoPhillips	USA	175.8 billion
Volkswagen Group	Germany	168.3 billion
General Electric	USA	162.4 billion
Fannie Mae	USA	154.3 billion

From Special Report: The World's Biggest Companies, edited by Scott DeCarlo 04.02.08, Forbes.com

From *The Plaid Avenger's World #6 Nuclear Insecurity Edition.* Copyright © 2008, 2009, 2010, 2011, 2012 by John Boyer. Copyright © 2006 by Kendall Hunt Publishing Company.

Bravely walking into a new world order and perhaps blunderingly assisting in the rise of powerful autocracies in Russia and China with well-intentioned military interventions, America's importance in the future is undoubtedly assured do to the blessings of relief, currents, the particulars of climate and their effects on agriculture as well as the rich soils of the east which served to lure and direct the movement of the first colonists west—a pattern that has continued almost to the present. Hopefully Americans have not forgotten the geographic basis for the prosperity that exists today nor the author of this land, which in large measure has shaped the culture of freedom we so enjoy today.

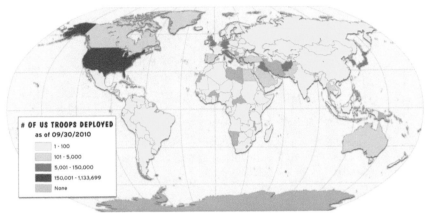

Map courtesy of Katie Pritchard

KEY TERMS TO KNOW

- longitudinally
- harbors
- cultural diffusion
- nodes
- easterly
- break-bulk point
- ecumene
- gateway city
- Manichean
- specie
- cultural land scape
- Manifest Destiny
- multinational corporations

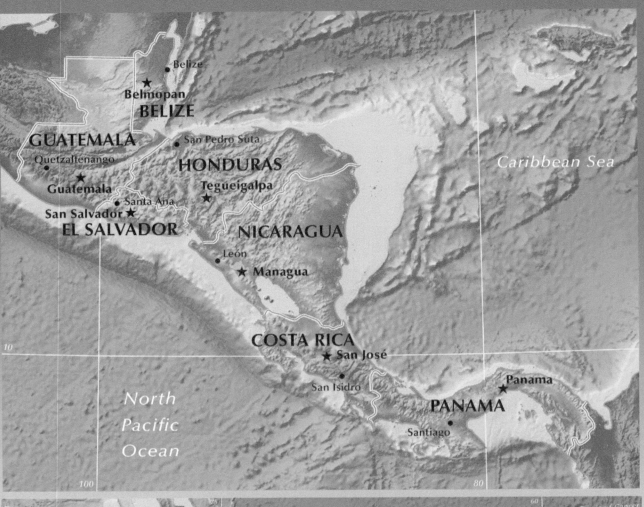

Belize
★ Belmopan
BELIZE
GUATEMALA
San Pedro Suta
Quetzaltenango
HONDURAS
Caribbean Sea
★ Guatemala
Tegueigalpa
Santa Ana
San Salvador ★
EL SALVADOR
NICARAGUA
León
★ Managua
COSTA RICA
10
★ San José
San Isidro
Panama
North
Pacific
Ocean
PANAMA
Santiago
100
80

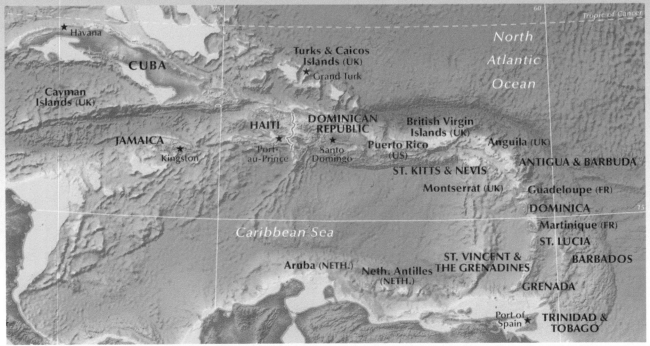

Tropic of Cancer
★ Havana
North
Turks & Caicos
Islands (UK)
Atlantic
CUBA
★ Grand Turk
Ocean
Cayman
Islands (UK)
DOMINICAN
British Virgin
HAITI
REPUBLIC
Islands (UK)
Anguila (UK)
JAMAICA
Puerto Rico
Port-
Santo
(US)
ANTIGUA & BARBUDA
Kingston
au-Prince
Domingo
ST. KITTS & NEVIS
Montserrat (UK)
Guadeloupe (FR)
DOMINICA
15
Martinique (FR)
Caribbean Sea
ST. LUCIA
ST. VINCENT &
Aruba (NETH.)
THE GRENADINES
BARBADOS
Neth. Antilles
(NETH.)
GRENADA
Port of
TRINIDAD &
Spain
TOBAGO

Maps courtesy of Katie Pritchard and NOAA

Middle America

But godliness with contentment is great gain, for we brought nothing into the world, and we cannot take anything out of the world. But if we have food and clothing, with these we will be content. But those who desire to be rich fall into temptation, into a snare, into many senseless and harmful desires that plunge people into ruin and destruction. For the love of money is a root of all kinds of evils. It is through this craving that some have wandered away from the faith and pierced themselves with many pangs. (1 Timothy 6:6-10)

Most Christians are aware of what Jesus taught when he said, "Therefore I say to you, do not worry about your life, what you will eat or what you will drink; or about your body, what you will put on. Is not life more than food and the body more than clothing?" (Matthew 6:25 NKJV) But fewer actually realize these things choke out our lives like weeds do crops in the garden. The loveliness of the Caribbean can hide a wounded spirit both geographically and culturally, while close to us; just below the border we can find desperation that needs more than a material solution. What are the aspects of our neighbors to the south that so invites us to spend money AND assist others?

The area we call Middle America consists of a triangular shaped **landform** that has acted as a narrowing land bridge largely located in the tropics between North America and South America. This landform is flanked on the west by the warm Caribbean Sea and the Gulf of Mexico. On the east is the enormous Pacific Ocean. As do most tropical areas, Middle America faces both a great deal of challenges and exciting opportunities. Because of the diversity of cultures experienced in this area, cultural terms such as Latin America are actually inaccurate when describing this region. Where exactly is Middle America? For the purpose of this work it is considered to be all of the areas with a coastline bordering the Pacific and Atlantic Oceans south of the United States and above the continent of South America. Let us examine how the physical geography of this region has affected many aspects of the human geography.

Careful with Those Plates

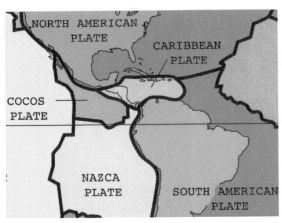

From *This Dynamic Earth: The Story of Plate Tectonics* (online edition) by W. Jacqueline Kious and Robet I. Tilling, prepared by U.S. Geological Survey

Besides an **attenuated** landform, much of Middle America is mountainous. In fact, without the mountains resulting from tectonic activity many of the islands in the Caribbean Sea would not exist at all! Geologists tell us the Caribbean plate is actually in contact with four other plates. The resulting stresses of the converging and divergence of these plates are instrumental in producing volcanoes and earthquakes as well as the mountain ranges running down the spine of Middle America. The climate as one might expect is warm. This warmth and the resulting precipitation can be a deadly mix. Erosion has long plagued farmers of Middle America especially since the high relief has been over grazed in large measure by the arrival of European domesticated animals.

Do not be deceived, however, though the majority of Middle America is tropical, the mountains and high relief can indeed lead to cooling. As you might expect in an area largely tropical, a majority of the climate, however, consists of warmth and heavy rains. With the high relief of the mountains and volcanoes, this cooling and the subsequent orographic effect of precipitation result in **windward** and **leeward** effects. This varying precipitation has given Middle America a range of climatic conditions—many ideal for particular crops. Previous discussions of North America revealed how important differing agricultural patterns can be to the development of societal culture and even ideology. Similarly, Middle America is an amazingly complex area with a diversity of agriculture.

The Coast with the Most

One can actually go from rainforests and warm-moist areas along the coast called the **Tierra Caliente** (sea level to 2500 feet elevation) to the moderate climates of the **Tierra Templada** (2500 to 6000 feet elevation) and then to the dryer and cold climates in the **Tierra Fría** (6000 to 1150 feet elevation) within relatively short distances, merely by taking a trip up the mountains. Each of these areas lends itself to fantastic arrays of crop potentials. The Tierra Caliente area near the coast is famous for its bananas and other tropical fruits. In fact, some geographers believe the tomato originated in the area between the Tierra Caliente and the Templada regions. For many years, Europeans and North Americans were afraid to eat a member of the nightshade family because this fruit had an infamous reputation as being a plant used to poison royalty. A great example of a type of inverted **hierarchical diffusion** actually occurred here when the lower classes would eat it and eventually it made its way up to the higher classes. Usually hierarchical diffusion works the other way around. Like when the author dresses up like his boss in another failed attempt to be promoted. Anyway, the Tierra Templada is famous for its coffee, wheat and maize (native corn), whereas in the harsher, drier and much colder highlands one can grow the tough potato from South America and many of the various grains such as barley and wheat that we are so accustomed to.

The biomes in Middle America lend themselves to a great deal of diversity in terms of animals and plants. In fact, of the millions of species on earth many of those yet to be discovered are in this region. Despite this wonderful diversity, however, risks exist. The cutting of the rainforests can contribute greatly to the loss of precious soils through erosion and by the percolation or **leaching** of valuable nutrients resulting from the tropical rains taking nutrients down into the soil away from the shallow roots of the tropical trees. Since we all want to be good stewards of God's resources, it is important to understand the nature of this area and the importance of good soil and forest management techniques.

Another **human-environmental** difficulty, associated with the arrival of Europeans into the Caribbean, resulted from a combination of mountains and tropical conditions that have unfortunately resulted in much **erosion** after the Europeans brought animals such as goats with them. In large measure, the poverty one might experience in various places is a result of the arrival of these Old World animals during the Columbian exchange often with catastrophic results. Feeding a growing world tropic population is going to be an increased challenge for farmers everywhere, and Middle America is no exception.

Hang Those Flags!

The **vexillology**, or study of flags of the Caribbean, abstractly reflects the cultures and physical geography of the Caribbean. The physical geography of the stars, the sun, and the sea are abstractly placed on the maps and reflect a strong symbolic meaning associated with the landscapes of this region. The cultural legacies of Africa are manifested often in green, yellow and black and these combinations offer interesting insights into the origins and history of many of the cultures here. Jamaica is a great example. Though relatively close to Spanish-speaking Cuba and Hispaniola in the Greater Antilles of the Caribbean, Jamaica is an English-speaking nation with the predominant

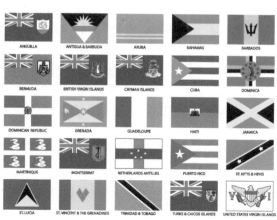

Image © Basheera Designs, 2013. Used under license from Shutterstock, Inc.

ethnicity being black. Looking at the flag of Jamaica, one can trace the African roots by viewing the green and yellow flag with the black colors. Flags can be a terrific addition to any classroom and by definition should be able to be drawn by a child from memory accurately. For these reasons, flags are excellent both anecdotally and colorfully and speak volumes of a culture's views and history. Many of the republics of the mainland in Middle America, for example, use varying degrees of blue and white in their flags, which are of a republican nature like the French and Spanish flags.

The unfortunate legacy of slavery that occurred in the southern United States has a spatial dimension you may not be aware of. The first slaves who were brought to the New World were probably bound for the Caribbean. South America and the Caribbean are where the preponderance of these slaves arrived because of the agricultural demands. The Portuguese initially used mostly west-African slaves as had Arabs previously in east Africa. The West Africans demonstrated a valuable ability to grow sugar cane initially on Sao Tome and the Principe Islands. And as we saw with Jamestown, the easterly currents brought them to the New World. Under terrible conditions, these unwilling travelers on slave ships crossed the **Middle Passage** of the Atlantic. The islands of the Caribbean sat waiting, perfect for growing sugar. Eventually, the plantation form of agriculture arose with its emphasis on profits. Ultimately, the Barbadian slave code, which would create perpetual slavery would diffuse north and be adopted into the slave markets of Charleston, South Carolina, and would manifest itself into the codified laws of Virginia and the other colonies of the South. Climate and currents worked together to create the largest forced movement of people in the world against their wills. The preponderance of the slaves (who would end up in the Caribbean) traveled to the Americas across the **middle passage** and worked in the sugar and tobacco industries.

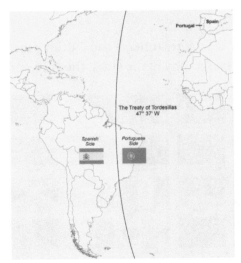

Map courtesy of Katie Pritchard

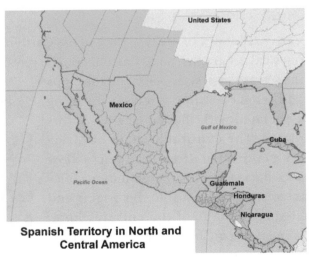

Spanish Territory in North and Central America

The World Factbook

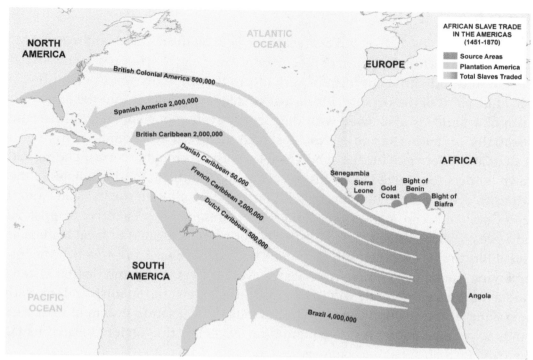

The World Factbook

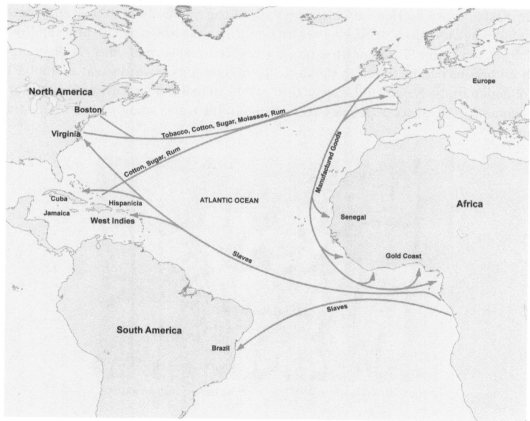

The World Factbook

Whose House is This?

The **hacienda** or "big house" is a characteristic item on the cultural landscape of Middle America. This livestock farm or precursor of American ranches represents an independent and self-sufficient form of agriculture that in many ways personified the individual spirit of the region. This diffusion of Spanish culture into the agricultural realm of America is associated with the **viceroy system** of colonial administration. Essentially, an authoritarian regime designed to govern autonomously from either Mexico City or Peru and further subdivided into districts roughly corresponding to the drawn borders recognized today historically made it difficult for the peoples of these regions to overcome the divisions which separated them. Both the hacienda and the viceroy system according to some authorities represented a breakup of Spanish rule and were characteristically absolute in the authority delegated to local leaders and their ability to rule over their subordinates. Under the **encomienda system**, a means of employing the labor of native-Americans, even powers of life and death existed in Middle America particularly within the relations between the Spanish and the Native Americans. The transition from an encomienda to a hacienda system of agriculture stands in marked contrast to the plantation system in this region, located usually where the English-speaking colonists settled.

The **plantation** is marked by a large-scale endeavor usually based on one or two cash crops. The plantation system is more reflective of the industrial age with its emphasis on production and efficiency. Both the hacienda systems represented attempts by capitalists to receive returns on their investments. The profitability of each, in somewhat different directions, gives us a measure of cultural diversity—whose origins can be found in the agricultural attempts toward sugar and tobacco production in the New World. Just as the Caribbean had unique forms of agricultural production, a diversity of peoples also existed in the warm tropics to the immediate south.

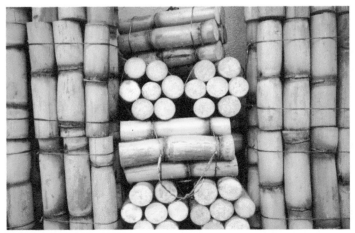

Image © Elena Kalistratova, 2013. Used under license from Shutterstock, Inc.

The ethnicities of the Caribbean are of a wide array ranging from Spanish-speaking people in the Dominican Republic who are descended from both the Spanish and Native Americans known as **Creole** to the descendants of African slaves brought to the New World with modified British speech accents such as in Jamaica. The French presence in the rich "sugar islands" manifests itself today in places like Haiti and into the Leeward Islands where the islands of Guadalupe and Martinique are still dependent on France. The mixture of African and Europeans are often referred to as **mulatto** and generally the differences in population are of little consequence to the peoples there. Notice on the map towards the south near the Gulf of Venezuela, the former Dutch islands of Aruba and Curacao sit strategically offshore of the oil rich areas of Maracaibo in Venezuela. Though you might think of Venezuela and Colombia as South American countries, in many ways they culturally share the same sunny and cheerful culture of the Caribbean, as does the gulf coast of the United States. What are the subregions or areas of Middle America?

Middle America can easily be separated into mainland and islands. **Mexico** is the largest nation on the mainland—an area easily lending itself to stereotypes. Contrary to the views of most North Americans, Mexico is actually a quite diverse landscape. Somewhat similar to the United States in that two mountain chains run basically north and south, it differs by virtue of possessing a huge plateau between them in the center of the nation. The rich legacy of the Spanish can be seen in the **plazas** and landscapes of Mexico. The movement of peoples and culture into the United States is reflected in large measure by the flat-roofed landscapes and the use of fountains whose tradition is in the plaza. Revolution has shaped Mexico and generally replaced the hacienda system previously mentioned. The control of public lands on the **Ejidos** continues however, and normally are public lands controlled by the government and run by 20 families or more. To the south in Mexico we find the state of **Chiapas** where centrifugal effects of ethnicity and even language pose a modest threat to the Mexican union. Further to the north in Mexico we see marked social-cultural differences.

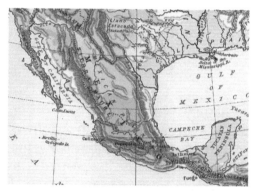

From *Historical Atlas* (1911) by William Shepherd, courtesy of University of Texas Libraries

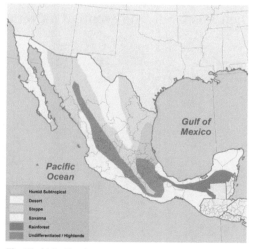

The World Factbook

Move Out!

To the north we find the **maquiladoras** or the factory areas along the border. Unlike the ecumene in Canada, this area is somewhat impoverished and tends to be a less

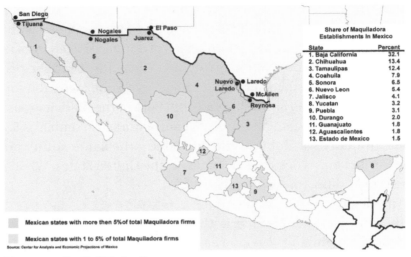

Map source: *The World Factbook*

permanent region. Initially, many of the "border towns" along the US and Mexican border were small but with the change in laws affecting manufacturing decades ago, factories became profitable on the border due to the relatively inexpensive labor available to the US companies. With the displacement of the American manufacturing sector, largely to Asia in the last generation, many of these towns faced massive unemployment and the result was the beginning of a movement pattern known as **chain migration** into North America. The movement into North America consisted of young males initially seeking work—**pulled**—and many desperate to leave an area where little work existed—**pushed**—and then eventually as wives moved to be with their husbands, the eventual movement of entire towns resulted. These patterns of movement are generally a global phenomenon, with most migrations occurring today from southern to northern latitudes. Many of these longitudinal travelers represent a **counter-movement** or reverse of earlier colonial era patterns. Interestingly, it is usually the intention of the migrants to travel only short distances when such moves are made as families. A much longer distance is the domain of the settler, usually young males. The colonization process described earlier in North America is a prime example of what has occurred in

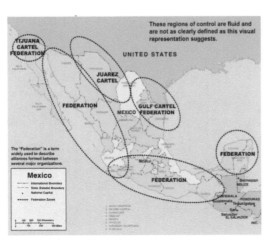

Source: U.S. Drug Enforcement Administration, adapted by CRS (P. McGrath 3/2/2007)

much of Middle America in the last generation. Although Mexico faces numerous challenges, including seemingly unending drug wars and gang activities, it is a mineral-rich nation with limitless potential. Tourism has been a leading industry in Mexico for obvious reasons. The beauty of God's creation in the people and in His beautiful natural world is hard to miss in the region of Middle America!

SOME MAQUILADORA COMPANIES YOU MAY KNOW

- 3 Day Blinds
- 20th Century Plastics
- Acer Peripherals
- Bali Company, Inc.
- Bayer Corp./Medsep
- BMW
- Canon Business Machines
- Casio Manufacturing
- Chrysler
- Daewoo
- Eastman Kodak/Verbatim
- Eberhard-Faber
- Eli Lilly Corporation
- Ericsson
- Fisher Price
- Ford
- Foster Grant Corporation
- General Electric Company
- JVC
- GM
- Hasbro
- Hewlett Packard
- Hitachi Home Electronics

- Honda
- Honeywell, Inc.
- Hughes Aircraft
- Hyundai Precision America
- IBM
- Matsushita
- Mattel
- Maxell Corporation
- Mercedes Benz
- Mitsubishi Electronics Corp.
- Motorola
- Nissan
- Philips
- Pioneer Speakers
- Samsonite Corporation
- Samsung
- Sanyo North America
- Sony Electronics
- Tiffany
- Toshiba
- VW
- Xerox
- Zenith

Fun in the Sun

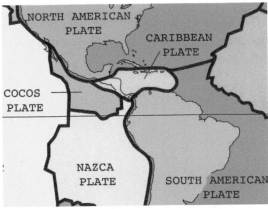

From *This Dynamic Earth: The Story of Plate Tectonics* (online edition) by W. Jacqueline Kious and Robert I. Tilling, prepared by U.S. Geological Survey

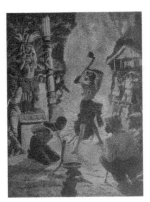

© 2007 JupiterImages Corporation

Incredibly beautiful but at times violent and harsh, the islands of the Caribbean Sea can be buffeted cruelly by hurricanes and other tropical storms. Traditionally, these areas consisted of highly contested areas sought by the empires of Europe for their enormous profit potential in the form of sugar and other crops such as tobacco. Nevertheless, life could be hard and fast with tropical diseases in large measure a function of the increased movement of the age of exploration and the Colombian exchange of animals and plants. Perhaps Cuba is a good example of the beauty and tumult that is the Caribbean.

As a member of the Greater Antilles with Jamaica, Puerto Rico and the Island of Hispaniola, these islands lay generally latitudinal across the areas that see many of the seasonal storms that wash them with moisture. The great nation of Cuba has seen itself the battleground of efforts by American force in the Spanish American War and the Cold War. Due to its proximity to the United States, Cuba both chafed under and received an advantage from its allies in the former Soviet Union. To American eyes, revolution seems to be the lay of the land in this land of extremes, but to the people attempting to survive it represents just another autocracy in the long history of totalitarian power to our south. Recent attempts by the son of the former dictator Fidel Castro to serve only two terms are

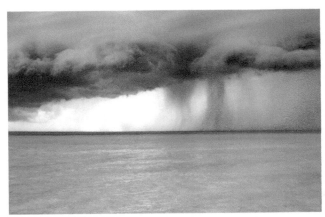

Image © Art_girl, 2013. Used under license from Shutterstock, Inc.

being watched carefully as an opportunity for this formerly great culture to shift back into a free market mode. Relations with Venezuela to the south and the growing autocracies of Russia and China may betray this lack of progress. Still, Cuba with certainty will be able to avoid the natural disasters facing the island of Hispaniola next door.

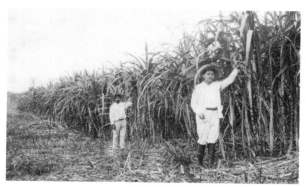

Photo by C.B. Waite, from Frank and Frances Carpenter Collection, Library of Congress

Country/Territory	Contribution of Tourism Economy to GDP (2002)
	Percent of GDP
Anguilla	58
Antigua and Barbuda	72
Aruba	47
Bahamas	46
Barbados	37
Bermuda	26
British Virgin Islands	85
Cayman Islands	31
Cuba	11
Dominica	22
Dominican Republic	18
Grenada	23
Guadeloupe	33
Jamaica	27
Martinique	10
St. Kitts and Nevis	25
St. Lucia	51
St. Vincent and the Grenadines	29
Virgin Islands (U.S.)	42

Most Christians are familiar with the earthquakes that hit Haiti in 2010, but very few statistics are available to document the total generosity displayed toward this poor island nation which is on the eastern half of the island of Hispaniola; a divided island like New Guinea in Indonesia. Millions of dollars and countless hours of time have been given to provide essential needs to the Haitians in recent years. The Dominican Republic next door actually occupied by US Marines for years earlier in the last century has so far escaped many of the challenges facing the former French colony of Haiti, but the Spanish-speaking nation of the Dominican Republic will continue to be persuaded by developments between the United States and Cuba. The island of Puerto Rico (the last major Island group in the greater Antilles) is in fact a territory of the United States as are the Virgin Islands next door.

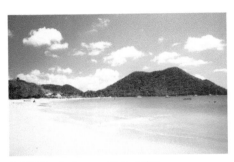

© 2007 JupiterImages Corporation

Puerto Rico has influenced the United States through migration and its contributions to the American nation through its contributions of military service and continued political support for continued membership with commonwealth status in the United States. Primarily, sugar is grown agriculturally and much of the American industry has moved to the island to take advantage of inexpensive labor. Jamaica historically provided aluminum ore (bauxite) to a world entering the age of air and space. The Virgin Islands next door actually was sold by the nation of Denmark to the United States! The US dollar is the medium of exchange in this nation, which is like other islands in the world considered being an insular part of the United States. The Virgin Islands is the first of the Lesser Antilles we will discuss in the Caribbean. Unfortunately, due to high demand in the United States, drugs are a valuable resource in the Caribbean. Narcotics trafficking can make people rich as they try to enter the United States. **Offshore banking** is a means of escaping the tax burden that has grown in the United States, for example, while maintaining close proximity to American businesses. Compared to the banks of Switzerland, drugs, tourism and offshore banking are all heavily influenced by the American economy.[1]

Two island chains coming from off the northern coast of South America—the Windward Islands that eventually become the Leeward Islands to the north, form the Lesser Antilles. Aptly named for their exposure to the sometimes violent storms emerging from the Atlantic Ocean, these beautiful islands actually share more than their local cultures. The entire region of the Gulf of Mexico and the Atlantic coasts of Venezuela and the countries of northern South America share a Caribbean-type regional culture. A visit to Charleston, South Carolina, or New Orleans will give a hint of this atmosphere.

---

[1] Plaid Avenger's World (Dubuque, Iowa: Kendall Hunt), 325.

Sugar has been an important resource of this area causing colonial competition throughout history and is partially responsible for an amazing diversity of people and cultures. The triangle of trade previously mentioned actually made the Caribbean the center of world trade (early globalization?) and in many ways was responsible for a series of world wars in the 18th century that were felt in North America. Perhaps inaccurately characterized as relaxed and laid back, the rhythms of this area seem to strongly suggest an indomitable joy despite the apparent challenges of the environment. Caribbean coastal cultures differing from the changing landscapes of Middle America and Mexico make this area potentially rich and important for the United States as we continue to view the areas in terms of opportunities for missions and enjoy the security of this southern area.

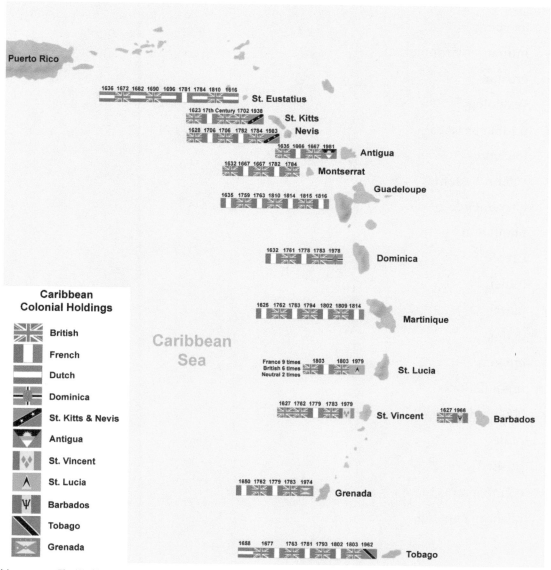

Map source: *The World Factbook*

KEY TERMS TO KNOW

- land form
- attenuated
- windward
- leeward
- Tierra Caliente
- Tierra Templada
- Tierra Fría
- hierarchical diffusion
- leaching
- human-environmental
- erosion
- vexillology
- middle passage
- hacienda
- viceroy system
- encomienda system
- plantation
- Creole
- mulatto
- plazas
- ejidos
- chiapas
- maquiladoras
- chain migration
- pulled
- pushed
- counter-movement
- offshore banking

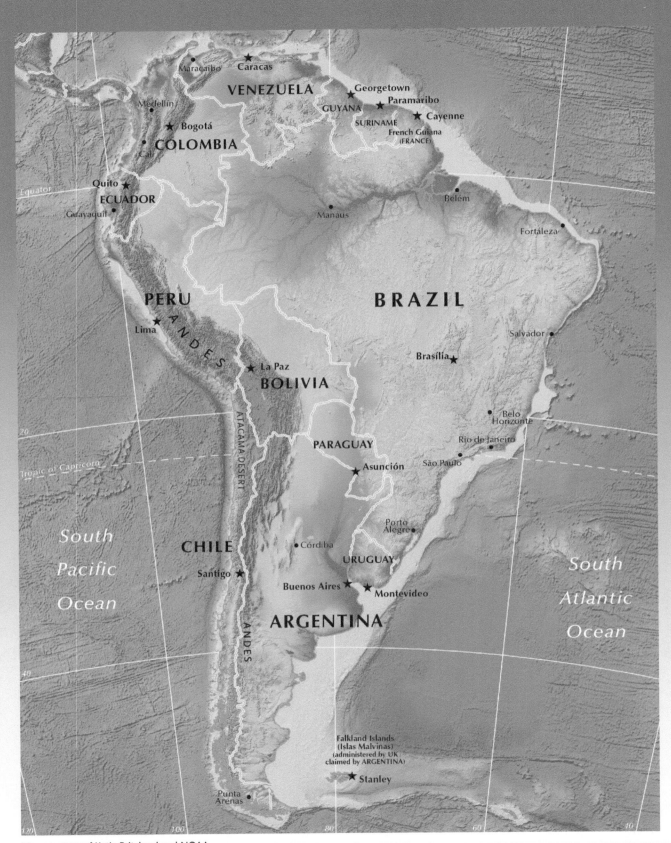

Map courtesy of Katie Pritchard and NOAA

South America

Praise the Lord, all nations! Extol him, all peoples! For great is his steadfast love toward us, and the faithfulness of the Lord endures forever. Praise the Lord! (Psalm 117:1–2)

Now the Lord is the Spirit, and where the Spirit of the Lord is, there is freedom. And we all, with unveiled face, beholding the glory of the Lord, are being transformed into the same image from one degree of glory to another. For this comes from the Lord who is the Spirit. (2 Corinthians 3:17–18)

"No matter what I do, I just can't seem to get an A in that class" are words frequently uttered by frustrated students. In fact, sometimes it seems we live on a treadmill and if we aren't careful we can spend a lifetime staying where we are and never "getting ahead." The scriptures remind us of the hardships of life and their temporal nature. The continent of South America has been described as a challenging one by most geographers, and sometimes it appears the situation is almost hopeless. Yet, hope never entirely leaves us if we simply give thanks for what we have. Blessed to see unlimited opportunity in South America, an entire continent waits for you to find your purpose in an area closer in many ways to North America than Europe!

The shape of South America resembles an ice cream cone with the majority of the continent in the tropics and a tapering cone transecting higher latitudes as it approaches the extremes of its southern limits. The size of South America is roughly three-fourths the size of North America, so it is a gigantic continent and one filled with an extreme diversity. From the hot humid rainforests of the interior to the cold dry windswept plains of Patagonia, South America offers an amazing array of animal and plant species—each reflecting a different biome and climate. To understand the climates one must understand the currents.

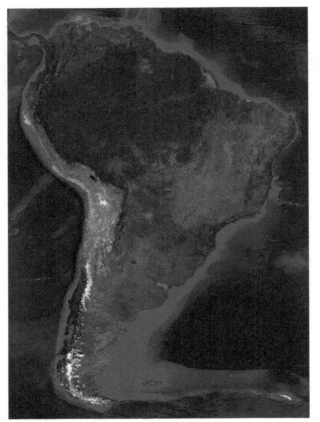

Adapted from *Blue Marble: Next Generation* image by Reto Stockli, NASA Earth Observatory (NASA Goddard Space Flight Center)

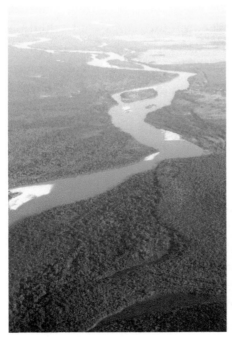

Image © Frontpage, 2013. Used under license from Shutterstock, Inc.

The currents of South America are moving in directions somewhat the opposite of what we would expect for the northern hemisphere. Since Earth's southern hemisphere is mostly water, it is easy to forget the change in direction of the water and atmospheric flows due to the Coriolis effect. These currents are important to understanding the climates of South America. The west-wind drift is responsible for the cold-water current commonly known as the Humboldt Current that proceeds up the coast of South America from the South. This cold water creates turbulence as it meets warmer water and as it rises up from the ocean floor. Similar phenomenon occurs off of the coast of Japan and North America and, like Peru and Ecuador, is key to understanding the excellent fishing resources and the subsequent effects on culture in these areas. Another aspect of the position of South America relative to the rest of the Earth's surface is El Niño.

The El Niño event is characterized by a shifting of the currents towards the west. The moving of the currents toward Australia, according to some, may have tended to increase dryness there. As these pressure changes periodically reverse and move the large circular patterns of the ocean to the east of the continent of South America, the Humboldt Current diminishes considerably. On other occasions, the currents of the southern Pacific move further to the east and this enhances the effects of the cold currents off the coast of South America. An integral aspect of the climate of South America and the history of the area is the relief.

Overcoming the "Curse"

South America is surrounded by high ground throughout much of the continent. The Andes Mountains actually extend from Venezuela westward through Colombia and Ecuador and then southward into Peru and Bolivia and even down to Chile and Argentina. The northern most parts of South America see the Guinea Highlands and to the south of the equator on the eastern side of Brazil are the Brazilian Highlands. These mountains had the effect of making settlement into South America a severe challenge, and this, in turn, has characterized what some geographers call the "Curse" of South America. One of the largest rivers in the world, the Amazon, pours into the ocean and due to its location on the equator makes traveling up the river very challenging. The Amazon is probably the most navigable of the rivers, yet its typically east west flow pattern generally insures that travel is restricted in this direction; moreover, there are no major cities serviced by the Amazon. Perhaps the most temperate climate in South America is found in Uruguay and northern Argentina, but even developments in this area were delayed due to the currents of the southern hemisphere and their counter-clockwise motion away from the continent. Obviously, the interaction of the continent of South America has had an important interaction with the global phenomenon of currents that create the climates, but the effect of relief also plays a key role in the rich diversity of the climates displayed and the biomes that survive there.

The climates of South America are—as you might expect—tropical. From the Caribbean to southern Brazil and Bolivia, the tropical, wet climate is encountered with the biome of the tropical rainforest. Throughout the southern cone-shaped area of South America, the humid subtropical climate is similar to the southeastern United States in terms of moisture but perhaps a bit cooler on average with seasons. As one

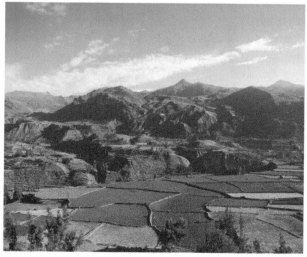

Image © ckchiu, 2013. Used under license from Shutterstock, Inc.

approaches the snow-covered mountains to the west, the land becomes much drier and grasslands appear. The biome here is similar to the American central plains and interestingly at one time, according to Alfred W. Crosby, supported herds of cattle equal in size to those of the great bison herds of North America.[1] It is little wonder that the Europeans eagerly brought their cattle with them to this short, grassland biome. As you would intuitively guess, the mountains of the Andes are very cold and dry and reflect the highland climate mentioned in this book's introductory chapter. As in Middle America, the varying relief patterns produce a varied agricultural outpouring depending on elevation. One particular type of produce that has changed the world is the potato. The potato originated in the central Andes, possibly in eastern Peru or northern Bolivia. Like the tomato mentioned in a previous chapter, this food item affected the culture and population of the world dramatically.

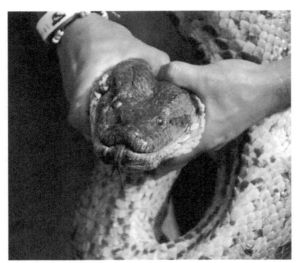

Image © Vadim Petrakov, 2013. Used under license from Shutterstock, Inc.

Anyone interested in biological diversity will not be disappointed by a study of South America. From the dendrobates frog—one of the most lethal creatures on Earth—to the electric eel, the Amazon basin presents wonders of creation. The huge anaconda as well as vampire bats have been unpleasant neighbors for the denizens of the basin for years and yet, the enormity for potential in South America has long been overlooked. Located in proximity midway between the North American continent and Europe, this example of relative place makes South America ideal for future development within the global economy.

Bolivia is an interesting case. As one of only two landlocked countries on the continent—the other being Paraguay—it really is two countries in terms of relief as are the other countries of the Andes Mountain sub regions of South America. The **Altiplano** to the west is a high plateau that contains the famous Lake Titicaca. This lake provides much needed moisture to the dry arid higher elevation of the Altiplano. Extremely high in elevation, this dry, often cold and snow-covered volcanic mountain landscape stands in sharp distinction to the eastern and northern parts of Bolivia. To the east of the Andes Mountains is the southern extreme of the Amazon watershed and in the east dropping from over 20 thousand feet to nearly sea level. Resources in Bolivia have represented the challenges politically facing the people of Brazil.

---

[1] Ecological Imperialism: The Biological Expansion of Europe, 900-1900 by Alfred W. Crosby (New York: Cambridge, 1997), 178.

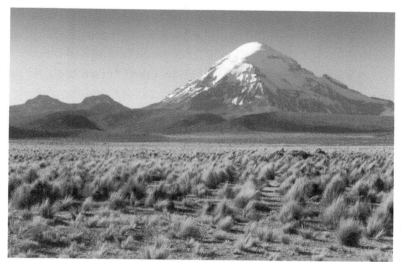

The altiplano of the Andes Region.

The Coloquiri mine near the capital city of La Paz has produced silver and tin for years. Recently President Evo Morales, one of the first Native American presidents to be elected in South America, has nationalized the mine amid discord that has brought rioting into the streets of the cities as rival mining workers fight for control. The economic divide is reflective of the ethnic divisions in Bolivia. The Native American or indigenous peoples of the highlands stand in contrast to the mestizo or people of mixed Spanish-speaking heritage in the Amazon basin or lowlands to the north. The loss of millions of dollars has done little to help the people economically. An attempt to export natural resources such as natural gas to the United States has been delayed due to the landlocked nature of the country. Attempts to export resources to the United States have initiated attempts to export through Argentina.[2]

Paraguay is the other landlocked country in South America. Recent interest in **Paraguay** has led numerous mission teams from various churches into the area. The Mormon Church has been very successful in this traditionally Roman Catholic area. The language of **Guarani** has attracted many scholars dedicated to developing scripture into this area. The **Gran Chaco** spreads through the center and west of Paraguay and is a hot plain that is quite dry and borders the **Piranha** and **Paraguay Rivers**, both flowing south into the **Rio de La Plata** off of the coast of Uruguay and the **Pampas**

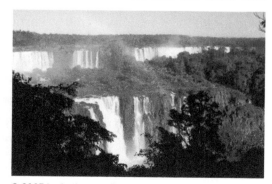

© 2007 JupiterImages Corporation

---

[2]Geography: Realms, Regions, and Concepts by deBlij, Muler and Nijman (USA: Wiley, 2012).

of Argentina. Another interesting area in Paraguay is known as the triple frontier area. This controversial **frontier** is partially claimed by Brazil, Argentina and Paraguay and has even seen the threatened use of military force in an attempt to control this powerful waterway project known as Hidrovia. The Hidrovia waterway project possesses an enormous potential for production of hydroelectric power and for obvious reasons is an area highly sought by the rival nations of the region. Recent economic developments to include the **Mercosur** trading bloc of South American nations has been a problem for Paraguay.

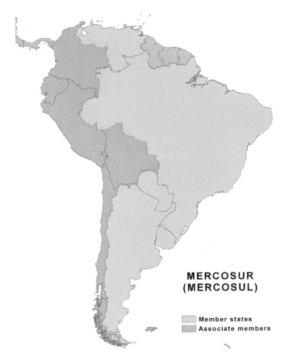

MERCOSUR (MERCOSUL)

Member states
Associate members

Map courtesy of Katie Pritchard

Resentment exists in this landlocked nation since its suspension from the trading bloc for political reasons recently. Particularly galling to the Paraguayans is the recent acceptance of Venezuela, which has been admitted for membership into the trading bloc, one of the largest in the world behind the European Union in terms of **GDP** (Gross Domestic Product)—the total value of goods and services produced within the state. Perhaps another example of the struggles of a landlocked nation is the fact Paraguay still utilizes the Mercosur system in its attempts to export products abroad as it needs to use transportation routes through surrounding countries in attempts to reach the ocean.

The Apex

The southern cone or apex of South America consists of Argentina, Chile and Uruguay. With an increasingly temperate and dry climate as one heads south, it is no surprise the cultural landscape of Uruguay has attracted numerous immigrants from Europe over the years. Uruguay possesses enormous potential as a developing economy with the valuable port city of Montevideo on the Rio de la Plata. Somewhat slowed in settlement by the direction of the currents in the southern hemisphere; nevertheless, Spanish culture continued to grow in this area and spread into Argentina. The famous Pampas region may be the cultural heart of such terms as ranch and lasso and other words reminiscent of the American west. The Argentines have seen their economy challenged in recent years by varying political successes. An inability to harmonize labor interests and the demands of various locals has tended to make foreign investment somewhat problematic for the hopes of developing Argentina. Sovereignty issues surrounding the Falkland Islands generally are concerned with the potential of offshore mineral resources.

Irridentism and Attenuation

Chile is perhaps the most **attenuated** nation on Earth. Its strangely elongated shape is a function of natural geography—the Andes Mountains! In recent years the mines of the Atacama Desert have produced valuable metals to include copper. Perhaps one of the strangest natural landscapes in the America's can be seen here with ancient monkey puzzle trees replicating our redwood trees, small Andean Mountain cats and tiny deer can be seen there. A mysterious and wonderful continent, South America offers unparalleled opportunities for serving others through whatever vocation one might choose—ministry, business or agriculture.

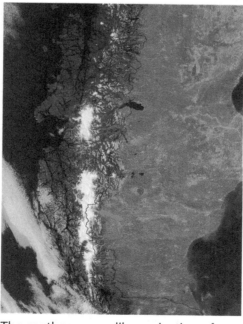

Blue Marble: Next Generation image by Reto Stockli, NASA Earth Observatory (NASA Goddard Space Flight Center)

The southern cone-like projection of South America.

Perhaps no greater opportunity to help South America comes in the sub region of the northwest or the high Andes Mountains. The Andes Mountains extend north as far as Venezuela and we see the familiar pattern of bifurcated climates as functions of relief. Standing in sharp contrast to the western cool mountain regions are the moist, hot Amazonian basin regions to the east of the countries of Peru, Ecuador and Colombia. Accusations of irredentism can be made when drawn borders do not necessarily reflect natural borders. When a government attempts to expand its borders into areas where there are perceived cultural similarities, **irredentism** can occur. This has not been a particularly large problem in South America, but much success has been made in recent years by the government of Colombia against the FARC insurgency.

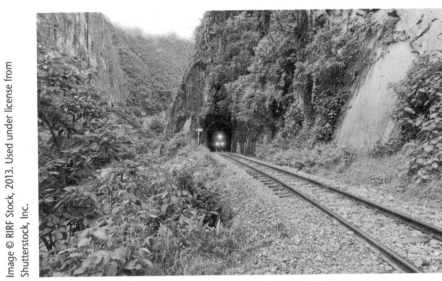

Image © RIRF Stock, 2013. Used under license from Shutterstock, Inc.

Transportation follows level terrain when possible.

Strategically important to the United States, these countries off the fertile Pacific coast have seen insurgencies as varying groups claim authority and potentially dangerous frontier areas such as between Colombia and Venezuela. The most important potential from a transportation viewpoint may be the recent attempts by the Colombian government to provide transportation nodes between the Caribbean Sea and the Pacific Ocean. Like Panama (formerly a state of Colombia), this relative location between two large bodies of water runs into the harsh realization of what seems to be a constant in South America—contrasting physical geography! The Cordillera Central and Cordillera Occidental and Cordillera Oriental mountains transect the industrial areas and Colombia's attempted development of transportation routes. Rainforests also stand in the path of attempts by the Colombian government to reduce shipping costs, which are notably higher for Colombia than Peru or Ecuador on the coast. Attempts to use railroads and investments in river dredging my eventually produce much potential for the nation of Colombia.

The sad legacy of drug use from South America through the Caribbean and into Mexico has led to the creation of a trail of misery, which is so preventable. The richest nation on Earth's high demand for drugs has produced armies recruiting boy soldiers and left gang wars in its path. Enormous profits at minimal investment have made drug production very profitable and have made many areas of the northern Andes very dangerous and frontier like. In their attempts to gain power, numerous gangs use the money obtained from their drug deals to achieve parity in power with the elected governments. Eventually the governments and these groups enter into relationships and finally a power struggle exists to clarify who is in charge. Too often it is the mission of the military in this country to maintain or enforce the structural order of the society. Life is indeed hard, but when one uses these illegal drugs they are not only hurting themselves, but others as well particularly in South America.

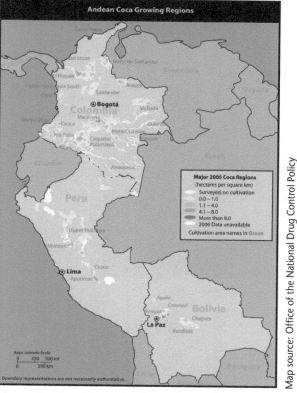

Map source: Office of the National Drug Control Policy

The agricultural hearth of cocaine.

The Caribbean coast of South America is somewhat different ethnically and culturally then other parts of South America. Oftentimes the descendants of slaves, the former European colonies of Suriname, French Guiana and Guyana enjoy access to the Atlantic Ocean. It is not surprising to meet people of various European and South Asian peoples. Besides amazing diversity, the European Space Port is actually located in French Guiana. The relative location in proximity to the equator allows spacecraft the ability to obtain speeds more easily, necessary to depart the atmosphere. A new resource perhaps in an age of space, nevertheless traditional resources such as gold has also been discovered there.

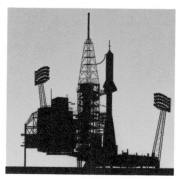

Image © VALIK-NOVIK, 2013. Used under license from Shutterstock, Inc.

No Habla Español

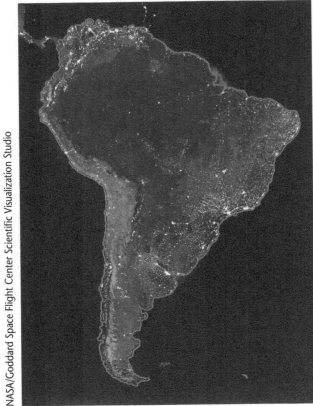

NASA/Goddard Space Flight Center Scientific Visualization Studio

South America at night. Note the majority of lights are coastal!

The huge nation-state of Brazil illustrates many of the geographic challenges facing South America. According to some sources it has about the fifth highest population of any nation in the world as well as about fifth in size of the world's nation-states. Speaking Portuguese, a legacy of the Treaty of Tordesillas itself reminiscent of the slow progress made in exploring South America due to the location of the specie required in the age of exploration and the challenges of the currents. Look at the locations of the major cities such as Rio de Janeiro and Sao Paulo and you will see how they are relatively near the coast. This coastal location of the cities of South America reflects a colonial pattern seen also in Africa and India to see opportunities of trade but perhaps not permanent settlements.

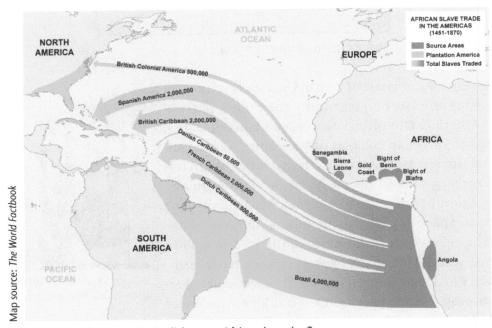

Map source: *The World Factbook*

Where in the America's did most African's arrive?

Recent attempts to settle into the interior of the continent have led the Brazilians to adopt a forward capital strategy similar to Pakistan's. The placing of Brasilia has been an attempt to reinforce the control of the wild interior region of Brazil. By placing the capital city there, people are forced to live in the area to work in the government and the hope is this will pull industry into the interior. The city of Manaus has demonstrated the human-environmental effect of settling into the interior. The precious and diversity of organisms in the rainforest have led to an appreciation of the great sensitivity of many of these specialized species. The southeastern region of Brazil is an industrial core where gold has been discovered in the past. To the far south, more European type agriculture prevails with crops ranging from grapes to rice. This wealthy area stands in contrast to the northeastern part of the country where a large percentage of the population occurs but where very little production occurs. The cities of Brazil are somewhat different from what you might expect to find in the United States.

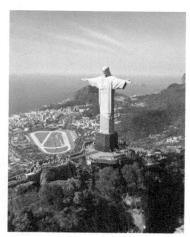

Image © Mark Schwettmann, 2013. Used under license from Shutterstock, Inc.

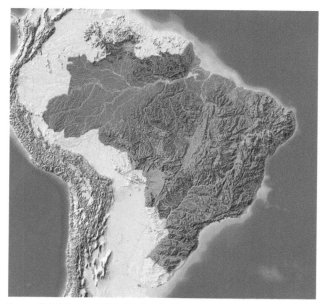

Image © AridOcean, 2013. Used under license from Shutterstock, Inc.

Unlike the United States, many of the more prosperous people in Brazil's huge cities live downtown. More properly, they probably live on an urban spine or main road that leads downtown. Again, whereas in the United States the more affluent tend to live in the suburbs, in South America generally and Brazil in particular we find the shantytowns of poor individuals who tend to live in the outskirts of the city where they must travel to get work. The cultural landscape can be quite different as well. Regardless, the opportunities for American ministry in Brazil remain despite the growing prosperity of the nation.

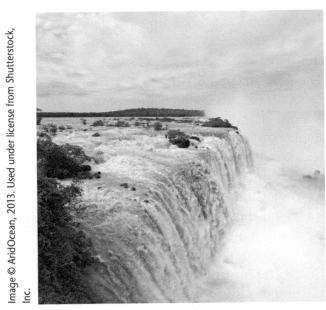

Image © AridOcean, 2013. Used under license from Shutterstock, Inc.

Brazil: Hydro-power house!

Sugar, Sugar

Brazil has led the way in recent years due to its production of alternative fuels. One fuel in particular is gasohol and is an extract from the sugar cane. This is a much more effective energy source than the ethanol used from corn. Brazil has had enormous potential for the future for several years and probably will continue to represent many opportunities for industry and missions in the years to come!

KEY TERMS TO KNOW

- Altiplano
- Paraguay
- Guarani
- Gran Chaco
- Piranha River
- Paraguay River
- Rio de La Plata
- Pampas

- frontier
- Mercosur
- GDP
- attenuated
- irridentism

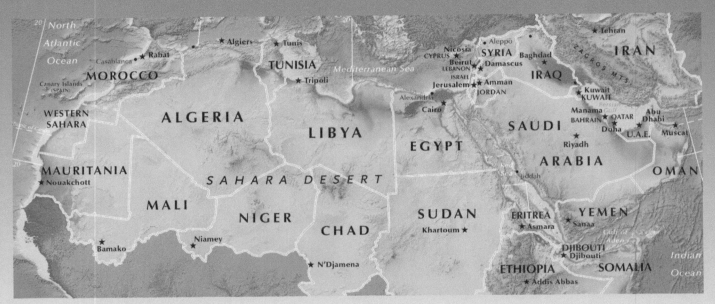

Map courtesy of Katie Pritchard and NOAA

North Africa and the Middle East

But the Lord sits enthroned forever; he has established his throne for justice, and he judges the world with righteousness; he judges the peoples with uprightness. The Lord is a stronghold for the oppressed, a stronghold in times of trouble. And those who know your name put their trust in you, for you, O Lord, have not forsaken those who seek you. (Psalm 9:7–10)

Have you ever felt your best just isn't good enough? This burdensome thought often pervades our thinking and can be a cruel fallacy that knows no boundaries. In the region we will cover in this chapter dwell various peoples, many of whom are doers of their religion rather than just spectators. The religiosity of this people can be treated with nothing less than respect. And yet, a loving relationship with a creator is an increasingly new experience for many of them. The part you might play in the future of this region by demonstrating your faith is unlimited. We can be cheerful in the realization our best is good enough for our Creator, thanks to His Son!

Why So Dry?

When Jesus said, "Don't worry about what you will eat or drink . . . " very few of us consider the drink part of the statement. In North Africa and what is referred to as the Middle East, this is a real problem however. In fact, it is not a stretch to identify the culture of this part of the world as a function in large measure of the paucity of fresh water. The rivers and melting snows of this part of the world have been instrumental in producing patterns of human distribution. With these distributions of population have emerged different outlooks and worldviews. Perhaps from these schools of thought come many of the news headlines we see today.

Rifts and Rafts

The first thing one notices about this region of the world is it is mostly arid. The obvious similarities in the shape and direction of the Red Sea and the Persian Gulf betray a pattern of tectonic activity that may, in part, explain this desiccation. In fact, the processes affecting the Earth's surface are largely responsible for the relief and mountains that both block precious moisture and yet unevenly distributes much of the valuable fresh water this area so desperately needs. Famous for trade, Arabs and Persians alike have traveled the Indian Ocean spreading trade and Islam as far as Indonesia. This "wet road" in many ways rivaled the famous overland route sought by the ancients called the Silk Road.

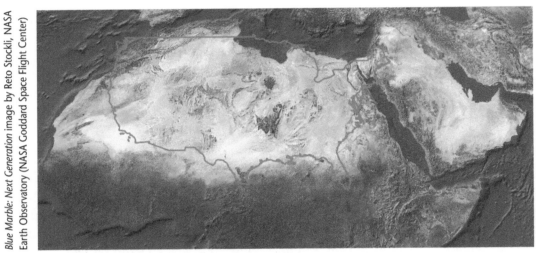

Blue Marble: Next Generation image by Reto Stockli, NASA Earth Observatory (NASA Goddard Space Flight Center)

The Sahara (Arabic for Great Desert) is great indeed!

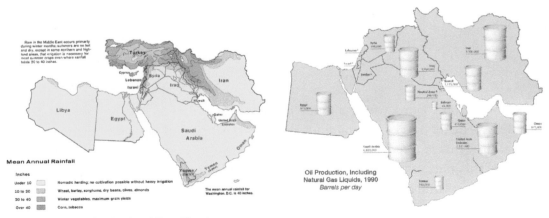

CIA maps courtesy of University of Texas Libraries

Water and Oil—both essential for survival and trade.

The precious fresh water initially in the form of mountain springs and eventually flowing as rivers are in different measures captured and distributed by the Atlas Mountains, the Zagros Mountains in Iran and the Caucasus Mountains to the north standing guard next to the Taurus Mountains in Turkey that also work in tandem with the Hadley Cells (see the introduction) to block moisture from entering the area. These rivers and their precious water help explain the earliest civilizations where Noah and his family settled down, and many Bible scholars believe Nimrod settled into this area. Fierce but ephemeral empires such as Assyria and Babylonia alternately rose and fell inevitably to be conquered by peripheral areas. The availability of fresh water in this area also explained how civilization occurred. Differentiation of labor—different jobs in a society—existed once a surplus of agriculture could be obtained. The resulting population and subsequent growth of cities brought into being an important dynamic in the human experience that remains with us today.

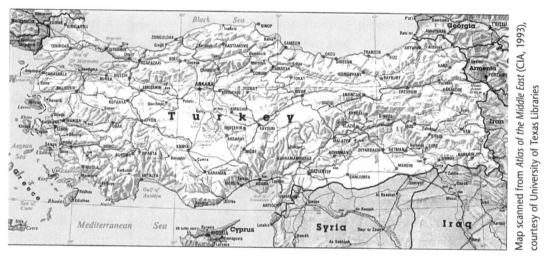

Map scanned from *Atlas of the Middle East* (CIA, 1993), courtesy of University of Texas Libraries

Asia Minor—Note the plateau that makes up most of the peninsula of Turkey—long a frontier between cultures.

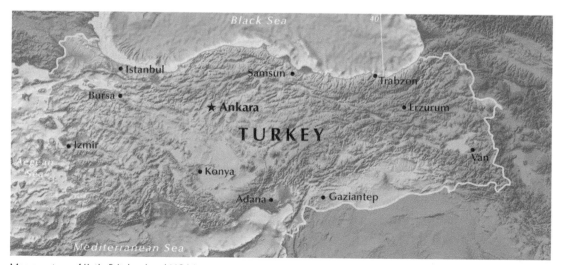

Map courtesy of Katie Pritchard and NOAA

Numerous empires have emerged in response to the availability of water, but why did they seem to fall and how does this relate to the tumultuous nature of the North African and Middle Eastern region today? The answer may lay in the concept of nomadism. **Nomadism** has been a powerful influence in the development of world civilizations generally but especially in this particular region. Nomads generally engage in what is known as movement, often somewhat cyclical in nature. This means basically they have to travel with the seasons to keep their livestock alive. Regardless, the coveted fresh water and soft life of the cities held a simultaneous appeal and repulsion that may in part explain the inherent totalitarianism that seems to exist throughout the region and the need for the state to remain vigilant against opposing ideas that may threaten it.

Modern day nomadism still continues to exist in North Africa along the coast of northern Africa and is responsible for a culture of nomadism that is referred to as **transhumance**. A popular expression, "heading to greener pastures," describes this well. As you might remember, nomads follow their herds of livestock since the wet or windward side of the mountains is moister. In a similar manner, the mountains of this region are responsible for the melting snows that flow into the Persian Gulf from the Euphrates and Tigris Rivers. Additionally, the Nile River branches into the Blue Nile with origins in the highlands of Ethiopia in the horn of Africa, and the White Nile, which originates in Kenya with Lake Albert in Uganda. So, the importance of tectonic plate activity over time and its effect on water supplies can easily be seen. How has this affected the Middle East today?

This Little Light of Mine

Some scholars believe the political systems of this region today reflect this disdain for softness correlated as wickedness and proof of irreligious or corrupting influences such as existed in harems and paradise gardens where water flowed and life was easy. To this day, political upheavals may occur when it is perceived the authorities are unable to defend their interests, or when it appears they have become dangerously close to the **Dar al Harb** or "house or land in rebellion" most often seen as the west. This idea is at odds with the **Dar al Islam** or idea of a world in submission to the "house or land of Allah." Perhaps a dualistic world-view of good vs. evil is in large part a perspective that can be correlated to the physical geography of the region of North Africa and the Middle East! We must respect the sometimes intense and conservative nature of Islam today. The very religious people who live in this region are without question sincere and this is proven by their adherence to the five pillars of Islam. It is important for Christians to bear this in mind when dealing with Muslims and amazing inroads of faith have been made in recent years. Religiosity can sometimes be wearying, as one can never be certain of obtaining salvation since one's works are never perfect. We do know through our God given faith that Jesus is God through his perfect obedience and submission to the father and His sinless life. This positive message of hope will always have an audience among our friends both in this part of the world and the entire globe!

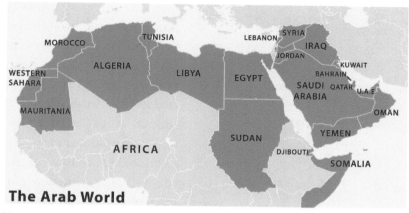

The Arab World

Map courtesy of Katie Pritchard

Submit

Generally we see three patterns of high population in this region. The North African Arabs are generally more sparsely populated over this area with the exception of Egypt. The aforementioned Nile River partly explains why Egypt is the demographic center of the **Arab** World. The Arab peoples share much in common to include ethnicity, language and culture, but perhaps the greatest single cultural factor uniting this part of the world is the religion of **Islam**. The ethnicity of Arabism is in large measure a function of language. From Iraq to Senegal the language of Arabic can be heard. This has given rise to the concept of pan-Arabism or a sense of pride based on an Arab identity. The wealthy states of the Persian Gulf with the power of oil money have according to some seen themselves as the leaders of the Arab World and may in some ways serve as opposing forces within modern Islam to the Turks and Persians.

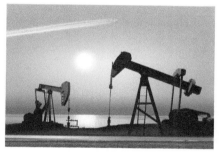

The religion of Islam is the primary unifying force in the Islamic world today. With its faith in what they call the one God Allah, the belief that his prophet Mohammed's writings have been preserved in the sacred text of the Koran and the various scholarly traditions associated with it. Muslims has successfully endured some of the harshest and most diverse climates on Earth. Still, differences do exist within the faith. It is particularly important not to overstate these differences, but they do exist. The Persians are generally of the **Shiite** form of Islam whereby the problems of the line of the succession from the Prophet extended to the son-in-law Ali. Most of the adherents of this form of Islam believe only God can choose the leader of their

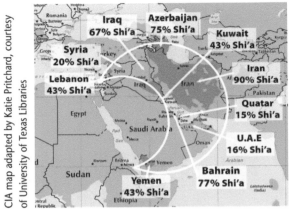

Shia and Sunni Islam in the Middle East.

religion. **Sunni** Muslims on the other hand, the predominant persuasion of the Arabs and Turks, believe that the succession from the Prophet should follow from the companion or father-in-law of Mohammed. Either way, though we as Christians are united by our faith and belief in the individual relationship we have with our Creator through his Son, we can certainly respect and appreciate the conviction of these people.

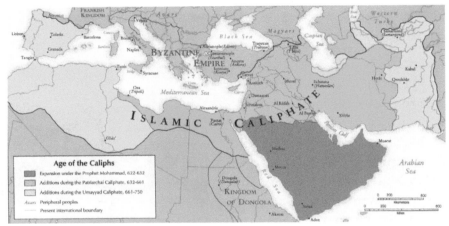

Map scanned from *Atlas of the Middle East* (CIA, 1993), courtesy of University of Texas Libraries

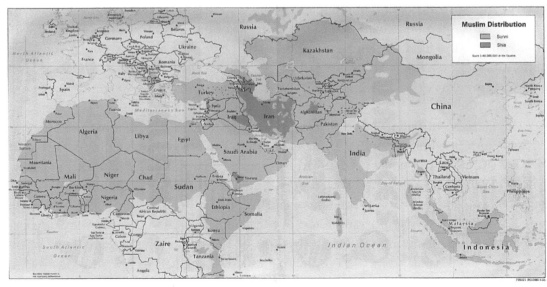

Map source: CIA map courtesy of University of Texas Libraries

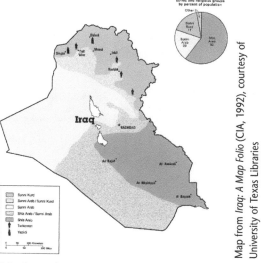

Map from *Iraq: A Map Folio* (CIA, 1992), courtesy of University of Texas Libraries

Ethnic and sectarian patterns in Iraq.

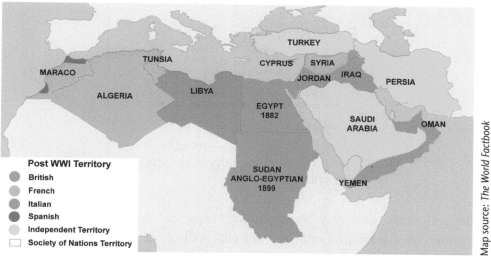

Map source: *The World Factbook*

How many borders do you recognize here?

Modest Trade

Another important aspect to the cultures of Islam is recognition of the social structures of gender. Women generally are to be respectful of men and a married woman of age covers her head in humility and submission. The men likewise see that the windows of the homes and the corridors leading into the home from the front door are maintained in this same spirit of modesty. There is much to be admired in the strength of the Muslim family and the increase in their population shows that fruitfulness abounds. In fact, the young increasingly inhabit cities in this part of the world. Some people believe the "Arab Spring" movement is a function of youth and social networks like Facebook.[1]

---

[1]Kaplan, Robert D. The Revenge of Geography (New York: Random House, 2012), 122.

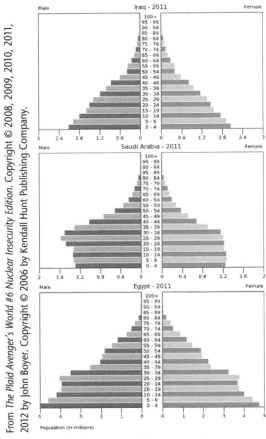

Population pyramids—note the number of young people in these Arab countries.

Trade has always been very important in this part of the world and the souks and bazaars generally are located near the old city walls or medinas of the cities. Trade through the Middle East existed in antiquity since Roman times and various empires of Europe have overtime sought access to the Euphrates and Tigris Rivers to gain access to the Persian Gulf as an alternative means of movement to China. Today we see a similar mixture of interests from both East and West in the Indian Ocean where China is attempting to gain access to valuable oil supplies. The western gateway to the Indian Ocean will continue to be an important region from a strategic viewpoint and one shared by Iranian and Arab peoples.

The cities in this region of the world tend to be similar to those in Europe in that a wall often exists reminiscent of ancient and medieval times when security remained a paramount aspect of life. The **medina** often contains the old section of the city and can be called a Kasbah. These aged roads are narrow and surrounded by high-walled buildings and are frequented by merchants in covered areas called **souks**. When the merchandisers are permanent and there is an enclosed area for their business dealings, it is referred to as a bazaar, which is a Persian word.

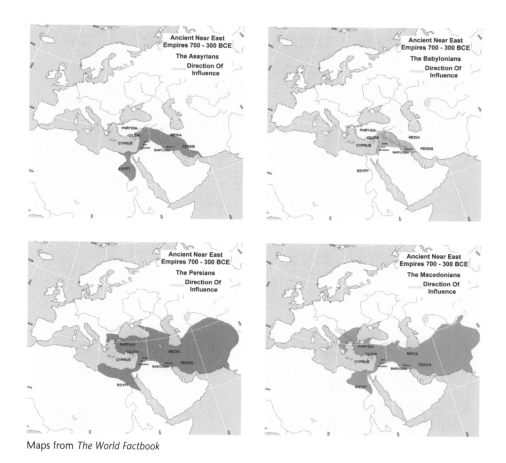

Maps from *The World Factbook*

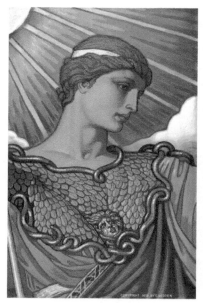

By Elihy Vedder, 1896, Library of Congress

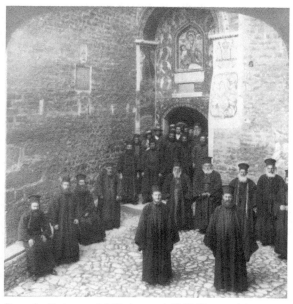

Stereo by Underwood & Underwood, 1907, Library of Congress

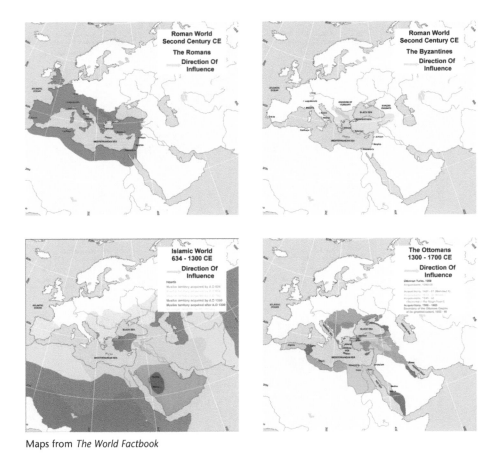

Maps from *The World Factbook*

It's Humanity's Fault (Line)

Two other important cultural zones of the North African/Middle East area are Turkey and Iran. These peoples have shared identity like the Arabs and tend to exist in greater numbers as a direct correlation to the amount of water available. The Turks today live on the Anatolian Plateau and share their nation-state with different peoples such as the Kurds. Water supplies are sufficient due to the elevation and the snow covered

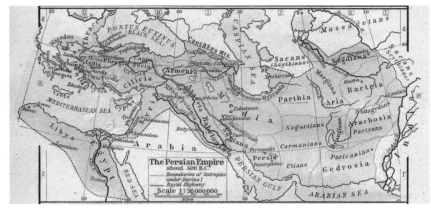

From *Historical Atlas* (1911) by William Shepherd, courtesy of University of Texas Libraries

mountains in winter that provide a checker-
board of high elevation lakes. The Turkish
people also are believed to have originated
as nomads in Central Asia and arrived on
the Anatolian Plateau in the last millennium, replacing the ancient Greeks and Persians before them. The Turkish language is
responsible for the many nations we see
with the suffix "-stan" on the end of their
names meaning "land of." The Turkish peoples have undergone many changes since
the First World War when they were a part of
the axis powers. Increased liberalization
throughout the 20th century may be changing due to increased conservatism in Mus-

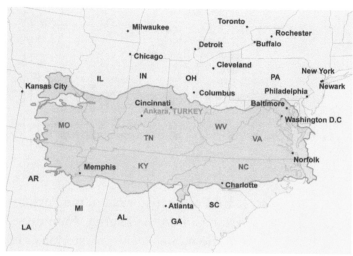

Map courtesy of Katie Pritchard

lim circles. We will see more about the Turks in the chapter of this book on Central
Asia. Another large nation with a high population that accompanies the headlines
these days is Iran.

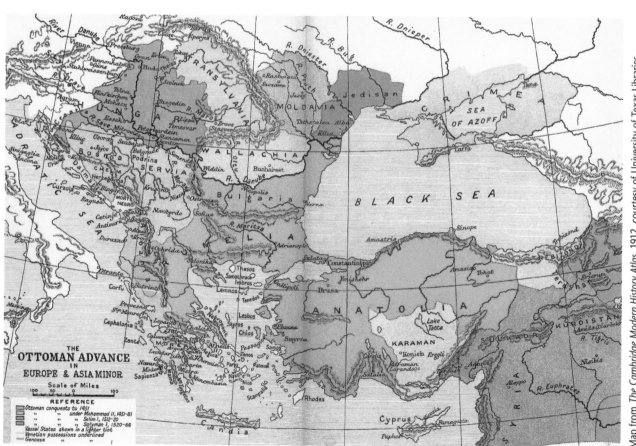

Note the Anatolian Plateau as a frontier region between east and west or Asia and Europe.

Map from *The Cambridge Modern History Atlas*, 1912, courtesy of University of Texas Libraries

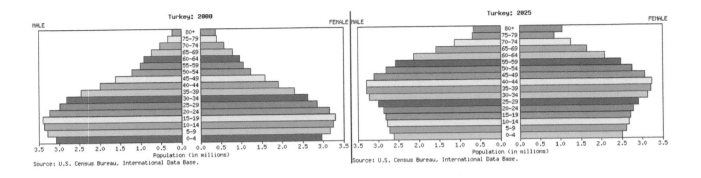

Iran or its historical name Persia is named for the region of Pars or Fars near the Persian Gulf in the Zagros Mountains. The term Iran is generally believed to be taken from the name **Aryan**, mysterious peoples believed by some to be from the cultural hearth of Eastern Europe or central Asia north of the **Caspian Sea**. Like so many other nomadic groups from this region such as the Scythians and Parthians, it is hard to be sure since written records are non-existent or at least very rare. The language of **Farsi**, the language mostly spoken in Iran today, originated or is named for this area. The

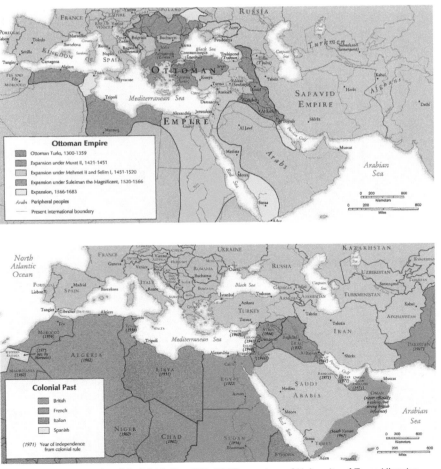

Maps scanned from *Atlas of the Middle East* (CIA, 1993), courtesy of University of Texas Libraries

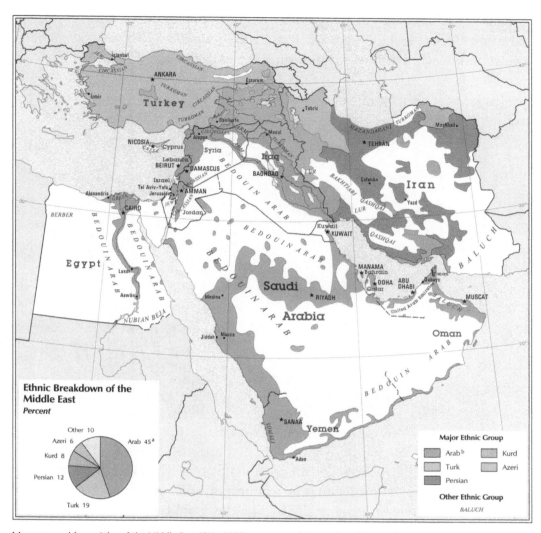

Map scanned from *Atlas of the Middle East* (CIA, 1993), courtesy of University of Texas Libraries

ancient city of Persepolis is located in Pars and was the ancient capital of the Persians who replaced the Medes and Elamites in controlling vital trade routes through the Zagros Mountains. The famous Persian bureaucracy consisting of expert bookkeepers managed a huge empire. Another example of a more dynamic people absorbing an established civilization, the Persians under Darius eventually would advance as far as Europe and India establishing a great civilization that traveled on roads and utilized post offices for transportation and communication. Many scholars believe the ideas of heaven and hell were first explained there with the dualistic religion of **Zoroastrianism**. In fact, Darius was able to convince his followers that foreigners were infidels in the words of Tom Holland and duty towards the King was in essence a religious requirement.[2] Regardless, the Iranian people have been a powerful influence in the world extending as far as Afghanistan to the west and to the eastern Mediterranean for

---

[2]Holland, Tom. Persian Fire (New York: Anchor, 2005).

thousands of years. It is fascinating to think of the prophet Daniel witnessing his faith to the king of Persia, and to watch the news headlines today as Iran again re-emerges as a power influencing the areas of its former ancient empire.

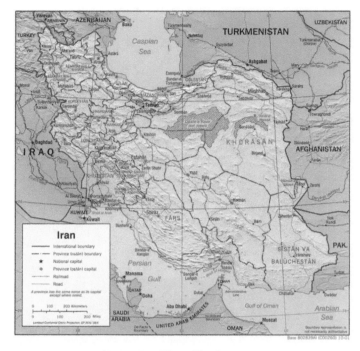

CIA map, courtesy of University of Texas Libraries

Wedged generally in-between the great states of Turkey and Iran is the area referred to as **Kurdistan**. Kurdistan is an example of a nation, but not a state. To be a **state** the borders should be recognizable to both the members (**citizens**) of that nation and others outside of the nation. **Nationalism**, the sense of shared history, culture and traditions is strong with the Kurds. While generally Muslims, there are Jewish

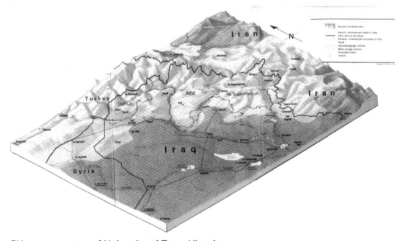

CIA map, courtesy of University of Texas Libraries

populations that claim their ancestry to the deportation of the Jews to Assyria that you may have read about in the book of II Kings in the Bible. The amount of faith required to maintain a culture when immersed into another is a testament to a disciplined and faithful scriptural study and the education or transmission of culture to subsequent generations. The employment of chemical weapons by Iraq accentuated the plight of the Kurdish people to the United States when chemical weapons were used against the population at the end of the Gulf War in 1991. A stateless people, the Kurds to this day are playing a very important role in the affairs of Arabs, Turks and Persians alike.

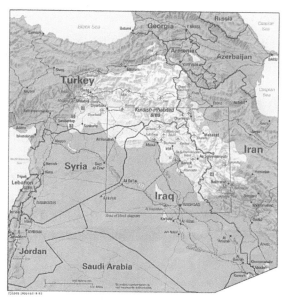

CIA map, courtesy of University of Texas Libraries

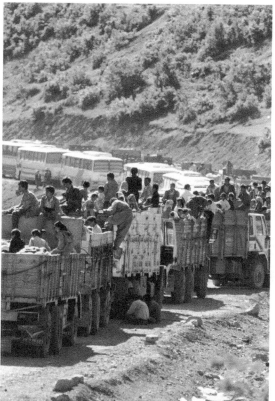

Dept. of Defense photo by PH₂ (AC) Mark Kettenhofen, U.S. Navy.

Kurdish refugees. All our families have been refugees or strangers at some time in the past.

Lone but Never Alone

The nation-state of **Israel** has survived against all odds in the Middle East and one with the only predominately Jewish population is Israel. On the border of the eastern Mediterranean Sea, the size of modern Israel is marginally larger than the state of New Jersey. The history of Israel in some ways seems to be a history of the world. Destroyed by the ancient Romans and then spread out during the diaspora, the ethnic religion of the Jews has survived against all odds and its existence is miraculous. Restored in large measure by British mandate after an unprecedented nearly two millennium diaspora or expulsion, the Jews returned under British authority after World War II while the world for a very brief period agreed to the existence of the state, partially as an outpouring of horror as the evils of the holocaust became known. The indigenous and now stateless peoples are the Palestinians who had been ruled by the Turks until the

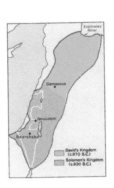 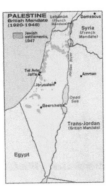 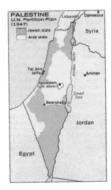 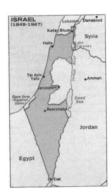 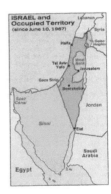

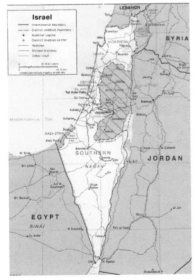

Maps from *The World Factbook*

end of World War I. After World War II, the United Nations in a rare display of unanimity agreed to recognize the state, but the age-old challenge of Jewish relations with the recently indigenous populations of Palestinians is reminiscent of the relations the Israelites had with the surrounding tribes at the end of the original Exodus you have read about. The United States remains a close ally with Israel and some believe the Israeli proficiency in technology has benefited this mutual relationship in terms of intelligence with the United States. Many Christians in the United States today sincerely hope the fate of the United States will continue to be intertwined with that of the nation-state of Israel, the only representative democracy in the Middle East today.

KEY TERMS TO KNOW

- nomadism
- transhumance
- Dar al Harb
- Dar al Islam
- Arab
- Islam
- Shiite
- Sunni
- medina
- Souks
- Aryan
- Caspian Sea
- Farsi
- Zoroastrianism
- Kurdistan
- state
- citizens
- nationalism

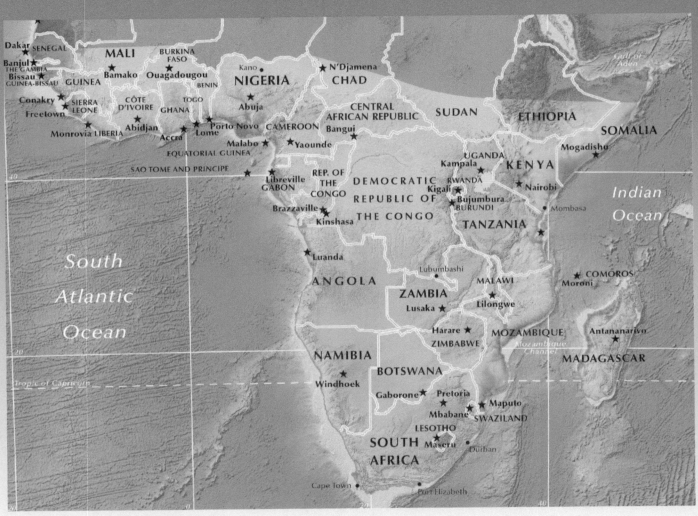

Map courtesy of Katie Pritchard and NOAA

Sub-Saharan Africa

Then children were brought to him that he might lay his hands on them and pray. The disciples rebuked the people, but Jesus said, "Let the little children come to me and do not hinder them, for to such belongs the kingdom of heaven." (Matthew 19:13–14)

Then the righteous will answer him, saying, 'Lord, when did we see you hungry and feed you, or thirsty and give you drink? And when did we see you a stranger and welcome you, or naked and clothe you? And when did we see you sick or in prison and visit you?' And the King will answer them, 'Truly, I say to you, as you did it to one of the least of these my brothers, you did it to me.' (Matthew 25:37–40)

Sometimes it seems we are drowning in wealth. A challenge for the author is simply to remain healthy by not eating too much! When sadness or depression strikes, as it inevitably does, we must immediately give thanks for what we have. Not everyone, however, is challenged to remember the blessings they receive, and consequently they can easily see the challenges around them. The continent of Africa is rife with problems like AIDS, and where so many families are not growing healthily from lack of a proper diet. Many children can become orphans or at least, not get the care they need. But God cares even for the children. When we begin to see the world through the eyes of Him who loves us, we can shake off our minor worries and concerns and be refreshed by serving those He also loves and who need some of our wealth and blessings. Where are the areas of need in Sub-Saharan Africa today?

Africa needs help just like the rest of the world! Its challenges like all of ours are primarily spiritual. To reach the continent with hope and to make a real difference, we must notice the uniqueness of the continent. Since the "great desert" or Sahara as it's called in Arabic is such a geographic barrier, we are dividing our discussion into two different regions—the area of the north that is predominantly dry and typically Islamic in culture and the southern part of the continent.

Notice the location of the continent of Africa on your globe. In addition to size, it is the most tropical continent on Earth. The equator runs midway through the continent

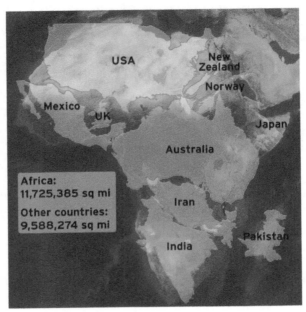

Adapted from *Blue Marble: Next Generation* image produced by Reto Stockli, NASA Earth Observatory (NASA Goddard Space Flight Center)

and as one might expect, this accounts for the warm moist climate of the interior. As one proceeds both north and south, the Hadley Cells discussed in the first section begin to reveal the phenomenon of wet-dry climates. These enormous areas of grasslands made famous in so many animal documentaries spread far and wide, but there are deserts as well. The deserts of the Kalahari and the Namib are a function of maritime influences below the equator where the cold waters of the Southern Ocean begin to spread into the Atlantic. It is the Atlantic Ocean that brought European explorers into contact with the Indian Ocean.

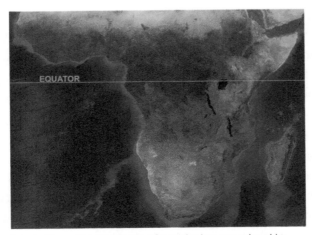

Adapted from *Blue Marble: Next Generation* image produced by Reto Stockli, NASA Earth Observatory (NASA Goddard Space Flight Center)

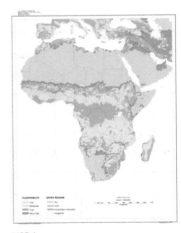

USDA map

Smooth and Groove

One of the challenges facing the student of geography is locating the numerous nations in Africa. One of the reasons there are so many small countries, particularly in West Africa, is because of the tendency of the explorers to trade from the coast. The explanation for this is simple; look at the coastline of Africa. It is one of the smoothest continents in the world. In fact, according to Robert D. Kaplan in the book, *The Revenge of Geography*: "Though Africa is the second largest continent, with an area five times that of Europe, its coastline south of the Sahara is little more than a quarter as long."[1] The additional problem is that the continent possesses few good harbors and very few navigable rivers from the ocean unlike Europe. The result was that European and Arab traders were forced to build temporary forts and deal with local chieftains. The arrival of the industrial revolution only intensified this hunger for resources and the manipulation of cultures to obtain them. The question then becomes: Did Europe progress technologically faster than the continent of Africa because of the paucity of ports, navigable rivers and smooth coastlines?

A deterministic perspective, or one that excludes a faith in God's power, would seek a geographical explanation. As Christians we should bear in mind, however, that God is the ultimate author of the Earth and all that is in it. Occasionally we get glimpses of patterns in His Creation. One interesting suggestion from the famous author Jared Diamond is that a lack of domesticated beasts of burden was instrumental in lower agricultural yields, which in turn prevented industry from prospering in Africa.[2] Another perspective explaining the challenges facing the continent historically and today is the landform. Essentially Africa is surrounded by escarpments from the coast and in the

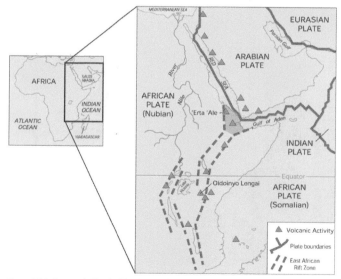

From *This Dynamic Earth: The Story of Plate Tectonics* (online edition) by W. Jacqueline Kious and Robert I. Tilling, prepared by U.S. Geological Survey

---

[1] Robert D. Kaplan, "The Revenge of Geography" (Random House, 2012), 31.
[2] Diamond, Jared. Guns, Germs, and Steel: The Fates of Human Societies, 91.

rift valley—a huge tectonic separation running from the horn of Africa in the northeast to Zambia. This difficulty penetrating the continent is reminiscent of South America and has been instrumental in the shaping of internal movements of various peoples, particularly from the west heading into the south. The European experience in Africa has been particularly important in shaping the political geography of Africa today.

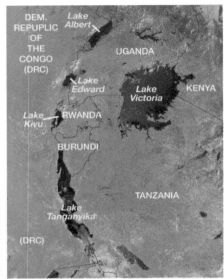

Jacques Descloitres, MODIS Land Rapid Response Team, NASA/ GSFC and Katie Pritchard

The lakes are representative of the rift caused by tectonic plates.

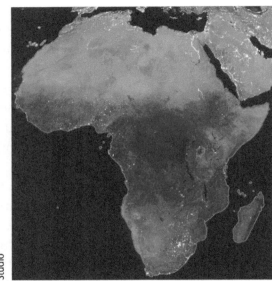

NASA/Goddard Space Flight Center Scientific Visualization Studio

Africa at night. The lights represent coastal-populated areas important for trade like in South America.

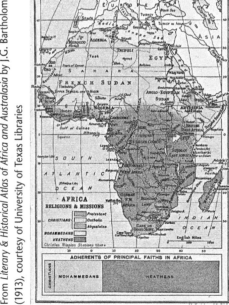

From *Literary & Historical Atlas of Africa and Australasia* by J.G. Bartholomew (1913), courtesy of University of Texas Libraries

The religious "fault line" of Africa.

Internally, we can see the effect on culture of the Great Rift Valley too. As you may remember from our discussion of North America, most movement of peoples and culture is often latitudinal in direction. When the Bantu-speaking peoples began to move, for example, from the western and central parts of the continent to the east, they encountered this famous rift valley. Note on the map the highlands and giant lakes such as Lake Victoria, Malawi and Tanganika. These lakes in large measure have the characteristic shape such as Lake Baikal in Siberia because they have also been formed by tectonic activity. So, the direction of water and high rifts or chasms tended to funnel travel towards the south where many of the peoples of western Africa eventually emerged. As late as the 17th century the Lundas continued this trend and the result has been a sort of geographic cul-de-sac on the southern end of the African continent! Once again physical geography has shaped the cultures and movements of people upon the Earth.[3]

Draw Mister!

Drawn borders in the south of Africa really represent European interests more as a genuine reflection of African political realities. Indigenous peoples travel the borders relatively freely, while those who are obviously of foreign ancestry will be carefully scrutinized. The legacy of colonial administration, the border often is drawn irrelevantly to the direction of most people's movement. The European powers for the

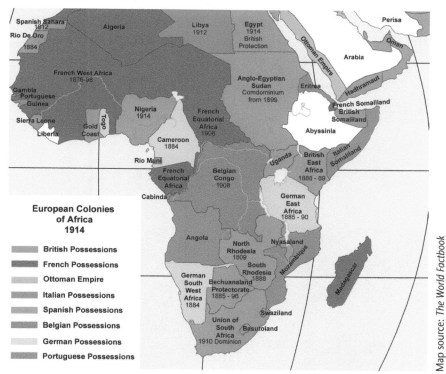

Map source: *The World Factbook*

Notice the "French Lake" in West Africa and the British attempt at a cape to Cairo railroad blocked by the Germans and Belgians.

---

[3]The Times Atlas of World History (United Kingdom: Hammond, 1984).

geographic reasons mentioned above tended to share and balance interests in Africa at various times. The French were particularly strong in western Africa while the British tended to be interested in areas adjacent to bodies of water important for naval purposes such as Egypt and South Africa. Even little Belgium claimed part of the action in the 19th century in the central part of Africa while the Germans and Italians nibbled at the eastern and Horn regions of the continent. These generalizations aside, the fact is today we are seeing a strong counter movement from the continent back to Europe.

Counter Movements

Many of those teeming and sometimes desperate folks attempting to arrive in Europe are attempting to escape terrible conditions and are seeking asylum. Many of these young people are heading to the countries that initially colonized the African countries, a type of counter movement. While the colonial experience is controversial, some saying hospitals, roads, and faith are good things to deliver, others point out that the exploitation of resources and the pitting of one group against another have more than compensated for the good deeds done by the colonial powers. Perhaps one of the most dire legacies of colonialism is the European tradition of drawn borders. These drawn borders do not correspond in most cases with ethnic groups and this has had fatal and horrific consequences. One relatively recent example of some of the problems resulting from colonization is the genocides that have plagued the continent. In particular the tendency to favor one tribe over another has tended to ignite tensions in places like Rwanda in the 1990's where the Belgium government had favored the Tutsis over the Hutus. When the Hutu tribes—people whom claim relationships on the basis of

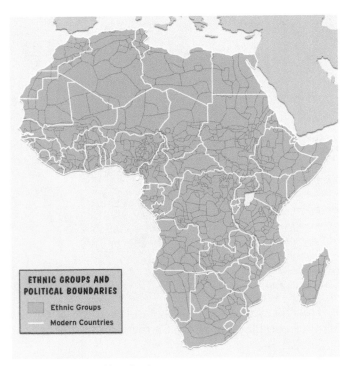

Map source: *The World Factbook*

ancestry or ethnicity—took power, retribution began. The outside intervention of Tutsi's from neighboring Uganda exacerbated the tensions and led to a fierce civil war claiming up to a million people. Retribution by the Hutu majority may have resulted in up to one million deaths.[4] This sad experience has been followed by genocides in the Sudan where countless numbers of Christians have dedicated their lives and money towards helping.

HELP! Hold the Line

In fact, Christians have held the line so to speak against Islam from Senegal to Ethiopia. It is of great interest to the geographer how this line representing the differing religions and cultures generally follows the Sahel—the dry area bordering the Sahara. Likewise, Christians have flocked to Uganda and Kenya over the years in an effort to help these countries obtain water and other vital resources. Because ministries are welcome here, the western nations have been able to donate time and money to these areas. Areas of Islam generally have been less friendly to Christian missions and simultaneously see intact family structures with high rates of childbirth. One area of opportunity will continue to be AIDS. In many regions of Sub-Saharan Africa this disease has reached gigantic proportions and the horror of AIDS shows itself in countries that often reflect an average age for males in the 40's as a result. Regardless of the need, Christians know Jesus loves the children and there is no better way to demonstrate His Love than to help His children in Africa today. But all is not bleak on the continent. Let us examine one of the richest areas—South Africa.

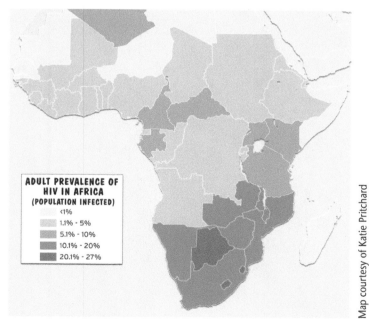

ADULT PREVALENCE OF HIV IN AFRICA (POPULATION INFECTED)
- <1%
- 1.1% - 5%
- 5.1% - 10%
- 10.1% - 20%
- 20.1% - 27%

Map courtesy of Katie Pritchard

A sad map of suffering in Africa.

---

[4]Prunier, Gérard (1995). *The Rwanda Crisis, 1959–1994: History of a Genocide* (2nd ed.). (London: C. Hurst & Co. Publishers), 4.

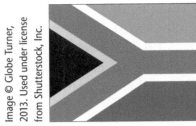

South Africa—one of only a few nation-states that have six colors in their flag!

Despite the relatively recent plague of AIDS, South Africa's GNP places it around roughly half that of Sub-Saharan Africa.[5] Blessed with numerous minerals and sitting in a strategic location on the southern point of Africa, this area of more moderate climates and mixed cultures ranging from European to indigenous peoples funneled south by the Rift Valley. South Africa is sitting on diamonds and gold as well as other less appreciated but nonetheless important resources like coal. Despite Africa's geographic handicaps and frustrating post-Colonial period, with faithful missionaries on the ground providing a genuine effort against diseases and loving a generation of children, the way could easily be set for the rise of an African revival of spirit and economy.

KEY TERMS TO KNOW

- Sahel

---

[5]http://www.tulane.edu/~internut/Countries/South%20Africa/southafricaxx.html

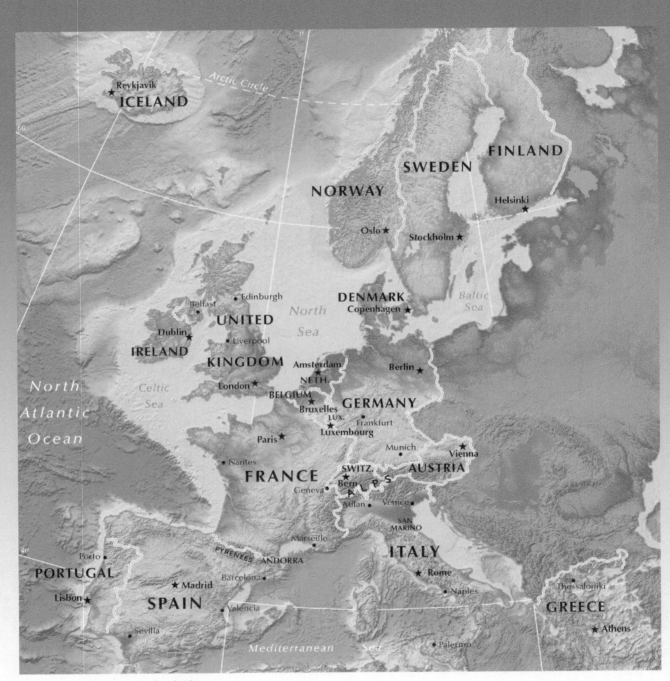

Map courtesy of Katie Pritchard and NOAA

Europe

But our citizenship is in heaven, and from it we await a Savior, the Lord Jesus Christ, who will transform our lowly body to be like his glorious body, by the power that enables him even to subject all things to himself. (Philippians 3:20)

For centuries people migrated from Europe in record numbers. A counter-migration is occurring today with people from the former colonies of the British Empire emigrating instead to the United Kingdom. Regardless of where people are, or where they are going, we must anticipate the opportunity to serve others where needs exist. The greatest need is—hope!

Peninsula of Peninsulas

Europe is an exciting **peninsula**! In fact, it is a series of peninsulas growing like tree branches out of a bigger peninsula. This series of landforms combines with the continent's relative location on the planet to reveal an amazing display of variety in cultures. These cultures have placed Europe on the cutting edge of changes from the Industrial Revolution to the growth of a supra-national government today. Europe is an exciting proof of the impact of physical geography on global cultures!

If you look at a globe and observe Europe from across your classroom, you will probably notice it is located to the extreme north of the world. In fact, New England in North America roughly corresponds with the region of southern France in terms of latitude. How is it that we see such differences in climate? The answer is simple, the gulf stream of currents travels from the warm sunny tropics and carries with it latent energy in the form of moisture. As this moisture precipitates, latent energy is released into the atmosphere and the result is warmth. This moisture is obviously an aid to the agriculture of the continent, but perhaps as important is the location of the seas and oceans that mark the borders of Europe.

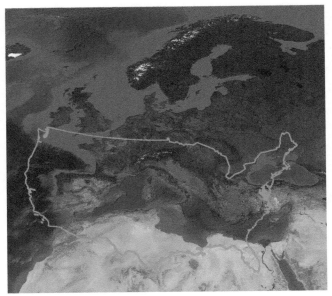

From *Blue Marble: Next Generation* image produced by Reto Stockli, NASA Earth Observatory (NASA Goddard Space Flight Center)

Going the Wrong Way–Naturally!

If you look at the map of Europe you will first notice the relatively east west pattern of the high mountains in the center—the Alps. As you look to the west, you will see the Carpathian Mountains that run in a semi-circular pattern through Romania, and as you follow the line of these mountains to the south, you notice the Dinaric Alps on the side of the generally longitudinally shaped Adriatic Sea. These mountains proceed south through the Balkan Peninsula and in effect mark the different plates, which come together to form Europe. In fact, if you look at all of the seas surrounding Europe

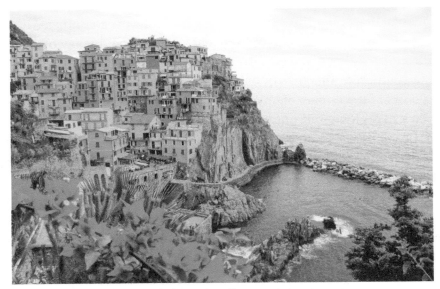

Image © JeniFoto, 2013. Used under license from Shutterstock, Inc.

they all seem to be flowing in distinct north-east-west patterns like the Black Sea and the Mediterranean, roughly parallel. Besides evidence of plate activity, the connection between these two seas has caused an interesting phenomenon of currents, which generally flow in a counterclockwise direction. Somewhat opposed to what one would expect the Coriolis Effect to display in the northern hemisphere, as explained by David Abulafia in his book *The Sea*; the Mediterranean Sea has a high evaporation of water. Because there are relatively few rivers to replenish the sea, the majority of the water comes flowing into it from the Black Sea.[1] This inflow and the subsequent phenomenon of a counterclockwise pattern in part, explain how the Apostle Paul and Christianity defused into the European continent from the Holy Land. It also explains some of the climactic differences we see in Europe, which also may in an indirect way help explain some of the challenges this continent confronts economically today.

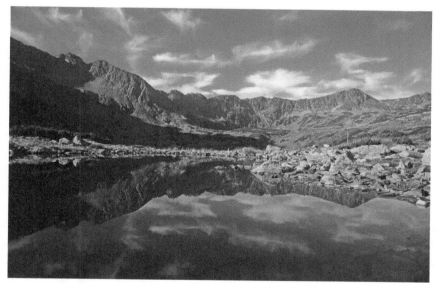

Image © falk, 2013. Used under license from Shutterstock, Inc.

Wet Skies/Dry Skies

The Mediterranean climate we described in the beginning of this book is certainly evident here! The warm, dry, sunny slopes of the mountainous regions of southern Europe no doubt contributed to the rise of a western civilization with a distinct culture. Many geographers believe the hills and mountains of the southeastern part of Europe lent themselves to independence and autonomy. These various city-states each had convenient climates for agriculture and enabled outdoor events to occur such as the Olympic races or events at the **acropolis**. Because the mountains tended to prevent any empire from taking control (such as ancient Persia), this tradition of the independent individual probably was a key to many of the freedoms Europeans were able to eventually develop. Contrasting with the cool, rainy, **maritime** climate of the northern

[1]Abulafia, David. The Great Sea (New York: Oxford, 2011), xxvii.

part of France, Britain and into Germany, in southern Europe, as one might expect, a warm, dry, Mediterranean climate exists.

Climatic differences in many ways may represent a **centrifugal** effect on the attempts to create a new European Union. Centrifugal effects are those that tend to pull peoples apart culturally. As you may know, **centripetal** forces pull us together. Examples of centripetal forces would be language, religion, ethnicity, etc. These forces can be illustrated as functions of changes in time over space historically.

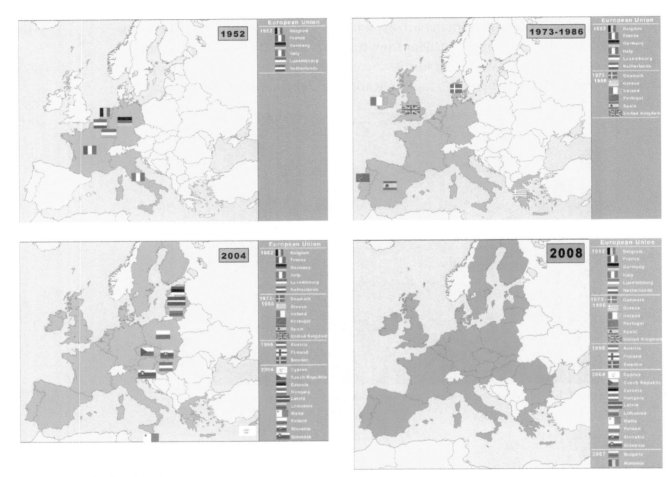

Maps courtesy of Katie Pritchard

Spread of Steam

A good starting point for discussing the effects of physical geography on European culture and how Europe is alternately pulled together and pushed apart is to note the spread or **diffusion** of the **industrial revolution**. The industrial revolution was a result of the agricultural advances (described in the third section of this book). With the advances in population and with a surplus of food, more manpower was available to be used in the burgeoning factories. The industrial revolution first appeared in Great Britain, which was spatially favored by an abundance of coal, iron and harbors for shipping. The rail lines, which quickly connected these resources, were instrumental in bringing people to the mines and factories where more machines were created. The development of steam engines continued to enable miners to dig deeper while the use of new iron smelting techniques utilizing purified carbon also known as coke to produce better grades of iron. Cities began to grow near the coalfields and the mines, and harbors enabled the goods to be shipped to a global market. This process would defuse to the continent of Europe.

The Belgians and Dutch were the next nations to receive the Industrial Revolution probably due to the proximity of the harbors to Great Britain, which delivered the machines and people to work on them. From the "low countries" the industrial revolution moved east and south into Germany and France. It is interesting to note that many of the debtor nations in the European Union today were some of the last to receive the revolution. It is quite possible that some of the cultural challenges we are seeing today are a result of the uneven spread of the industrial revolution. The urban landscape of Europe is also somewhat unique and reflects the history of Europe.

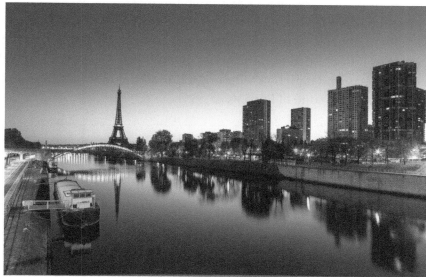

Image © Crobard, 2013. Used under license from Shutterstock, Inc.

The unique cultural landscape of Paris on the Seine River.

Generally the **CBD** or central business district of Europe's great cities presents relatively unimpressive skylines, at least compared to those of the bright shining cities of East Asia and even North America. With small narrow roads often designed to be negotiated on foot or by horses, the Europeans with only a few exceptions do not see the need to see their buildings becoming increasingly tall because of the high cost of land. These large, low, sky lined cities are generally surrounded by **greenbelts** or park areas where nature can be seen in contrast to the often somewhat denuded cities. The urban pattern of European cities often is centered on a river such as Paris with the Seine or London on the Thames. These **gateway cities** essentially represented portals to the world at various times from during the age of exploration until the scramble for colonies. So how do gateway cities and the diffusion of steam relate to European unity and dissension today?

With the European Union's emergence we have begun to see what is known as **supranationalism.** This is when people of various **nation states** (see Chapter 19) begin to work together to form a sort of supra state. Interestingly, because of Europe's history, and because of the strong influence of Middle Eastern and central Asian invaders through the valleys and plains of southern Europe, there seems to be a different view held of the individual's relationship to the state as compared to views held in northern Europe. Today, we see Germany attempting to persuade the Mediterranean nations of Portugal, Spain, Greece, and Italy to control their social spending programs. These recent attempts at unifying a **Eurozone** have run into some problems in recent years.

Push Me/Pull Me

One of the major challenges facing Europe as it attempts to unite in a spirit of supranationalism is the **demographics** of the continent. The population is increasingly seen as aging and this brings with it many consequences. One of the consequences of a population's aging is the paucity or lack of available labor. This causes friction because many of the immigrants arriving into Europe are doing so through what is known as the **periphery**. By periphery we refer to an area outside of the **core**, or more industrial area. In the case of Europe, this periphery is generally Eastern Europe, and this area with its relative poverty and high rate of immigration from lower latitudes threatens to put a halt to the Schengen Zone of Europe.

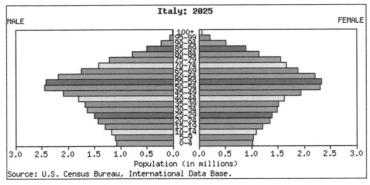

Map by Katie Pritchard

Europe has what can be described as various sub regions within the continent. These various differences in physical geography and climate have been demonstrated historically and are apparent today in areas of borders and in economic matters. In an attempt for example, to control illegal immigration and to protect indigenous or local labor, the Europeans have created a zone that allows border controls to be lifted called the **Schengen Zone.** Romania and Bulgaria are currently unable to enter the Eurozone and are sensing a second-class status by not being able to enter this Schengen Zone. The states of northern and western Europe are increasingly separated into a regional and cultural block from those of southeastern Europe because of their desires to protect the various social programs that protect their peoples. These sensitivities to economic concerns are not merely limited to the borders, however. One change that has tended to supersede borders has been recent attempts to lift air border controls.[2] Easier travel amongst these nation-states in Europe will no doubt have cultural ramifications and may serve to continue building transnational unity (centripetally), pulling the continent closer together.

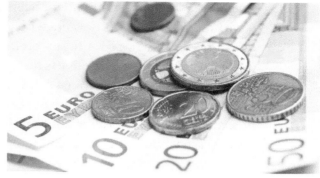

I owe, you owe—Euro!

The attempt to create a European Union has also created restrictions on who can enter this supranational organization, particularly in the economic downturn that occurred after 2008. The resulting austerity measures, resulting from this recession, have seen Germany attempting to pressure various southern European countries into controlling their amounts of spending for the purposes of keeping the **Euro** strong. Since Germany is the largest economy of Europe in many ways, it stands to lose if the credit it has given to southern European countries such as Italy, Spain, Portugal and Greece are not repaid. The countries of the Mediterranean region are more likely to feel exploited by what they perceive to be unfair austerity measures designed to force them into paying out to what they could perceive as conquering-type powers. Besides interregional problems between the creditor states of northern Europe and the emerging economies of the south, there are other regional considerations as well.

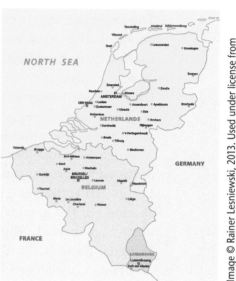

The vital ports of "Benelux" are easily seen in this map.

Where Does the Core End?

A major area of population in Europe is referred to today as the core. This **core** region consists of huge populations in the Low Countries of **Benelux**. Here we see Belgium with its famous port of Antwerp—so highly sought in World War II to supply invading allied forces—to Amsterdam in the Netherlands, the most populous city there. Relatively close to the great **gateway city** of London, these areas are the densely populated cores of Europe. Moving west from the "low countries" on the continent, we come to the Ruhr Valley with over eight million people. It is a massive urban agglomeration connected by a huge river. When the industrial revolution **diffused** from England to the mainland Germany is considered by some historians to have received the technology and associated social changes after Britain and the Dutch had embarked upon the quest for resources from colonies. This particular model would explain in part why the

---

[2]http://www.stratfor.com/situation-report/eu-shengen-area-enlargement-be-completed-march-30

Axis powers in World War I might have attempted to contest established borders out of a partial frustration in a new era with an aggressive world-view. Regardless, the population necessary to sustain any civilization is generally considered to be around 2.3 children per couple. Europe is not sustaining this rate of childbirth in an even manner. Poland currently has one of the highest rates of population on the continent followed by some of the other more peripheral countries. Without question, by tracing the diffusion of the industrial revolution from the island of Great Britain to the mainland, we also see areas of high population.

Members Only

Turkey has attempted to enter the **European Union** unsuccessfully for many years. The exclusion of one of the more liberal middle-eastern countries has caused some backlash as a result of perceived discrimination on the basis of religion. European exclusivity has not been confined to Turkey alone, however. The Baltic States recently were accepted into the European Union but states like Moldova, Belarus and the Ukraine have been excluded and there is very little prospect of these eastern European states or Russia being allowed to join the union anytime soon. It will be interesting to see if the supranationalism of Europe will be a centripetal force pulling the various **nation-states** together or if it will begin to come apart under the pressures arising between the creditor regions of northern Europe and the debtor regions of southern Europe. Only time will tell whether this continent—that at one time squabbled in the shadows of the greater empires of the Middle East and Far East—will maintain the advantage it received in the industrial revolution and the spread of capitalism and Christianity, or if it will decline into a multitude of different regions and peninsulas.

Remember Proverbs 14:4 —"Righteousness exalts a nation, but sin is a reproach to any people." (KJV)

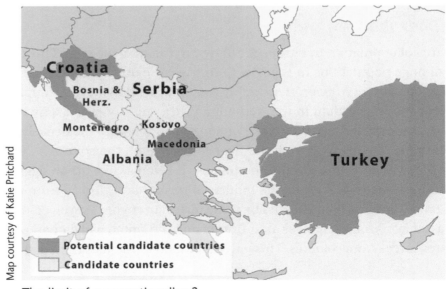

Map courtesy of Katie Pritchard

The limit of supranationalism?

KEY TERMS TO KNOW

- peninsula
- acropolis
- maritime
- centrifugal
- centripetal
- diffusion
- industrial revolution
- CBD
- greenbelts
- gateway cities
- supranationalism
- nation states
- Eurozone
- demographics
- periphery
- core
- Schengen Zone
- Euro
- Benelux
- gateway city
- diffused
- European Union
- nation-states

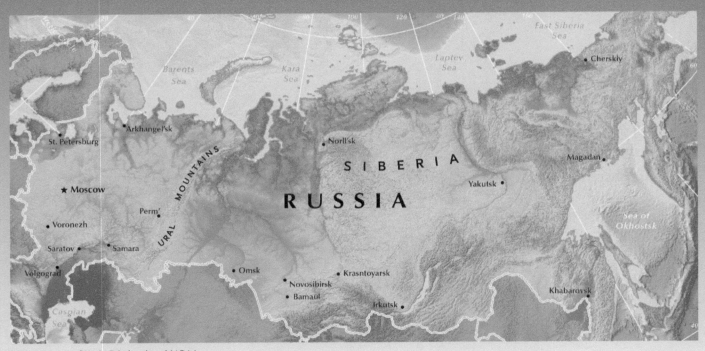

Map courtesy of Katie Pritchard and NOAA

Russia

Therefore I tell you, do not be anxious about your life, what you will eat or what you will drink, nor about your body, what you will put on. Is not life more than food, and the body more than clothing? Look at the birds of the air: they neither sow nor reap nor gather into barns, and yet your heavenly Father feeds them. Are you not of more value than they? But seek first the kingdom of God and his righteousness, and all these things will be added to you. Therefore do not be anxious about tomorrow, for tomorrow will be anxious for itself. Sufficient for the day is its own trouble. (Matthew 6:25–26; 33–34)

The Russians are a testament to endurance. They have persevered through challenges. What makes them so resilient, and will this resiliency continue is the question many geographers ask as they see the transformations occurring in Russia today. In Romans 5:3 we see where Paul tells us tribulation produces perseverance. Are you able to discern geographic challenges and lessons learned by the Russians that can apply to your own life?

Frozen Chosen

Russia is huge! The vastness and topographic relief of Russia have implications both for the cultures and the greatness of the nation-state on this largest landmass on the

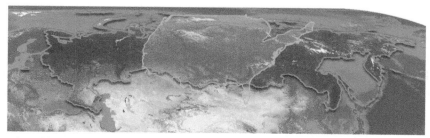

Adapted from *Blue Marble: Next Generation* image produced by Reto Stockli, NASA Earth Observatory (NASA Goddard Space Flight Center)

planet. Unparalleled in terms of resources, the effects of the human interaction with the environment are increasingly evident today.

The sun literally never sets on the nation-state of Russia. In many ways a harsh landscape greets the Russian peoples as they endure the hardships of life and perpetuate a great and powerful culture. Essentially, this huge landmass spreads longitudinally about 170 degrees. Essentially flat in the northern parts of the nation, the ground is in a state of **permafrost** for much of the year. Unlike Scandinavia in Europe, which receives a great deal of snow, there is no maritime or ocean current to provide the requisite moisture for snow. The result is a very cold and dry continental climate. Just as climate is a long-term effect of proximity to oceans and latitude, Russia not only has the ocean currents, but also is extremely northern in latitude.

Distance and Longitude

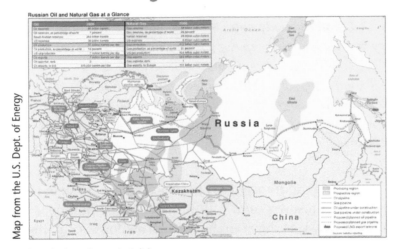

Russia is mineral rich!

When one considers the southern areas of Russia are generally corresponding to those along the **ecumene** of Canada, one has a great appreciation for the coldness and hugeness of Russia. Still, it is important for one to remember that the effects of **topography** play a very important part in creating climate.

High mountains both block and trap water as the clouds tend to become cool through a process known as the adiabatic lapse rate that sees orographic uplifting, or the rise of warm air that cools (see the introductory chapter). In the case of Russia, the only real topography that blocks moisture producing a windward and leeward effect is the Caucuses. They tend to provide a natural border for the Russians and play an extremely important role psychologically in the minds of the Russian peoples. The Ural Mountains go generally north to south and are the dividing range between what is generally considered European Russia and Asian Russia. The other important areas of relief include the ranges from the Pamirs through the Tien Shan and from the Altay Mountains to the Sayan Mountains to Lake Baikal. Perhaps these mountains are important not just in how they provide natural borders for Russia to the south but how they affect the hydrography of the region.

If you look at the map and find Lake Baikal, you will see that it is generally in the shape of the southern mountain chains too. Like the lakes in East Africa that follow the rift valley, this huge lake also is a function of the folding of the Earth's surface. Some experts believe about one-fifth of the freshwater on Earth is in this deep lake. Unfortunately as we shall see, there are some environmental risks inherent in this. Anyway, the largest lake in the world is the Caspian Sea. Why is this large body of water not a sea and yet another smaller body in central Asia, the Aral Sea, is? This is debatable, but remember this, the definition of a sea is that its salinity levels correspond to the world's oceans. Both the Aral Sea and Lake Baikal do have salt in them but it is much less than the world's oceans because of the input of rivers flowing down from both the Pamir's and the Tien Shan Mountains. Since the definition of a sea is that it has salt water, and since according to Mikhail S. Blinnikov the Caspian Sea only has one-third the salt water of the world's oceans, it is therefore a lake![1]

Most of the rivers of Russia flow from south to north because of the southern topography previously described. The area of Russia today referred to as Siberia is neatly divided by two major rivers flowing north. Between the Yenisey and the Ob Rivers is the West Siberian Plain. This area is generally very swampy when the permafrost begins to melt in spring. The next major river to the east is the Lena River and this begins what is referred to as the Russian Far East.

Got Gas?

An aspect of major importance to the Russian economy now is the decision to depend upon the export of natural resources. Energy of course is a major component of these exports. In particular, natural gas from the region of western Siberia bound for energy starved Europe. Coal is another resource the Russians have historically utilized. Next to the United States, Russia is the premier producer of coal in the world. Taken as a whole, the Russians have a huge area they call home that is cold and crossed by rivers and bordered by mountains. Rich in mineral resources, they lack one thing: harbors.

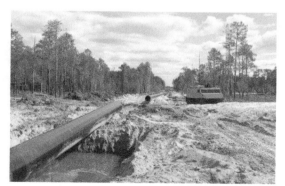

Image © Leonid Ikan, 2013. Used under license from Shutterstock, Inc.

It's not that Russia doesn't have harbors, but it is an unfortunate aspect of their geography that only one major ice-free port near the Atlantic Ocean is adjacent to the Barent's Sea and lay in Murmansk where it receives the benefits of the Atlantic

[1] Mikhail S. Blinnikov, "A Geography of Russia and Its Neighbors" (New York: Guilford), 17.

currents; the same currents that bring rain and warmth to Scandinavia and northern Europe. Nevertheless, with temperatures barely above zero degrees Fahrenheit during the winter, Murmansk is no picnic. Note also the distance in relative location from the Norwegian Sea, which in addition to being largely above the Arctic Circle is greatly separated from the ice-free port in Vladivostok on the Pacific Ocean. This enormous distance leads population geographers to wonder about the future of Russia and its ability to control its far east possessions.

Babies Anyone?

Of increasing interest to **demographers**—or students of population and changes in it—is to include statistics and distribution in the population of Russia. Like Europe, the **population pyramids** are increasingly inverted. This inverted population graph increasingly reveals an aging population. Additionally, women outlive men in many areas by enormous amounts. (For more information on population geography, see Appendix H.) Of historical concern to Russians is their ability to maintain control of the Russian Far East, an area increasingly broached by fast growing populations from Muslim Central Asia. Many experts say a population to be sustained must increase by at least 2.1% merely to continue to exist. If this is the case, the Russians with their 1.6% annual growth rate are in a similar situation with Europe. The government of Russia now pays $10,000 to parents if they have a second child to increase birthrates.[2]

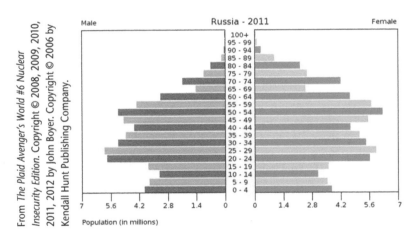

From *The Plaid Avenger's World #6 Nuclear Insecurity Edition.* Copyright © 2008, 2009, 2010, 2011, 2012 by John Boyer. Copyright © 2006 by Kendall Hunt Publishing Company.

An inverted pyramid the opposite of the arab countries shown in Chapter 4 page 72.

How Cold I Am

Unfortunately, like in the United States, many Russians have turned to alcohol because it is cheap and available, and it helps them sustain the toughness of life. While hope can seem far away at times when one studies the Russian peoples and their histories,

[2]Blinnikov, Michael S., "A Geography of Russia and its Neighbors" (New York: Guilford Press, 2011), 140.

the truth is God has a special plan for all of us. He is in control of Russia just as he is the United States. Even though life can be hard and very discouraging and frightening at times, one thing we can be sure of is that his love for us remains intact. In the Bible we see the verse, "For I know the thoughts that I think toward you," says the Lord, "thoughts of peace and not of evil, to give you a future and a hope." (Jeremiah 29:10–12 NKJV)

KEY TERMS TO KNOW

- permafrost
- ecumene
- topography
- demographers
- population pyramids

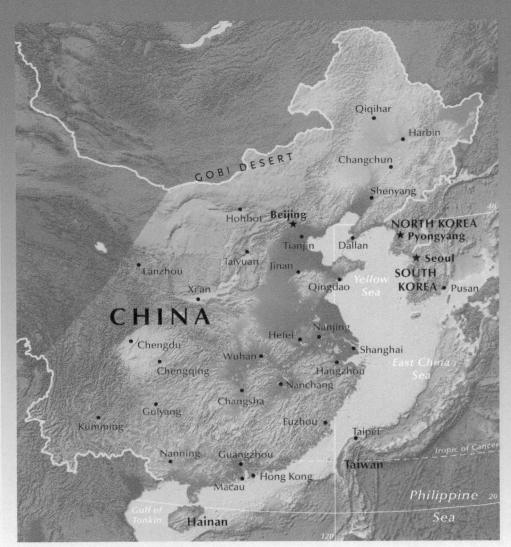

Map courtesy of Katie Pritchard and NOAA

CHAPTER

8

East Asia

As for the rich in this present age, charge them not to be haughty, nor to set their hopes on the uncertainty of riches, but on God, who richly provides us with everything to enjoy. They are to do good, to be rich in good works, to be generous and ready to share, thus storing up treasure for themselves as a good foundation for the future, so that they may take hold of that which is truly life. (1 Timothy 6:17–19)

China has emerged as an industrial giant like the United States. Similarly to the US boom, times have created certain "growing pains" that provide a ripe opportunity for us as servants of the Lord. One important aspect of this is providing equal rights—life amongst these and the blessings of justice. Remember Psalmist taught in Psalm 72:2 when he said, "He will judge your people with righteousness, and your poor with justice." (NKJV)

SEZ Who?

"A totally unique world with a culture so different from ours" was the statement the author heard one day from a veteran of Asian service who was describing his experiences in East Asia. When asked to give specific examples the answer was, "everything, the plants, the animals even the food!" Indeed East Asia is a region of fascinating landscapes and historical extremes of both beauty and darkness. Cut off from much of the western world for so long, this enormous part of the Asian continent indeed developed separately from the western world while creating various unique cultures whose resources and productivity continuously beckoned the west with trade and commerce opportunities. At times it seemed the west's cravings for the products of the orient and its money was pulled to the east as it continues to be today. It is believed a Christian revival as well as unprecedented economic growth is occurring in China today. No doubt this exotic area will continue to make the headlines, and who knows—you or your future family members may live or even marry someone from there.

Landlocked Countries in Asia

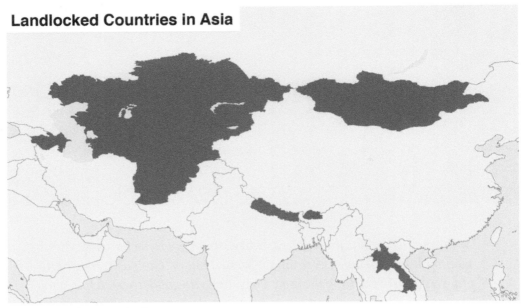

Map courtesy of Katie Pritchard

The area under observation consists of the Islands of Japan, the peninsula of Korea and the large island nation of Taiwan. To the far north are the windswept plains of Mongolia. By good fortune, this generation is alive at a time of great excitements as we see East Asia emerging on the world scene during one of its periodic forays out into the world. Considered by many to be the richest area of the 21st century world

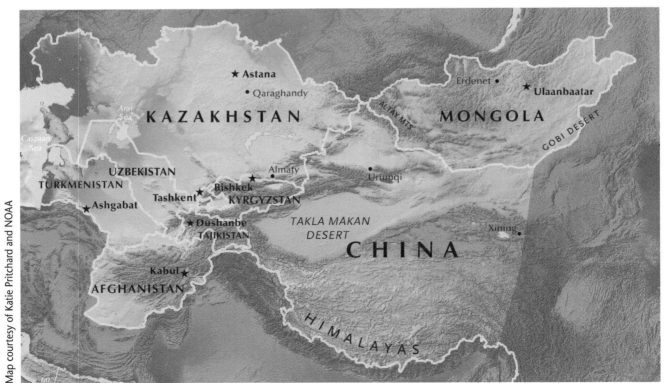

Map courtesy of Katie Pritchard and NOAA

CENTRAL ASIA

economically, the opportunities for service abound, but first one must understand the culture. And to understand the culture development and dispersion, we must study the topography and other various aspects of physical geography.

To the north of China are the cold and dusty deserts of the Gobi and the Takla Makan Desert. Standing like a cold sentry to the north are the Pamir Mountains, and to the northwest the fabled Tien Shan or mountains of the clouds. Further, surrounding China to the southwest are the Pamir's and the Karakorum Range as we travel counterclockwise. To the south are the mighty Himalayas and the furrowed brow of numerous north-south flowing mountain ranges with valleys channeling fast-flowing rivers pushing south taking cultures and people with them.

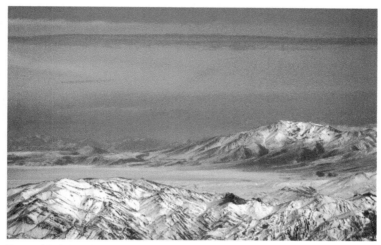

Dept. of Defense photo by SSgt. Cherie A. Thurlby, U.S. Air Force.

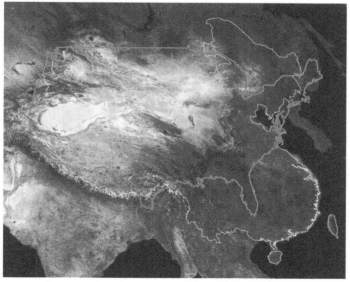

From *Blue Marble: Next Generation* image produced by Reto Stockli, NASA Earth Observatory (NASA Goddard Space Flight Center)

These high-mountain chains stand as a bulwark against the seasonal tropical rains of the monsoon and leave China isolated like a turtle behind a shell of physical geography. Occasionally over time this culture has "come out of its shell" and has ventured abroad only to withdraw itself behind its isolating geography when it felt endangered. This pattern of alternating expansion and contraction from and behind these natural borders has not only protected and sustained China during its long history but also has tended to both protect and limit China's prospects for growing at sea.

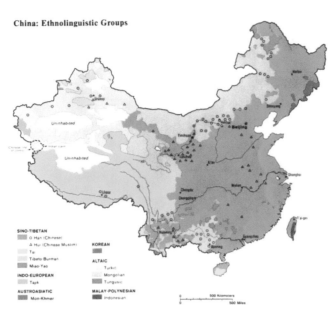

China: Ethnolinguistic Groups

SINO-TIBETAN
○ Han (Chinese)
△ Hui (Chinese Muslim)
Tai
Tibeto-Burman
Miao-Yao
INDO-EUROPEAN
Tajik
AUSTROASIATIC
Mon-Khmer

KOREAN

ALTAIC
Turkic
Mongolian
Tungusic
MALAY-POLYNESIAN
Indonesian

CIA map, courtesy of University of Texas Libraries

A term frequently heard in recent years is **globalization**. Simply stated, globalization is the increasing interconnectedness of what would seem to be a smaller world. *Smaller* is a relative term but refers to the speed with which one can communicate or travel to distant parts of the world. Globalization has caused many environmental problems, for example, numerous species of East Asian animals and plants have come to the United States with varying degrees of impact on local populations. If you have seen bamboo or kudzu in the American south growing on the sides of the road, you have seen an impact of globalization. The ability to communicate rapidly with people in the different corners of the Earth is another reason to study languages and obey the Great Commission of Jesus Christ. As we shall discuss later on, much progress has been made in this regard in recent decades.

SEZ Who?

As far back as the Roman Empire we know efforts were made to obtain Chinese silk and other luxury products. Quite possibly, attempts to dredge the Euphrates and Tigris rivers and various disastrous military endeavors were initiated by the desire to find a water route through the Indian Ocean in an attempt to bypass the land routes called the **Silk Road**. Later, the Portuguese would exploit the growing weaknesses of the Persian and Turkish empires by what essentially was a maneuvering around or flanking of those empires to gain access to trade. The terminus of this trade was China and some historical geographers even believe the westward expansion of the United States in many ways was a continuation of the search for the elusive "northwest passage" into Asia. The capitalist nations of Western Europe and the Americas continued to see their

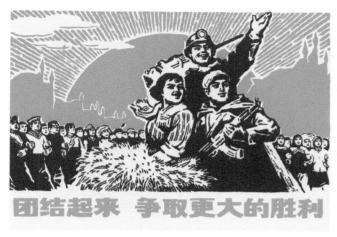

Image © John Lock, 2013. Used under license from Shutterstock, Inc.

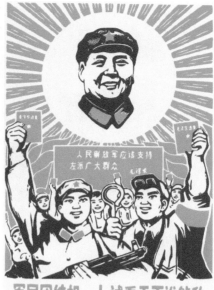

Image © Johny Keny, 2013. Used under license from Shutterstock, Inc.

monies drained by buying Asian products. Reciprocity, however, did not occur, as western products seemed to be not so sought after. Recent economic trends have tended to reinforce this general inequality.

In the 1970's, for example, the Chinese began to initiate a system of reforms, which in many ways reversed the intensely centralized economic planning characteristic of the powerful leader Mao Tse-Tung. Upon Mao's death, a series of five-year plans occurred that had previously been called **The Great Leap Forward**. These utilized the collectivization impulse typical of Asian nationalism into groups of **communes** for the production of agriculture and iron. In many ways disastrous, nevertheless the Chinese nation survived a mercurial dictator and the Korean War (in its infancy) to become an economic powerhouse. The reforms instituted seemed to anticipate the British release of Hong Kong and began a re-characterization of the coastal areas into **Special Economic Zones** or **SEZ's**. These areas offering tax incentives for foreign investments are one reason the skyline of Chinese cities are remarkably fresh and new. As China's economy has taken off so has its tendency to come "out of its shell" and directly influence the wider world for the purpose of seeking resources and influence.

Hemmed In

The famous geographer and traveler Robert D. Kaplan refers to what strategists today call a "First Island Chain" and a "Second Island Chain" when discussing the various islands that ring around China. The United States has essentially dominated the First Island Chain closest to China consisting of Taiwan, Luzon (the northern island in the Philippines) and the Ryuku Island chains as well as the Japanese home islands. These islands tend to funnel Chinese attempts at exploration into the Pacific. A secondary

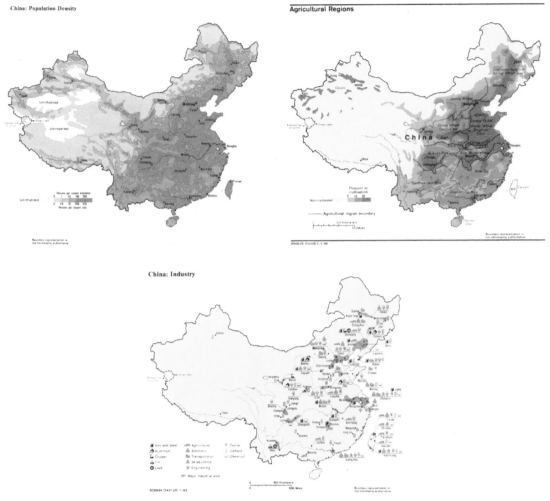

China: Population Density

Agricultural Regions

China: Industry

CIA maps, courtesy of University of Texas libraries

island chain consists of Guam and the Marianas Islands.[1] These islands tend to constitute a barrier similar to those on land, which will tend to protect China and yet remain a challenge to China as it seeks to emerge from its shell in the future. Mr. Kaplan is cited here again, as it is Kaplan's contention that China today is a reflection in part of the Great Wall and its role in the varying interactions between China and the nomads of Inner Asia.[2] China has periodically grown in varying impulses or dynasties throughout its history and now seems to be emerging again in large measure because it feels secure. China and much of East Asia has also been sought after by various western traders who have attempted to reach it across mutually forbidding geographies of land and the distance by water. China's unique culture despite its geographic isolation has continued to diffuse in unique ways. Religion is a terrific example of a cultural expression that has pierced China's isolating physical geography.

---

[1] Kaplan, Robert D., "Monsoon" (New York: Random House), 286.
[2] Kaplan, Robert D., "The Revenge of Geography" (New York: Random House), 195.

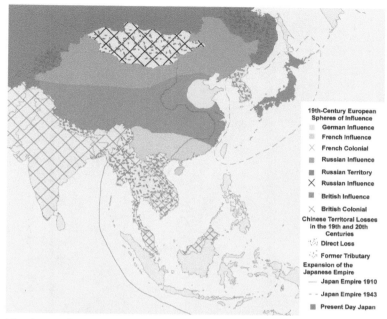

Map source: *The World Factbook*

Lights Please!

Historically **Confucianism** has provided an ethical system promoting societal order and concerned with establishing proper relationships. The importance of tact and preventing conflict within a traditionally high-populated area is obvious. The religion of **Buddhism** has also historically been a powerful source of hope and today remains an important aspect of East Asian cultures, where it spread to from India. The type of Buddhism known as **Mahayana** believes in a savior that can be the Buddha or any of the **enlightened beings** or **Bodhisattva** who have decided not to go into **Nirvana** or what we as Christians would call heaven, because they want to help other individuals achieve their exalted state. As you might expect, the geography of China and the direction of the mountains and rivers have helped diffuse Buddhism into Southeast Asia but in a form slightly different, which we will discuss in that chapter. Another interesting aspect of culture as it has related to China is agriculture.

Today's Christianity has tended to take hold only in a few places as a consequence of the colonial experience when Christians followed the capitalists of Europe to these far-off shores. To many colonial minds, the faithful displayed little difference from the greedy outsiders and were of the same ilk. One such area of Christian expansion is perhaps the most Christian nation in East Asia today, Korea.

The Harvest is Great

Today the Korean peninsula stands guard over the northeastern region of China close to the mineral riches of Manchuria and the capital city of Beijing. Divided at the end of World War II, almost on a whim by military staff officers tasked with organizing occupation forces from the conquering American army, the line reflected the first major

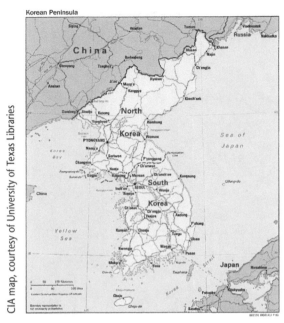

Korean Peninsula

CIA map, courtesy of University of Texas Libraries

The Korean Peninsula.

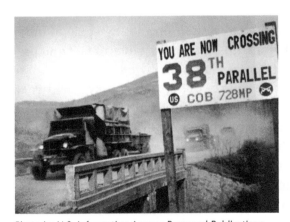

Photo by U.S. Information Agency Press and Publications Service Visual Services Branch, from National Archives and Records Administration

latitude above Seoul and the Han River Valley where the victorious American Army headquarters was with the former Japanese headquarters. The Soviets honored this line, similar to lines drawn in Germany and Austria and similar to what would occur in Southeast Asia soon thereafter. Both the Soviets and the Americans thus divided Korea with little consideration of long-term consequences to the Korean Peninsula.[3] The Korean Peninsula now consists of a totalitarian North, somewhat of a cold war relic, and a proudly confident and energetic South, which is much closer to being a democratic republic. With its high GDP, South Korea joins Hong Kong, the Republic of China, Taiwan and the tiny city-state of Singapore as some of the newest producers of manufactured goods. Despite nearby bellicosity, the South continues to prosper and is a very important factor in spreading the Good News of Jesus Christ to the rest of East Asia. It has been suggested in the past that South Korea could overtake the United States in terms of the numbers of missionaries sent to the field.

---

[3]The War for Korea: 1945–1940 "A House Burning" by Allan R. Millett (Lawrence, Kansas: The University Press of Kansas, 2005), 45.

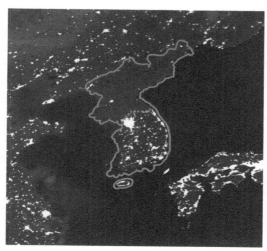

NASA/Goddard Space Flight Center Scientific Visualization Studio

An amazing contrast at night on the Korean Peninsula.

Though such ideas have proven a bit overly optimistic, the truth remains—the Korean Peninsula has been faithful![4]

To the south of Korea is the island of Taiwan. Taiwan, though small in size, represents the exiled former government of the mainland and is on the island of Formosa. Though only slightly smaller than Maryland and Delaware combined, this nation state of 25 million is a powerful force. At one time, the tallest skyscraper in the world jutted defiantly towards the mainland. Taipei 101 indeed had 101 floors and though recently surpassed as the tallest building in the world, it remains a testimony to the energetic peoples who dwell there. Taiwan appears to represent a major thorn in the side of the People's Republic of China. Just as we in America often feel burdened by our past, the Chinese are very sensitive to the presence of a national government claiming authority over the mainland. The emergence of a communist government in China over half a century ago represented a nationalistic impulse that still is extremely emotional today. This emotion can be seen over areas of contention that both appeal and exacerbate racial and national tensions in various frontier areas.

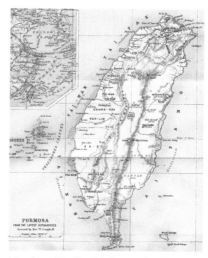

Map from *The Scottish Geographical Magazine* (Volume XII: 1896), courtesy of University of Texas Libraries

[4]http://www.christianitytoday.com/gleanings/2013/july/missionaries-countries-sent-received-csgc -gordon-conwell.html

Hemmed In?

A legitimate interest in procuring safe routes by sea for vital resources is increasingly causing a shift in relations with China with various nations of the world, particularly in the East and South China Seas and the Indian Ocean. Frontier areas off of the coast of China include the Senkaku Islands (Japanese name) or Daiyou Islands (Chinese name).

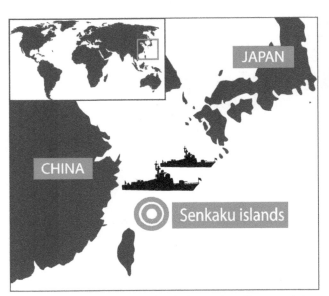

These islands represent what may be only the beginning of what are becoming different areas of contention as Chinese Sea power increases and a simultaneous decline of an American commitment in the South China Sea continues. China's growth has produced another area of contention in recent years as well—the oil-rich Spratley Islands off of the coast of the Philippines and Vietnam. Such maritime areas of contention demonstrate a somewhat subtle transition occurring as China begins to flex its international muscles. The original route

Image © vadimmmus, 2013. Used under license from Shutterstock, Inc.

intended to circumvent the Silk Road has become a series of sea bases known as a String of Pearls strategy by China and naval bases are being built at Gwadar Pakistan and in Sri Lanka by the Chinese in an attempt to help secure their access among other things to Middle Eastern oil and the vital **Strait of Malacca**.

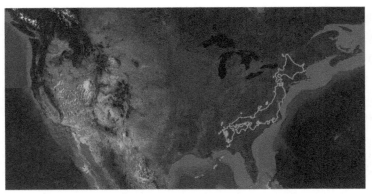

Map courtesy of Katie Pritchard and NOAA

Finally to the north of the economic colossus of China is Mongolia. Mongolia was originally the home of fierce nomadic peoples who were walled out of China. These nomads dwelt on horseback upon the semi-arid plains and grasslands to the north of China. Dwelling in round tents, or yurts, modern Mongolia is a study in contrasts

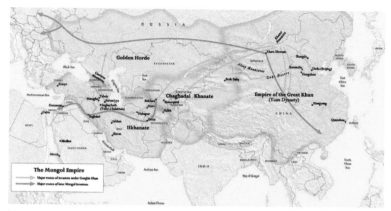

Map source: *The World Factbook*

today as electric lights cast shadows on traditional tent cities. Mongolia is in a delicate situation today. A few generations ago, Mongolia was firmly in the grip of a powerful Soviet neighbor. In fact, the capital city of Ulaanbaatar means "Red Hero" after the early communist leader there. In recent years, however, China has been moving ever closer to controlling Mongolia, and as China finds less of a threat from its North, it is increasingly emboldened to take to sea and explore. Seeking oil and minerals from around the world, the security of a modern China will continue to draw the world to it as it has since ancient times. This increasingly globalized planet will offer us great opportunities to live out our faith and to be living testimonies of hope and faith in a busy world that is preoccupied with riches and security.

KEY TERMS TO KNOW

- globalization
- The Great Leap Forward
- communes
- Special Economic Zones (SEZ's)
- Confucianism
- Buddhism
- Mahayana
- enlightened beings
- Bodhisattva
- Nirvana
- Strait of Malacca

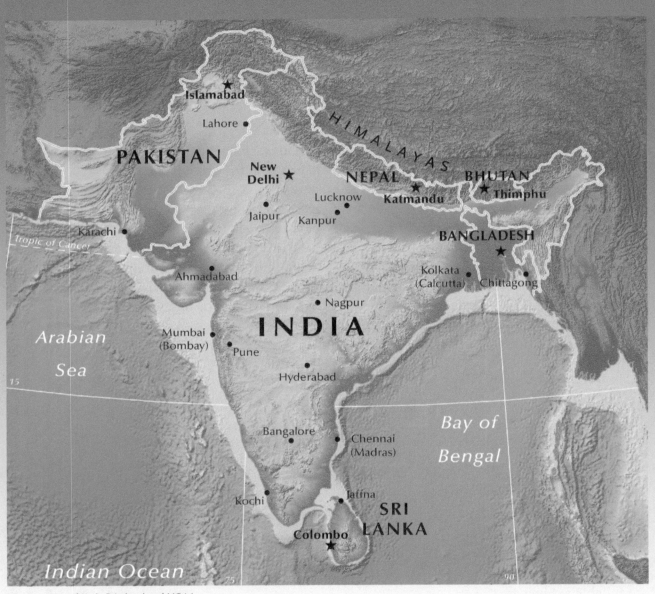

Map courtesy of Katie Pritchard and NOAA

South Asia

For by him all things were created, in heaven and on earth, visible and invisible, whether thrones or dominions or rulers or authorities—all things were created through him and for him. And he is before all things, and in him all things hold together. And he is the head of the body, the church. (Colossians 1:16–17)

I n the book of Proverbs (Proverbs 23:10 NKJV), we are exhorted to respect ancient landmarks and to respect the poor. South Asia is a vibrant and wonderful culture and civilization with a terrific potential future. You have many opportunities as a geography student to recognize how these borders, many recently drawn, have provided opportunities for those who would be peacemakers in one of the most populous areas on the planet, and one rife with needs on both sides of India's borders!

Roughly one-third the size of the United States, India is the world's largest democracy. Soon to be the world's most populous nation, it is a reflection of the location and past of its people. Christianity is growing remarkably fast there, and the future of India is exciting and bright!

Located in the center of the Indian Ocean, India is a large, triangular peninsula jutting into the Indian Ocean separating the roughly equally large Arabian Sea and the Bay of Bengal. This relative location has been important over the ages as nations seeking to trade with China have used it as a way station along the route as well as used it as a very important source of natural resources. Located on the southern rim of the gigantic Asian continent, the **subcontinent** of greater India is greatly affected by the Indian Ocean—essentially a watery frontier on its southern border. India has seen various land empires, such as Persia and the Mongols, generally from the north and east move down the elevation (like a highway off-ramp) into it occupying as far as New Delhi in the Ganges plain south to the Deccan Plateau. Simultaneously, the monsoons have created a type of buffer region for trade.

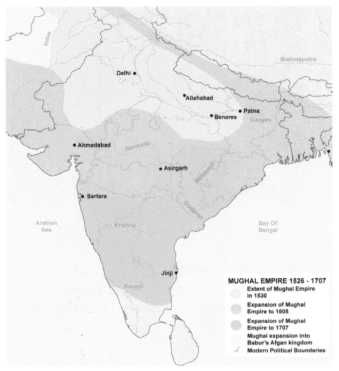

Map courtesy of Katie Pritchard

Here Comes the Rain Again

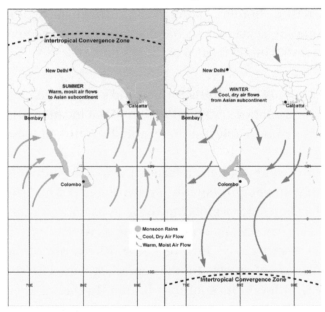

Map courtesy of Katie Pritchard

Because of temperature differences during the year, the Indian Ocean has consistently been a predictable route of travel because of the **monsoon** winds. The monsoon winds are drawn off of the Indian Ocean and toward land in the summer because of atmospheric pressure disparities and bring with them extensive seasonal rains. In the winter, the winds reverse direction blowing from the north and resulting in a drier season. The tilt of the Earth and the disparity of temperatures and pressure systems over continents and oceans ultimately create these special conditions and when high relief such as the Himalayan Mountains become involved, these can be catastrophic such as is often the case in Bangladesh with flooding and consequent disease epidemics due to its tropical nature. In fact, according to Robert D. Kaplan, "The population of Bangladesh is roughly half that of the United States and greater than that of Russia and packed into an area about the size of Iowa."[1] During the Age of Sail, this seasonally consistent wind pattern from the north and south enabled explorers and traders to either sail into the wind or travel with the wind behind them as they engaged in trans-regional trade between the Middle East and Southeast Asia, and ultimately globally between Europe and East Asia.

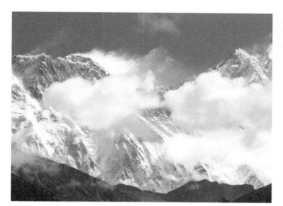

© JupiterImages Corporation

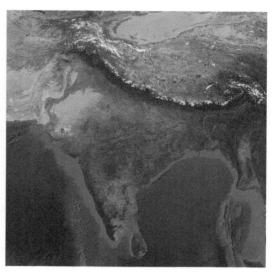

From *Blue Marble: Next Generation* image produced by Reto Stockli, NASA Earth Observatory (NASA Goddard Space Flight Center)

As globalized trade continued to develop through history—from the Ancient Greeks to Alexander, to the Romans, to the Arabs and Persians—all have mingled along the coasts of the subcontinent that can still be seen to this day. India will surely continue to be an extremely important state in the future, for it is situated between the valuable oil supplies of the Persian Gulf and its correspondingly Persian culture and the vital Strait of Malacca to the east, which is China's lifeline to the Gulf. Standing on guard towards the eastern approaches to Indonesia is the Andaman Island chain, the possession of India. So what we have described as greater India is actually one of many cultures spread over the rim of the continent on the Indian Ocean. Between the volatile Arab and Persian cultures to the west and the exploding economy of China to the east, India will continue to be of extreme importance to the United States.

India has defined natural borders. The term **Greater India** is used to describe these natural borders, which according to some scholars have spread from modern day Afghanistan in the west across the inclined elevations of Pakistan to the mountains of Burma in the east. High natural borders in the form of mountains ring Greater India from the Karakorum Range to the Himalayas along the northern flank. Only a few

---

[1] Robert D. Kaplan, "Monsoon: The Indian Ocean and the Future of American Power" (New York: Random House, 2010), 140.

passes functioning as gates from the higher elevations from the west of central Asia have served as invasion routes for centuries—most notably from the Aryans. The coastal areas of southern Iran and Pakistan have been instrumental in the spread of culture laterally from west to east corresponding to the rivers.

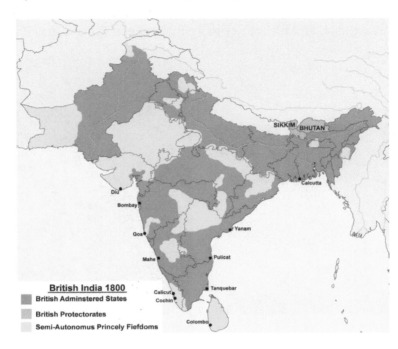

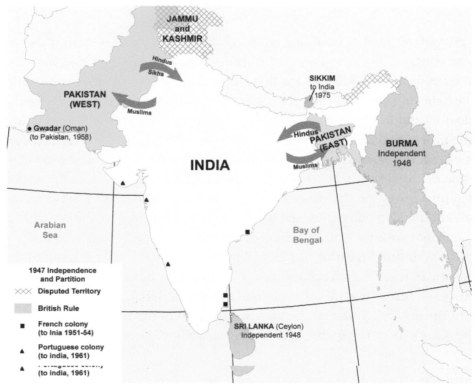

Maps courtesy of Katie Pritchard

The great River of India flowing generally from the mountains of the North with their spring thawed flows and eventually turns east. Ringed to the Northeast by the Thar Desert, the city of Delhi generally seems to be the western limit of many of these historical empires that to spread into India. The other key river, the Brahmaputra, continues this general pattern of East-Western Trade beginning in the northeast as its source in the mountains of China and continues to become clearer. Generally isolated but still surrounded by vibrant neighbors, the world's largest democracy today still remains greatly divided between North and South and has seen a renewal of post-colonial nationalism.

Do What You Can Do!

A renewed sense of being Indian is called **Hindutva**. Temples on the cultural landscape today mark the identity of religion as a key aspect of India. A relatively new film industry called Bollywood shows the confidence of Indian culture in an uncertain world. Still the world's largest democracy faces challenges from abroad. Since the Great Partition of 1947, where greater India was divided into Pakistan to the east and west of India during the British withdrawal from the subcontinent, India has since had several armed confrontations with its neighbor Pakistan. Pakistan was originally intended to be a Muslim land that was set aside by the British as they withdrew from India. Originally successful, Pakistan has since become what some would call a failed state. The development of nuclear weapons has only increased the tensions between the former residents of greater India. The primary area of tension surrounds the regions of **Jammu and Kashmir**. Located at the head of the river that serves as the key artery of Pakistan, the Indus River is a point of contention only increased by Pakistan's relation with the emerging power of China.

China has also caused some strategic headaches for India with recent Maoist insurgency efforts in Nepal and smaller

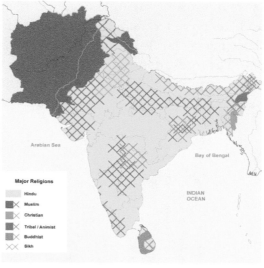

Map source: *The World Factbook*

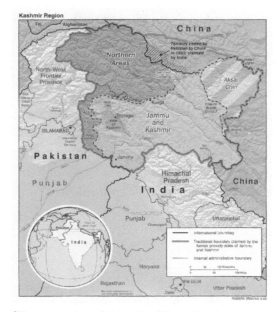

CIA map, courtesy of University of Texas Libraries

Bhutan to the northeast. The view from India is increasingly one of a sense of vulnerability by Islam extremists supported in large measure by China. This security concern has been most pronounced since the massive terrorist attack in India's largest city of Mumbai in 2008. Challenged from abroad, India continues to develop technologically. Many have identified the peninsula of Gujarat—the home of the Patel or business families of the nineteenth century—as the seat of Hindu nationalism today.

Many jobs in the technology sector have been located in recent years to India. Interestingly, as Christianity has spread in the southern areas of India so have technological opportunities for the Indian people. Many of the people of southern India are of Dravidian background—these people tend to have darker skin. This pattern of skin color has fit into the traditional ethnic religion of India and is known as a defining factor of the **caste system**. Though technically illegal, this system still perpetuates itself and has provided many opportunities for evangelical outreach, particularly among those people in the past considered to be untouchables. It is exciting to see India, the world's largest democracy, continuing to grow and becoming stable in uncertain times. Still, as anyone who has served there can tell you, India has a long way to go to become a secure and gigantic democracy!

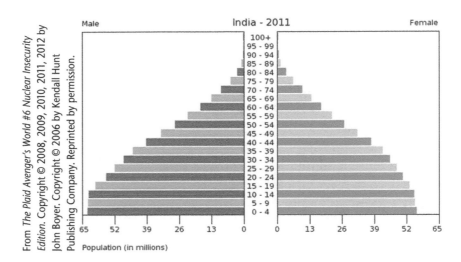

From *The Plaid Avenger's World #6 Nuclear Insecurity Edition.* Copyright © 2008, 2009, 2010, 2011, 2012 by John Boyer. Copyright © 2006 by Kendall Hunt Publishing Company. Reprinted by permission.

A perfect pyramid indicating the challenges of population growth and the challenges of life in India.

The population of India is on the verge of surpassing China in terms of numbers. It is indeed a terrific time to consider the admonition of scripture and to learn more about the rich and ancient cultures of the "subcontinent" to make a real and eternal difference.

KEY TERMS TO KNOW

- subcontinent
- monsoon
- Greater India
- Hindutva
- Jammu and Kashmir
- caste system

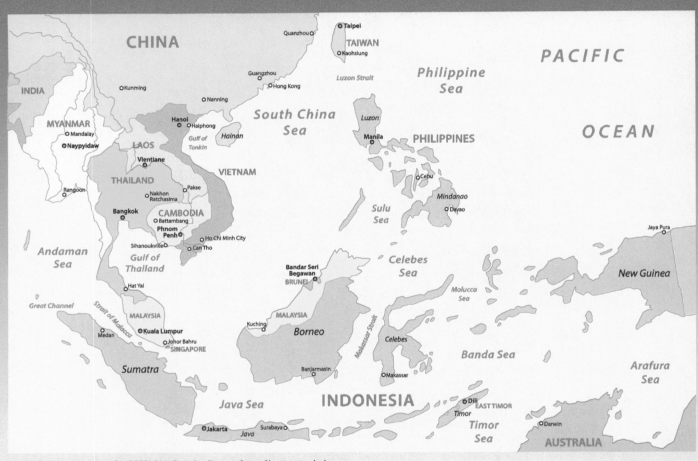

Southeast Asia

And it is my prayer that your love may abound more and more, with knowledge and all discernment, so that you may approve what is excellent, and so be pure and blameless for the day of Christ, filled with the fruit of righteousness that comes through Jesus Christ, to the glory and praise of God. (Philippians 1:9–11)

If we want to reach others with our hope we must share the faith we have been given. Despite the numerous opportunities the world provides to share this hope, we must be on our guard to be the salt we see mentioned in Matthew 5:13 (NKJV). Paying close attention to living a pure life, one without hypocrisy is instrumental in demonstrating genuine hope to the people of Southeast Asia, many of whom are dedicated Buddhists and Muslims. One thing is for sure; everyone knows when his or her food is salted. So will they notice you when you live as blame free of a life as possible!

The key to understanding Southeast Asia is to see it as a bridge between east and south Asia. Like the rapidly flowing rivers flowing generally in a southeastern direction from southern China, ethnically and culturally much of Southeast Asia represents a tradition common to East Asia. In both Buddhism and business, Southeast Asia has roots in China and population flows continue to demonstrate this historical pattern. Southeast Asia is of terrific importance to the United States in particular and to the world in general. A true mosaic of cultural influences can be seen in this vital region.

Call Your Mommy!

The map of Southeast Asia will demonstrate the key physical aspects that have molded a culture of patience and calm acceptance of the difficulties and joys of life. Positioned between the great and ancient cultures of China and India, this continent consists of mostly water on a series of tectonic plates that have caused terrific ocean rifts. A recent **tsunami** in 2004 claimed hundreds of thousands of lives. Fierce tropical storms called typhoons and tsunamis are just some of the challenges facing an area often consisting

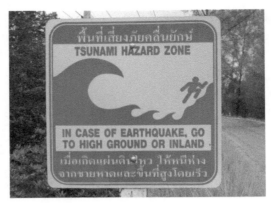

Image © AJE44, 2013. Used under license from
Shutterstock, Inc.

mainly of high terrain and volcanic cones. The tsunami gave the United States an incredible opportunity to demonstrate good will and its traditionally Christian nature because the United States was the only nation possessing the fleet assets to provide medical care and emergency services nearby. In an era (see below) where China is working hard to make cultural and economic inroads into this strategically vital region, the United States was well-served by its powerful effort to help these tsunami victims and their families with seaborne medical aid and supplies.

The climate is of course tropical, and the region is nearly all within the tropic lines of latitude. As you might expect of the location, the rainforest (one of the largest in the world) prevails, and the monsoons bring plenty of rains to the area as discussed in the previous chapter.

So what are the aspects of culture that show an acceptance of the somewhat predictable fate associated with the regular seasonal monsoons?

Be Good

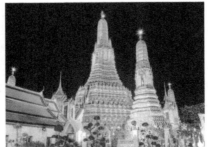

Image © Ko.Yo, 2013. Used under license from Shutterstock, Inc.

Buddhist landscape.

Cultural diffusion from India and East Asia is manifested in the Buddhism of the area. **Theravada** type of Buddhism though different from the Buddhism of East Asia is still grounded in the peaceful teachings of the great Buddha. Unlike the Mahayana Buddhists of the north, the dedication of the monks and the bright clothing and colorful temples of this sub-region place a great emphasis on good works and is generally considered to be more concerned with achieving instant insights. The use of nuns and monks appears to suggest the idea that salvation or escape from the samsara cycle can be achieved by good deeds and personal growth. Angels of enlightened beings called bodhisattvas can guide the faithful in their attempts to achieve an escape from life. We would perhaps consider this to be similar to the workings of the Holy Spirit in our lives as Christians. The

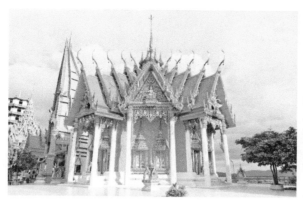

Image © Paul Clarke, 2013. Used under license from Shutterstock, Inc.

Note the Oceanic influence here on the architectural landscape.

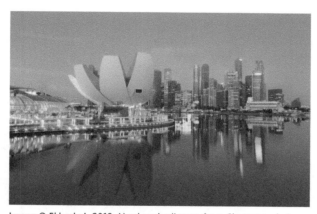

Image © Ekkachai, 2013. Used under license from Shutterstock, Inc.

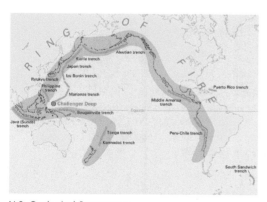

U.S. Geological Survey map

religion and the people of Southeast Asia seem to reflect the pastel colors of the clothing and the lovely tropical flowers surrounding them. This peaceful Buddhism seems to transition into a more peaceful form of Islam than many of us have been led to believe by listening to the news.

Evidence of Islam is obvious. Indonesia, the most populous Islamic nation in the world along with neighboring Malaya and Singapore, are a dynamic people whose religion seems to provide a great measure of stability. The sultanate of oil-rich Brunei on the island of Borneo demonstrates the synchronism of the area and the merging of different religions and traditions. The name sultanate itself is of Turkish or central Asian origin, so much history can be gained merely by observing the **cultural landscape**, the human imprint on the horizon, and the **toponyms** or place names. Despite the influence of Islam, other religious influences can be felt in this region culturally.

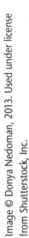

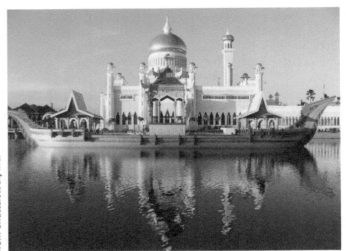

The Sultanate of Brunei—the toponym reflects a Turkish past while the landscape synchronistically reveals Islam and Pacific influences.

Cultural Mosaic

The ubiquitousness of Hindu temples demonstrates the importance of the monsoon winds historically to this area. Today the Andaman Islands located on your map by the Andaman Sea are an Indian possession and reminds the world of the importance India has paid in the past and present due both to trade and the diffusion of Islam. Going to the west to the Philippines, this huge archipelago of over 7,000 islands is overwhelming Roman Catholic due to Spanish forays during the age of sail in history.

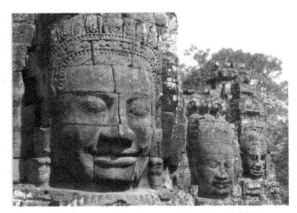

The greatest population of the followers of Islam is in Indonesia in southern Southeast Asia. This is fortunate for the United States for a couple of reasons: strategically and economically. From a business standpoint, it is hard not to see the export of manufacturing jobs to Southeast Asia. Although Japan is probably the undisputed leader in transnational corporations globally, the rise of developing economies in the world seem to be creating a prospective boom in Southeast Asia. Numerous manufacturing firms and transnational corporations (TNC's) from developing countries have continued to move to Asia and Southeast Asia is no exception. Of the world's largest fifty TNC's from developing countries, thirty-eight are located in Asia. As one might expect, a large number of these are in

Southeast Asia and include seven in Singapore alone.[1] The urban skyline of Southeast Asia with its famous Patrones towers in Kuala Lampur in Malaysia reflects the growing economic strength of Southeast Asia as well.

Pearl Power

Perhaps of more immediate importance to the United States in these uncertain times is the strategic importance of Southeast Asia militarily. When one considers the Philippines with over seven thousand islands and the legacy of American military involvement there, one begins to see why the scope of a strategy has been developed in recent years with Southeast Asia as the nexus of interest of the United States, China and India.

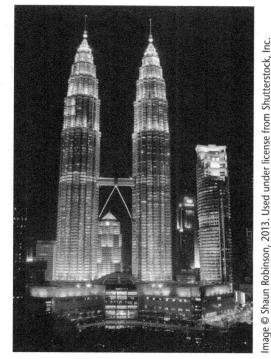

The Petronas Towers in Kuala Lumpur, Malaysia.

Image © Shaun Robinson, 2013. Used under license from Shutterstock, Inc.

The United States originally became involved in the Philippines with the Spanish-American War. While most Americans were aware of the importance of Cuba, with the overwhelming success of Commodore George Dewey the United States found itself with an archipelago of islands under its charge. American military leadership fought against the Muslims in the southern island of Mindanao and Special Forces troops are still there today. The importance of a secure Philippines to the United States goes back to earlier in the last century. With the rise of Japan in World War II, the northern Island of Luzon in the Philippines drew American armies like a magnet. Why? For the similar reason of forming a launching point into China and for the purpose of trade and today as a means of restraining the Chinese as mentioned above, the Philippines are of enormous importance as is Taiwan. General Douglas MacArthur likened the island of Luzon to an "unsinkable aircraft carrier." Today, another geographic location—the Straits of Malacca—is of vital importance to China as it pursues its "String of Pearls" strategy across the Indian Ocean.

The "String of Pearls" strategy is essentially a focused attempt by China to establish a series of ports for the purpose of transporting oil from the Persian Gulf where approximately one-fourth of the world's oil supply flows. To get to this oil, an enormous expenditure of effort has been focused on the Iranian Makran Coast and the island of Sri Lanka to the south of India. Perhaps most important of all has been the

---

[1]United Nations Report on Trade and Development, "The Universe of the Largest Transnational Corporations." (2007). http://unctad.org/en/Docs/iteiia20072_en.pdf

demonstrated need to keep the Strait of Malacca open and to prevent any foreign power from blocking the free flow of shipping through the strait and the adjacent micro nation-state of Singapore. Any obstruction to this vital area would certainly result in a near catastrophic situation for oil-hungry China. As such, Southeast Asia has seen an attempt by the Chinese to build a canal across the Isthmus of Kra in Burma. This attempt to build a canal has been compared by Robert Kaplan to America's creation of the Panama Canal, an act presaging a great superpower. Without question, from a Chinese standpoint alone, Southeast Asia will be of vital strategic importance. This makes this business intense climate equally important to the United States who is greatly interested in supporting India.

KEY TERMS TO KNOW

- tsunami
- Theravada
- cultural landscape
- toponyms

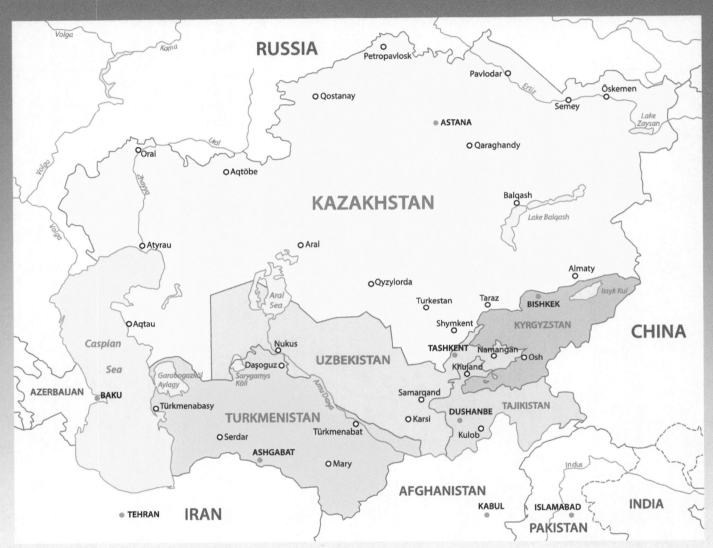

Central Asia

*Blessed is the man who trusts in the L*ORD*, whose trust is the L*ORD*. He is like a tree planted by water, that sends out its roots by the stream, and does not fear when heat comes, for its leaves remain green, and is not anxious in the year of drought, for it does not cease to bear fruit. (Jeremiah 17:7–8)*

Even though this area does not receive much rain, the people of Central Asia can still be prosperous by rooting themselves in the Lord. He will provide for those who trust Him. These nations are troubled by many powerful neighbors, but worshipping God will dissolve the violence. When Jesus spoke to those around him, he was able to reach them where they were. We likewise can understand a culture if we honestly attempt to understand it for the purpose of sharing our hope. Central Asia is, indeed, a thirsty land where water is needed and the agricultural aspects of Jesus' word can reach fertile ground!

Water Please

A common theme you may have noticed throughout this book is how physical geography appears to shape culture. How God created the physical world has without question made a mark on human societies. For this reason the student of geography must be simply amazed at how important the amount of rainfall in the region we call Central Asia has impacted the world. While much of this region only receives about eight inches of rain per year, the impact on livestock caused dramatic movements throughout history affecting empires from the ancient to the present. In particular, the Turkish Empire represented in some ways the apogee of a Muslim insurgence into Europe until circumstances enabled the Europeans to emerge as the preeminent power on Earth. Today we see this region again becoming extremely important in terms of oil.

Moving to the east from the Caspian Sea, you will see the states of Turkmenistan and Uzbekistan and to the far north Kazakhstan. The small mountainous states of

Kyrgyzstan and Tajikistan stand between China's ambitions and one of the world's great oil supplies. Rivaling the Persian Gulf oil fields and the oil fields of North Africa are those of the Caspian Sea basin. As important as these oil fields are, so are the pipelines they are connected to. To understand how the Western powers came to have the technology to tap these reserves and the tenuous business relationships and strategic possibilities of these areas, it is important to understand how and why the Western powers gained a technical advantage of the peoples of central Asia and what the future might hold there.

Another area we will touch upon in this chapter is the region known as the Trans-Caucasus area between the Black Sea and the Caspian Sea. Here the nations of Georgia, Armenia and Azerbaijan stand valiantly against growing encroachments from the north from Russia. As mentioned before, geography is a highly subjective discipline and the definition for a region is a loose one. It is felt that past associations with the former Soviet Union have given these regions a flavor somewhat peripheral to the nation-state of Russia today.

Going Green

Over time, several nomadic peoples dependent upon the thin belt of green grasses in the central Asian steppes engaged in various movements over time on the basis of their needs for increased fodder for their horses and livestock. The rises and declines of the ancient civilizations in large measure was a function of trade and the ability to exchange with the Chinese. The attempts to exploit the manufacturing capabilities and to receive the items created in the Far East led the Egyptians and Mediterranean powers of Greece and Rome to attempt to traverse the Red Sea and the Persian Gulf for the purposes of bypassing the land "silk road" used for trade. The Romans in fact, may well have weakened themselves in their attempts to control Babylonia or present day Iraq in various military operations possibly intended to keep the supply routes through the Euphrates and Tigris Rivers open. As the great empires of the west and east in concert prospered and declined a cycle of conditions that were probably favorable for expansion, or **push-pull factors** that encouraged the various central Asian societies to infringe upon these trade routes. Many groups emerged from central Asia to dramatically crash into the various civilizations throughout history: the Huns, Mongols, and Avars etc. The one group we want to focus on is the Turks. Grouped on the basis of perceived similarities in language, the Turks at various times proved instrumental in taking over the central Asian area and nearly destroyed late-medieval Europe on the verge on the modern. Why they didn't succeed and how the West

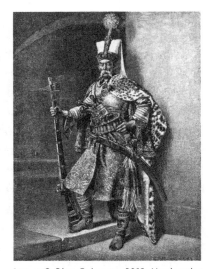

Image © Oleg Golovnev, 2013. Used under license from Shutterstock, Inc.

gained the advantage in technology can be viewed geographically in terms of land and sea. Just as the water is necessary to sustain life on the Steppes, it appears to be as important to an empire on land.

Floating on By

The water instrumental in marking the apogee of the Turkish Empire is salt water. The Battle of Lepanto between rival galleys demonstrated the affinity to land, which marked the central Asian empires and one that brought into conflict the dynamism of the merchant class into conflict with the military or warriors toward the seventeenth century, the Janissaries. The Janissaries grew in strength as the state relied increasingly upon them for loyalty. Initially called the Sipahis or military-nobles, they were a landowning class and represented a type of feudal power. When the Turks were unable to acquire more land however, the Sultan's were unable to procure additional loyalty by dispensing of property. In other words, a feudal system was perpetuated.[1] At the Battle of Lepanto, the Turk commanders demonstrated the increasingly rigid or ossifying nature of the Turkish civilization when they claimed their bows were superior to the arquebuses of the infidels.[2] The reluctance to explore new ideas also reflected in the lack of support for a middle-class of merchants or creators of capital. So, while the Turks lost the battle of Lepanto, more importantly they ceded a waterway from the Mediterranean and across the Indian Ocean preferring instead the conservative leadership of the Janissaries (military class). So, while the West developed trade with East Asia and the development of capital ensued and with it the opportunity for profits and upward social mobility, the Turks would begin a slow road to relative insignificance in terms of technology.[3] By the end of the seventeenth century, the industrial revolution would be underway in Great Britain where it would defuse to the continent.

It's Too Oily!

Today the technology of the West is quite interested in the vital oil fields of the areas around the Caspian Sea. The pipelines for this oil in many ways represents a type of circulatory system for the greater core or industrialized regions of the world. One very important oil pipeline crosses Georgia today and in part explains the decision of Russia to intervene militarily into this country in 2008. It appears the Russian decision to enter northern Georgia translated into an ability to reach one of the few oil pipelines from the Caspian region that did not go through Russian held territory. Now within range of artillery, Russia has further monopolized its ability to control this vital area again. Moving to the east, one leaves Christian Georgia where the Georgian Orthodox Church is the predominant faith. To the south is Armenia, a nation still

---

[1] Getz, Trevor R. and Streets-Salter, Heather. "Modern Imperialism and Colonialism: A Global Perspective" (Boston: Prentice Hall, 2011), 122.

[2] Rodgers, W. L., "Naval Warfare Under Oars: 4th to 16th Centuries" (Annapolis, Maryland: Naval Institute Press, 1967), 187.

[3] Kaplan, Robert D., "Monsoon" (New York: Random House, 2010), 50.

administratively at least in control of part of Jerusalem and at one time a bulwark for the Christian faith against advancing Islam. To the east we come to Muslim Azerbaijan, which has the vital break-bulk point of Baku, which overseas much of the important oil reserves from the aforementioned areas around the Caspian Sea. Using a type of Persian dialect, Azerbaijan like Georgia and Armenia have been mountainous areas demonstrating a propensity to avoid the orthodoxy of the adjacent great powers throughout history attempting to dominate them. The reason is simply mountains! Towering over Georgia, Armenia and Azerbaijan are the mighty Caucasus Mountains. This natural border between Russia and the former empires of Turkey and Iran seem to be a psychological border for the Russian peoples who for the most part live in a relatively flat open area.

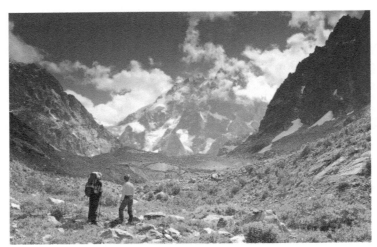

Image © My Good Images, 2013. Used under license from Shutterstock, Inc.

The Caucasus Mountains, one of Russia's few natural land borders.

The Aral Sea makes an environmental problem. Due to a tendency to utilize the valuable resource of fresh water for irrigation in neighboring Kazakhstan and Uzbekistan, the stage has been set for an environmental disaster of titanic proportions. Anytime humans alter the landscape, they run the potential risk of damaging the environment and precautions should always be taken. Good stewardship will remain a challenge for the various emerging economies and nations of Asia.

KEY TERMS TO KNOW

- push-pull factors

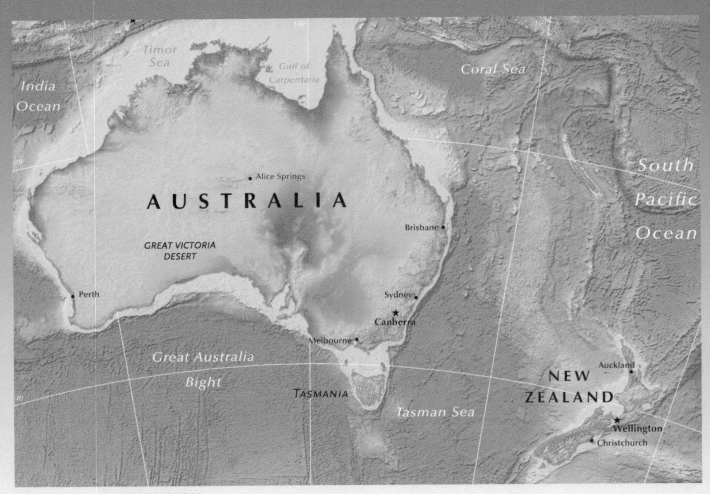

Map courtesy of Katie Pritchard and NOAA

Australia

So that we may no longer be children, tossed to and fro by the waves and carried about by every wind of doctrine, by human cunning, by craftiness in deceitful schemes. Rather, speaking the truth in love, we are to grow up in every way into him who is the head, into Christ, from whom the whole body, joined and held together by every joint with which it is equipped, when each part is working properly, makes the body grow so that it builds itself up in love. (Ephesians 4:14–16)

Almost everyone wants to go to Australia! It is such a wonderfully exotic continent and so far away. Despite the terrifically unique land that is Australia and New Zealand, challenges there are both obvious as in environmental, and perhaps not quite so obvious as involving immigrants and social changes. Like the United States, Australia is learning from its past, and a large part of the wisdom that comes from any lesson learned is to know God is ultimately to judge harshly our actions if we are not committed to our faith in His Son's purpose and not

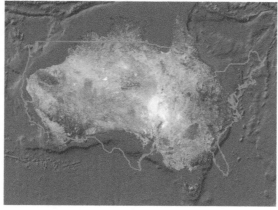

From *Blue Marble: Next Generation* image produced by Reto Stockli, NASA Earth Observatory (NASA Goddard Space Flight Center)

about His business! You can never escape the love and authority of God, and you can't travel further from the United States to do his work than Australia! Remember Job 28:24 (NKJV). For He looks to the ends of the earth, *And* sees under the whole heavens.

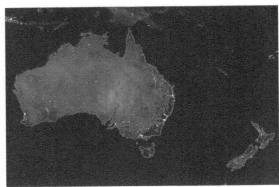
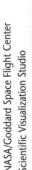

NASA/Goddard Space Flight Center Scientific Visualization Studio

Note the coastal locations of Australian and New Zealand cities.

Australia is three things: an island, a nation and a continent. This is a good time to review some basic terms. An **island** is a body of land surrounded on all sides by water. A **nation-state** consists of two terms: a **state** and a **nation**. A nation is a location that has a shared history and culture. This is a more human concept, whereas a state has defined borders recognized both within by the citizenry and without by other nations. As you recall, a **citizen** is a member of the state.

Outback, Mate

Regarding physical geography, Australia is a **continent**. It has its own tectonic plate it consists of, unlike other huge islands like Greenland. Within this continent is a diversity of varying topography that interacts with the southern currents to create a unique watershed in southeast Australia called the Murray-Dingly watershed in New South Wales. The vast interior is of varying colors—most noticeably red. The Japanese and Chinese covetously harvest the mineral-rich interior. To the north are the crocodile strewn tropical swamps, to the south is the cooler island of Tasmania and to the southeast are the major islands of New Zealand. Australia is tangential to the Great Barrier Reef, perhaps the greatest remaining coral reef popularized in a recent children's movie. This brings us to the colorful origins of Australia.

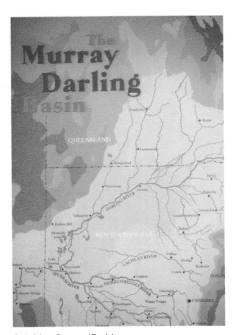

© Ashley Cooper/Corbis

From Prison to Production

As Niall Ferguson says in the book "Empire," "Small wonder the early settlement of Australia required compulsion."[1] When one considers how far Australia is from the rest of the world, the very remoteness of this wonderful continent is revealed. Even with high-speed jet aircraft, it will take about fifteen hours to go from Los Angeles, California to Melbourne, Australia. So why did the early pioneers come to Australia? As Mr. Ferguson points out, many of the early people came to Australia in an attempt to avoid floggings and branding as punishment for crimes. Ferguson again points out in his book the remarkable differences between the American experiment where a Puritan Utopia and plantation system in North America became a rebellious republic, but Australia, initially colonized at Botany Bay by prisoners, mostly shoplifters exiled into a penal colony ultimately became a loyal British colony.[2]

I Will Be a Bilby

Perhaps the thing that most amazes us about Australia are the wonderful wildlife and plants there. The **biomes** here are truly unique. Everyone knows about kangaroos, but have you ever seen a wombat or a bilby? Such strange creatures epitomized by the "confused" duck-billed platypus which lays eggs and has a beak like a bird, and yet is fur-bearing and possesses reptilian-like poison glands on the rear legs, capable of delivering a nasty sting! But the uniqueness doesn't stop here. Even the snakes are different. There are no boas, just pythons. The turtles are side-necked not like ours in North America, and the lizards are totally different as well. Most of the snakes are venomous, again at odds with our experience, while instead of monkeys or apes, we see the koala bear in the mighty eucalyptus forests. These stately trees like columns holding up the sky are similar in size to our American redwood trees.

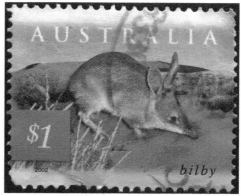

Image © IgorGolovniov, 2013. Used under license from Shutterstock, Inc.

The imagination of the Creator's handicraft is evident in this Bilby!

Drawing the Animal Line

Why is the wildlife so different in Australia? This is a good question and one for which there is no easy answer. Wallace's Line runs generally from southwest to northeast between the islands of Sulawesi and Borneo in Indonesia. Above the line, one tends to find a plethora of mammalian orders. Below it we find generally marsupials or mammals that tend to give birth to premature young, which must negotiate into a pouch to

---

[1] Niall Ferguson, Empire. (Basic Books: New York, 2002), 84.
[2] Ibid., 85.

be carried by their mother. Biogeography aside, Australia is a fascinating place from a human perspective as well.

Stewardship

An unfortunate aspect of globalization is the increased travel of people to areas previously ignored due to distance such as Australia. Australia has indeed faced a plethora of natural disasters ranging from the famous fences to contain rabbits or the mice infestations. The incredible damage of invasive species is a frightening aspect of the curse on the planet. Australia's ecosystems seem particularly vulnerable because of the unique niches or positions various animals occupy. In addition to increased travel is the abundance of technological devices that quickly alter the environment such as chainsaws. The lumber industry actually relies on helicopters to lower lumberjacks into forests where they can then cut themselves to nearby roads. Granted mankind has been given stewardship over the Earth, but better stewardship will be required in years ahead by you and other committed Christians. The non-Christian world seems to feel we believe we are to exercise domination over the Earth when in fact, we have been granted **dominion**. Just as we are to be good stewards of our bodies we, likewise, must be considerate of our environment.

No Fear Here!

One of the oldest tricks in the world is for a religious class in conjunction with a political leader to use the element of fear as a means of controlling a population. Whether it is the Aztecs with their fear of the sun burning out, or the fear of a celestial object hitting the Earth, we must remember our Lord told us not to worry. We are not given to a spirit of fear, and therefore we can be better stewards of those things we have been given responsibility for because we do not feel the need to hoard or consume more resources than we need. Concerns of global warming due to the industrial revolution, or the proliferation of **chlorofluorocarbons** believed to be responsible for the hole in the **ozone layer** may or may not be caused by humans, but regardless, we can study these phenomenon and search for solutions not out of a spirit of fear but because we have been granted a spirit of confidence through the peace we have in a loving God who created the Earth and sustains it!

The study of climate change often depends on such diverse sources as wine keeper's diaries and the fascinating study of dendrochronology (tree rings) to observe changes in moisture and temperature through history. Many environmental geographers even believe changing climate patterns have been instrumental in the expansion and movement of various nomads such as we mentioned in the earlier chapter of the Middle East. Again, we see how various elements of human culture are, in fact, in large measure a function of physical geography.

KEY TERMS TO KNOW

- island
- nation-state
- state
- nation
- citizen
- continent
- biomes
- dominion
- chlorofluorocarbons
- ozone layer

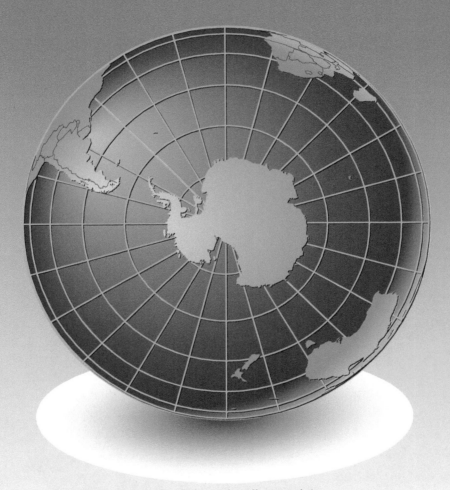

13

Antarctica and Oceania

Jesus said to her, "Everyone who drinks of this water will be thirsty again, but whoever drinks of the water that I will give him will never be thirsty again. The water that I will give him will become in him a spring of water welling up to eternal life." (John 4:13–14)

Most people think water is a cheap and easily procured resource. When our Lord spoke to the multitudes in Matthew 6:25, telling them not to worry about what they would eat or drink, they more than likely understood the reference to water in an intense way that might elude us today. An arid climate can indeed be a worrisome existence and life can be harsh. A tough existence is the calling of many Christians throughout the globe and we have a duty to encourage and support them in any way we can. No place on Earth is likely to be more extreme than Antarctica or more pleasant than much of Oceania. Just like our lives have peaks and valleys, we can be consistent in our approach towards our loving and eternal Father who loves us without qualifications. Remember, regardless of the extremes we face in this life; the Lord's admonition not to worry is always a good one to reflect upon. Let us, therefore, get about the works He considers important now without delay!

Commonly known as the South Pole, Antarctica is really a continent. Famous for its severe conditions and interesting animal life, few people know what potential it really holds. Even less people know that it is surrounded by one of the newest described geographic areas. So why is Antarctica a continent?

Antarctica is actually part of a tectonic plate and as such is a continent. Largely unexplored, it is nevertheless one of the most peculiar places on Earth. Severe cold and the accompanying wind and dryness make it seemingly uninhabitable. There are, however, a few sea mammals that have proliferated in the area as well as birds. Specially adapted to the cold, these generally large and bulky creatures depend on the fish rich seas for their diets. Whales, seals and penguins are generally what one thinks about when they think of the animal life on Antarctica. Other than simple plant life that appears on the tundra, these are the most noteworthy life forms on the continent. The newest geographic body to be described surrounds the continent.

Whale Tale

The Southern Sea is the name of the sea that flows around Antarctica. Continually flowing eastward, this ocean is one of the most tumultuous in the world. Its northern boundary empties into the other oceans of the world and there is a marked difference between the contrast of the icy continent of Antarctica and the relatively warmer (but still cold!) waters surrounding it. This contrasting temperature accounts for the roughness of the seas and this in turn seems to provide nutrients to the abundant whale populations of the world. With little resistance from landmasses, this current flows fast and can be littered with icebergs of varying sizes. So what resources does Antarctica hold?

Although many mineral resources including coal and oil have been found in Antarctica, it remains a continent of untapped potential. Preventing any meaningful exploration are numerous international treaties designed to prevent greedy people from competing with one another to be the first to tap these potentially valuable areas. Isn't it amazing how God continually provides us with the resources we need, such as heat, food, clothing and water? Unfortunately we seem to never have enough and often fail to give thanks. Perhaps if we were more thankful we would need less, and then there wouldn't be so much difficulty finding more resources without being burdened by regulations and restrictions. Perhaps you will be the one to find a resource and you will be able to share it providing a Christian testimony in the process.

Drowning in Thirst

Speaking of oceans and water. Imagine living where water is everywhere but not enough to drink. This is the situation faced by the early travelers throughout the Pacific Ocean region we now refer to as Oceania. Where these people came from is still a mystery with conflicting theories arguing the movement of peoples originated in China or Siberia and others (less commonly) have argued that the peoples of Oceania originated in South America. The truth is there is a terrific amount of mystery here. What are not in question are the remarkable accomplishments of those men and women who migrated across half of the Earth's surface to create unique cultures on islands of varying hospitality. Some writers believe this circumnavigation may be the single greatest accomplishment in the history of mankind and one of the most recent.[1] With simple catamarans or boats with outriggers to provide additional support, it is a terrific accomplishment and one no doubt contingent upon understanding currents both atmospheric and at sea.

---

[1] Borthwick, Mark, "Pacific Century" (Boulder, Colorado: Westview Press, 2014), 11.

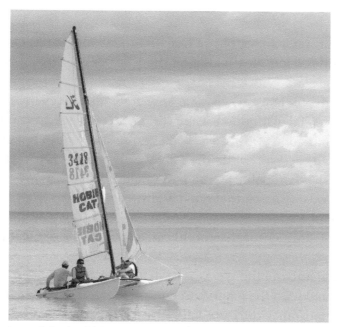

Image © Kamira, 2013. Used under license from Shutterstock, Inc.

Going Nuts

A quick look at a selection of flags will reveal the importance the people of this region place on celestial objects such as stars and the sun. These might be insights into the deep-seated awareness of the environment that led these early explorers. Another common color is the blue of the ocean. Without question, the physical environment can be seen in the vexillological (flag) displays on the human landscape today.

A biological aspect of the biomes of this region is the simple coconut. Able to float on the ocean for great distances, in many places the coconut obviously came ashore and was an important aspect of soil creation enabling life forms to thrive. Thrive is exactly what some of these creatures have done. The Christmas Island crab covers the streets with bright red shells as they run to and fro. Crabs have even developed that are dependent upon the crab for their source of food and have specially adapted bodies for this purpose. So, the lowly coconut floating across the open ocean riding the ocean currents in many cases probably served to sustain human life and enable the early travelers to cross this amazing area.

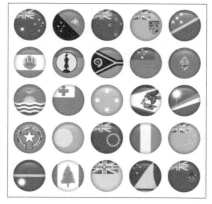

Image © Luca_Luppi, 2013. Used under license from Shutterstock, Inc.

Miles of Isles

Some of the important sub-regions of Oceania today include Melanesia, Micronesia, and Polynesia and are loosely divided on the basis of varying interpretations of language and ethnicity and because of the relationship of tectonic activities and the resulting landforms and volcanoes. The enormous distances involved make this an extremely controversial distinction. The people of Melanesia appear to be very similar to those on the island of New Guinea. The Micronesians may appear in many ways to be descendants of East Asia, while the Polynesian peoples are best characterized by the Hawaiians. As you probably learned, the Columbian exchange or age of discovery unleashed numerous diseases that make it difficult today to draw distinctions of origins on the basis of ethnicity. Since we all came from the Ark, it is probably best to reflect on the strategic significance of this area to the world's great powers in the last century.

America in general and the West Coast in particular have been viewed as increasingly interconnected with the Pacific Rim, particularly in terms of business. This area was of extreme importance during an age of steam as ships required coaling and supply bases every thousand miles or so. Various developing nations attempted to stake

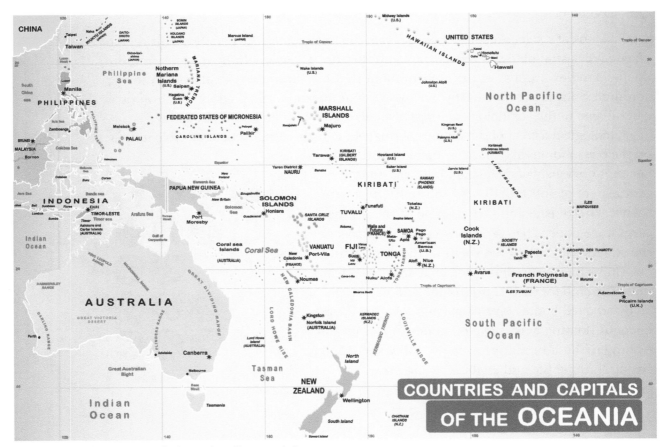

out "turf" across the Pacific for the purpose of developing secure transport routes in an attempt to fulfill that ancient yearning—trade with China! The United States became involved in the Philippines at the beginning of the last century in the Spanish American War and this would bring it into conflict with the Japanese in World War II initially in Polynesia when Pearl Harbor erupted into flames. The Central Pacific drive by the Naval forces of the United States would bring American interests in a type of continuing "manifest destiny" or westward expansion to the areas of Melanesia where they would fight to defend Australia and through Micronesia in an effort to bring force to bear on the Japanese home islands. American involvement in the Pacific continued through the Vietnam War and into the present, and in fact the recent Presidential administration has attempted to "pivot" in its efforts to capitalize on American interests in the areas adjacent to East Asia. This will no doubt continue to make the Pacific Ocean a road to the back door of the United States in years to come.

UNIT TWO

HUMAN GEOGRAPHY

Introduction: Main Ideas and Thematic Structure

"Beloved, you do faithfully whatever you do for the brethren and for strangers." (3 John 1:5)

God created the world. Despite the many problems, despair, and fears we may confront, we can rest assured His Love for us is unceasing. In Genesis 9:1–3, God blessed Noah's descendants and instructed them "to be fruitful and multiply, and replenish the earth." Furthermore, God provided mankind the resources necessary to spread across the Earth. In Mark 14:62 and Rev 19:11–16, Jesus promises to return, thereby giving us both hope and a reason to be faithful in attempting to reach the world with the truth and to serve the needs of a lost and suffering world. A spatial perspective in general, and knowledge of human geography in particular, can better enable us to serve the various peoples of the Earth, armed with the truth of the Great Commission. Any goal for service must, however, have as its basis a strategy. Any strategy should be compatible with concepts of human geography. To understand the concepts of human geography, we will examine the nature of geography and the themes governing a geographic perspective. A world system analysis can delineate the areas of the world most capable of serving others, as well as identify areas particularly in need.

In This Chapter:

- The Nature of Geography
- Unifying Themes in Geography
- World-Systems Analysis
- Development and Underdevelopment in the World-Economy
- Key Terms to Know

- Study Questions
- Further Reading

THE NATURE OF GEOGRAPHY

Most Americans relate the term geography to the rote memorization of trivial facts associated with various countries of the world: capitals, imports and exports, highest mountains, largest lakes, most populous cities, climates and the like. This trivialized impression of the subject matter with which geography is concerned most likely stems from the fact that until recently, geography was not taught as a distinctive subject in most American elementary schools and high schools. Even today, it is often taught as a marginalized part of "social science" courses in elementary schools and civics or history courses in high schools. As a result, most Americans think of geography as a collection of trivial factoids rather than a distinct academic subject such as history, economics, mathematics or physics are. But within academia, geography is a thriving, diverse discipline with its own set of theories, research methods, terminology and subject matter and with a unique way of looking at the world. Indeed, the Association of American Geographers, the largest professional society of geographers in the world, counts over 5,000 professors, students and professionals as members.

So what is it that geographers do? What is their method of analysis? What questions do geographers ask about the world? These questions, as it turns out, are not easily answered. Indeed, any two geographers might answer them in very different ways, for geography is not unified by subject, but rather method. This is yet another reason for misconceptions about what geography is on the part of the lay public and, indeed, on the part of many academicians themselves. Geography does not seem to "fit" into academe the same way that other subjects do because the discipline is not unified or defined by the subject matter with which it is concerned. Rather, it is unified and defined by its method and approach, its mode of analysis. This mode of analysis (or approach or perspective) involves a **spatial perspective**. In this way geography can be conceptualized as a way of thinking about the world, about space and about places. This spatial (geographical) perspective involves the fundamental question as to how both cultural and natural phenomena vary spatially (geographically) across the earth's surface. As such, it is quite literally possible to study the geography of almost any phenomenon that occurs on the earth's surface. Employing these ideas, we may define the academic discipline of geography as *the study of the spatial variation of phenomena across the earth's surface*. So, geographers do not study a certain "thing" or subject. Instead, they study all sorts or "things" and subjects in a specific way—spatially.

The 18th century German philosopher Immanuel Kant understood very well the unique position that geography held within academia. Kant argued that human beings make sense of and organize the world in one of three ways, and human knowledge, as well as academic departments in the modern university, is arranged or organized in the same way. First, Kant wrote, we make sense of the world *topically* by organizing knowledge according to specific subject matter: biology as the study of plant and animal life, geology as the study of the physical structure of the earth, sociology as the study of human society, and so on. Each of these fields is unified by the subject matter with which it is concerned. Second, according to Kant, we make sense of the world *temporally* by organizing phenomena according to time, periods and eras. This is the sole domain of the discipline of history. Finally, Kant argued that we make sense of the world *chorologically* (geographically) by organizing phenomena according to how they vary across space and from place to place. This is the sole domain of the discipline of geography. The disciplines of history and geography are similar in that they are both unified by a method rather than the study of a specific subject matter. The region (discussed below) in geography is analogous to the era or period in history—they are the main units of analysis in each of the respective disciplines.

Figure 1.1 represents a generalized model for understanding the nature of the academic discipline of geography. This figure illustrates the field's three main subfields: physical geography, human geography and environmental geography. The description and analysis of patterns on the landscape unites each of these subfields. When most people think of the term landscape they think of something depicted in a painting, or perhaps a garden. But when geographers employ the term landscape, they are referring to the totality of our surroundings. In this sense, the **physical landscape** refers to the patterns created on the earth's surface as a result of natural or physical processes. For example, tectonic forces create continents and mountain chains. Long term climatic processes create varying vegetative realms. Wind and water shape and modify landforms. **Physical geography**, then, is the subfield of geography that is concerned with the description and analysis of the physical landscape and the processes that create and modify that landscape. The various subfields of physical geography such as biogeography, climatology and geomorphology are natural sciences, allied with such fields as botany, meteorology and geology, and, like these allied fields, research in physical geography is undertaken largely according to the scientific method.

Human geography is the subfield of geography that is concerned with the description and analysis of cultural landscapes and the social and cultural processes that create and modify those landscapes. While physical geography is concerned with the natural forces that shape the earth's physical landscapes, human geography analyzes the social and cultural forces that create cultural landscapes. The **cultural landscape**, then, may be conceptualized as the human "imprint" on the physical landscape resulting from modification of the physical landscape by human social and cultural forces. Given the power and influence of human technology and institutions, many human geographers see human beings as the ultimate modifiers of the physical landscape. The various subfields of human geography, such as historical geography, economic geography and political geography are social sciences, allied with such fields as history, economics and political science. In addition to their own research methodologies, human geographers often employ research methods from these allied fields. Traditionally, human geography has been concerned with how cultural processes such as religion, language and world-view affect the cultural landscape. More recently,

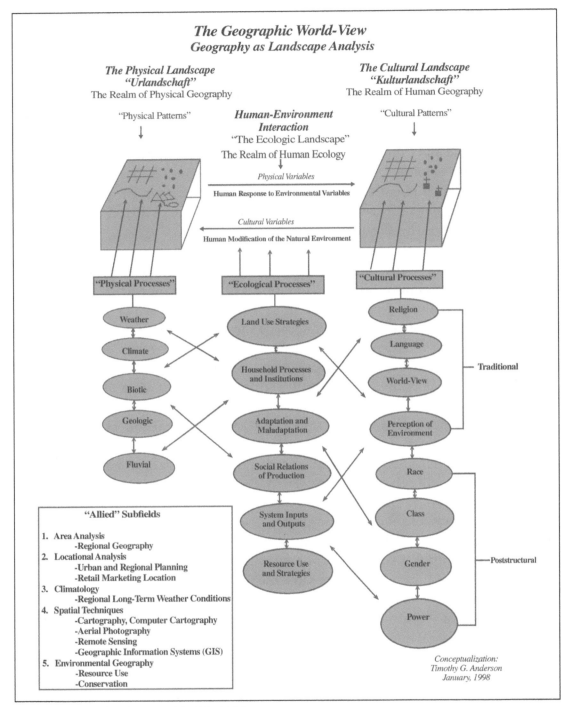

Figure 14.1 The Geographic World-View

however, cultural geographers have begun to question traditional ideas about how cultural landscapes are created by focusing on so-called post-structural processes to reevaluate the nature of cultural landscapes. In such research, the cultural landscape is conceptualized as a stage upon which social struggles dealing with such concepts as race, class, power and gender are played out. In this sense, the cultural landscape is the product of such struggles.

Although all geographers do not recognize it as such, it can be argued that **environmental geography** is a third major subfield of geography. Environmental geography is concerned with the interrelationships between humans and the natural environments in which they live, or nature-society relationships. Environmental geographers study the patterns created on the landscape by such interactions and the processes involved, such as social relations of production, cultural adaptations or maladaptations to particular environments, modifications to the environment wrought by human economies and technologies, and the use (or misuse) of natural resources.

UNIFYING THEMES IN GEOGRAPHY

The discussion in the previous section illustrates the diverse nature of the academic discipline of geography. In spite of this diversity, however, we can identify some common themes with which most geographical studies are concerned and which unify the field. Three common concepts have already been identified: pattern, process and landscape. In addition, we can delineate five unifying themes in geographic research:

Location

This theme addresses the question, "where is it at?" We can think of location in two primary ways. **Absolute location** refers to a specific point on the globe—latitude and longitude, for example. On the other hand, **relative location** refers to the location of a place or phenomenon with respect to other places or phenomena around it. For example some places may occupy a more central role with respect to the economy of a country. Such places may be said to occupy a more central relative location.

Place and Space

This theme refers to the description and analysis of the patterning of phenomena in a certain place or across space. This patterning can be analyzed in terms of the distribution, density and concentration of phenomena.

Human-Environment Interaction

This theme explores the complex relationships between human beings and their natural environment, how people interact with the environment around them, the nature of that interaction and the influence of the natural environment on human culture. Interpretations of the role played by the environment in human affairs and the nature of human-environment interaction have changed substantially over time. The ancient Greeks, for example, attributed observed cultural differences around the world to the climates in which people lived. It was argued that African cultures differed from

European cultures because African societies evolved in a hot climate. That is, they argued that the environment plays a deciding role in terms of shaping cultural values, ideals and traditions—certain environments and climates create certain cultures. This supposition is known as **environmental determinism**. Surprisingly, this argument continued to be used by many social scientists to account for cultural differences around the world well into the 20th century. Some prominent American geographers in the early 20th century, for example, argued that a unique subculture punctuated by poverty, subsistence agriculture and a distinctive folk culture (food, music, social systems, etc.) developed in Appalachia because of the region's mountainous terrain and geographical remoteness. But under close scrutiny, of course, environmental determinism is an untenable supposition that does not explain reality. Culture is not created by the climate of a place or by mountains—culture is learned behavior passed on from generation to generation. By the 1940s the use of environmental deterministic arguments to explain culture began to wither under close scientific scrutiny. Led by French human geographers beginning in the 1930s, the idea of **possibilism** began to replace determinism. This supposition argued that the environment surrounding us offers certain possibilities, but what people do with those possibilities is determined by cultural values and traditions which are learned and which evolve over time. Today, geographers have modified possibilism into a workable hypothesis that may be termed **environmental perception**. This hypothesis argues that different cultures perceive or conceptualize the environment in which they live in different ways. These differences in perception may be attributed to differences in cultural values and traditions, which result in the creation of varying cultural landscapes. In this way, it is argued, any cultural landscape can be "read", analyzed and deconstructed to understand the values, ideals and traditions (the "culture") of the people that created that landscape.

Movement

This theme seeks to understand how and why observed phenomena move through space—"how did this pattern or distribution come to be?" The central concept employed by geographers to explain the movement of people, ideas and innovations from place to place is **diffusion**. In this sense, cultural diffusion may be thought of as the movement of ideas, traditions and innovations through space. Three different kinds of movement can be employed to explain how diffusion takes place. *Hierarchical diffusion* describes the movement of ideas and innovations in stair-step fashion from person to person: one person tells two people and they tell two people and they tell two people, and so on. This kind of diffusion is relatively slow and it may take weeks, months or years for ideas to move from one place to another. Before the advent of mass communication technology in the early 20th century, most diffusion was hierarchical in nature. A second type of diffusion is *contagious diffusion*. Contagious diffusion refers to the rapid movement of innovations and ideas through space in the same manner that a contagious disease spreads through a population. Many people (perhaps in the millions) become aware of an idea or innovation at the same time. In today's age of globalization, the internet and highly-evolved methods of mass communication, contagious diffusion is the primary way in which ideas move from place to place. A third type of diffusion is known as *relocation diffusion*. Relocation diffusion describes the movement of ideas over long distances in a relatively short time, usually attributed to mass migrations of people from one place to another place. The fact that the majority of North Americans speak English as a mother tongue and practice some form of Christianity can most likely be attributed to the migration of millions of Europeans to North America over some 400 years (relocation diffusion) and the subsequent movement across the continent (contagious diffusion).

Regions

The **region** is the primary unit of analysis for the geographer. A region is simply an area within which there is homogeneity of a certain phenomenon or certain phenomena—that is, homogeneity through space. Both physical and human geographers use the concept of region to describe and analyze places and subject matter. In this sense, a **culture region** is a place within which a certain culture is predominant. Geographers identify three primary types of regions. A **formal region** is a region that is easily identified through the use of verifiable data. The distribution of German speakers in Europe or the region in the United States in which winter wheat is grown is an example of a formal region. A **functional region** is a place within which there is movement. The predominance of a certain kind of movement in that place defines the region itself. The best example of a functional region is a trade area or a market area. Finally, a **perceptual region** is a region that is not easily identifiable, the parameters of which may vary from person to person. The "Midwest" and the "South" in the United States are examples of perceptual regions. The location of both of these regions is not exact and may vary from person to person based on their own perceptions.

WORLD-SYSTEMS ANALYSIS

The main goals of this text are to give students a basic understanding of the human geography of the world, to delineate the world's major culture regions, to illustrate how human culture and cultural landscapes vary across space, and to examine the phenomenon of economic "development" and "underdevelopment". In order to accomplish these goals effectively we will employ the concepts of pattern, process and landscape, as well as the five themes outlined above. In addition, **world-systems analysis** is used as a thematic context around which the book is structured. World-systems analysis is best described as a distinctive approach to the study of social change developed by the American sociologist Immanuel Wallerstein in the early 1970s. This approach combines economic, political, sociological, geographical and historical aspects in a holistic historical social science that is based on three different research traditions: dependency theory, the French *Annales* School of history (especially the work of Fernand Braudel), and Marxist theory.

World-systems analysis is chiefly concerned with analysis of the nature, development and structure of the capitalist world economy and provides a useful context within which to compare and contrast regions of relative "development" and "underdevelopment" in the world's economy through time and space. In his three-volume work *The Modern World-System*, Wallerstein maintains that there have been only three fundamental ways, or **modes of production**, in which societies throughout history have been organized in order to sustain production. These **modes of production**, these societies, can be distinguished by determining the division of labor in production that is dominant in these societies.

The *reciprocal-lineage mode of production* refers to a society in which production is differentiated mainly by age and gender, and exchange is merely reciprocal in nature (that is, barter exchange dominates the economy). Wallerstein calls such systems **mini-systems**, and there have been countless numbers of these throughout history. Such societies are usually small in terms of population and geographical area and there are few, if any, class divisions (anthropologists refer to such societies as *tribes*).

The *redistributive-tributary mode of production* describes a society that is class-based and in which production is performed by a large agricultural underclass that pays tribute to a small ruling class (anthropologists refer to such societies as *chiefdoms*). Wallerstein calls these societies **world-empires**, and there have been many of them since the Neolithic Revolution around 10,000 B.C. (examples would include the ancient kingdoms of Mesopotamia and the Nile Valley, the Mayan and Aztec societies in Middle America, various kingdoms in western and southeastern Africa, the ancient dynasties of China, and the Ottoman and Roman empires). World-empires were very large in terms of population and geographical size.

Finally, the *capitalist mode of production* also refers to a class-based society, but is distinguished by the goal of a ceaseless accumulation of capital operating within a market logic and structure (capitalism). Wallerstein calls such societies **world-economies**. According to Wallerstein, there has been only one successful world-economy. It originated in Western Europe around the middle of the 15th century and spread to encompass the entire world through long-distance sea trade, colonialism and world conflicts by the beginning of the 20th century. World-empires and world-economies are called *world-systems* by Wallerstein because the divisions of labor operating within them are larger than any one local grouping.

In world-systems analysis, then, the world is seen as a single entity—a capitalist world-economy. Wallerstein argues that in order to meaningfully understand the nature of the global economy and of social change one must not consider the role of individual countries so much as the entire world-system. To do so is to commit the fundamental **error of developmentalism**, which dominates current liberal studies of development and Marxist analyses, both of which see individual countries progressing through stages of "development".

DEVELOPMENT AND UNDERDEVELOPMENT IN THE WORLD-ECONOMY

One of the most useful aspects of world-systems analysis with respect to understanding the human geography of the world and its division into "developed" and "underdeveloped" realms is its delimitation of the spatial, political and economic structure of the current capitalist world-economy. According to Wallerstein the capitalist world-economy that has developed since the mid-15th century has three primary structural features:

1. A single world market which operates within the context of a capitalist ideology and logic; this logic and ideology effects economic decisions throughout the entire world-system.

2. A "multiple-state" system in which no single state ("country") is able to dominate totally and within which political and economic competition among various states is structured and defined.

3. A three-tiered economic and spatial structure of stratification in terms of the degree of economic "development" and "underdevelopment" of the world's various states. In this textbook, this basic three-tiered structure is employed as the primary tool, as a model and a theory, for understanding basic differences in the human geography of the world today and in the past. In place of terms like "developed world" and "developing world", or "first world" and "third world", we will use the terms *core*, *semi-periphery* and *periphery* that are employed in world-systems analysis to differentiate between regions of varying economic "development" in the world. This text argues that an understanding of the differences between these regions is fundamental to a meaningful appreciation of the differences in such things as the nature of cultures, the structure of economies, political organization and population issues and problems around the world.

Table 14.1 employs widely available socio-economic statistics for selected countries to illustrate general socio-economic differences between core, semi-peripheral and peripheral regions. It should be noted that while the terms "core" and "periphery" are employed to indicate geographical location in common usage, in world-systems analysis they do not *necessarily* refer to a state's geographical location on the globe. Rather, they are used to refer to a state or region's "location" in the world-economy, that is on the "inside" (core), on the "outside" (periphery), or somewhere in the middle (semi-periphery) of the world-economy in terms of relative control. Those states in the core control and direct the world-economy, while those in the periphery are most often controlled and directed by the core states. Further, history shows us that it is clear that "core" and "periphery" are not geographically or temporally static—states move up and down within this hierarchy over time at a non-constant rate. A recent excellent example of this rule is the former Soviet Union. Before its breakup in late 1991, one could argue (using socio-economic data) that the Soviet Union was a core state. Since

Table 14.1   World Demographic/Socio-Economic Indicator Data, 2009

Country	POP	BR	DR	NI	IM	TFR	<15	>65	GNI/PPP
World	6,810	21	8	1.2	46	2.6	27	8	$10,090
More Dev.	1,232	11	10	0.1	6	1.6	17	16	$32,320
Less Dev.	5,578	22	8	1.4	50	2.7	30	6	$5,170
Least Dev.	828	35	11	2.4	80	4.6	40	3	$1,230
Selected Core States									
Germany	82.0	8	10	−0.2	3.9	1.3	14	20	$35,940
Japan	127.6	9	9	0.0	2.6	1.4	13	23	$35,220
USA	306.8	14	8	0.6	6.6	2.1	20	13	$46,970
Norway	4.8	13	9	0.4	2.7	2.0	19	15	$58,500
Spain	46.9	11	8	0.3	3.5	1.5	14	17	$31,130
Selected Semiperipheral States									
Russia	141.8	12	15	−0.3	9	1.5	15	14	$15,630
South Africa	50.7	23	15	0.8	45	2.7	32	5	$9,780
Costa Rica	4.5	16	4	1.3	9.7	1.9	27	6	$10,950
Argentina	40.3	18	8	1.0	12.9	2.4	26	10	$14,020
Mexico	106.5	21	5	1.7	24	2.4	32	75	$11,330
China	1,331	12	7	0.5	21	1.6	19	8	$6,020
Malaysia	27.2	23	5	1.8	10	2.9	33	62	$11,300
Saudi Arabia	27.6	30	3	2.7	16	4.1	38	81	$16,620
Selected Peripheral States									
Pakistan	180.8	30	7	2.3	67	4.0	38	4	$2,700
Laos	6.3	28	7	2.1	64	3.5	39	4	$2,060
Bolivia	9.9	29	8	2.1	50	3.5	38	4	$4,140
Congo	68.7	44	13	3.1	92	6.5	47	3	$3,090
Nigeria	152.6	41	15	2.6	75	5.7	45	3	$1,940

POP = Population (millions)

BR = Births/1000 persons/year

DR = Deaths/1000 persons/year

NI = Natural Increase/annum (%)

IM = Infant Mortality Rate (deaths of infants under 1 per 1000 live births)

TFR = Total Fertility Rate (average number of children born to a woman during her lifetime)

<15= Percentage of population less than 15 years of age

>65 = Percentage of the population greater than 65 years of age

GNI/PPP = Gross national income in purchasing power parity/population (US $) (2008)

Source: Population Reference Bureau, 2009 World Population Data Sheet http://www.prb.org

the breakup, however, economic conditions have deteriorated to the point that Russia is now clearly a semi-peripheral state. Further examples would include several countries in Southeast Asia such as Indonesia, Thailand, Malaysia and Singapore. Peripheral states until the 1980s, they all are now part of the semi-periphery due to surging manufacturing economies and greater political and economic stability.

Core States

The **core states** of the world-economy today include most states in northern, western and southern Europe, the United States and Canada, Japan, and Australia and New Zealand (see Map 1 on the CD that accompanies this text). It is from here that the world-economy is directed and where its primary command and control centers, such as New York, London, Paris, Frankfurt, and Tokyo, are located. Western Europe emerged as the first core region of the capitalist world-economy in the mid-15th century and remained the primary core until the 20th century, when the United States, Canada, Japan and Australia and New Zealand joined its ranks. The wealth of the core stemmed at first from highly efficient agricultural production and control of merchant capitalism through long-distance sea trade in valuable tropical agricultural products (such as tea, coffee, sugar, tobacco, cotton and spices) during the era of colonialism. Portugal, Spain, the Netherlands and the United Kingdom were the successive **hegemonic powers** (dominance in economic, political, military and cultural affairs of the world) of this early world-economy from the mid-15th century until the early 20th century.

The United States emerged as the primary hegemonic power after World War II. From this period until the early 1970s, the wealth of the core was based primarily on dominance in industrial capitalism focused on heavy industry (cars, ships, chemicals, manufacturing and the like). The United States, Canada, the Soviet Union, Germany and Japan all emerged as the major players in world industrial production during this era. With the exception of the Soviet Union, all of these states remain in the core today. Since the early 1970s, post-industrial restructuring in the core economies has taken place, with a switch away from a reliance on heavy industry to a focus on service industries and information technologies. This era is generally referred to as the era of "globalization" that is characterized by a pronounced international division of labor (this will be discussed further in Chapter 15).

In comparison with semi-peripheral and peripheral locations, the core states all have highly developed economies that are oriented toward service industries and post-industrial technologies such as information technology and computer software production. These advanced economies enjoy a very high standard of living, high gross national products and per capita incomes, and are generally the "richest" countries in the world. Other characteristics of the core states include stable, democratic governments with large militaries, low infant mortality rates and high life expectancies (measures of relative health and availability of adequate health care), low birth rates, fertility rates and rates of natural increase (all signs of very low population growth rates), and large urban (as opposed to rural) populations.

Peripheral States

The **peripheral states** of the world-economy today are located primarily in Sub-Saharan Africa, South Asia (Pakistan, India and Bangladesh) and parts of Southeast Asia (e.g. Papua New Guinea, Cambodia, Laos) and some parts of Middle and South America (e.g. Guatemala, Bolivia, Haiti). The peripheral states all have several things in common. Historically, they are all former colonies of core states and, accordingly, are generally located in either subtropical or tropical areas. During the era of merchant capitalism and colonialism, these areas were assigned a specific role in the world-economy by the dominant core powers: producers of valuable tropical agricultural goods such as sugar, tea, coffee, cotton and spices. As colonies, these areas lost political sovereignty to colonial governance by the core powers and traditional economies and societies were replaced by a colonial economy focusing on plantation agriculture linked heavily with the core. Slavery and peonage were employed by the core powers as the primary form of labor control in the periphery. Most of these former colonies regained political sovereignty after the end of the colonial era beginning in the late 19th century but have struggled since then to rebuild economies and societies that were heavily disrupted by colonialism.

Today, the economies of the periphery remain largely agricultural. The majority of the populations in these countries rely on subsistence farming, low-wage labor on agricultural plantations or low-skilled, low-wage service positions in urban areas. Compared with the core and the semi-periphery, living standards are relatively low, as are per-capita incomes—these areas are among the "poorest" countries in the world. Peripheral regions are plagued by a myriad of problems today: weak, inefficient and often corrupt governments, political instability, ethnic conflict, weakly-developed economies and a lack of public services taken for granted in core regions such as regular electric service, availability of clean water and public sewage services. High infant mortality rates and relatively low life expectancies belie weakly-developed health care systems and a susceptibility to epidemics and chronic problems with diseases such as malaria and AIDS. While core states have very low rates of natural increase (or even negative population growth in some countries), the peripheral populations are the fastest growing populations in the world. Compared with the core and semi-periphery, the peripheral states have very high birth and fertility rates and "young" populations—a significant proportion of these populations is younger than fifteen years of age. If core populations can be described as "old" with stable growth rates, then peripheral populations can be characterized as "young" and growing rapidly.

Semi-Peripheral States

The **semi-peripheral states** today include many of the countries of Middle and South America (e.g. Mexico, Costa Rica, Chile, Brazil, and Argentina), Eastern and Southeastern Europe (e.g. Russia, Poland, Bulgaria, and Hungary), Southwest Asia (e.g. Turkey, Saudi Arabia, and Iran) and Southeast and East Asia (e.g. Indonesia, Malaysia, Thailand, China and South Korea). Other semi-peripheral "outliers" include such countries as South Africa and much of Saharan Africa (e.g. Tunisia, Algeria, and Libya). As the term implies, the semi-periphery occupies a "middle" place in the hierarchy of "development" in the world-economy. If one considers socio-economic indicators and demographic data, it is clear that the data for semi-peripheral countries are midway between the extremes of the core and periphery—per capita incomes, birth and fertility rates, and rates of natural increase in the semi-periphery are neither the highest nor the lowest in the world, but rather somewhere in between. Accordingly, many world-systems analysts characterize semi-peripheral countries as not the richest, but certainly not the "poorest" countries in the world.

Many, but not all, of these countries are also former colonies. But since the 1960s most of them have managed to achieve some amount of economic and political stability, largely with loans from the World Bank and foreign aid from the core countries. But as a result, many are saddled with large debts to the World Bank and banks in the core. Economic stability in these countries was largely achieved through a focus on heavy industry and manufacturing as central features of the economy under the authority of rather strong (and sometimes corrupt and heavy handed) central governments. At the same time, most semi-peripheral economies are still heavily dependent upon the agricultural sector. Indeed, one of the most characteristic aspects of the semi-periphery is a mixed economy dependent upon agriculture (largely for export to the core), heavy industry and manufacturing, and a small but growing service sector. Social stratification in semi-peripheral societies reflects this mixed economy: a large rural agricultural lower class; a relatively large urban blue collar manufacturing class; and a small, wealthy urban professional class.

This intense social stratification—a vast difference between the richest and poorest members of society—is one of the hallmarks of the semi-periphery. According to Wallerstein, the most pronounced and acute class struggle occurs in the semi-periphery. This class struggle is often accompanied by chronic political and economic instability. The semi-periphery is also the focus of periodic restructurings of the world-economy during times of economic stagnation, which provide the necessary conditions for this restructuring. For example, it is usually the semi-periphery that is most adversely affected by crises in the world-economy. During the Industrial Revolution in the late 18th and early 19th centuries, for example, traditional agricultural and artisan economies in places such as Germany and Ireland (part of the semi-periphery at that time) were upset by the changes wrought by industrialism in Great Britain. Many farmers and artisans who could no longer make a living at home moved to core regions like Great Britain and the United States in order to take jobs in urban factories, thus supplying the core with a needed industrial workforce. In today's world-economy a similar situation is occurring in the semi-periphery. This time around traditional economies are being reordered by the current restructuring usually referred to as "globalization". This restructuring involves the outsourcing of manufacturing jobs by multi-national firms from the core to the semi-periphery, especially in the textile industry (the manufacturing of clothes, shoes and the like). At the same time, this economic reordering has again resulted in traditional economies being upset and phased out. One of the consequences of this has been a renewed large-scale migration of low skilled farmers and laborers from the semi-periphery (Latin America, East and Southeast Asia, Southwest Asia) to the core (Western Europe, North America, Australia).

This has resulted in a pronounced **international division of labor** characterized by economic specialization in each of the three regions of the world-economy. Peripheral economies are dominated by subsistence agriculture, plantation agriculture and natural resource extraction, all mainly for export to the semi-periphery and core. While local, low-wage labor is employed in the production of these resources and products, the capital and management is often controlled from or by the core in the form of multi-national corporations. Semi-peripheral economies specialize in small-scale commercial agriculture, heavy industry and manufacturing (steel, chemicals, etc.) and textile production, the latter for export primarily to the core. Core economies are highly diversified but are primarily service-based. That is, most workers are employed in the service sector of the economy, which includes everything from retain sales to real estate, banking, health care, education, government and high-tech industries such as computer software production. Commercial agriculture is an important part of the economy in all of the core countries, but relatively few people make a living wholly as farmers (typically less than 10% of the population). While heavy industry and manufacturing was the mainstay of the industrial economies of the core from World War II until the 1970s, employment in this sector of the economy and its overall importance to the economies of the core have declined dramatically over the past twenty years.

Summary

This chapter has discussed the nature of the discipline of geography, outlining its main themes, its place in academia, and its distinctive way of looking at the world around us. It has also introduced some of the main themes with which this text is concerned and outlined its primary goals, namely general patterns in the human geography of the world, with an emphasis on the following:

- A basic understanding of the major culture regions of the world, where these regions are located, their general characteristics, and their attendant cultural landscapes

- An appreciation of how populations vary from place to place around the world, what populations "look" like, how they are structured, and various problems and policies related to population in different parts of the world

- A comprehension of the various ways in which people make a living around the world, how economies and societies are structured in different parts of the world, and the nature of the world-economy today and in the past

- An understanding of the concepts of economic "development" and "underde-velopment" and how critically important these are in understanding the nature of economies, societies, and ways of life around the world both today and in the past

This chapter has also introduced the basic premises of world-systems analysis and presented it as a general model for understanding the development of capitalism in the world-economy and for comprehending its nature and structure today. The three-tiered spatial and economic hierarchy of core, semi-periphery, and periphery will be used as a thematic context and as a model, within which various regions of the world might be placed. It is argued throughout the text that virtually all aspects of differ-ences in the human geography of the world, especially with respect to the goals out-lined above, can be more fully understand within the context of this world-systems model. As is the case with any model, it must be understood that this model simplifies reality to a certain extent. The model is useful in understanding *general*, global pat-terns and differences, especially at the regional level. It is hoped that through the application of this model, students will gain a fuller comprehension of the myriad ways in which the human geography of the world varies from place to place and from region to region.

KEY TERMS TO KNOW

- Spatial Perspective
- Physical Landscape
- Physical Geography
- Human Geography
- Cultural Landscape
- Environmental Geography
- Absolute Location
- Relative Location
- Environmental Determinism
- Possibilism
- Environmental Perception
- Diffusion
- Region
- culture region
- Formal Region

- Functional Region
- Perceptual Region
- World-Systems Analysis
- Modes of Production
- Mini-Systems
- World-Empires
- World-Economy
- Error of Developmentalism
- Core States
- Hegemonic Powers
- Peripheral States
- Semi-Peripheral States
- International Division of Labor

STUDY QUESTIONS

1. With what themes is the academic discipline of geography concerned? What are the five unifying themes of geography? In what important ways does geography differ from most other academic disciplines in terms of its subject matter and method of analysis?

    _____

    _____

    _____

    _____

    _____

    _____

    _____

    _____

2. Discuss the concept of "landscape" and its importance in the discipline of geography.

    _____

    _____

    _____

    _____

    _____

    _____

    _____

    _____

3. What are the fundamental features of world-systems analysis? Discuss the basic structure of the world-economy using the terms core, semi-periphery and periphery. How does world-systems theory conceptualize and explain economic "development" and "underdevelopment"?

_____

_____

_____

_____

_____

_____

_____

4. What opportunities for service exist in the periphery today? How might goals for Christian service in the periphery differ from those you might pursue in the semi-periphery?

_____

_____

_____

_____

_____

_____

_____

FURTHER READING

Christopher Chase-Dunn and Thomas D. Hall, eds., *Rise and Demise: Comparing World-Systems* (Boulder: Westview Press, 1997).

Saul Cohen, *Geopolitics of the World System* (Lanham: Rowman & Littlefield, 2003).

Harm De Blij, *The Power of Place: Geography, Destiny, and Globalization's Rough Landscape* (Oxford: Oxford University Press, 2009).

James S. Duncan, Nuala C. Johnson, and Richard H. Schein, eds., *A Companion to Cultural Geography* (Oxford: Blackwell, 2004).

Derek Gregory et al, eds., *The Dictionary of Human Geography* (Oxford: Blackwell, 2009).

Thomas D. Hall, ed., *A World-Systems Reader* (Lanham: Rowman & Littlefield, 2000).

Geoffrey J. Martin, *All Possible Worlds: A History of Geographical Ideas* (New York: Oxford University Press, 2005).

Donald Mitchell, *Cultural Geography: A Critical Introduction* (Oxford: Blackwell, 2000).

Peter Taylor, *Political Geography: World-Economy, Nation-State and Locality* (Essex: Longman, 1993).

Immanuel Wallerstein, *World-Systems Analysis: An Introduction* (Durham: Duke University Press, 2004).

Peter N. Stearns, *Globalization in World History.* (New York: Routledge, 2010).

Web Sites

Population Reference Bureau (http://www.prb.org).

United Nations (http://data.un.org).

The World Bank (http://data.worldbank.org).

Four Revolutions: The Evolution and Dynamics of Global Core-Periphery Relationships

[1]Now the whole earth had one language and one speech.[2] And it came to pass, as they journeyed from the east, that they found a plain in the land of Shinar, and they dwelt there.[3] Then they said to one another, "Come, let us make bricks and bake them thoroughly." They had brick for stone, and they had asphalt for mortar.[4] And they said, "Come, let us build ourselves a city, and a tower whose top is in the heavens; let us make a name for ourselves, lest we be scattered abroad over the face of the whole earth." (Genesis 11:1–5)

In This Chapter:

- The Neolithic Revolution

- The Merchant Capitalist "Revolution"

- The Industrial Revolution

- The Post-Industrial (Post-Modern) Revolution

- Key Terms to Know

- Study Questions

- Further Reading

Since the goal of this text is to aid the student in understanding the basic characteristics of the human geography of the world today, especially with respect to development and underdevelopment and global core-periphery relationships, then it is altogether appropriate that we understand the evolution of these relationships over time. We must start at the beginning; we must know from where we have come, before we can know where we are today. What are the historical processes that have resulted in present global geographical patterns? Toward these ends, this chapter introduces general, long-term, global-scale trends in the development of the world-economy.

The chapter argues that there have been four significant "revolutions" in human history that have successively shaped and reordered the world's economies, political geographies, cultures and landscapes. Each revolution represents a clear break with what had come before with respect to dominant modes of production, forms of labor control, social relations of production, dominant technologies in use, and the types of natural resources exploited. Each revolution resulted in a significant increase in the amount of power that could be harnessed per person per year. Further, each revolution resulted in substantial changes in the ways in which human beings conceived of the world around them, how humans perceived of themselves in the world and their place in it, and how certain natural resources could be used and exploited. Over time, the effects of these revolutions resulted in the alteration of the world's cultural landscapes into what they are today. The cultural landscapes of today reveal these past changes. They reveal changing cultural traditions, ideals, and values. They reveal social, political, and economic struggles that have taken place over time and space. The world's cultural landscapes are, in short, a palimpsest of the last 12,000 years of human history.

THE NEOLITHIC REVOLUTION

What Was It?

The first revolution to significantly alter the ways in which human beings viewed and used the natural world around them was what anthropologists refer to as the **Neolithic Revolution**. This term refers to the period in human history about 10,000–12,000 B.C. when the first large-scale urban settlements began to appear, together with concomitant changes in the structure and nature of societies, modes of production, and social relations of production. The most important feature of the Neolithic Revolution, however, and what engendered most of these changes, was the domestication of plants and animals. **Plant and animal domestication** refers to the gradual genetic change of plants and animals through selective breeding such that they become dependent upon human intervention for their reproduction. Certain plants and animals or certain varieties of plants and animals were selected for particular qualities such as taste or caloric value or nutritional value, while other varieties were left behind. These selected varieties of plants and animals were nurtured, protected and cared for in gardens and fields and continuously reproduced. Over many generations this caused genetic change, resulting in plants and animals with distinctive characteristics found to be helpful to human beings (again, characteristics such as taste or resistance to pests and drought). Today, this process occurs in the form of scientific genetic breeding of plants and animals carried out at laboratories and universities.

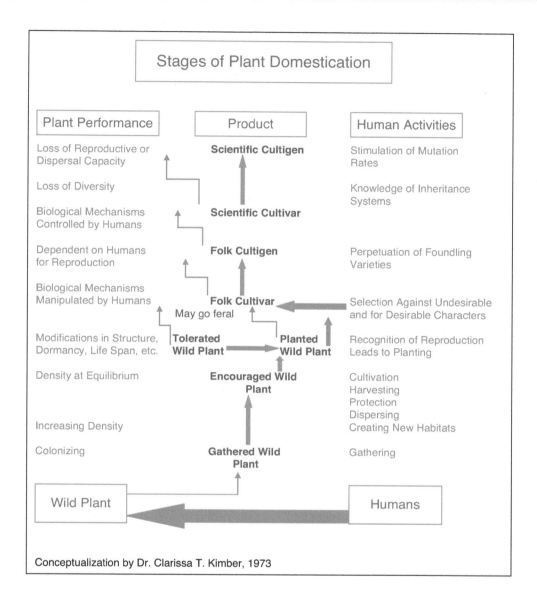

Stages of Plant Domestication

Plant Performance	Product	Human Activities
Loss of Reproductive or Dispersal Capacity	**Scientific Cultigen**	Stimulation of Mutation Rates
Loss of Diversity		Knowledge of Inheritance Systems
Biological Mechanisms Controlled by Humans	**Scientific Cultivar**	
Dependent on Humans for Reproduction	**Folk Cultigen**	Perpetuation of Foundling Varieties
Biological Mechanisms Manipulated by Humans	**Folk Cultivar**	Selection Against Undesirable and for Desirable Characters
	May go feral	
Modifications in Structure, Dormancy, Life Span, etc.	**Tolerated Wild Plant** → **Planted Wild Plant**	Recognition of Reproduction Leads to Planting
Density at Equilibrium	**Encouraged Wild Plant**	Cultivation Harvesting Protection Dispersing Creating New Habitats
Increasing Density		
Colonizing	**Gathered Wild Plant**	Gathering
Wild Plant		Humans

Conceptualization by Dr. Clarissa T. Kimber, 1973

Without a doubt, the most important and far-reaching result of plant and animal domestication was the advent of agriculture on a scale that had not been seen before. Before the advent of large-scale agriculture, the vast majority of societies all over the world could be described, in world-systems analysis language, as mini-systems, with social relations of production and social and political organizations that were tribal in nature. Exchange in these mini-systems was basically reciprocal, social classes were weakly developed, and their geographic extent was very small, amounting to little more than a claimed "homeland" or hunting territory. Agriculture, however, wrought social and economic changes that changed the world forever. Where it occurred, much more "complex" societies quickly developed, with highly stratified societies, vast increases in food production, and despotic forms of political organization that claimed and defended large territories by force. That is, where plant and animal domestication first occurred, where agriculture first originated, mini-systems gave way to the development of world-empires.

Why and Where Did It Occur?

There are two primary theories about when, where, and why agriculture first originated. The first, what we might call the orthodox theory of domestication, is agreed upon by most historians and anthropologists. The second was proposed by the geographer Carl O. Sauer in the mid-20th century. The orthodox theory, that which is most widely accepted by social scientists and for which there is the most archaeological evidence, argues that plant and animal domestication occurred independently in several areas of the world at about the same time in history—from about 8,000 to 12,000 B.C.—through a process of **independent invention**. That is, populations in different parts of the world "invented" agriculture on their own without contact from outside populations, without "learning" it from others. Most experts argue that some sort of ecological stress—overpopulation or climate change, for example—forced these populations to move from a nomadic hunting and gathering type of lifestyle to a more sedentary lifestyle more and more dependent upon agriculture to feed burgeoning populations.

This revolutionary change did not happen overnight, or even in a few generations, but rather most likely occurred over hundreds of years and over many human generations. But where it did occur, in the following so-called **culture hearths** of innovation and invention, societies began to look very different, the hallmark of which was the first urban civilizations. Table 15.1 lists some of the earliest culture hearths and gives dates by which world-empire types of civilizations had developed. The dates for the domestication of various plants and animals are not given here, but radiocarbon dating of plant and animal remains suggests that plant domestication occurred as early as 12,000 to 15,000 years ago in Southwest Asia and the Nile Valley and 5,000 years ago in Middle America and the Andean Highlands of South America.

Another less widely accepted theory of the development of agriculture was proposed by the American geographer Carl O. Sauer in his book *Agricultural Origins and Dispersals* in 1952. Sauer suggested that agricultural first developed in Southeast Asia as early as 20,000 years ago and from there diffused to the other areas of the world. This theory is thus one based on the idea of **cultural diffusion** from an original hearth area to all other regions of the world. Sauer reasoned that agriculture would have developed first in an area where the richest array of different kinds of useful plants naturally occurred, most likely a tropical region, and in a place where people were not under any kind of ecological stress. Such populations, Sauer argued, would have not been *forced* to invent agriculture, but rather would have had ample time over many generations to experiment with growing different varieties of useful plants. This theory, however, is at most a thought experiment and there is little archaeological evidence to support it. It also presupposes that populations in certain parts of the world were not "advanced" enough to invent agriculture on their own and that they therefore

Table 15.1   Major Culture Hearths

Culture Hearth	Location	Date	Domesticates
Mesopotamia	Southwest Asia	by 5,500 B.C.	wheat, barley, rye, grapes, oats, cattle, horses, dogs, sheep
East Africa	Nile Valley	by 3,300 B.C.	barley, coffee, cotton, millet, wheat
Incan	Andean Highlands	by 2,500 B.C.	potato, tomato, llama, guinea pig, alpaca
Mediterranean	Crete, Greece	by 2,500 B.C.	barley, grapes, goats olives, dates, garlic
Indus Valley	Pakistan	by 2,300 B.C.	wheat, cattle, dog, rye, sheep, horse
North China	Huang He Valley	by 2,200 B.C.	soybeans, buckwheat, cabbage, barley, plum
Southeast Asia	Vietnam, Cambodia, Thailand	by 1,500 B.C.	bananas, chicken, pig, tea, dog, rice, taro, water buffalo, yams
Meso-America	Mexico, Guatemala	by 1,250 B.C.	maize, beans, taro, chile peppers, dog
West Africa	Ghana, Mali	by 400 B.C.	arrowroot, millet, pigs, rice, oil palm

must have been shown how by invading populations with such knowledge. For these reasons Sauer's theory is not widely held to be true.

What Changes Did It Engender?

An agricultural lifestyle had the effect of radically altering the nature and structure of societies and economies in each of the various culture hearths. Aside from new innovations and techniques that increased crop yields and food production, such as crop rotation and large-scale irrigation projects, the most revolutionary change was the development of highly stratified, agriculturally-based societies with codified class structures, a class-based division of labor, and a redistributive-tributary mode of production. Anthropologists refer to such societies as *chiefdoms*, and in essence this describes a *feudal* social and economic order. In the world-systems perspective, Wallerstein refers to these societies as *world-empires*.

At one end of the socio-economic spectrum in these societies an agricultural underclass comprised up to 90% of the population. This peasant underclass produced agricultural surpluses, the storage and redistribution of which was controlled and directed by an aristocratic (title by blood birth) royalty at the other extreme of the socio-economic spectrum. These rulers also directed the building of vast agricultural projects such as irrigation schemes (in North China and the Nile Valley) and the construction of monumental structures (such as the Great Wall and the pyramids). Such rulers (known as kings, emperors, pharaohs and the like) are often called **god-kings** by anthropologists because they often claimed to possess supernatural powers and to have achieved communion with the gods. These rulers surrounded themselves with other elite classes such as scribes and priests. These ruling elite lived in a central urban location known as a city-state, the basic political unit of world-empires. The presence of distinctive elite classes points to the development of other revolutionary changes first witnessed in each of these culture hearth that set the stage for the development of vastly more complex societies and economies that forever changed the ways in which humans interacted with the natural world around them:

- Written languages to keep records of agricultural surpluses and the redistribution of surpluses

- The development and use of calendars to track the seasons and to predict planting and harvesting times

- The development of an organized military under the command of the ruling elite in order to defend a claimed political territory

- Significant population increases as a result of more stable food supplies

THE MERCHANT CAPITALIST "REVOLUTION"

What Was It?

Although it is not always referred to as a "revolution", the development of merchant capitalism in northwestern Europe in the mid-15th century and its diffusion around the world over the ensuing 400 years engendered changes in societies, economies and cultures that shaped the modern world-economy more than any other event. If we define **capitalism** as the production and exchange of goods and services for private money profit, then most historians would agree that it has existed for millennia in many places around the world. **Merchant capitalism**, however, arose in only one region of the world at a specific point in history—Holland and England in the mid-15th century. Merchant capitalism was an altogether new version of capitalist production and exchange because it was based heavily on long-distance sea trade in exotic products from the tropics and subtropics.

Because such products were rare and costly to acquire (it took five years to travel by ship from Holland to the southeast Asian spice islands in the 16th century) the high relative value of such trade meant great wealth to the countries and individuals that controlled it. Before the advent of merchant capitalism, most trade was merely regional in nature and used land-based caravans or shipping routes that plied coastal regions.

Merchant capitalism involved the use of new sailing and navigation technologies to strike out into the oceans out of sight of land on risky overseas ventures in search of rare tropical goods for which Europeans were willing to pay high prices (such as sugar, cotton, tea, coffee, pepper, and other spices). In short, merchant capitalism ushered in the era of colonialism and global trade that radically altered the world forever. It was the first step toward creating the "globalized" world that we live in today.

Why and Where Did It Occur?

Why did merchant capitalism develop in a relative backwater spot in the world at the particular time that it did? Compared to the great civilizations of China, South Asia and Southwest Asia, Europe in the early Middle Ages lagged far behind in terms of technology and scientific know-how. Earlier, traditional theories attributed the development of merchant capitalism in northwest Europe to such things as Protestant Christianity (Weber's "Protestant work ethic") or European racial superiority. While Weber's theory is still held by some to be of explanatory value, nobody still believes that Europeans were somehow "better" or "smarter" than other world civilizations and "invented" capitalism due to this superiority. Instead, most historians today argue that a series of events happened first in Europe, effecting societies there in more drastic ways than others and resulting in a fundamental reordering of European societies and economies.

The most important of these events was most likely the **Black Death**, the Bubonic plague that ravaged Europe from 1340–1440. The Black Death struck elsewhere around the world, but nowhere with such far-reaching consequences. Anywhere from one-third to one-half of the population of Europe died during this period. Most of those that died came from the peasant classes, in a feudal society that part of the population with the lowest caloric intake and the highest susceptibility to such respiratory diseases. This had drastic repercussions for European economies because with so much of the peasantry gone, labor was now in very short supply. As a result, those peasants that remained acquired something that they had never possessed before—bargaining power over their aristocratic landlords. Peasants began to demand something for their labor, either payment in kind or money wages. In short, the Black Death precipitated a **crisis of feudalism** in Europe. The ancient feudal organization of labor and production could no longer keep up with the demand for food, especially as populations began to increase rapidly again after the plagues subsided. World-systems analysts argue that the replacement of a feudal organization to societies and economies with a different form of production and exchange based on individual money profit—capitalism—was the solution to this crisis in the feudal order.

Along with the reordering of economies came a fundamental reordering of societies as well, the most important aspect of which was the emergence of a new class of people—a middle class. Because production was now based on profit and competition, those that could produce the most reaped the most profit. This spurred technological innovations, especially in agricultural production. The use of steel plows, the draining of marshlands and crop rotation schemes, for example, led to higher agricultural surpluses than ever before. This also meant that more and more of the European population did not have to farm because agriculture had become more efficient and more productive. Many people began to move to towns and cities and became shopkeepers, merchants, and artisans (weavers, blacksmiths, millers, tailors, bakers, etc.). Over ensuing generations this new middle class rose in social, economic and political importance and they began to pass wealth on to successive generations. Such dynastic, wealthy urban merchant families came to dominate the social and economic life of coastal towns in northwestern Europe, especially in Holland and England, by the 16th and 17th centuries. By the late 16th century, these powerful urban merchants began to sponsor overseas trading ventures to newly "discovered" tropical regions in order to supply the new and growing demand for rare, expensive tropical agricultural products by the expanding middle class. Colonialism—the political, economic and social control of tropical peripheral regions by European core powers using coerced labor—was invented by northwestern European urban merchant capitalists in order to more efficiently supply this demand. It was this new merchant capitalist colonial order that created the European-centered capitalist world-economy with its characteristic tripartite global economic geography of core, semi-periphery and periphery.

What Changes Did It Engender?

In summary, the development and expansion of merchant capitalism based on long-distance sea trade resulted in the following revolutionary developments:

- The replacement of feudal, agricultural societies with economies dominated by merchant capital interests involved in long-distance sea trade

- The invention and domination of colonialism

- The birth and dominance of a middle class of urban merchant entrepreneurs

- The creation of a capitalist world-economy dominated by a few nation-states in Europe

- The creation of a "core" of relatively high economic and technological development and a "periphery" of relatively low economic and technological development

- The creation of the use of varying labor control systems in the different part of the world-economy: slavery in the periphery, wage labor in the core, tenant farming in the semi-periphery

- The increased use of non-human and non-animal sources of energy; a drastic increase in the amount of energy harnessed per capita, per year

- The initiation of a capitalistic logic in the world-economy; since capitalism rewards innovations that make production cheaper, it engenders constant technological innovation

THE INDUSTRIAL REVOLUTION

What Was It and Where Did It Occur?

The **Industrial Revolution** represents a third major break with the past with respect to far-reaching societal changes around the world, especially in the core countries of the world-economy during the 19th and 20th centuries, whose wealth was built on the backs of economies focused on heavy industry and manufacturing. Most significantly, the Industrial Revolution ushered in vastly different methods and modes of industrial production, systems of labor control, and social relations of production. These changes occurred first in the Midlands of central England beginning in the early- to mid-18th century but spread very quickly to the rest of Europe (Belgium, Holland, France, Germany, and Russia) and North America (especially the northeast United States) by the mid- to late-19th century. The Industrial Revolution ushered in the Machine Age.

The Industrial Revolution radically altered societies and economies in two important ways. First, modes of production were revolutionized with the introduction and application of new labor-saving technologies and machines. The earliest of these new technologies was the steam engine. Steam engines were first put to use in the British Midlands running pumps to remove excess water from coal mines, but the technology was soon put to use running all types of machines that heretofore had employed human or animal power such as mills and looms. The first industry to be completely revolutionized by the machine age was the textile industry. Steam engines that spun and wove yarn into textile goods replaced traditional cottage textile industries in the rural countryside of Europe, where such goods had for millennia been produced by hand. The mode of production that came to dominate regions that became industrialized was the urban factory staffed by low-wage, low-skilled workers running steam-driven machines.

Many of these workers were women and children from the rural hinterlands of emerging industrial cities who came to the cities in search of work as traditional ways of making a living were being radically altered. This represents the second major change wrought by the Industrial Revolution—a new form of labor control characterized by the factory organization of low-wage, low-skilled laborers. Such laborers lived in housing, often built by the factory owners, very near to the factories in which they worked. Long working hours (production could take place around the clock with the advent of gas lighting and, later, electricity), poor living conditions, and exposure to hazardous environmental pollutants (coal smoke, chemicals) characterized the lives of the earliest factory workers. Workers often performed the same menial tasks hour after hour in cramped and hot conditions. In the United States, the industrialist Henry Ford mastered the factory mode of production and labor control with the innovation of the assembly line, where workers performed the same task hour after hour as cars traveled down an assembly line (this mode of production is often referred to as **Fordism**).

The factory mode of production built around urban factories staffed by low-skilled wage laborers and powered by petroleum-based fuels (first coal, then oil products like gasoline) revolutionized production. The countries that industrialized first, like Great Britain, Germany, and the United States, soon outpaced and out produced their competitors. Although industrialization came to different countries at different times, the economies of all of the core powers of today were built upon heavy industrial production between the mid-18th century and 1960. Industrialization brought immense wealth and power to these core countries, especially in the early 20th century when steel production, shipbuilding and automobile manufacturing became the hallmark of the core economies. Many semi-peripheral areas did not "industrialize" until the 1960s and 1970s, while large-scale industrialization has yet to appear in most areas of the periphery. The semi-peripheral economies hope that a strong manufacturing and heavy industry base will also bring the same wealth that it brought to the core economies, but it remains to be seen whether this will happen or not.

THE POST-INDUSTRIAL (POST-MODERN) REVOLUTION

The **Post-Industrial Revolution** describes revolutionary changes in societies, economies and cultures that have taken place since the early 1970s, predominately in the core regions of the world-economy. But because changes that take place in the core affect all regions of the world-economy, this revolutionary period in which we now live is fundamentally transforming societies, economies, and cultures all over the world. This period has seen the development of new modes of production, the advent of so-called "new information technologies" such as the internet (these have ushered in the "computer age"), and a pronounced global division of labor in the world-economy.

Perhaps the most significant development during this latest revolution is the process of **globalization** in the world-economy, directed from the core by multi-national conglomerates employing rapidly-evolving forms of information technology to increasingly expand the scope of *interconnectedness* among the parts of the world-economy. Such interconnectedness has led not only to a fundamental restructuring of the world-economy. This post-industrial or "postmodern" age has also ushered in an era in which people and places all over the world are linked and tied together to a degree never before seen in human history. Rapidly-evolving forms of mass communication, faster and cheaper forms of travel between continents, and large-scale international migrations are all in part responsible for such international linkages.

In terms of modes of production, a central feature of the post-industrial era has been a restructuring of the world-economy characterized by globalization and a marked international division of labor. In the core regions of the world-economy this restructuring involved a move from economies based on heavy industry and manufacturing between World War II and the early 1970s, to service-based economies from the 1970s until the present. Manufacturing jobs and manufacturing-based industries (such as steel production and automobile assembly plants), once the cornerstone of core economies, have increasingly moved to the semi-periphery and in some instances to peripheral locations. This process many be referred to as **global outsourcing**, and it has occurred primarily due to lower costs of labor (wages) in semi-peripheral and peripheral locations such as Mexico, Indonesia, Malaysia, and much of Latin America. This geographical outsourcing has led to the movement of manufacturing-based industries and jobs (especially those in which the costs of labor are very high, such as textile production and automobile assembly) to such semi-peripheral locations. In the core regions themselves a new mode of production, called "just-in-time" or **post-Fordist production**, has replaced traditional factory organizations of labor. So-called "blue collar" low-wage and low-skilled jobs have rapidly declined in number with the decline in the number of manufacturing industries. In their place, a new kind of worker has emerged: highly-skilled, high-wage labor in which brains rather than brawn matter the most. This is especially true in the new information technologies like software production and computer assembly that are an increasingly important part of the core economies in the post-industrial era.

In the end, the post-industrial era has led to a reinforcement of the core—semi-periphery—periphery structure of the world-economy and made the differences between them greater than ever before. That is, life in the core for the average person is vastly different than it is in the periphery. Today, the core controls the flow of wealth and information in the post-industrial world-economy. The core contains the nodes, or nerve centers, of the world-economy (places such as New York, London, and Tokyo) and it is here that the largest multi-national companies in the world are located. Core economies are primarily service-based and information-based in nature. The semi-peripheral regions today are the places where much of the world's manufacturing now takes place. Agriculture is still an important part of these economies, especially the production of plantation products for export to the core. A small but expanding service sector is also characteristic of many of the semi-peripheral economies. Peripheral economies remain largely dependent upon traditional subsistence agricultural economies and plantation agriculture for export to the core. The service and manufacturing sectors of the economy in the periphery are both still rather weakly developed.

Finally, **post-modernism** has significantly altered traditional ways of life and forms of artistic expression such as art, literature, music, and poetry, as well as philosophy and other scientific endeavors. These alterations have been most conspicuous in the core regions of the world-economy, but their effects have trickled down to the semi-periphery and periphery as well, albeit to a lesser extent. Post-modern expression is characterized by a lack of faith in absolute truths, a mélange of forms and styles, a rejection of order, and a deconstructionist ideology in which traditional ways of articulation are continually questioned. This post-modern "condition" has resulted in a reordering of societies, economies, and modes of production, especially in the core, and is characterized by the following conditions:

- Increasing globalization of the world-economy

- The development of a "frenetic" international financial system

- The development of, and reliance upon, new information technologies

- A world-economy more and more reliant upon the flow of information

- A world-economy that is increasingly *illegible* to the average person; interconnections are so complex that the world is harder to comprehend, global capitalism is harder to "locate"; a world of confused senses and order

- A world that is increasingly "*hyper-mobile*"; a world-wide informational economy with telecommunication technology as its foundation; a "space of flows" that dominates sense of place; a perception of the world through the medium of information technologies

- A world increasingly effected by *time-space compression*; a marked increase in the pace of life; a seeming collapse of time and space that affects our abilities to grapple with and comprehend the world

Unfortunately, after the flood, mankind disobeyed God's instructions to Noah to spread over the Earth. In Genesis 11:1, we begin to see the marks of civilization on the cultural landscape and the beginning of civilization with its consequent characteristics. Without adequate food supplies, however, urban growth would have been as impossible then as it would be now, and civilization thwarted. Adequate agricultural production is likewise inseparably connected to the rise of technology. A series of agricultural and industrial revolutions has resulted in an increasingly globalized, technologically connected world today. An increasingly efficient planet-wide "assembly line" of production requiring practically zero inventories, and accompanied by time-space compression, will probably result in decreased loyalties. There has never been a greater opportunity for leadership through service than today. Our role model during these hectic times is the Savior. Jesus said, in John 12:26, "If any man serve me, let him follow me; and where I am, there shall also my servant be: if any man serve me, him will my Father honor."

KEY TERMS TO KNOW

- Neolithic Revolution
- Domestication
- Independent invention
- Culture hearth
- Cultural diffusion
- "god-kings"
- Capitalism
- Merchant capitalism
- The Black Death

- "Crisis of Feudalism"
- Colonialism
- Industrial Revolution
- Fordism
- Post-Industrial Revolution
- Globalization
- Global Outsourcing
- Post-Fordist Production
- Post-Modernism

Name _____ Date _____

STUDY QUESTIONS

1. What are the primary characteristics of the Neolithic Revolution? When, why and where did it occur?

    _____

    _____

    _____

    _____

    _____

    _____

    _____

    _____

2. What are the defining characteristics of the Merchant Capitalist Revolution? When and where did it occur? What fundamental changes in societies and economies and modes of production resulted from this revolution?

    _____

    _____

    _____

    _____

    _____

    _____

    _____

3. Define and describe the main characteristics of the Industrial Revolution. When and where did it occur? What revolutionary changes in industrial modes of production did it engender?

_____

_____

_____

_____

_____

_____

_____

_____

4. Define the Post-Industrial Revolution. When and where did it occur? What fundamental changes in societies, economies and modes of production resulted from this revolution?

_____

_____

_____

_____

_____

_____

_____

_____

FURTHER READING

Hans Bertens, *Literary Theory: The Basics* (New York: Routledge, 2001).

J. M. Blaut, *The Colonizer's Model of the World: Geographical Diffusionism and Eurocentric History* (New York: Guilford Press, 1993).

Fernand Braudel, *Civilization and Capitalism, 15th–18th Century*, Vol. I, *The Structures of Everyday Life* (New York: Harper & Row, 1981).

Carlo Cippola, *The Fontana Economic History of Europe: The Industrial Revolution, 1700–1914* (London: Fontana, 1976).

Phyllis Deane, *The First Industrial Revolution* (Cambridge: Cambridge University Press, 1979).

Jared Diamond, *Guns, Germs, and Steel: The Fates of Human Societies* (New York: W. W. Norton & Co., 1997).

Michel Foucault, *The Order of Things: An Archaeology of the Human Sciences* (New York: Vintage Books, 1994).

Marvin Harris, *Good to Eat: Riddles of Food and Culture* (Long Grove: Waveland Press, 1985).

David Harvey, *The Condition of Postmodernity* (Oxford: Blackwell, 1989).

J. David Hoeveler, Jr., *The Postmodernist Turn: American Thought and Culture in the 1970s* (Lanham: Roman & Littlefield, 1996).

David Landes, *The Unbound Prometheus: Technological Change and Industrial Development in Western Europe from 1750 to the Present* (Cambridge: Cambridge University Press, 1969).

William McNeill, *The Rise of the West: A History of the Human Community* (Chicago: University of Chicago Press, 1963).

Sidney W. Mintz, *Sweetness and Power: The Place of Sugar in Modern History* (New York: Penguin, 1985).

Lewis Mumford, *Technics and Civilization* (San Diego: Harcourt Brace & Co., 1963).

Carl O. Sauer, *Agricultural Origins and Dispersals* (New York: The American Geographical Society, 1952).

Wolfgang Schivelbusch, *Tastes of Paradise: A Social History of Spices, Stimulants, and Intoxicants* (New York: Vintage Books, 1992).

Peter Stearns, *The Industrial Revolution in World History*, 3rd ed. (Boulder: Westview Press, 2007).

Immanuel Wallerstein, *The Modern World-System I: Capitalist Agriculture and the Origins of the European World-Economy in the Sixteenth Century* (San Diego: Academic Press, 1981).

The Concept of Human "Culture"

"Go therefore and make disciples of all the nations, baptizing them in the name of the Father and of the Son and of the Holy Spirit, teaching them to observe all things that I have commanded you; and lo, I am with you always, even to the end of the age." (Matthew 28:19–20)

To be obedient to Jesus' command, we must understand principles of human culture. Culture is a dynamic activity that changes over time and spreads over space. By defining culture and understanding the global variations of culture, we can better create a "sense of place." An increasingly detached world seeks security and authenticity; it is our job to provide it!

In This Chapter:

- Varying Definitions and Critiques of "Culture"
- Core-Periphery Relationships
- Key Terms to Know
- Study Questions
- Further Reading

VARYING DEFINITIONS AND CRITIQUES OF "CULTURE"

Traditional Definitions

Culture is one of those words that many of us often use without thinking very deeply about what it exactly means. In the post-industrial era, punctuated by the so-called "culture wars" and post-modern dialogue, it is often used as a catch-all term to describe attributes relating to such things as race, ethnicity, and gender. Today, "culture" is a highly-elusive term that means a lot to some social scientists but nothing at all to others. That is, its meaning and importance is highly debated, and in academia today it is one of those ideas that is being rigorously critiqued and deconstructed. But however one might approach or define human culture, there is no denying that the study of how it varies geographically and how it shapes and influences cultural landscapes is central to the field of human geography. It is altogether necessary, then, to have a basic understanding of what culture is, how different academic traditions define it, and how it is expressed in the landscape in different parts of the world-economy.

Although the concept of human culture in its various forms is a central focus of most of the humanities and social sciences, it tends to be defined in different ways by various academic disciplines. In sociology, for example, a stress is placed upon the codes and values of a group of people. Sociologists would argue that if you really want to know the "culture" of a group, whether it be an ethnic group or a class of people or an entire society, one must understand the rules of conduct that have been agreed upon by members of that group. These rules of conduct might include laws, social mores and traditions, and codes relating to family and societal structure. Sociologists tend to look at how order is achieved and how society is organized in order to understand the values and traditions of that society. Anthropology, a discipline defined as the study of human cultures, tends to focus on the everyday ways of life of a group or society. Such ways of life might include linguistic norms, religious ideals, food, dress, music, and political structures. In order to uncover and understand the cultural values and traditions of a group or society, anthropologists study these ways of life.

While there is a long tradition of debate about the meaning and nature of culture in the academic literature of many of the social sciences, cultural geographers, until recently, have traditionally spent little time defining what culture is. Instead, traditional human and cultural geography in the United States focused on how culture was expressed in the landscapes of places—the landscape, especially its physical manifestations such as houses, fields, settlement patterns, neighborhoods, etc., were "read" and analyzed in order to uncover clues as to the cultural values and traditions of the people that built them. Until post-modern thought began to influence the field in the 1970s, most cultural geographers were content to rely on definitions of culture that had been developed by sociologists and cultural anthropologists in the 20th century. For these cultural geographers, then, human culture consists of many aspects of a group or society that, when combined together, results in a distinctive way of life that distinguishes that group or society from others:

- Beliefs (religious beliefs and political ideals, for example)
- Speech (language and linguistic norms and ideals)
- Institutions (such as governmental and legal institutions)
- Technology (skills, tools, use of natural resources)
- Values and Traditions (art, architecture, food, dress, music, etc.)

As such, cultural values and traditions are not biological in nature. Such traditions are learned, not genetically inherited (that is, we are not born with these values), and are passed on from generation to generation through a mutually intelligible language and a common symbol pool or iconography. For cultural geographers, who seek to identify the spatial expression of culture, a **culture region** is an area in which a distinctive way of life (as defined above) is dominant.

The New Cultural Geography

Post-modern thought has had a dramatic effect on the field of cultural geography over the past twenty years, especially in Great Britain and the United States. In what has come to be known as **The New Cultural Geography**, a new generation of scholars is turning traditional notions of culture and its expression on the landscape on its head. Heavily influenced by post-modern literary and philosophical traditions and by neo-Marxist thought, one of the leading voices in this new movement has gone so far as to argue that culture does not even exist and that we learn little about the nature of the world and of the societies in it by approaching culture in the traditional ways outlined above. Rather, it is argued by the new cultural geographers that what we might call "culture" for lack of a better term is not a thing, but rather a process that shapes values, traditions, and ideals. These processes and their accompanying values and traditions differ significantly not from society to society or country to country, but from person to person and are influenced by such things as an individual's class, gender, race, and sexuality. In this line of thought it follows that our perception of the world is influenced by the same factors, and it is argued that cultural landscapes hold clues to such factors working in society. They can be read and deconstructed and analyzed in the same way that a literary text can. The cultural landscape, then, is not seen as simply the built environment or the human imprint on the physical landscape. Instead, the New Cultural Geography conceptualizes it as a place or a "stage" upon which, and within which, societal problems and processes are worked out, especially with respect to struggles relating to class, race, ethnicity, gender, and politics.

CORE-PERIPHERY RELATIONSHIPS

Folk Cultures

Both traditional and post-modern conceptualizations are valuable for a broad understanding of how "culture" varies around the world. Employing these ideas alongside the core, semi-periphery, periphery model of the world-economy from world-systems analysis, we can understand basic, general differences in ways of life around the world. It should be noted that these basic differences do not translate well down to the local or individual level. To understand the cultural processes at work at such scales one must analyze cultural processes and patterns at those scales. Here, we are concerned with broad global patterns.

At the global scale, and in a broad sense, we can distinguish between two primary "types" of culture operating today. At one end of the spectrum are so-called folk cultures. This term describes human societies and cultures that existed in most parts of the world until the Industrial Revolution. At this point, as the core, semi-peripheral, and peripheral areas of the modern world-economy became better defined, a major divergence occurred. Folk cultures remained the norm in the periphery and parts of the semi-periphery, but in the core, and today in some parts of the semi-periphery, cultural values and traditions came to be increasingly modified by "popular" tropes, fads and ideas (this is discussed in more detail below).

A **folk culture** refers to a way of life practiced by a group that is usually, rural, cohesive, and relatively homogeneous in nature with respect to traditions, lifestyles, and customs. Such groups and societies are characterized by relatively weak social stratification, goods and tools are handmade according to tradition that is passed on by word of mouth through tales, stories and songs, and non-material cultural traits (e.g. stories, lore, religious ideals) are more important than material traits (e.g. structures, technologies). The economies of folk societies are most characteristically subsistence in nature—farming or artisan activities are undertaken not to necessarily make a profit, but rather to simply survive—and the markets for such products are usually local or regional in nature. Finally, order in folk cultures is based around the structure of the nuclear family, ancient traditions, and religious ideals. If we define a folk culture by these characteristics (and this is a very "conservative" definition), then such cultures and societies are practically nonexistent in the core of the world-economy. Instead, they describe most societies that are tribal or "traditional" in nature in the periphery and in some remote, rural parts of the semi-periphery (the Amazon Basin of Brazil, for example, which is part of the semi-periphery). Even so, some folk culture traits almost always persevere even in the post-industrial societies of the core; they are "holdovers" of our folk cultural roots from hundreds or even thousands of years ago. Some examples would include the popularity of astrology or tarot card reading, the fairy tales that each of us learns as children, and folk songs from long ago that are still passed on today ("Auld Lange Syne" or "Yankee Doodle").

Popular Cultures

While folk cultural traditions dominate most societies in the periphery, the societies of the core and parts of the semi-periphery today are best described by the term popular culture. Although some ethnic groups in core regions of the world-economy attempt to live in a "traditional" or folk manner, or practice a "traditional" lifestyle, it is nearly impossible for such groups do so in the core because popular culture is so pervasive and far-reaching. For example, even though many Americans see the Amish as a distinctively "folk" society, closer inspection reveals that compared to true folk cultures in the periphery Amish society today is not truly folk in nature. Although most Amish do not use electricity and employ rather simple machinery in their agricultural systems, that machinery is mass-produced, material for barns and houses is purchased from retail stores, and their agricultural endeavors are capitalistic, profit-making undertakings.

Compared with folk cultures, **popular cultures** are based in large, heterogeneous societies that are most often ethnically plural, with a concomitant plurality of values, traditions, and ideals. While folk cultures are by definition conservative (that is, resistant to change), popular cultures are constantly changing. This is due to the power and influence of fads and trends that change rapidly and often in core societies, as well as to the dominance and influence of mass communication in the core. While ideas and trends are slow to move from place to place in folk cultures (usually through hierarchical diffusion), they can move around the planet instantaneously by means of mass communication technology (satellites, the internet, television, radio, etc.) in a popular culture (by means of contagious diffusion). This, in fact, is the central defining characteristic of popular cultures—such fast change and quick diffusion is what makes a culture subject to "popular" (read trends and fads) ideas. In the post-modern era, such trends and fads have significantly shaped how people in core societies receive news, what music they listen to, what books they read, what movies they see, what food they eat, and what clothes they wear. In a folk culture, such things are dictated by tradition that has been passed on by word of mouth over many generations.

Other characteristics of popular cultures include the use of material goods that are invariably mass-produced, and societies in which secular institutions (government, the film industry, MTV, multi-national corporations employing advertisements to entice people to buy their products) are of increasing importance in shaping the "look", the landscapes and ways of life in core societies. The power of such popular fads, trends, and ideas is expressed in the standardized landscapes that are a hallmark of the core and parts of the semi-periphery. That is, popular culture tends to produce standardization that is reproduced *everywhere* in such societies. This can be seen in styles of architecture, music, clothing, dialects, etc., that are the same throughout large, populous societies and over large distances. Currently, the strongest popular culture in the world stems from the United States. Things "American" (music, food, films, styles and the like) affect nearly every place on the planet, including even traditional folk societies in the periphery. Because the diffusion of popular ideas and fads occurs via mass communication, even traditional societies in far corners of the "developing" world are not immune to the influences of popular culture from the core.

Delimiting and defining the geography of popular culture presents a challenge to human geographers because such cultures tend to produce "placelessness" that challenges unique regional expression. For example, ranch style homes became popular in the United States in the 1950s. Although the style probably originated in the eastern part of the country, such houses became so popular so fast that they soon could be found everywhere around the country, including Alaska and Hawaii. Another example would be popular music. When a song goes out over the radio or on television it is heard by millions of people at once, all over the country, or even the world. That song, then, becomes known by millions of people of varying ethnicities, cultures, and nationalities—it has become a song known to millions, not just a few members of a specific tribe or ethnic group as is the case with a folk song. In this way, popular culture fads and trends are extremely powerful. Popular culture supersedes ethnic and national boundaries and spreads rapidly across large distances, often at the expense of local or regional folk cultures. Even so, regional expression often still exists in the form of such things as regional dialects, accents, and food preferences, even in societies such as the United States where strong popular cultures predominate. For example, many people in the South today continue to speak English with a strong regional accent in spite of the fact that most people there are exposed to standardized, accent-neutral English in schools and on television news programs and the like.

The post-industrial world-economy of today is punctuated by stark divisions within it. In the previous chapters we have seen how this plays with respect to vast differences between the core, semi-periphery, and periphery in such things as standards of living, population structure, modes of production, and social relations of production. This chapter has demonstrated that these differences are also seen in the types of "cultures" operating in the world-economy: popular cultures in the core, folk cultures in the periphery, and a mix of each in the semi-periphery. The following chapters will address a variety of other aspects of culture and argue that these too vary with respect to "location" in the world-economy.

Perhaps the greatest contribution any of us can make is to create or contribute to "a sense of place." This can begin in our own homes and on campus as we attempt to create and reinforce a cultural hearth. A loving and safe place is analogous to a military base of operations and is vital for the security of those we see sent out into the world. A **cultural hearth** is the source of a unique way of life and is the area serving as a source of cultural diffusion. **Cultural diffusion** is the process of spreading the aspects of culture from the cultural hearth. Cultural diffusion can spread in unexpected ways and at different speeds. It is absolutely essential that the cultural hearth we build be like the home in Matthew 7:24: built on solid rock.

What services and encouragement are you providing your family and school, thereby creating a genuine cultural hearth capable of changing the world? Remember Jesus' admonition in Matthew 5:13, "You are the salt of the earth; but if the salt loses its flavor, how shall it be seasoned? It is then good for nothing but to be thrown out and trampled underfoot by men." As we turn to the study of language and religion, we see concrete examples of how a cultural hearth can be instrumental in cultural diffusion.

KEY TERMS TO KNOW

- Culture
- Culture Region
- The New Cultural Geography
- Folk Culture
- Popular Culture
- Cultural Hearth
- Cultural Diffusion

STUDY QUESTIONS

1. How has the field of geography traditionally addressed and defined the concept of culture?

_____

_____

_____

_____

_____

_____

_____

_____

2. How does the New Cultural Geography conceptualize human "culture" and how does this differ from traditional treatments of the subject by human and cultural geographers?

_____

_____

_____

_____

_____

_____

_____

3. What constitutes a folk culture and where would one most likely find a true folk culture in the present world-economy?

    _____

    _____

    _____

    _____

    _____

    _____

    _____

4. How does your personal testimony, or that of your family, church, or school, affect others around you in your community? What is it about the customs, manners, and traditions that provide a Christian witness to others and meets the requirement of being the salt and the light written about in Matthew 5:13?

    _____

    _____

    _____

    _____

    _____

    _____

    _____

FURTHER READING

Jeff Chang and D. J. Kool Herc, *Can't Stop Won't Stop: A History of the Hip-Hop Generation* (New York: Picador, 2005).

Henry Glassie, *Pattern in the Material Folk Culture of the Eastern United States* (Philadelphia: University of Pennsylvania Press, 1968).

Marvin Harris, *Cows, Pigs, Wars, and Witches: The Riddles of Culture* (New York: Vintage Books, 1989).

Marvin Harris, *Theories of Culture in Postmodern Times* (Lanham: AltaMira Press, 1998)

Alan Light, ed., *The Vibe History of Hip-Hop* (New York: Plexus, 1999).

D. W. Meinig, ed., *The Interpretation of Ordinary Landscapes: Geographical Essays* (New York: Oxford University Press, 1979).

Donald Mitchell, *Cultural Geography: A Critical Introduction* (Oxford: Blackwell, 2000).

S. Craig Watkins, *Hip Hop Matters: Politics, Pop Culture, and the Struggle for the Soul of a Movement* (New York: Beacon Press, 2006).

Wilbur Zelinsky, *Exploring the Beloved Country: Geographic Forays into American Society and Culture* (Iowa City: University of Iowa Press, 1994).

The Geography of Language and Religion

"For I say to you, that unless your righteousness exceeds the righteousness of the scribes and Pharisees, you will by no means enter the kingdom of heaven." (Matthew 5:20)

In Chapter 2, we discussed Genesis 11:9 and the fruit of man's disobedience. Instead of spreading upon the Earth, we saw mankind settle into an urban existence. The creation of languages resulted from God's punishment for building the tower of Babel. The development of languages is important to the geographer because it is often integral to both ethnic and nationalistic identifications. Just as languages have diffused, so have the world's religions. Religions like language reflect world view and identify deeply held perceptions of ultimate existence. Indeed, a backward reconstruction of both language and religion demonstrate the truth of Acts 17:26a: "From one man he created all the nations throughout the whole earth."

In This Chapter:

- The Classification and Distribution of Languages
- The Classification and Distribution of Religions
- Key Terms to Know
- Study Questions
- Exercises
- Further Reading

Students in an introductory human geography course might wonder why the analysis of the distribution of languages and religions is such a prominent component of most such courses given that language is the central theme of linguistics and religion is a major theme of philosophy and history. The answer is really very simple: language and religion are the defining cornerstones of human culture (at least as it is traditionally defined) and identity (ethnic and national or even individual identity). They are two of the most important characteristics that distinguish human beings from all other animals given that no other species possesses the capacity for speech or the ability to perceive of one's own mortality in a spiritual sense (at least as far as most biologists know). Many other kinds of animals have the ability to communicate with each other, sometimes in very complex ways, but none possess the capacity for language. Likewise, it is clear that many other species exhibit emotions and "feelings" but so far as we know no others can think and philosophize about what is going to happen to them when they die. So, if a main goal of human geography is to delineate and understand how human cultures vary over space, then it behooves us to know how the two major facets of culture vary over space. That is, a map of religious and linguistic regions is in many ways a map of culture regions.

THE CLASSIFICATION AND DISTRIBUTION OF LANGUAGES

Classification of Languages

Language is defined as an organized system of spoken and/or written words, words themselves consisting of symbols or a group of symbols put together to represent either a thing or an idea, depending on the kind of writing system in use. In **syllabic languages**, the symbols that are used (e.g. "letters") represent sounds. German, English, Arabic and Hindi are examples of syllabic languages. **Ideographic languages** employ ideographs as symbols to represent an idea or thing. Examples of ideographic languages include Chinese, Japanese, and Korean. All human beings are biologically "hardwired" for language. This means not that we are born knowing a language, but rather that we are born with the *ability* to learn a language or languages because it is imbedded in our genetic makeup. The linguist Noam Chomsky calls this "deep structure."

With respect to other forms of animal communication, human language is unique in two primary ways. First, human languages are *recombinant*. This means that words and symbols can be taken out of order in a sentence and recombined to form a different sentence and thus communicate a completely different, or even subtly different, idea. Dogs, for example, are not capable of arranging barks in different orders to communicate extremely intricate ideas. Second, word formation in all human languages is almost completely *arbitrary*. This means that there is really no rhyme or reason as to why a certain word, symbol or ideograph is used to stand for something. There are, of course, exceptions to this rule. One is *sound symbolism*, in which the pronunciation of a word or the shape of an ideograph suggests an image or meaning. For example, many words in English that begin with "gl-" have something to do with sight (glimmer, glow, and glisten). Another exception to this rule is *onomatopoeia*, an instance in which a word sounds like something in nature that it represents (e.g. cuckoo, swish, cock-a-doodle-doo). But such exceptions are very rare. The vast majority of words in all languages have simply been made up and then passed down over generations although, to be sure, words and languages change over time.

There are roughly 6,700 different languages in use around the world today. But the vast majority of these languages are spoken by a relatively small number of people. This means that a relatively small number of languages have thousands or even millions of speakers. Consider the following list of the top ten languages by number of native (mother-tongue) speakers in 2009 according to SIL International, one of the leading organizations that collect and publish linguistic data (www.ethnologue.com):

Language	Primary Locations	Number of Speakers
Chinese	China	1.213 billion
Spanish	Middle America, Latin America, Spain	329 million
English	North America, British Isles, Australia, New Zealand	328 million
Arabic	Southwest Asia, North Africa, South-Central Asia	221 million
Hindi	India	182 million
Bengali	Bangladesh	181 million
Portuguese	Brazil, Portugal	178 million
Russian	Russia	144 million
Japanese	Japan	122 million
German	Germany, Austria, Switzerland	90 million

Of the nearly 6,700 languages in use today, 389 (about 6%) account for 94% of the world's population. The remaining 94% of languages in the world are spoken by only 6% of the world's population.

Linguists have devised classification schemes that describe and account for similarities and differences between and within different languages. At the broadest level, a **proto-language** describes an ancestral language from which several language families (described below) or languages are descended. No proto-languages are spoken today, but they are theorized to have been in use thousands of years ago. For example, Proto Indo-European was the language theorized to have been spoken in eastern Anatolia (present-day Turkey) and the Caucasus Mountain region 5,000 years ago. These people were the "original" Indo-Europeans (probably some of the first "Caucasians") and the language they developed became the basis for all of the languages that are classified by linguists as Indo-European. If we use the analogy of a tree to represent a group of languages that are linguistically related, then a proto-language is the roots and trunk of the tree.

In this analogy, each branch of the tree represents a **language family**. A language family is a group of languages descended from a single earlier language whose similarity and "relatedness" cannot be the result of circumstance. How do we know that certain languages are "related" to each other? Linguists employ two main methods to determine linguistic relatedness. One is genetic classification, in which it is assumed that languages have diverged from common ancestor languages (proto-languages) and therefore languages that diverged from the same proto-language will have inherit similarities. Compare, for example, the following words for "mother" in selected Indo-European languages:

English	*mother*
Dutch	*Moeder*
German	*Mütter*
Irish Gaelic	*mathair*
Hindi	*mathair*
Russian	*mat*
Czech	*matka*
Latin	*mater*
Spanish	*madre*
French	*mére*

It is obvious that all of these words sound very similar to each another. Given the rule that word formation is arbitrary, it is impossible that such strong similarities are the result of mere coincidence, especially given the fact that some of these populations are separated by thousands and thousands of miles. When we add to this list hundreds or thousands of other words that display such similarities it is clear that these languages have a common ancestor, common linguistic roots. When languages are shown to have a common ancestor, such as those above, they are said to be **cognate languages**.

Reviewing the list above once again it is also clear that some of the languages have even more commonalities to others in the list. Compare, for example, the even more clearly defined similarity between Latin and Spanish, English and Dutch, and Russian and Czech. These groupings of languages whose commonality is very definite are called **language subfamilies**. Think of these groupings as twigs of larger branches on the language tree, while individual languages are the leaves of the tree. Proceeding even further with respect to similarity, linguists recognize **dialects**. A dialect is defined as a recognizable speech variation *within the same language* that distinguishes one group from another, both of which speak the same language. Sometimes these differences are based on pronunciation alone (the different varieties of English spoken around the world or a "southern" or "New England" accent) and sometimes they are based on slightly different words for the same thing (British English "lorry", American English "truck"). Similarly, **pidgins** are languages which develop from one or more "mother" languages that have highly simplified sentence and grammatical structures compared to the mother languages. When such a language becomes the native language of succeeding generations, it is referred to as a **creole language**. Most creoles are either English-, French-, or Spanish-based and are spoken in the periphery of the world-economy, in former colonial areas, where two or more groups of people speaking mutually unintelligible languages were forced to communicate with each other during the colonial era.

Political and ethnic fragmentation is characteristic of many former colonial regions in the periphery of the world-economy. In Nigeria, for example, at least 500 different tribal languages are spoken, many of them not even in the same language family. In such places, governments and businesses often make use of a *lingua franca* to carry out official business. A lingua franca refers to a language that is used habitually among people living in close contact with each other whose native tongues are mutually unintelligible. English and French are common lingua francas in much of sub-Saharan Africa, Arabic is the lingua franca of much of North Africa and Southwest Asia, and English can be thought of as the lingua franca of the internet and of air traffic control and airline pilots around the world.

Linguistic Diffusion and Change

Why does the map of world language families (Map 2 on the accompanying CD) look the way it does? What spatial processes have led to the present-day distribution of languages? How do languages change over time and space? In general, cultural diffusion (both hierarchical and relocation diffusion) and geographical isolation over time and space have resulted in the linguistic patterns we observe today. Relocation diffusion on a massive scale since the advent of the capitalist world-economy in the 15th century, together with the displacement and subjugation of native populations, has resulted in very large linguistic regions, especially in the Americas.

These two processes (relocation diffusion and displacement) explain the fact that the vast majority of populations in North, South and Middle America speak one of three languages (all of them Indo-European languages): English, Spanish, and Portuguese. Before Columbian contact, there were probably as many as 30 million people living in the Americas, speaking literally hundreds of distinctive languages in at least a dozen different language families. In other words, the linguistic map was highly complicated and extremely diverse. Massive relocation from Europe and the decimation of native populations over a 300-year period resulted in a vastly "simplified" and less complex linguistic map in the Americas. This is not to say that no Native American languages survive. Many do, but with few exceptions the number of people who speak these languages is very small compared to the number of English, Spanish and Portuguese speakers. The colonial era also ushered in a period in which many European languages, such as English, Spanish, Portuguese and French, acquired many more new speakers in their overseas colonies than they ever had at home. In part this was a result of the outright extermination of African and Native American languages in the Americas through either severe population decline or cultural subjugation through slavery. In the process, European languages were of course deemed to be "superior" to others, and Europeans forced Africans and Native Americans to learn the language of the colonizers. This was the case not only in the Americas, but in colonial sub-Saharan Africa as well.

The present-day world linguistic map also is the product of centuries of linguistic change over time and space. In the pre-industrial era, for example, migration and spatial isolation and segregation gave rise to separate, mutually unintelligible languages. As populations diverged over time and space, populations became isolated from each other. And as these migrating populations encountered new natural environments and human societies they were forced to invent new words to describe new circumstances, places, and things. It has also been shown that languages change naturally in place over time, even in the absence of outside cultural forces such as immigration or hostile invasion. Take, for example, the case of English and how significantly the language changed between the 9th and 17th centuries. The Old English of 9th-century Britain (*Beowulf* is the most famous literary example) would hardly be recognizable to most English speakers today. But 500 years later, due to influences from Latin, French, and Danish, as well as to natural linguistic evolution over time, the language had evolved into the Middle English of Chaucer (*The Canterbury Tales*), a language that most English speakers today can understand. By the 17th century the language had evolved into the Modern English of Shakespeare. As one of the world's most widely-spoken languages and as a world-wide lingua franca, English is changing more rapidly today than ever before as it incorporates words from a variety of different cultural sources around the world.

The Distribution of the World's Major Language Families

In conjunction with Map 2 on the CD-ROM this section lists the world's major language families and important subfamilies and maps the distribution of their speakers.

1. **Indo-European Family (386 languages) (about 2.5 billion speakers)**

   - Albanian Subfamily—Albania, parts of Yugoslavia and Greece

   - Armenian Subfamily—Armenia

   - Baltic Subfamily—Latvia, Lithuania

   - Celtic Subfamily—parts of western Ireland, Scotland, Wales, Brittany

   - Germanic Subfamily—northern and western Europe, Canada, USA, Australia, New Zealand, parts of the Caribbean and Africa

   - Greek Subfamily—Greece, Cyprus, parts of Turkey

   - Indo-Iranian Subfamily—India, Pakistan, Bangladesh, Afghanistan, Iran, Nepal, parts of Sri Lanka, Kurdistan (Iran, Iraq, Turkey)

   - Italic (Romance) Subfamily—France, Spain, Portugal, Italy, Romania, Brazil, parts of western and central Africa, parts of the Caribbean, parts of Switzerland

   - Slavic Subfamily—eastern Europe, southeastern Europe, parts of south-central Asia

2. **Sino-Tibetan Family (272 languages) (about 1.1 billion speakers)**

   - Chinese Subfamily—China, Taiwan, Chinese communities around the world

   - Tibeto-Burman Subfamily—Tibet, Myanmar (Burmese), parts of Nepal and India

3. **Austronesian Family (1,212 languages) (269 million speakers)**

   - Formosan Subfamily—parts of Taiwan

   - Malayo-Polynesian Subfamily—Madagascar, Malaysia, Philippines, Indonesia, New Zealand (Maori), Pacific Islands (e.g. Hawaii, Fiji, Samoa, Tonga, Tahiti)

4. **Afro-Asiatic Family (338 languages) (250 million speakers)**

   - Semitic Subfamily—North Africa (Arabic), Israel (Hebrew), Ethiopia (Amharic), Middle East

   - Cushitic Subfamily—Ethiopia, Kenya, Eritrea, Somalia, Sudan, Tanzania

   - Chadic Subfamily—Chad, parts of Nigeria, Cameroon

   - Omotic Subfamily—Ethiopia

   - Berber Subfamily—parts of Morocco, Algeria, Tunisia

5. **Niger-Congo Family (1,354 languages) (206 million speakers)**

   - Benue-Congo Subfamily—central and southern Africa

   - Kwa Subfamily—bulge of west Africa

   - Adamaw-Ubangi Subfamily—northern part of central Africa

   - Gur Subfamily—between Mali and Nigeria

   - Atlantic Subfamily—extreme western part of the bulge of west Africa

   - Mande Subfamily—western part of the bulge of west Africa

6. **Dravidian Family (70 languages) (165 million speakers)**

   - Four Subfamilies—southern India, parts of Sri Lanka, parts of Pakistan

7. **Japanese Family (12 languages) (126 million speakers)**

8. **Altaic Family (60 languages) (115 million speakers)**

   - Turkic Subfamily—Turkey, Uzbekistan, Turkmenistan, Kazakhstan, Azerbaijan, eastern Russia (Siberia)

   - Mongolian Subfamily—Mongolia, parts of adjoining areas of Russia and China

   - Tungusic Subfamily—Siberia, parts of adjoining areas of China

9. **Austro-Asiatic Family (173 languages) (75 million speakers)**

    - Mon-Khmer Subfamily—Vietnam, Cambodia, parts of Thailand and Laos

    - Munda Subfamily—parts of northeast India

10. **Tai Family (61 languages) (ca. 75 million speakers)**

    - Tai Subfamily—Thailand, Laos, parts of China and Vietnam

11. **Korean Family (1 language) (60 million speakers)**

12. **Nilo-Saharan Family (186 languages) (28 million speakers)**

    - Nine Subfamilies—southern Chad, parts of Sudan, Uganda, Kenya

13. **Uralic Family (33 languages) (24 million speakers)**

    - Finno-Ugric Subfamily—Estonia, Finland, Hungary, parts of Russia

    - Samoyedic Subfamily—parts of northern Russia (Siberia)

14. **Amerindian Languages (985 languages) (ca. 20 million speakers)**

    - As many as 50 different language families, hundreds of subfamilies

    - North America = ca. 500,000 speakers; 150 languages (top languages = Navajo and Aleut)

    - Central America = ca. 7 million speakers; (top language = Nahuatl)

    - South America = ca. 11 million speakers; (top language = Quechua)

15. **Caucasian Family (38 languages) (7.8 million speakers)**

    - Four Subfamilies—Georgia, surrounding region on western shore of the Caspian Sea

16. **Miao-Yao Family (15 languages) (5.6 million speakers)**

    - Southern China, northern Laos (Hmong), northeast Myanmar

17. **Indo-Pacific Family (734 languages) (3.5 million speakers)**

    - The most linguistically complex place on earth—Papua New Guinea and surrounding islands

18. **Khoisan Family (37 languages) (300,000 speakers)**

    - Three Subfamilies—parts of Namibia, Botswana, Republic of South Africa

19. **Australian Aborigine (262 languages) (ca. 30,000 speakers)**

    - Only five languages have over 1,000 speakers

    - At time of European contact, 28 language families, 500 languages spoken by over 300,000 people

20. **Language Isolates (296 languages) (ca. 2 million speakers)**

    - Languages which have not been conclusively shown to be related to any other language; some examples are:

    - Basque (Euskara)—southern France, northern Spain

    - Nahali—5,000 speakers in southwest Madhya Pradesh in India

    - Ainu—island of Hokkaido, Japan; now probably extinct

    - Kutenai—less than 200 speakers in British Columbia and Alberta

The Classification and Distribution of Religions

Classification of Religions

Together with language, religion is a human characteristic that distinguishes us from every other animal species on the planet. As with language, we are also most likely biologically "hard-wired" with the capacity for abstract thought about spiritual matters, our own mortality, and the nature of the universe and our place in it. We are born with these capacities, but not with a certain set of beliefs concerning these things—these beliefs are learned. By definition, a **religion** is a system of either formal (written down and codified in practice) or informal (oral traditions passed from generation to generation) beliefs and practices relating to the sacred and the divine. Who am I? Why am I here? What is my purpose in life? What is my place in the universe? What will happen to me when I die?

These are questions that every human being ponders because we have the biological capacity to think about and philosophize about such things. Human religions attempt to answer such questions through systems of beliefs, practices and worship. As the answers to these questions vary so do religious belief systems; as the answers to these questions vary from place to place, to a large extent so does human culture. As is the case with human languages, there are literally thousands of religions practiced around the world today. In most of the peripheral regions of the world-economy there are as many religions as there are ethnic groups and can vary substantially over relatively short distances. For human geographers, religion is an extremely important aspect of the cultural landscape because religious beliefs and customs have a significant physical manifestation in the form of religious structures. Although religious practices, beliefs and traditions vary substantially around the world, most religions share the following characteristics in common:

- Belief in one or many supernatural authorities

- A shared set of religious symbols (iconography)

- Recognition of a transcendental order—offers a divine reason for existence and an explanation of the inexplicable

- Sacraments (prayer, fasting, baptism, initiation, etc.)

- Enlightened or charismatic leaders (priests, shaman, prophets)

- Religious taboos

- Sacred structures (temples, shrines, cathedrals, mosques, etc.)

- Sacred places (pilgrimage sites, holy cities, etc.)

- Sacred texts

Human religions can be divided into two broad categories and two narrower sub-categories. At the broadest level, we can distinguish between monotheistic and polytheistic religions. **Polytheistic religions** involve a belief in many supernatural (that is, not of this world) beings that control or influence some aspect of the natural or human world. The vast majority of human religions, in terms of number, are polytheistic in nature, numbering in the thousands. Such religions usually, but not always, have a very small geographic distribution, often coinciding with tribal or ethnic boundaries. For most of human history, polytheistic belief systems have been by far the most common. **Monotheistic religions** appeared on the human stage quite late, probably not until around 1,500 B.C. Monotheism involves the belief in one omnipotent, omniscient, supernatural being who created the universe and everything in it and thus controls and influences all aspects of the natural and human world. There are in effect only three monotheistic religions today: Judaism, Christianity, and Islam. In terms of number of adherents and believers, however, two of these (Christianity and Islam) have over one billion adherents each. That is, out of a total world population of around 6.5 billion, fully one-third are either Christians or Muslims. The geographic boundaries of Christian and Islamic beliefs, then, do not coincide with political boundaries but rather supercede and overlap them. We can account for such distributions in much the same way that we can account for the very large distribution of Indo-European speakers around the world: relocation diffusion on a massive scale during the colonial era, and the acquisition of new members either by force or through missionary activities.

We can also identify two sub-categories of religions. First, **Ethnic religions** are those in which membership is either by birth (you are "born into" the religion) or by adopting a certain complex ethnic lifestyle, which includes a certain religious belief system. That is, an ethnic religion is the religious belief system of a specific ethnic or tribal group and is unique to that group. Most (but not all) of these kinds of religions are polytheistic in nature and have very small geographical distributions, sometimes no larger than a village or group of villages. These religions, therefore, have very strong territorial or ethnic group identity. In most such religions, there is no distinction between made between one's ethnic identity (i.e. one's culture) and one's religion: one's religion is one's culture. Examples of ethnic religions include Judaism, Hinduism and various tribal belief systems that are ubiquitous throughout the periphery of the world-economy. Second, **universalizing religions** are those in which membership is open to anyone who chooses to make a solemn commitment to that religion, regardless of class or ethnicity. Membership in these religions *is* usually relatively "easy", and usually involves some sort of public declaration of one's allegiance to the belief system (baptism, for example). Universalizing religions are also distinguished by the fact that they are often characterized by strong evangelic overtones in which members are admonished to spread the faith to non-believers. For these reasons universalizing religions have very large geographic distributions that cover vast regions of the world, the boundaries of which overlap the political boundaries of individual states. There are only three universalizing religions: Christianity, Islam, and Buddhism, although Buddhism rarely carries with it evangelic activities and therefore has a much smaller distribution than Christianity and Islam.

Finally, it should be noted that the influence of popular culture and post-modern thought and philosophies in core regions of the world-economy, have significantly influenced the growth of secularism. **Secularism** refers to an indifference to, or outright rejection of, a certain belief system or religious belief in general. In its extreme such "beliefs" may become like a religion itself. It is an increasingly characteristic of many post-industrial societies, and thus influences core societies more than any other societies around the world. At least one-fifth of the world's population, by this definition, is secular, and this figure is even higher in parts of northern and western Europe, where the figure approaches 70 percent in some instances.

Attributes and Distributions of the World's Major Religions

In conjunction with Map 3 on the accompanying CD-ROM, this section lists the world's major religions, identifies their major characteristics, and maps the distribution of their adherents.

1. **Hinduism (ca. 740 million adherents concentrated in India, Nepal, and Sri Lanka)**

   - One of the world's oldest extant religions

   - The ethnic religion of the Hindustanis

   - Hearth in the Indus Valley ca. 1500 B.C., then spread to India, Nepal, Sri Lanka and parts of SE Asia

   - Beliefs and practices:

     - A common doctrine of *karma*, one's spiritual ranking, and *samsara*, the transfer of souls between humans and/or animals

     - A common doctrine of *dharma*, the ultimate "reality" and power that governs and orders the universe

     - The soul repeatedly dies and is reborn, embodied in a new being

     - One's position in this life is determined by one's past deeds and conduct

- The goal of existence is to move up in spiritual rank through correct thoughts, deeds and behavior, in order to break the endless cycle and achieve *moksha*, eternal peace

- Life in all forms is an aspect of the divine—hundreds of gods, each controlling an aspect of the natural world or human behavior

- One need not "worship" a god or gods

- **The Caste System**—a social consequence of the Hindu belief system

  - The social and economic class into which one is born is an indication of one's personal status

  - In order to move up in caste one must conform to the rules of behavior for one's caste in this life

  - This thus highly limits social mobility

- Sacred texts

  - The *Rig Vedas*, hymns composed by the Indo-Aryans after the invasion of the Punjab; the oldest surviving religious literature in the world, written in Sanskrit

  - *Brahmanas*, theological commentary, defined different castes

  - *Upanishads*, defines karma and nirvana, etc.

- Cultural landscapes

  - Shrines, village temples, holy places and rivers (the Ganges), pilgrimage sites and routes

2. **Buddhism (ca. 300 million concentrated in East and Southeast Asia)**

- Founded by Gautama Siddharta in the 6th century B.C. in northeast India

- Diffusion was mainly to China and Southeast Asia by monks and missionaries

- The primary religion in Tibet, Mongolia, Myanmar, Vietnam, Korea, Thailand, Cambodia, Laos; mixed with native faiths in China and Japan

- A universalizing religion

- Beliefs and practices:

  - Retains the Hindu concept of *karma*, but rejects the caste system

  - More of a moral philosophy than a formal religion

  - The ultimate objective is to reach nirvana by achieving perfect enlightenment

  - The road to enlightenment, Buddha taught, lies in the understanding of the four "noble truths": 1. to exist is to suffer 2. we desire because we suffer 3. suffering ceases when desire is destroyed 4. the destruction of desire comes through knowledge or correct behavior and correct thoughts (the "eight-fold path")

- Sects:

    - Theravada (Sri Lanka, Myanmar, Thailand, Laos, Cambodia)

    - Mahayana (Vietnam, Korea, Japan, China, Mongolia)

    - Zen (Japan)

    - Lamaism (Tibet)

- Cultural landscapes:

    - Shrines and temples

    - Holy locations where the Buddha taught

3. **Chinese Faiths (ca. 300 million adherents in China)**

- Two main forms: Confucianism and Taoism, both date from the 6th c. B.C.

- The goal of both is moral harmony within each individual, which leads to political and social harmony

- Chinese religion combines elements of Buddhism, Animism, Confucianism, and folk beliefs into one "great religion"; each element services a different component of the self

- The Taoist approach to life is embodied in the Yin/Yang symbol; stresses the oneness of humanity and nature; people are but one part of a larger universal order

- Confucianism is really a political and social philosophy which became a blueprint for early Chinese civilization; it teaches the moral obligation of people to help each other, that the real meaning of life lies in the here and now, not in a future abstract existence; Kong Fu Chang taught that the secret to social harmony is empathy between people

4. **Judaism (ca. 18 million adherents mainly in N. America and Israel)**

- The ethnic religion of the Hebrews

- The oldest religion west of the Indus (ca. 1,500 B.C.)

- Founder regarded as Abraham (the patriarch)

- Sacred text = the Torah (the five books of Moses)

- Beliefs and practices:

    - God is the creator of the universe, is omnipotent, but yet merciful to those who "believe" in Him

- God established a special relationship with the Jews, and by following his law they would be special witnesses to His mercy

- Emphasis is on ethical behavior and careful, ritual obedience

- Among the traditional, almost all aspects of life are governed by strict religious discipline

- The Sabbath and other holidays are marked by special observances and public worship

- The basic institution is the Synagogue, led by a rabbi chosen by the congregation

- Cultural landscapes:

  - Synagogues

  - Holy sites (e.g. the wailing wall, Jerusalem, sites of miracles, etc.)

5. **Christianity (ca. 1.6 billion adherents worldwide, but especially in Europe, N. America, Middle and South America)**

- A universalizing religion

- A revision of Judaic belief systems

- Founder regarded as Jesus, a Jewish preacher believed to be the savior of a sinful humanity promised by God; his main message was that salvation was attainable by all who believed in God (died ca. 30 A.D.)

- Sacred text = the Bible; Old Testament is based on the Hebrew Torah and is the story of the Jews; New Testament is based on the life of Jesus and his teachings

- Mission: conversion by evangelism through the offering of the message of eternal life and hope

- Reform movements:

  - Split in the 5th century between the western church at Rome (Catholicism) and the eastern church at Constantinople (Orthodoxy)

  - Protestant Reformation in the 15th and 16th centuries, led mainly by northern Europeans over moral and political issues

  - Protestantism took hold in northern Europe and spread to North America, Australia and New Zealand

- Cultural landscapes:

  - Churches, cathedrals, graveyards, iconography

6. **Islam (ca. 1 billion adherents worldwide, but especially in N. Africa, SW Asia, South-Central Asia, Indonesia, Malaysia)**

- Founder: Muhammad ("Prophet"), born 571 A.D.; believed to have received the last word of God (Allah) in Mecca in 613 A.D.

- Diffusion: rapidly throughout Arabia, SW Asia, North Africa, then to South and Southeast Asia

- Organization: theoretically, the state and the religious community are one in the same, administered by a caliph; in practice, it is a loose confederation of congregations united by tradition and belief

- A universalizing religion

- Sacred Text: the Koran—the sayings of Muhammad, believed to be the word of God

- Divisions: two major sects—Sunni (Orthodox) and Shi'ah (Fundamentalist); Shiites mainly in Iran and parts of Iraq and Afghanistan; Sunni are the majority worldwide

- Beliefs: mainly a revision of both Judaic and Christian beliefs; those who repent and submit ("Islam") to God's rules can return to sinlessness and have everlasting life; religious law as revealed in the Koran is civil law; smoking, gambling and alcohol are forbidden

- The faithful are admonished to practice the five "**pillars of Islam**":

  - Public profession of faith

  - Daily ritualistic prayer five times per day

  - Almsgiving

  - Fasting during daylight hours during Ramadan

  - A pilgrimage to Mecca at least once in one's lifetime if physically and economically possible

- Cultural landscapes:

  - Mosques, minarets, religious schools, iconography

The study of both languages and religion reveals key ingredients to human culture. We should study the religions of the world in an attempt to find common ground, whereby we can present the liberating good news of the Gospel of Jesus Christ. While we may not understand the religious actions of others, we can certainly respect other's convictions, since we ourselves have experienced at some time the rejection of truth in our increasingly secular society.

KEY TERMS TO KNOW

- Language
- Syllabic Languages
- Ideographic Languages
- Proto-Language

- Language Family
- Cognate Languages
- Language Sub-Family
- Dialect
- Pidgin Language
- Creole Language
- *Lingua Franca*
- Religion
- Polytheistic Religion
- Monotheistic Religion
- Ethnic Religions
- Universalizing Religions
- Secularism
- The Caste System
- The "Pillars of Islam"

STUDY QUESTIONS

1. Why are language and religion important in understanding the distribution of world culture regions?

   _____

   _____

   _____

   _____

   _____

   _____

   _____

   _____

2. Compare and contrast ethnic and universalizing religions. What are the distinguishing characteristics of each and how do they differ in terms of geographic distribution of adherents?

   _____

   _____

   _____

   _____

   _____

   _____

   _____

   _____

3. Some characterize Christianity as a faith rather than a religion. How then does the example of the thief on the Cross in Luke 23:42–43 prove or disprove this characterization?

_____

_____

_____

_____

_____

_____

_____

_____

FURTHER READING

Melvyn Bragg, *The Adventure of English: The Biography of a Language* (London: Hodder & Stoughton, 2003).

Noam Chomsky, *On Language* (New York: New Press, 1998).

David Crystal, *The Cambridge Encyclopedia of Language*, 2nd ed. (Cambridge: Cambridge University Press, 1997).

Mircea Eliade, *The Sacred and the Profane: The Nature of Religion* (San Diego: Harvest Books, 1957).

Susan Tyler Hitchcock, *Geography of Religion: Where God Lives, Where Pilgrims Walk* (Washington: National Geographic Society, 2004).

William James, *The Varieties of Religious Experience* (New York: Penguin, 1958).

M. Paul Lewis, ed., *Ethnologue: Languages of the World*, 16th ed. (Dallas: SIL International, 2009).

Chris Park, *Sacred Worlds: An Introduction to Geography and Religion* (London: Routledge, 1994).

Steven Pinker, *The Language Instinct: How the Mind Creates Language* (New York: Harper Collins, 1995).

Ninian Smart, ed., *Atlas of the World's Religions* (Oxford: Oxford University Press, 2009).

Huston Smith, *The World's Religions*, 50th Anniversary Edition (New York: HarperOne, 2009).

Roger W. Stump, *Boundaries of Faith: Geographical Perspectives on Religious Fundamentalism* (Lanham: Rowman & Littlefield, 2000).

Roger W. Stump, *The Geography of Religion: Faith, Place, and Space* (Lanham: Rowman & Littlefield, 2008).

Nicholas Wade, *The Faith Instinct: How Religion Evolved and Why it Endures* (New York: Penguin, 2009).

Web Sites

Ethnologue (www.ethnologue.org).

Sacred Sites: Places of Peace and Power (www.sacredsites.com).

Sacred Destinations (www.sacred-destinations.com).

SIL International (www.sil.org).

The Geography of World Population

"Then they also brought infants to Him that He might touch them; but when the disciples saw it, they rebuked them. But Jesus called them to Him and said, "Let the little children come to Me, and do not forbid them; for of such is the kingdom of God. Assuredly, I say to you, whoever does not receive the kingdom of God as a little child will by no means enter it." (Luke 18:15–17)

"Jesus loves the little children" is how the song goes. If the Lord Jesus Christ did not see children as interruptions; and compared them to the Kingdom of God so should we. The study of population geography is of vital interest to the human geographer. We see a terrific opportunity during this time of unprecedented population growth to fulfill a purpose of eternal consequence. In John 4:34–35 it says, "Do you not say, 'There are still four months and *then* comes the harvest'? Behold, I say to you, lift up your eyes and look at the fields, for they are already white for harvest!" Life is indeed short, let's get busy!

In This Chapter:

- World Population Distribution
- Factors in World Population
- Core-Periphery Population Patterns
- Population Theory
- Key Terms to Know
- Study Questions
- Further Reading

In Chapters fourteen and fifteen we outlined the development, structure and geography of the present-day capitalist world-economy. These chapters argued that the tripartite structure of the world-economy (core, semi-periphery, and periphery) is a useful model for understanding the human geography of the world. The two previous chapters were mainly concerned with "cultural" issues and how cultures, in a broad sense, vary from core to periphery. The remaining chapters address in greater detail how the geography of the world-economy varies with respect to social and economic factors such as population, political structure, and economies. We begin in this chapter with how the human population varies across the planet, especially with respect to distributions, structures, and core-periphery relationships. We are often reminded by the news media and various international organizations that population "problems" confront our world today. Invariably these problems are presented as having something to do with either overpopulation or how the growing world population affects the supply and use of various natural resources. If there are "problems" related to population, what are they? Do such issues vary between the core and periphery? How do the structures of populations differ in the zones of the world-economy? How is population distributed around the world? These are the questions that are addressed in this chapter.

WORLD POPULATION DISTRIBUTION

If one examines a map of global population distribution one of the first things that is readily apparent is that the world's population is not evenly distributed. While some regions are very densely populated (Europe and much of Asia, for example), there are large parts of the earth that are very lightly populated (such as the arctic regions, Australia, and Siberia). In general, if indeed there are "problems" relating to overpopulation, those problems are not found everywhere around the world; it is not that there are too many people on the planet (that is a value judgment), but that there are too many people in certain places. The densest population clusters tend to be located in two main types of natural environments around the world. The first is the fertile river valleys of the tropics and sub-tropics and the second is the coastal plains of the mid-latitudes which are in general temperate regions. More precisely, it is possible to identify four major concentrations of population:

- East Asia (China, the Koreas, Vietnam, and Japan)
- South Asia (India, Pakistan, and Bangladesh)
- Europe (The British Isles to western Russia)
- North America (Boston to Washington, D.C.; West Coast)

Roughly 75 percent of the world's population lives in these four areas; four out of ten people in the world live in just two: East and South Asia. Other smaller concentrations of dense populations occur on the island of Java (part of Indonesia), the Nile Valley of Egypt, central Mexico, and southeastern South America (southern Brazil and eastern Argentina).

FACTORS IN WORLD POPULATION

Density

We have alluded to the fact that the way populations "look", the way they are structured and their rates of growth, vary significantly between the core and the periphery. It is possible to compare and contrast different populations by comparing various statistics (examples of these statistics for various countries are listed in Table 1.1). One of the most elementary of these factors is population density. Density can be measured as **crude population density**, the total number of people per unit area of land in a place or region, or as **physiologic population density**, the total number of people per unit area of *arable* (agriculturally productive) land. The latter is actually a more telling figure because it measures the density of populations with respect to how much of the land on which they are living is productive enough to produce enough food for that population. When the difference between a country's crude and physiologic densities is very large, it is a sure sign that that country has quite a bit of marginally productive agricultural areas. This can be observed in the following list:

Table 1.1

Country	Crude Density/km²	Physiologic Density/km²
Japan	862	6,637
Bangladesh	2,124	3,398
Egypt	142	7,101
Netherlands	1,041	4,476
USA	67	335

Growth Rates

A second method for comparing populations is by examining population growth rates. Map 9 on the accompanying CD-ROM illustrates rates of natural increase around the world by country. Since the Industrial Revolution, the world's population has been growing at an exponential rate (2, 4, 8, 16, 32, 64 . . .). Currently, the world rate of natural increase is about 1.8 percent per annum. This means that 1.8 percent of the current population is being added each year. This figure translates into a current **doubling rate** of 40 years, but this doubling rate will decrease with added population each year. Given this growth rate, the world's population likely reached 7 billion in 2011. Comparing Map 9 with Map 1, it is clear that peripheral populations are growing at a much faster rate than those in the core and semi-periphery. That is, at a broad global scale, there is a direct correlation between economic "development" and population growth rates:

Table 1.2

Country	Rate of Natural Increase	Doubling Time
Poland	0.5%	141 years
Australia	0.75%	94 years
China	1.5%	46 years
Kenya	4.0%	17 years

Structure

A third way of comparing populations around the world is by observing differences in the "structure" of populations. By structure we mean the relative number of men and women in different age cohorts in a population. A population's structure is most clearly seen by constructing a **population pyramid** that charts both male and female populations in five-year age cohorts on a y-axis and percentage of total population on an x-axis. The term population pyramid is used to refer to such age-sex diagrams because the shape of these diagrams is pyramidal in developing countries, that is, in the peripheral regions of the world-economy. This pyramidal shape indicates a population that is "young" and growing. Birth rates and fertility rates (discussed below) are relatively high and life expectancies are relatively low. Thus, a substantial proportion of the population in the peripheral countries is very young, under 15 years of age, while the number of people in higher age cohorts, above 60, is very low. These young and growing populations in the periphery are clearly visible on Map 4 on the accompanying CD-ROM. By contrast, in the core and parts of the semi-periphery, age-sex diagrams tend to have a rectangular shape. These countries have low birth and fertility rates, higher life expectancies, and thus the population is more evenly distributed among age cohorts. These populations are "old" and stable.

Demographic Cycles

If we examine past patterns of population growth rates in different parts of the world it is possible to identify demographic "stages" through which populations tend to pass. Where a country is at with respect to this cycle (that is, what "stage" the country is in) tends to mirror economic "development". These cycles and stages can be discerned by examining the relationship between three major indictors: the **crude birth rate**, defined as the number of live births per 1000 persons per year; the **crude death rate**, defined as the number of death per 1000 persons per year; and the **total fertility rate**, defined as the average number of children born to women of childbearing age (roughly 15–45) during their lifetimes. It is possible to compute the **rate of natural increase** for a given country by subtracting the crude death rate from the crude birth rate. For example, if the crude death birth rate of a country is 20/1000 and the crude birth rate is 5/1000, then the natural increase is 15/1000, or a rate of 1.5% per annum. Death rates do not vary substantially from core to periphery. Indeed, some core countries have higher death rates than some of the poorest countries in the world (see Table 1.1). Only in areas of famine or economic and political unrest (and such occurrences are usually short-lived) are death rates inordinately high. This is largely due to advancements in medical technology, especially immunizations for diseases that used to kill millions of people every year. Such technology has become available even in some of the poorest countries in the world in the last 50 years. On the other hand, as can be seen in Table 1.2, birth rates and fertility rates, and thus rates of natural increase, vary substantially between the core and periphery.

CORE-PERIPHERY POPULATION PATTERNS

As mentioned above, populations tend to pass through stages, and these are revealed by comparing long-term historical patterns with respect to the relationship between birth rates, death rates, and rate of natural increase. This historical model of population change is usually referred to as the **Demographic Transition Model**, of which there are four stages (Figure 18.1). In Stage 1, birth rates and death rates are both very high, resulting in relatively low or fluctuating rates of natural increase. Until the Industrial Revolution, when societies around the world were still agricultural in nature, all populations around the world were in Stage 1, but today there are virtually no populations in this stage. In Stage 2, death rates fall off substantially but birth rates remain high, resulting in very high rates of natural increase. In Europe, this stage began around the middle of the 18th century, as economies and societies began to industrialize. New medical technology greatly reduced death rates, but birth rates and fertility rates remained very high due to advances in medicine and improved agricultural yields as a result of more efficient agricultural techniques and tools. With enough food to go around, most people saw little need to alter traditional conceptualizations and norms with respect to reproduction. This rapid and exponential growth in population in Stage 2 is the "transition" in populations that is referred to in the Demographic Transition Model. Today, most countries in the periphery, and some in the semi-periphery, are in Stage 2 of this demographic transition.

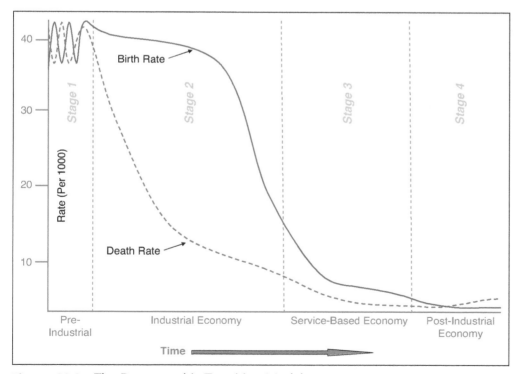

Figure 18.1   The Demographic Transition Model

In Stage 3 of the Demographic Transition Model, death rates remain quite low and birth and fertility rates begin to drop dramatically, resulting in decreasing rates of natural increase. Most of Europe and North America went through this stage during the late 19th and early 20th as these regions developed mature industrial economies. Today, most of the semi-periphery of the world-economy is currently in Stage 3. By Stage 4, which began sometime in the late 20th century in most of the core, birth rates had fallen so much that some countries have approached **zero population growth**. Indeed, in a handful of core countries today (mainly in northern and eastern Europe) populations are actually declining. The populations in the core regions of the world-economy have passed through each of these stages, and today they are the only regions in Stage 4 of the model.

Why is there such a strong correlation between economic "development" and fertility, and what factors account for these global patterns? These are extremely complex questions, for which there are few easy answers. It is possible, however, to identify some of the most probable explanations. To be sure, traditional values and customs concerning reproduction and conceptualizations of femininity and masculinity, as well as traditional religious customs, in the folk cultures of the periphery are part of the explanation. Access to modern forms of birth control (expanded in the core, more limited in the periphery) may also help to explain these patterns. But it can be argued that both of these explanations fail to take into account the power that women have in most societies around the world with respect to reproductive choice. They also fail to address differences in economies and lifestyles between the core and periphery. The most likely and most plausible explanation for the correlation between fertility and economic development is that the role of women in the societies of the core and periphery are quite different. In the subsistence agricultural societies of the periphery the role of a woman is often what we might call "traditional"—they are not only mothers, but also farmers. In such societies, traditional conceptualizations of women and children predominate and in these traditional economies children are an economic asset—the more hands for the fields, the better. On the other hand, in the core regions of the world-economy, post-modern ideas have led to radical critiques of such traditional roles for women. In most of the core societies, the role of a woman is not seen as just a mother, but also a breadwinner. So too, in these post-industrial economies in which very few people farm for a living and where the costs of living are substantial, children are in fact an economic liability. In the core, then, women have embraced other roles and put off having children until later in life. This has resulted in drastically lower fertility rates, since waiting to have children until later in life statistically reduces the number that a woman could have.

In summary, population "problems" in the periphery and parts of the semi-periphery involve those of an ecological nature. These populations are in Stage 2 of the demographic transition, with very high rates of natural increase. But at the same time, these are precisely the places that are least able to cope with young and growing populations, mostly due to weakly developed political and economic infrastructures. In short, there are increasingly too many people and not enough resources to go around—not only food resources, but other resources such as fuel and clean water. In the core and parts of the semi-periphery the "problems" are quite different. These societies are in either Stage 3 or Stage 4 of the demographic transition, with low birth and fertility rates and increasingly "older" populations. While the advanced post-industrial economies of the core would be able to cope with larger populations, they are precisely the places where rates of natural increase are the lowest. Here, the most pressing issues related to population involve questions of how to cope with an aging population in which more and more older people who are not working must be supported by fewer and fewer people of working age. This is an especially significant problem in core societies with substantial social welfare systems in which governments are in charge of funding retirement and pension plans.

Different societies are approaching such problems in different ways, with varying results. In India, for example, the population is now over 1 billion and is growing quite rapidly, at just under 2% per annum. In the 1970s India's federal government attempted to take an active role in population reduction by opening family planning clinics, dispersing contraceptives, and appealing to the patriotism of the population through public relations campaigns and advertisements. These efforts, however, have been met with much public resistance because they do not dovetail well with traditional Indian ideas about reproduction and the family. The results of the government's efforts have been mixed at best and India's population continues to grow rapidly. Another example of governmental intervention in population growth is China. In the early 1980s the Chinese government, a very powerful one-party system, took an active and rather forceful role in population reduction. Laws were enacted that gave tax breaks and other incentives to couples who chose to have no children. A one-child-only policy was also enacted and rigidly enforced that limited each couple in the country to only having one child. The government also used public relations campaigns and advertisements to appeal to the patriotism of its citizenry. The results of such policies were quite different than those in India. In 1970 the rate of natural increase was 2.4%, but it had dropped to 1.2% by 1983 and 1.0% in 1997. This success, however, came with some significant social costs. For example, a heavy male gender imbalance now exists in China as a result of an increase in abortions of female fetuses due to traditional Chinese ideals with respect to inheritance.

POPULATION THEORY

The issue of population has attracted the attention of large numbers of writers and social scientists over the past two centuries. Probably the most famous of these was the English writer **Thomas Malthus**, whose *Essay on the Principle of Population* (1798) set in motion a long-running debate regarding population growth that continues to this day. Malthus was writing at a time when England was in Stage 2 of the demographic transition and was experiencing exponential population growth. Malthus argued that while population was growing exponentially, food supplies were only growing arithmetically, and therefore would not be able to keep up with the demand for food. This, he wrote, would at some point result in a crisis punctuated by famine and social collapse.

Obviously, the crisis that Malthus predicted did not come to fruition, for he failed to predict new agricultural technologies and techniques that revolutionized agriculture in the 19th and 20th centuries. These new technologies (such as crop rotation schemes, irrigation technologies, and scientific genetic hybrids) greatly increased the amount of food that could be produced, even in some of the poorest countries in the world. Malthus' failings attracted many critics. Marxist thinkers, for example, argue that the real problem facing the world is not overpopulation, but the fact that the world's resources are not equally shared or distributed and are co-opted by the capitalist class. Another critic, **Esther Boserup**, has argued that population growth does not *necessarily* produce significant problems; it could in fact stimulate economic growth and better food production technology as it did in Europe in previous centuries. But populations in peripheral countries are increasing at unprecedented rates and many of these countries have more poor people than ever even though food production has in general increased substantially over the past few decades. These alarming trends have caused some experts to reevaluate Malthus' theory, taking into account not just food, but a variety of other natural resources. These so-called **Neo-Malthusians** argue that Malthus erred in the sense that he wrote only of food and not other natural resources but that his overall idea was correct. They contend that population growth in the developing world is a very real and very serious problem because the billions of very poor people that will be added to the world's population in the coming centuries will result in a ever-increasing desperate search for food and natural resources punctuated by more wars, civil strife, pollution, and environmental degradation.

Children are a blessing not a burden. Despite calamities we are reminded in 2 Timothy 1:7, "For God hath not given us the spirit of fear; but of power, and of love, and of a sound mind." We must also be confident in facing the present opportunities we have to reach the world for the purposes of helping children with our talents and treasure. As His obedient children, we may model His love demonstrated for us on the cross.

KEY TERMS TO KNOW

- Crude Population Density
- Physiologic Population Density
- Doubling Rate
- Population Pyramid
- Crude Birth Rate
- Crude Death Rate

- Total Fertility Rate

- Rate of Natural Increase

- Demographic Transition Model

- Zero Population Growth

- Thomas Malthus

- Esther Boserup

- Neo-Malthusians

STUDY QUESTIONS

1. Compare and contrast the structure of populations in the core, semi-periphery, and periphery of the world-economy today.

   _____

   _____

   _____

   _____

   _____

   _____

   _____

   _____

2. What are the main issues with respect to population that affect the core regions of the world-economy? What issues affect the peripheral regions?

   _____

   _____

   _____

   _____

   _____

   _____

   _____

   _____

3. What main factors account for differences in birth rates, fertility rates and rates of natural increase between the core and the periphery today?

_____

_____

_____

_____

_____

_____

_____

4. What is the primary argument of the neo-Malthusians? What do they argue the mistake in Malthus' logic is?

_____

_____

_____

_____

_____

_____

_____

FURTHER READING

Stephen Castles and Mark J. Miller, *The Age of Migration: International Population Movements in the Modern World*, 4th ed. (New York: Guilford Press, 2009).

Paul R. Ehrlich and Anne H. Ehrlich, *The Population Explosion* (New York: Touchstone, 1991).

W. T. S. Gould, *Population and Development* (New York: Routledge, 2009).

Michael R. Haines and Richard H. Steckel, eds., A *Population History of North America* (Cambridge: Cambridge University Press, 2000).

Richard Jackson and Neil Howe, *The Graying of the Great Powers: Demography and Geopolitics in the 21st Century* (Washington: Center for Strategic and International Studies, 2008).

Massimo Livi-Bacci, *A Concise History of World Population*, 4th ed. (New York: Wiley-Blackwell, 2006).

T. R. Malthus, *An Essay on the Principle of Population* (Dover: Dover Publications, 2007).

Laurie Mazur, ed., *A Pivotal Movement: Population, Justice, and the Environmental Challenge* (Washington: Island Press, 2009).

K. Bruce Newbold, *Six Billion Plus: World Population in the Twenty-First Century*, 2nd ed. (New York: Rowman & Littlefield, 2006).

Fred Pearce, *The Coming Population Crash: And Our Planet's Surprising Future* (London: Beacon Press, 2010).

Web Sites

U.S. Census Bureau (www.census.gov).

The World Bank (www.worldbank.org).

Population Reference Bureau (www.prb.org).

World Political Geography

"And hath made of one blood all nations of men for to dwell on all the face of the earth and hath determined the times before appointed, and the bounds of their habitation..." (Acts 17:26)

n an era of increasing globalization, we see the significance of the borders of the various nation-states somewhat superseded as various supra and sub-states emerge. A study of world political geography demonstrates the ongoing and dynamic nature of the changes occurring across the globe.

In This Chapter:

- Types of Historical Political Organization
- Core-Periphery Patterns of Political Cohesiveness
- Key Terms to Know
- Study Questions
- Further Reading

For most people the term *political* brings to mind things like elections, political parties, and vigorous partisan debates about various issues that dominate the airwaves and that are so much a part of our popular culture these days. While these concepts are each certainly political in nature, in an academic sense *political* refers largely to the structure and function of governments, issues related to territoriality, and power structures in various types of societies. **Political geography**, then, is the sub-field of human geography that is concerned with the analysis of the spatial expression of these issues. How do people govern themselves and how has this changed over time? How are governments structured in different parts of the world-economy? What are the spatial characteristics of different types of political organization around the world? This chapter addresses these and other issues.

TYPES OF HISTORICAL POLITICAL ORGANIZATION

In Chapter One we outlined the world-systems model of social and political change over time. World-systems analysts argue that historically there have been only three types of political, social, and economic organization: mini-systems, world-empires, and the capitalist world-economy. We can more fully understand such historical change by coupling the world-systems model with descriptions of societal structure borrowed from the fields of anthropology and political geography. Anthropologists and political geographers generally identify five different types of political organization that have occurred throughout human history, four of which can still be observed in societies today:

Band Societies

A **band society** is one in which the there are no formal positions of power and in which members of the society are united by ethnicity, cultural traditions, and kinship. Bands are usually quite small, perhaps only a few dozen extended families, and order is based in and around these extended nuclear families. Such societies exhibit no formal political claim to territory, with the exception, perhaps, of a claimed hunting territory. There is, however, strong territorial identity that is often associated with cultural identity. Until the Neolithic Revolution, most human societies were organized in such a manner, but few examples survive today. Band societies are limited to a few populations in southwest Africa, parts of tropical Southeast Asia, and some tropical rainforest regions such as the Amazon river basin of South America.

Tribal Societies

A **tribal society** is comprised of a few, perhaps many, bands of people united by common descent, linguistic similarity, and cultural values and traditions. Political leadership in these societies is usually transitory and is usually determined by virtue of perceived courage, bravery, or wisdom. Tribes are largely egalitarian in nature with respect to the communal use of resources and with respect to formalized class structures. Tribes usually claim a home "territory", but the defense of this territory is rarely undertaken with organized military power. Nevertheless, as is the case with band societies, tribal societies exhibit a very strong identity with a specific territory that is often conceived of as a people's "homeland." There are today many societies around the world that can be described as tribal in nature. The vast majority of these societies are located in the periphery and in some parts of the semi-periphery of the world-economy: much of sub-Saharan Africa, parts of tropical Southeast Asia, parts of Southwest Asia, and parts of Middle and South America. In world-systems analysis, both band and tribal societies are considered to be *mini-systems* in which production and exchange (mode of production) is largely egalitarian and reciprocal in nature. Tribal societies today, however, are also part of the capitalist world-economy, whose economies and societies are increasingly influenced by it.

Chiefdoms

A **chiefdom** describes a feudal social and economic order in which a powerful royal and aristocratic elite in a centralized control center controls the production and redistribution of agricultural products from different parts of a claimed political territory. World-systems analysis refers to this organization as the *redistributive-tributary* mode of production. Leadership in such societies is hereditary (by blood birth) and they often claim special divine authority to rule. Chiefdom societies are highly stratified by royalty and occupation, and social rank is largely determined by birth. Agricultural surpluses are generated by coercion of a large peasant class through peonage, serfdom, or slavery. These surpluses are then collected, controlled, stored and redistributed to the rest of the society by the royalty and aristocracy living in a central urban control center. Chiefdoms usually claim large territories, from which natural resources and agricultural products are extracted, and raise large, organized militaries to defend these territories by force. The central geographical feature of the societies is the *city-state*. World-systems analysis refers to this type of political and social organization as a *world-empire*. Today there are no surviving examples of chiefdoms. They were at one time, however, found all over the world as emerged after the Neolithic Revolution in the various so-called culture hearths: Mesopotamia, the Nile Valley, lowland Middle America, West and Southeast Africa, northern China, and the Indus Valley. This political and social organization also describes the situation in feudal Europe and Japan.

States

A **state** is an independent political unit occupying a defined, well-populated territory, the borders of which are recognized by surrounding states and militarily defended. All of the countries of the world today are in this sense states. This type of political organization represents a significant departure from that of bands, tribes, and chiefdoms for territory rather than cultural or ethnic affiliation is the basis of organization. Most of the world's states are multi-ethnic and multi-cultural in nature, and thus they are not "defined" by a certain culture or language or religion, but rather by place, by a territory. This basis of political organization developed in several areas around the world as feudal orders ended, especially in Europe and East Asia.

All states have a government, within which political institutions of the state function in order to exert control over the state's population and territory. Through such political power, governments are empowered to impose laws, exact taxes, and wage wars. The structure of this empowerment is basically found in two different forms of internal state political structure today. In **unitary states** governmental power and authority is centralized in a very strong central government operating from the state's capital city. The vast majority of the nearly 200 states in the world today are unitary states. A handful of states today, however, are **federal states**, in which governmental power and authority is vested in several different "levels". There is thus a hierarchy of power from the national level (federal governments) to the regional level (state or provincial governments) to the local level (city governments). Authority and control in states are vested in governments, but for those governments to have *political legitimacy* they must have some sort of ideology behind it that unites disparate groups within the society. Brute force, through the use of the military for example, may work in the short run, but without some central integrating philosophy behind it (such as "freedom" or "democracy" in the United States), a state's government can lose legitimacy and find its right to govern questioned by those it governs.

Nation-States

The idea of the nation-state emerged in Europe in the 18th and 19th centuries. By definition, a **nation-state** is a state (a territory) that is inhabited by a group of people (a nation) bound together by a general sense of cohesion resulting from a common history, ancestry, language, religion, and political philosophy. A *nation* in this sense refers not to a country, but to a group of people, and a *state* refers to a political territory. The ideal of the nation-state, then, combines these two concepts. As such, this type of political organization involves very strong allegiance to nationality and to territory on the part of the nation-state's citizenry. This political ideal probably first emerged after the Industrial Revolution in Europe as improved communication and transportation technologies enabled more efficient control of large territories. All of the major European colonial powers developed a strong nation-state ideal of political organization in the 18th and 19th centuries and by later exported this ideal all around the world as European power and influence grew very strong during the colonial era.

CORE-PERIPHERY PATTERNS OF POLITICAL COHESIVENESS

Today, all of the countries of the world-economy are politically organized as a *state*, but most aspire to the ideal of the *nation-state*. In practice, however, there are very few true nation-states as the term is defined above: one *nation* of people living in and claiming a defined political territory as its homeland. Why is this? To begin with, even in the strongest nation-states there are always threats to national cohesion. Economic inequality, racial and/or ethnic hostilities and injustices, or perceived disenfranchisement on the part of certain groups in a society may threaten national ideals. But the biggest obstacle to the ideal of the nation-state is the increasingly globalized world that has emerged since the Merchant Capitalist Revolution. Large-scale migrations (some voluntary, some involuntary) during this era, and continue today, have resulted in the creation of states that are fundamentally multi-national in nature, plural societies in which a variety of ethnic and national groups count themselves as citizens.

Some of the strongest (politically speaking) of such **multi-national states** have developed a strong sense of nationality in spite of the plural nature of the society. In some instances this occurred by "happenstance" as a result of a group or groups of people occupying a large territory over a long period (e.g. the European nation-states). In other instances, strong central governments sought to foster nationality overtly through public education systems and the development of a strong sense of patriotism (e.g. the United States, the Soviet Union, and China).

At the other end of the spectrum, multi-national states without a central organizing "principal" can sometimes degenerate into civil war or ethnic conflict in which there is a struggle on the part of the various nations of a state for political power (the former Yugoslavia and present-day conflicts in Africa, for example). At the same time, nations of people without their own state often engage in violence in order to achieve their own state and thus their own political power. On-going examples of such conflicts include the struggle of Palestinians, Kurds, and Basques to forge independent governments and states. Most such struggles, civil war, and political instability in general occur today in the periphery and parts of the semi-periphery of the world-economy. While the core states are not without their conflicts, such states usually have very strong central governments which may seek to quell such conflicts. Ethnic problems and conflicts are also usually worked out in the core through democratic processes or through public debate, both of which are relatively peaceful methods compared to the civil wars and military coups that are common in the periphery.

Political cohesiveness in most states today is influenced by two main types of "forces" working in society. **Centripetal political forces** are those that tend to bring together disparate groups in multi-ethnic, multi-national states. Such forces might include:

- Nationalism—identification with the state and acceptance of its national goals, ideals, and way of life

- Iconography—symbols of unification (flags, national heroes, rituals and holidays, patriotic songs, royalty, etc.)

- Institutions—national education systems, armed forces, state churches, common language

- Effective state organization and administration—public confidence in the organization of the state, security from aggression, fair allocation of resources, equal opportunity to participate, law and order, efficient transportation and communication networks

On the other hand, **centrifugal political forces** are those which tend to destabilize a society and pull disparate groups apart in multi-ethnic and multi-national societies. Examples of centrifugal forces might include:

- Internal discord and challenge to the authority of the state which can lead to **political devolution** in which national or ethnic groups seek to form separate political authority

- Ethnic separatism and regionalism—this is often seen in states where disparate populations have not been fully integrated, (nations without states); this can lead to **Balkanization** in which multi-national states break apart along ethnic lines

- Trouble integrating peripheral locations—this is especially a problem where disparate rural populations are located far away from the capital

- Social and economic inequality—this is most often seen in multi-nation states where the dominant group is seen to exploit minority groups in terms of control of wealth and social services, etc.

Borders are of extreme significance to the human geographer. Boundaries were used in the ancient world; in fact, the Bible exhorts us, in Deut. 19:14, not to remove the ancient landmarks. After the Middle Ages and during the Age of Discovery, with its subsequent process of colonization, the technologically advanced Europeans tended to fight among themselves for control of the world's resources and peoples. Drawing borders was a solution to the resulting chaos. Many feel the origins of the nation-state after the treaty of Westphalia in 1648 reflected the process of European borders reflecting local nationalism. French people, for example, began to not see themselves in a medieval way, as vassals to a particular local authority in a nearby castle; rather, the French began to see themselves as members of a larger group of people with whom they felt a commonality. The centripetal forces of sharing languages, religion, history, and money manifested themselves politically with the settling of boundaries. Borders are extremely tenuous concepts, but important ones subject to change. **Natural borders** such as the Pyrenees Mountains between Spain and France tend to divide people into linguistic and ethnic differences naturally and served as natural barriers to diffusion. Many historical geographers point out the relative autonomy of the city-states of Greece in antiquity, and the Cantons of Switzerland as examples of how natural borders tend to separate and can affect independence, identity, and even political processes. Irredentism is the source of much of the world's conflicts today. Irredentism can result when **drawn borders** separate a people who share identities. This frustrated nationalism or persecution can have terrible results, such as has been witnessed in the Caucasus mountains in the last decade, or the horrible genocide in Rwanda. Hopefully, by recognizing the importance of borders and their relationship to centrifugal and centripetal forces within a nation-state, we can serve as peacemakers and prevent violence.

We participate in organizations with various loyalties: states, communities, clubs, and churches. How these different social groupings make decisions politically is a fascinating study and of great importance to the geographer. Understanding the variations in these societal patterns is vital to seizing the opportunity we now have to share our faith. Peter said, in 1 Peter 3:15, "But sanctify the Lord God in your hearts, and always be ready to give a defense to everyone who asks you a reason for the hope that is in you, with meekness and fear...."

KEY TERMS TO KNOW

- Political Geography
- Band Society
- Tribal Society
- Chiefdom
- State
- Unitary State
- Federal State
- Nation-State
- Multi-National State
- Centripetal Political Forces
- Centrifugal Political Forces
- Political Devolution
- Balkanization
- Natural borders
- Drawn borders

STUDY QUESTIONS

1. Compare and contrast the term *nation* with the term *nation-state*. How are these two types of political organization different?

   _____

   _____

   _____

   _____

   _____

   _____

   _____

   _____

2. Based on discussions in class and on the material in this chapter, can the United States be considered a nation-state? Why or why not?

   _____

   _____

   _____

   _____

   _____

   _____

   _____

   _____

3. What kinds of political forces are most dominant in the three regions of the world-economy today?

_____

_____

_____

_____

_____

_____

_____

_____

FURTHER READING

John Agnew, *Hegemony: The New Shape of Global Power* (Philadelphia: Temple University Press, 2005).

John Agnew, Katharyne Mitchell, and Gerard Toal, eds., *A Companion to Political Geography* (New York: Wiley-Blackwell, 2007).

John Agnew, *Globalization and Sovereignty* (New York: Rowman & Littlefield, 2009).

Saul B. Cohen, *Geopolitics of the World System*, 2nd ed. (New York: Rowman & Littlefield, 2008).

Kevin Cox, *Political Geography: Territory, State, and Society* (New York: Wiley-Blackwell, 2002).

Jason Dittmer, *Popular Culture, Geopolitics and Identity* (New York: Rowman & Littlefield, 2010).

Wilma Dunaway, Colin Flint and Peter Taylor, *Political Geography: World-Economy, Nation-State and Locality*, 5th ed. (New York: Prentice-Hall, 2007).

Francis Fukuyama, *State Building: Governance and World Order in the 21st Century* (Ithaca: Cornell University Press, 2004).

Derek Gregory, *The Colonial Present: Afghanistan, Palestine, Iraq* (New York: Wiley-Blackwell, 2004).

Gerry Kearns, *Geopolitics and Empire: The Legacy of Halford Mackinder* (Oxford: Oxford University Press, 2009).

Baldev Raj Nayar, *The Geopolitics of Globalization: The Consequences for Development* (Oxford: Oxford University Press, 2007).

Edward Said, *Orientalism* (New York: Vintage, 1979).

Joanne Sharp, *Geographies of Postcolonialism* (London: Sage Publications, 2008).

The Geography of the World-Economy

"Now the great city was divided into three parts, and the cities of the nations fell. And great Babylon was remembered before God, to give her the cup of the wine of the fierceness of His wrath." (Revelations 16:19)

Although the scriptures are replete with warnings against idolatry, the Bible states that at the tower of Babel, mankind attempted to become greater than God. Interestingly, we see in the above verse that the generally accepted interpretation for the world-system is Babylon, and it will be brought down when the Lord returns. Today, we see the globalization of the world's economy unlike anything ever seen in history. It is imperative that we study the economy for the purpose of obedience. In Psalm 41:1–3, we read, "The Lord cares for the poor." We can help people by carefully investing our talents and treasure in locations that will return profit and create wealth enabling us to fulfill these instructions.

In This Chapter:

- The Classification of Economic Activities
- Factors in Industrial Location
- Economies of the Semi-Periphery and Periphery
- Economies of the Core
- Key Terms to Know
- Study Questions
- Further Reading

In previous chapters we have discussed the structure of the world-economy and defined the core, semi-periphery, and periphery. This chapter examines the nature of economic activities in the three regions of the world-economy in greater detail. How do people make a living in different parts of the world? How has globalization influenced the structure of the world-economy? What factors determine what kind of economic activities are undertaken in certain places? These are the primary questions addressed in this chapter.

THE CLASSIFICATION OF ECONOMIC ACTIVITIES

Economists identify five different types of economic activities, usually referred to as "sectors" of an economy. This classification of the various sectors of an economy will be employed in this chapter to compare and contrast economic activities, modes of production, and social relations of production in the various regions of the capitalist world-economy of today. The **primary sector** of an economy refers to activities related to the extraction of natural resources. This includes fishing, hunting, lumbering, mining, and agriculture. The **secondary sector** describes so-called "heavy" or "blue-collar" manufacturing industries that involve the processing of raw materials (usually natural resources) into finished products. This includes such activities as steel production, automobile assembly, the production of chemicals, food processing industries, and paper production. The following three sectors are defined as service industries, those businesses that provide services to individuals and the community at large. The **tertiary sector** refers to financial, business, professional, and clerical services, including retail and wholesale trade. The **quaternary sector** of an economy describes jobs and industries that involve the processing and dissemination of information, as well as administration and control of various enterprises. These jobs are often described by the term "white collar," and consist of professionals working in a variety of industries such as education, government, research, health care, and information management. Finally, the **quinary sector** refers to high-level management and decision-making in large organizations and corporations.

FACTORS IN INDUSTRIAL LOCATION

The location of various types of industrial activities is influenced by a variety of geographical factors. These factors are at work not only at the regional scale, but at the national and global scale as well. Among these factors are the following:

- The Costs of Production
  - **Geographically fixed costs**—costs relatively unaffected by location of the enterprise (e.g. capital, interest)
  - **Geographically variable costs**—costs that vary spatially (e.g. labor, land, power, transportation)

- Capitalist Ideology and Logic

  - Since the goal of almost all industries is the minimization of costs and the maximization of profit, the location of an industry is most likely to be where the total costs of production are minimized

- Complexity of the Manufacturing Process

  - The more interdependent a manufacturing process is, the more its costs of production are affected by location (e.g. steel production)

- Type of Raw Materials Involved in the Manufacturing Process

  - Raw materials that are bulky and heavy, perishable, or undergo great weight loss or gain in processing have the greatest effect on siting

  - Examples: pulp, paper and sawmills; fruit and vegetable canning; meat processing; soft drink canning

- Source of Power

  - Important when a source of power is immovable (e.g. the aluminum industry)

- Costs of Labor (Wages)

- The Market for the Product

  - **Market orientation**—placing the last stage of a manufacturing process as close to the market for that product as possible; products that undergo much weight gain during the manufacturing process (e.g. soft drink canning and bottling)

  - **Raw material orientation**—locating the manufacturing plant as close to the raw material that is used as possible; usually applies in industries that use very heavy or bulky raw materials (e.g. paper production)

- Transportation costs

  - Water—the least expensive for of transportation for bulky and heavy goods

  - Rail—also relatively inexpensive for bulky and heavy goods but with less flexible routes

  - Trucking—relatively expensive but carries the advantage of very flexible routes

  - Air—the most expensive form of transportation; employed usually for transporting very valuable goods or those that are time-sensitive (e.g. overnight mail service)

ECONOMIES OF THE SEMI-PERIPHERY AND PERIPHERY

The economies of the periphery and parts of the semi-periphery are dominated by primary economic activities. The vast majority of people in the periphery live in rural areas and make their living from **subsistence farming**. Subsistence farming systems involve agricultural activities that are undertaken not necessarily for money profit, but rather for daily sustenance. Three main types of subsistence agricultural systems are dominant in the peripheral regions of the world-economy today:

Shifting Cultivation

Shifting cultivation, sometimes called *slash and burn agriculture*, involves a complex set of farming practices employed in tropical wet regions where environmental conditions (heavy annual rainfall and very poor soils) are delicately balanced. It is an ancient practice that probably dates back to the earliest stages of the Neolithic Revolution and represents a rather sound ecological solution to the vagaries of life in such an environment. Shifting cultivation cannot support very large populations because tropical soils do not support the kinds of crops that can feed very large populations (such as grain crops). Rather, it involves the use of low technology tools such as machetes, hoes, digging sticks, and fire to harvest crops such as bananas, taro, cassava, and manioc. It is practiced by very small groups (bands and tribes) practicing a nomadic or semi-nomadic lifestyle in which a small area is cleared of brush with a machete, covered to allow it to dry, and burned, which fixes nitrogen into the soil. Plants that reproduce vegetatively (like those listed above) are then planted in the ashes. After one or two growing cycles the soils are exhausted and the group moves on to another site. This lifestyle is practiced mainly in tropical rainforest regions today by a relatively small number of people in locations such as the Amazon and Orinoco basins of South America, parts of Java and other Indonesian islands, parts of tropical central Africa, and parts of Middle America and the Caribbean islands.

Pastoral Nomadism

Pastoral Nomadism, sometimes referred to as *extensive subsistence agriculture*, describes the practice of following or hunting herds of game or herding domesticated animals. It is practiced by large numbers of people in tropical grassland environments (savannahs) in central and east-central Africa and some mid-latitude grasslands regions in south-central Asia. Pastoral nomadism involves an almost wholly nomadic lifestyle that is extensive in its use of land since livestock like cattle, sheep, and goats require much land per animal in order to thrive. Contrary to popular belief, most pastoral nomads each meat very infrequently because the animals they heard are the main source of wealth and income. Such societies are usually tribal in nature and the lifestyle involves seasonal movements to "greener" grazing lands. As such, there are few permanent settlements in the areas where pastoral nomadism is the dominant economic activity.

Intensive Subsistence Farming

Intensive Subsistence Farming refers to the subsistence production of a variety of grains and vegetables on small, permanent plots that are farmed intensively the year round. This is possible because such farming activities are undertaken mainly in wet regions of the sub-tropics. The most important of these regions and the most important crops are: China, India, and southeast Asia (Vietnam, Thailand, Cambodia, Laos, Myanmar), where rice is the most important crop; Middle America, where beans and corn are dominant; Southwest Asia from Syria to Pakistan, where wheat and rice are most widely grown; and central Africa, where millet, sorghums, and peanuts are very important. This is not to say that these are the only crops grown in these areas. In fact, intensive subsistence agriculture usually involves the production of a large variety of fruits, grains, and vegetables, but at a relatively small scale. Intensive subsistence agricultural systems employ relatively low-technology tools and innovations such as animal-drawn plows, manure for fertilizer, terracing systems, and not a small amount of human muscle power. These farming systems are undertaken by literally millions of people in much of the periphery and semi-periphery. Indeed, rice, the most important grain crop in the world, sustains at least half of the world's population on a daily basis.

Plantation Agriculture

A final important type of agricultural system undertaken primarily in the periphery and semi-periphery of the world-economy today is **Plantation Agriculture**. While all of the other forms of agriculture in these regions of the world-economy are subsistence in nature, plantation agriculture is a form of **commercial farming**, in which the main goal is the maximization of profit per unit area of land under cultivation in order to sell the products in the international marketplace. Plantation agriculture involves the commercial production of tropical and sub-tropical products such a tropical fruits, sugar, coffee, tea, and cocoa. A plantation is a large farm on which only one crop is normally grown. Most plantations are owned and managed by large multi-national corporations in the core but employ local low-wage labor. The capital input, as well as the main market for the crops grown on such plantations, is in the core regions of the world-economy. Thus, most plantation products are grown explicitly for export to the core. A British and Dutch innovation, the idea of the plantation dates from the colonial era when British, French, and Dutch companies established sugar plantations using African slave labor in the Caribbean. Plantations were also established in other colonial areas to produce a variety of valuable tropical agricultural crops: tea in India, spices in Indonesia, coffee in Africa and parts of Middle and South America. Today, most plantations are found in the Caribbean, Central America, and tropical central Africa.

Manufacturing

As discussed in Chapter One, the globalization of the post-industrial era has created a global economy that is punctuated by an international division of labor in which the periphery and the semi-periphery play an increasingly important role. In the semi-periphery, the post-industrial era ushered in an era in which manufacturing activities have become an important element of most economies. Semi-peripheral economies today are characterized by a mix of subsistence and commercial farming (mostly plantation agriculture) and light and heavy manufacturing activities that employ low-wage, low-skilled urban workers. Most manufacturing enterprises and plantations, however, are owned and managed by multi-national corporations in the core—the United States, Japan, and Europe. This pattern has developed over the past 30 years as a result of evolving service economies in the core and the movement of manufacturing activities out of the core in search of lower costs of production, especially with respect to wages. Some of the industries most effected by this are textiles (clothing and shoes), inexpensive retail goods (toys, for example), and automobile assembly. Thus, an international division of labor punctuated by multi-national companies in the core has evolved into what characterizes it today: high-wage service sector labor in the core; low-wage, low-skilled secondary sector (manufacturing) jobs in the semi-periphery; and low-wage, low-skilled primary sector jobs (subsistence agriculture and plantation enterprises) in the periphery.

ECONOMIES OF THE CORE

Primary Activities

Commercial agricultural activities in the core regions of the world-economy are punctuated by several distinguishing characteristics. First, agriculture employs a very small number of people but it is nevertheless very productive and remains an important part of core economies. But agriculture has undergone immense changes in the core over the past fifty years: the number of farmers has drastically declined, the average farm size has risen substantially, and many agricultural activities are increasingly being controlled by large corporations (this is known as **agribusiness**). Farming in the core today is characterized by high inputs of capital, heavy mechanization, the heavy use of hybrid crop and animal varieties, chemical fertilizers, and relatively low inputs of human labor. While such innovations have put many farmers in the core out of work or made them redundant, agricultural production in the core is the highest in the world in terms of crop and animal yields per unit area.

Five main types of farming systems dominate the agricultural economies of the core. First, **commercial dairying** involves the production of milk and milk products, primarily for large urban markets. While fresh milk production is located in the urban hinterlands of most large metropolitan areas in the core (because it is perishable), the production of milk products like cheese, yogurt, and butter is concentrated in the northern United States and northern and Alpine Europe. Second, **market gardening**, sometimes referred to as "truck farming," involves the commercial production of fruits, vegetables, or other specialized crops, again mainly for large urban markets. Market gardening is concentrated along the Atlantic coast of the United States from New Jersey to Florida to Texas, parts of coastal California, northwestern Europe (especially the Netherlands), parts of coastal Japan, and parts of Australia and New Zealand. Third, **mixed livestock and grain farming** refers to the production of livestock for human consumption alongside the production of grains (mainly corn and wheat) for use as livestock fodder. This describes the agricultural systems dominant in the Great Plains (wheat and cattle) and Midwest (corn, soybeans, hogs, and cattle) of the United States, the Pampas of Argentina (wheat, corn, and cattle), much of central Europe (sorghum, corn, cattle, and hogs), and the interior grasslands of Australia (wheat and sheep). Fourth, **livestock ranching** involves the commercial production of livestock (mainly cattle) for large urban markets and for international export. Ranching takes place mainly in semi-arid grassland environments of the mid-latitude regions of the core: the interior West of the United States, interior Australia, southern Brazil, parts of Argentina, and parts of Spain and Greece. Finally, **Mediterranean agriculture** involves the production of highly specialized Mediterranean crops like grapes, figs, dates, olives, and citrus fruits. Such activities are undertaken in regions around the world with the distinctive Mediterranean climate (hot, dry summers and cool, wet winters): southern California, the circum-Mediterranean, southwest Australia, parts of southwestern Africa, and parts of Chile.

Service Activities

The economies of the core regions of the capitalist world-economy were built upon a factory organization of labor and a reliance on heavy manufacturing industrial activity during the 19th and early 20th centuries. But the last 30 years have witnessed a vast shift in how core economies are structured. In search of lower costs of labor, many large corporations have spearheaded the development of an international division of labor in which manufacturing activities (and manufacturing jobs along with them) have been moved to semi-peripheral locations. Today, the vast majority of the population in core regions is employed in the service sector of the economy, especially the tertiary and quaternary sectors. Core economies are also increasingly information-based: some of the largest companies in the world, like AT&T and Microsoft, are in the business of perfecting and selling the access and dissemination of information.

This has resulted in revolutionary changes in the industrial landscape of the core countries and the geography of industry and manufacturing in these places. The once-dominant industrial centers such as the Great Lakes region in the United States, the British Midlands, and the German Ruhr district have now become "rust belts." Entirely new manufacturing centers have now developed in places in which the main resource for new information technologies, human brain power, is nearby. Examples of these new manufacturing regions include Silicon Valley in northern California, the Research

Triangle of North Carolina, and the "Golden Triangle" of central Texas. In Europe, such centers have been developed in many areas of eastern Europe such as eastern Germany, the Czech Republic, Hungary, and Poland.

Agricultural Revolutions

In Chapter 15, we discussed the importance of the Neolithic Revolution. Subsequent advances in agriculture have also been instrumental in supplying the population necessary to contribute to the world economy, and in many ways, may be responsible for many of the lines we see on maps and the exponential population growth we see on graphs today. These "Agricultural Revolutions" are described in the book "Human Geography: People, Place and Culture by Erin H. Fouberg and Alexander B. Murphy and H.J. de Blij.[1]

The **Second Agricultural Revolution** was important because of its association with **the Enclosure Movement**. This use of fencing limited pastoral lifestyles and may have been instrumental in large measure for the surplus population in some of the Puritan areas of England. Resulting unemployment may have led many to come to America. Besides fencing the land, the idea of personal property ownership, as symbolized by the burgeoning fences on the landscape, may have contributed in some measure to the capitalism accompanying the Industrial Revolution.[2] The psychological effect of land ownership may also explain why borders became increasingly drawn by the same European powers first affected by the enclosure movement and so often misunderstood by aboriginal peoples even today. For example, in the current U.S. conflict in Afghanistan, the Durand Line is viewed as a relic of bygone days of British power by the Pashtun peoples who just walk across the border to do business with those with whom they feel more ethnically or linguistically and culturally closer. Similarly, the pioneers who came to America operated under systems respecting private property ownership at odds with the ideas of the Native-Americans, who had never viewed the land as something to be owned.

The **Third Agricultural Revolution** is marked by the increased use of agrichemicals, modern farm equipment, and the use of food packaging.[3] These innovations together have made food much more abundant as a result of increased productivity and lower loss due to spoilage. A lessened need for farm hands as a result of reapers and combines in the north-western U.S. demonstrated an important aspect of modern farm equipment in the American Civil War, where numbers of farm boys were freed to fight against a Confederacy lacking this equipment and thereby restrained by manpower needs at home.

Look in a grocery store. Many people don't realize how many foods are not nearly in their original form. Potato chips, for example, do not grow on vines; they are manufactured. Despite the increased availability of **organic foods**, products generally free of

---

[1] Human Geography 9th ed. by Fouberg, Murphy and De Blij, Wiley Pub Hoboken NJ 2009 p. 353
[2] Ibid p. 360
[3] Ibid, 362–363

chemicals and **GMO's** -genetically modified organisms, these foods nevertheless constitute a small part of the offerings and foods purchased by the consumer. Generally, for better or worse, the American people rely largely on manufactured foods that generally are not in their original form as a large portion of their diet.

In Job 31:24, we read, "If I have made gold my hope, Or said to fine gold, '*You are* my confidence'; by verse 28, he draws the conclusion, "This also *would be* an iniquity *deserving of* judgment, For I would have denied God *who is* above." We must never confuse money with wealth; likewise, we should subordinate our own selfish interests to those of God, as stated in His Word. Any strategy of service in light of the above scripture should take the economic aspects of geography into account when developing a strategy for service. Despite wonderful technological advances, hundreds of thousands of people in the world still suffer from the effects of starvation. With an appreciation of the historical relationships between technology and agriculture, one can discern potential opportunities to meet the needs of others and, in the process, share our faith. By sharing our blessings with others, we demonstrate the love of Jesus Christ for all mankind and fulfill James' exhortation, "But be ye doers of the word, and not hearers only, deceiving your own selves." (James 1:23)

KEY TERMS TO KNOW

- Primary Sector
- Secondary Sector
- Tertiary Sector
- Quaternary Sector
- Quinary Sector
- Geographically Fixed Costs
- Geographically Variable Costs
- Market Orientation
- Raw Material Orientation
- Subsistence Farming
- Commercial Farming
- Shifting Cultivation
- Pastoral Nomadism
- Intensive Subsistence Farming
- Plantation Agriculture
- Agribusiness

- Commercial Dairying
- Market Gardening
- Mixed Livestock and Grain Agriculture
- Livestock Ranching
- Mediterranean Agriculture
- The Second Agricultural Revolution
- The Enclosure Movement
- The Third Agricultural Revolution
- Organic foods
- GMOs

STUDY QUESTIONS

1. Compare and contrast agricultural systems in the periphery, semi-periphery, and periphery.

   _____

   _____

   _____

   _____

   _____

   _____

   _____

   _____

2. Compare and contrast the defining characteristics of the economies of the core, semi-periphery, and periphery today.

   _____

   _____

   _____

   _____

   _____

   _____

   _____

   _____

FURTHER READING

Jason Clay, *World Agriculture and the Environment: A Commodity-by-Commodity Guide to Impacts and Practices* (Washington: Island Press, 2004).

Paul K. Conkin, *A Revolution Down on the Farm: The Transformation of American Agriculture Since 1929* (Lexington: The University Press of Kentucky, 2009).

Thomas L. Friedman, *The Lexus and the Olive Tree: Understanding Globalization* (New York: Anchor, 2000).

Anthony Giddens, *Runaway World: How Globalization is Reshaping our Lives* (New York: Routledge, 2002).

David Grigg, *An Introduction to Agricultural Geography* (New York: Routledge, 1995).

David Harvey, *The Limits to Capital* (London: Verso, 2006).

Paul Knox and John Agnew, *The Geography of the World-Economy*, 3rd ed. (New York: John Wiley & Sons, 1998).

Joel Kotkin, *The New Geography: How the Digital Revolution is Reshaping the American Landscape* (New York: Random House, 2001).

Marcel Mazoyer and Laurence Roudart, *A History of World Agriculture: From the Neolithic Age to the Current Crisis* (New York: Monthly Review Press, 2006).

Jan Nederveen Pieterse, *Globalization and Culture: Global Mélange* (New York: Roman & Littlefield, 2009).

Stephen Nottingham, *Eat Your Genes: How Genetically Modified Food is Entering Our Diet* (London: Zed Books, 2003).

Michael Pollan, *The Omnivore's Dilemma: A Natural History of Four Meals* (New York: Penguin, 2007).

Pietra Rivoli, *The Travels of a T-Shirt in the Global Economy* (New York: John Wiley & Sons, 2005).

Robert K. Schaeffer, *Understanding Globalization: The Social Consequences of Political, Economic, and Environmental Change* (New York: Rowman & Littlefield, 2009).

Eric Schlosser, *Fast Food Nation: The Dark Side of the All-American Meal* (New York: Harper, 2009).

Jan Aart Scholte, *Globalization: A Critical Introduction*, 2nd ed. (New York: Palgrave Macmillan, 2005).

Jennifer Thompson, *Genes for Africa: Genetically Modified Crops in the Developing World* (Cape Town: Juta Academic, 2004).

B. L. Turner and Stephen Brush, eds., *Comparative Farming Systems* (New York: Guilford Press, 1987).

World Bank, *World Development Report 2008: Agriculture and Development* (New York: World Bank Publications, 2008).

Urban Landscapes of the World-Economy

"Again, the devil took Him up on an exceedingly high mountain, and showed Him all the kingdoms of the world and their glory. And he said to Him, 'All these things I will give You if You will fall down and worship me.'" (Matthew 4:8)

As man settled into cities, we saw the creation of languages in Genesis 11. Likewise, when Satan sought to tempt Jesus, he attempted to use the glory of the cities. Truthfully, most of the human population lives in urban areas now, and we must be able to reach out to them there. To do our Lord's Will and to fulfill the Great Commission stated in Matthew 28:18–20, we must recognize the importance of urban landscapes and spaces to the world economy today.

In This Chapter:

- Global Patterns of Urbanization

- The Nature of Cities

- Urban Landscapes of the Core

- Urban Landscapes of the Semi-Periphery and Periphery

- Key Terms to Know

- Study Questions

- Further Reading

The previous chapters have outlined the basic structure of the world-economy, especially with respect to relative levels of "development" and "underdevelopment" in the core, semi-periphery, and periphery. This final chapter discusses global patterns of urbanization, especially during the post-industrial era of the late 20th and early 21st centuries, within this world-systems context. Although urbanization has been a phenomenon associated with many cultures for thousands of years (since the Neo-lithic Revolution), the highest rates of urban growth have materialized during the most recent industrial and post-industrial eras. As a result, there are now more people living in cities than ever before in human history. Where are the most urbanized places in the world? Where are urban populations growing the fastest? What are the potential consequences of high rates of urban growth in different regions of the world-economy? What are some of the distinguishing characteristics of cities and urban landscapes in the post-industrial era? How do urban landscapes differ in the different regions of the world-economy? These and other questions are addressed in this chapter.

GLOBAL PATTERNS OF URBANIZATION

A logical place to begin this discussion is with an overview of some general global patterns of urbanization. Map 15 on the accompanying CD-ROM, which illustrates the percentage of the population living in urban regions by country, clearly shows that the most urbanized populations today are in core and semi-peripheral regions. Indeed, of the regions of the world in which seventy percent or more of the population lives in urban areas, all are either in the core or semi-periphery of the world-economy:

- North America (The United States and Canada)

- Mexico

- Northern and Western Europe

- South America (with the exception of the Andean highlands)

- Australia and New Zealand

- Japan and South Korea

- Parts of Southwest Asia and North Africa (Libya, Saudi Arabia, Israel, Jordan, United Arab Emirates)

At the same time, however, data compiled over the last ten years indicate that urban populations are growing the fastest in the periphery and parts of the semi-periphery. This trend is dramatically illustrated on Map 13, which shows the average annual rate of change in urban populations by country between 2000 and 2005. The overall global trend in the post-industrial, then, has been stagnant or negative rates of urban growth in the core but very high rates of urban growth in the semi-periphery and periphery. The growth of urban populations in the semi-periphery and periphery is cause for concern because it is precisely these economies that can ill afford the social and economic pressures resulting from ever-increasing urban populations. Such pressures might include:

- Housing—to shelter newly arrived migrants (most such migrants in the semi-periphery and periphery have moved from rural areas to urban areas in search of jobs

- Food—urban dwellers do not produce food, but rather consume food produced in rural areas by fewer and fewer farmers

- Natural Resources—clean air and water

- Public Services—water and sewage services, trash collection, communication and transportation infrastructures, security (police), social services

- Social Problems—crime, ethnic conflict, economic inequalities, unemployment

- Jobs—to provide a living for newly-arrived migrants from the rural countryside

In order for an urban region to function smoothly, each of these must be addressed or provided. While similar problems plague all cities worldwide, including those in core regions, core economies are much better equipped to handle large urban populations. In many parts of the periphery and in parts of the semi-periphery such services are woefully inadequate at best and nonexistent at worst. Large and growing urban populations, then, present such areas with a myriad of issues and problems, and only add to the many economic and social problems that afflict these areas of the world-economy.

The growth of large cities in the semi-periphery and periphery of the world-economy during the late industrial and early post-industrial eras is illustrated in the following list of the world's largest metropolitan areas in 2005 according to the United Nations:

1. Tokyo-Yokohama, Japan (33.2 million) [*core*]

2. New York, USA (17.8 million) [*core*]

3. São Paulo, Brazil (17.7 million) [*semi-periphery*]

4. Seoul-Inchon, South Korea (17.5 million) [*core*]

5. Ciudad Mexico, Mexico (17.4 million) [*semi-periphery*]

6. Osaka-Kobe-Kyoto, Japan (16.4 million) [*core*]

7. Manila, Philippines (14.8 million) [*semi-periphery*]

8. Mumbai, India (14.4 million) [*periphery*]

9. Jakarta, Indonesia (14.3 million) [*semi-periphery*]

10. Lagos, Nigeria (13.4 million) [*periphery*]

11. Calcutta, India (12.7 million) [*periphery*]

12. Delhi, India (12.3 million) [*periphery*]

13. Cairo, Egypt (12.2 million) [*periphery*]

14. Los Angeles, USA (11.8 million) [*core*]

15. Buenos Aires, Argentina (11.2 million) [*semi-periphery*]

16. Rio de Janeiro, Brazil (10.8 million) [*semi-periphery*]

17. Moscow, Russia (10.5 million) [*semi-periphery*]

18. Shanghai, China (10.0 million) [*semi-periphery*]

19. Karachi, Pakistan (9.8 million) [*periphery*]

20. Paris, France (9.6 million) [*core*]

As late as the mid-20th century, nearly all of the most populous cities in the world were located in Europe or North America. Today, however, of the twenty largest cities in the world only six are located in core regions of the world-economy. Eight are in semi-peripheral locations and six are in the periphery. Thus, while large cities are associated with the wealthiest countries in most people's minds, it is clear that large urban populations are increasingly phenomena of the semi-periphery and periphery as well. Indeed, experts speculate that Mexico City will overtake Tokyo as the world's largest metropolitan area by 2025 and that only two or three cities in core regions (Tokyo-Yokohama, New York, and perhaps Osaka) will remain on the list of the twenty largest cities in the world.

THE NATURE OF CITIES

Why do cities exist in the first place? What advantages are offered by the agglomeration of large populations in a certain place? What functions do cities perform? The answers to these questions are extremely complex and may differ from place to place, not only within the same country, but within the different regions of the world-economy as well. But we can begin to understand the nature of cities by pointing out a few basic caveats concerning urban regions agreed upon by most experts:

1. *Cities perform certain basic economic functions*
   This is the reason that cities exist at all: for the efficient performance of functions that could not be adequately or efficiently carried out if a population were randomly dispersed through space. For example, producers are nearer to the consumers of their products, and workers are nearer to their places of employment. Time, money, and efficiency is saved by the agglomeration of people in space.

2. *Cities function as markets*
   This has been the case since the earliest Neolithic Revolutions. As such, they have close reciprocal relationships with their rural hinterlands. For example, cities consume food that is produced primarily in rural areas. Cities are also the places where raw materials from rural areas (such as agricultural products or natural resources) are processed into consumable goods. Cities dispense goods and services not only for their own urban populations, but rural populations as well.

3. *Cities tend to be efficiently located*
   Cities are most commonly located at certain advantageous sites:

   - Sites that offer security and/or defense such as a hilltop or island (many Neolithic and Medieval cities occupy such sites)

   - Sites that are economically advantageous, such as a **head of navigation site** on a river, a river fording or portage site, or a railhead site

4. *Cities function as "central places"*

The idea of cities as "central places" stems from the work of the German geographer Walter Christaller, who in 1933 published a theoretical study concerning the distribution of service centers. Christaller wanted to understand the theoretical spatial patterns that would result when rural residents traded with a central market town providing goods and services. The results of this study are referred to as **Central Place Theory** by human geographers. The theory has been applied in many different places around the world in order to more fully understand urban patterns and appears to have stood the test of time in terms of its explanatory value. Christaller was concerned with why cities are located where they are, why some cities grow while others do not, and why there is an apparently non-random pattern with respect to the location of cities with respect to other cities. Central Place Theory holds that the importance of a market city is directly related to its centrality—the relative importance of a place with respect to its surrounding region.

The central concept of Central Place Theory concerns the "range" of a good or service—the distance that people are willing to travel to obtain a certain good or service. Some goods and services, such as bread or food in general, are **low-range goods**, those for which people are not willing to travel far to obtain. Others, such as cars or furniture, are **high-range goods**, for which people are willing to travel long distances to buy. Christaller argued that the "centrality", or relative importance, of a market town or city is directly proportional to the types of goods and services offered there, and that a natural hierarchy of size will arise with respect to market locations based upon what types of goods or services are offered there. This central place hierarchy ranges from low-order places that offer only low-range goods, to high-order places that offer both low- and high-range goods and services. Central Place Theory thus gives us insight into the functions that cities perform, why some cities grow and others do not, and why there are many small central places but only a few very large central places.

URBAN LANDSCAPES OF THE CORE

The following sections list the distinguishing characteristics of urban regions in selected locations in the core, semi-periphery, and periphery of the world-economy:

The core regions of the world-economy contain some of the largest cities in the world. Several of these cities developed into the nodes or "command and control centers" of the world-economy and remain so today. These so-called **world cities** are distinguished by the following characteristics:

- Financial centers—head offices, stock market locations
- Command and control centers of world capitalist economy—corporate headquarters of multi-national firms
- Political centers
- Cultural centers
- Nodes of international linkages

Western European Cities

Medieval Origins   One of the most striking features of most western European cities today is the juxtaposition of pre-industrial and post-industrial features in the region's urban landscapes. Many western European urban centers can trace their origins to the medieval era (from the 10th to the 15th century), when they emerged as high-order places in the central place hierarchy due to economic and/or political importance. The siting and the pre-industrial landscapes of many western European cities reflect these medieval origins, as well as their early roles as transportation centers and economic and political centers. Many of the largest western European cities, for example, are located either on the coast or on a large, navigable river. Some occupy early head-of-navigation sites (London, for example) or river crossing sites (Frankfurt, Germany). Others occupy "defensive" sites, such as hill-top or island locations, and are often associated with the sites of medieval-era castles and fortifications (Edinburgh, Scotland and Heidelberg, Germany, for example). Another medieval feature of many western European urban landscapes is the seemingly haphazard arrangement of streets, reflective of a lack of centralized city planning and growth by "accretion" over long periods of time. It was only in the 19th and 20th centuries that many western European cities began to enact city planning schemes that began to alter ancient medieval urban city plans. The presence of straight, ceremonial boulevards, such as the Champs Elysées in Paris and Unter den Linden in Berlin, reflect this kind of centralized city planning.

Abundant "Green" Spaces   Also reflective of the more modern trend toward centralized urban planning is the presence of relatively large areas set aside for public use. Such spaces include pedestrian zones, public markets and parks. Many western European cities are surrounded by large tracts of forests and parks located at the urban-rural fringe on the outskirts of urban areas; these tracts are collectively known as **greenbelts**.

Dense Public Transportation Networks   Modern western European cities are characterized by well-developed, efficient urban transportation networks. These networks usually include bus, tram (streetcar), subway and light rail transportation.

"Low" Profiles   Compared to many North American cities, most large western European cities have relatively few tall skyscrapers. With the exception of London, Paris and Frankfurt, all of which have downtown central business districts with prominent skyscrapers, most European cities have a comparatively "low" landscape profile comprised of many square miles of multi-unit housing structures and retail services.

Emerging Post-Industrial Multiethnic Cities   Although most western European states emerged from the colonial era as very strong nation-states with ethnically homogeneous societies, the late 20th and early 21st centuries have been characterized by significant influxes of ethnic minorities, primarily from southern and eastern Europe, Asia and Africa. From Moroccans and Algerians in Spain and France, to

Indians and Pakistanis in England, to Serbs and Africans in Germany and the Scandinavian countries, the larger urban centers of western Europe have received the largest number of these immigrants and their presence has fundamentally altered the ethnic makeup of the region such that most western European societies can now be characterized as fundamentally multiethnic in nature. Increased immigration has altered European societies in many positive ways, but it has also not occurred without some significant social issues. For example, many of these new immigrants are refugees escaping political and economic turmoil in their home countries, and arrive in European cities without jobs or housing. Given the immigrants' need for jobs and housing, some cities have experienced significant strains in dealing with large influxes of unemployed immigrants. In response, many cities have constructed large numbers of immigrant housing developments in specific areas set aside for such housing, often on the outskirts of urban regions. This has created **ethnic enclaves**, neighborhoods that are numerically dominated by specific ethnic groups, with businesses, such as restaurants and retain shops, catering to those groups.

North American Cities

Changing Forms of Transportation   Historically, the most significant factor that has influenced the structure and size of North American cities has been changing dominant forms of transportation over time. In the pre-industrial era—from the colonial period until the late 19th century—most cities were oriented toward pedestrian and/or animal transportation. These pedestrian cities tended to be rather compact, with zones of varying land use forming concentric circles around a **central business district** nucleus dominated by retail services and high-rent residential housing. During the early industrial period, between roughly 1880 and 1940, urban transportation came to be dominated by streetcars, subways and railways. As a result, cities expanded dramatically in size as commuters could now live further from the central business district due to faster and more efficient forms of public transportation. Zones of varying urban land use expanded outward from the central business district along these public transportation arteries. These "streetcar cities" came to resemble a wheel, with the central business district as the hub and railway and streetcar lines as the spokes radiating outward from the center. After World War II, the widespread use of the automobile as the dominant mode of transportation engendered even more radical changes in the size and shape of American cities. With the construction of interstate highway systems, commuters began to live further and further away from the central city, leading to the development of intense **suburbanization** at the urban-rural fringe dominated by upper-income residential housing and services catering to that income group. Cities expanded dramatically in size such that most American urban regions can now be characterized as being comprised of multiple "cities within cities" covering hundreds of square miles and connected via a dense and efficient network of large highways.

Spatial Differentiation Based on Ethnicity, Race and Income   One of the most distinctive characteristics of North American cities today is the development of conspicuous sectors of varying residential land use that reflect societal differences in ethnicity, race, class and income. This has led to the development of distinctive ethnic and class-based neighborhoods within American urban regions. This trend began in the 19th and early 20th centuries with the immigration of millions of Europeans, especially those coming from southern and eastern Europe who settled in the large industrial cities of the Northeast, and the migration of hundreds of thousands of African-Americans from rural areas of the South to industrial cities of the North. Many of these immigrants and migrants settled among one another in distinctive ethnic neighborhoods near central business districts, downtown areas that were abandoned by upper-income whites in favor of suburban locales at the urban-rural fringe.

Zoning   Zoning refers to the detailed urban land use planning that city governments in the United States undertake; it is yet another distinguishing characteristic of American cities. Through the use and enforcement of zoning laws, city governments have the power to authorize and enforce what types of economic activities can take place in certain areas and what kind of structures can and cannot be built in certain areas. Such areas are said to be "zoned" for certain activities or kinds of structures. Such zoning laws have had a significant impact on the spatial differentiation of American cities with respect to both residential and business land use.

Gentrification   Gentrification refers to the revitalization of formerly abandoned properties in the central business district of American cities, a trend that is increasingly characteristic of American cities in the post-industrial era of the late 20th and early 21st centuries. As upper-income whites moved to suburban areas from the central city during the 1950s, 60s and 70s, and as warehousing and light industry activities also moved to urban peripheral regions during the same period, downtown areas in many American cities fell into disrepair. In order to revitalize downtown areas and to entice suburbanites back to the central business district, city governments began to support the efforts of wealthy investors in purchasing and revitalizing formerly abandoned downtown properties. These gentrification schemes often involve the construction of pedestrian malls dominated by expensive restaurants and specialty shops that cater to upper-income customers. While these activities have given many downtown areas a second life and contributed to economic revitalization, gentrification does not occur without some social costs. For example, as downtown areas were abandoned during the era of rapid suburban growth they were often repopulated by lower-income residents and recent immigrants. Because such residents lack the political and economic power of wealthy investors and developers, gentrification schemes often result in such residents being forced to move.

URBAN LANDSCAPES OF THE SEMI-PERIPHERY AND PERIPHERY

Latin American Cities

An Iberian Colonial Imprint   The most conspicuous urban landscape features of Latin American cities reflect the Iberian (Spanish and Portuguese) colonial imprint that is common throughout the region, from the southwestern United States in the north to the southern tip of South America. Spanish colonial goals were focused on the expansion of empire, the expansion of Christendom, and the extraction of valuable natural resources such as gold and silver, and distinctive urban landscape features reflect these colonial goals. For example, in order to accomplish these goals the Spanish instituted a centrally-planned and ordered network of urban centers that was built upon pre-existing networks of Native American towns. By law and in practice, all Spanish colonial towns were constructed on a rectilinear grid of streets oriented to the cardinal directions surrounding an open, public *plaza*. Almost all colonial towns were associated with *presidios*, forts of garrisoned military troops that exerted political and military control, and cathedrals staffed by Jesuit priests who were charged with converting Native Americans to Christianity. Other Iberian landscape features common in Latin American cities include Spanish architectural features such as *adobe* construction and red tile roofs.

Spatial Differentiation Reflecting Strong Class Differences   Like other semiperipheral areas of the world-economy, Latin America is a region characterized by relatively intense social stratification based upon class, race, ethnicity and income. The urban landscapes of the region reflect this stratification. In contrast to American cities, the wealthiest members of Latin American societies often live very near city centers, in elite sectors or neighborhoods. These elite sectors are surrounded by distinctive neighborhood sectors according to race, ethnicity and income. The poorest members of Latin American societies, especially those that are homeless, live in so-called **squatter belts** in urban-rural fringe areas on the outskirts of cities in very poor conditions devoid of urban services such as running water, electricity and sewage and trash disposal.

Southeast and South Asian Cities

A Western European Colonial Imprint   In contrast to Iberian colonial goals, the goals of western European colonial powers (such as Holland, England and France) in South Asia (e.g. Pakistan, India and Sri Lanka) and Southeast Asia (e.g. Vietnam, Myanmar and Malaysia) were decidedly merchant capitalist in nature. That is, profit based on the establishment of privately-financed plantations specializing in the production of tropical and subtropical agricultural products (such as tea, coffee, sugar, rubber and spices) was more important than the expansion of empire. After politically securing a colonial area, private companies typically established plantations in interior areas and warehousing and port facilities on the coast, often at the mouth of a major river. These port cities, which existed prior to European colonialism, came to be "remade" into European colonial outposts with distinctive European urban landscape features. Such features included European architectural styles employed in the construction of public buildings and the dwellings of European plantation managers, retail services catering to a European clientele, and European schools and churches.

Residential Segregation Based on Income and Class   As is the case in most urban centers around the world, South Asian and Southeast Asian urban residential sectors reflect differences in income and class. Colonial port cities (such as Mumbai and Calcutta in India and Hanoi, Vietnam) are usually characterized by three distinct types of residential zones: 1) an elite, European sector surrounding old warehousing facilities near port zones where European colonial managers and civil servants lived, worked, shopped and sent their children to school; 2) a sector of low-income housing also near historical port and warehousing zones numerically dominated by lower and middle class workers; and 3) a sector on the outskirts of cities dominated by low-income landless families. These sectors, called shantytowns, resemble the squatter belts that can be found on the outskirts of many Latin American cities and like squatter belts lack basic services such as running water, public sewage systems and electricity.

Cities are strictly organized into separate zones and neighborhoods. An understanding of the part transportation nodes have played in the historical development of urban areas is a fun study for developing a strategy designed to reach these areas consisting of the majority of the world's population. Understanding the linguistic and ethnic associations of human activity enables us to respect and identify political leadership to further our ultimate aims of sharing our faith through service. Human geography is a subject "made to order" for the purpose of seizing the opportunities available to us to make eternal differences on this enchanted planet. Remember what Luke said in Chapter 12:48b: "For everyone to whom much is given, from him much will be required; and to whom much has been committed, of him they will ask the more." We have indeed been given much. Let us not cease giving thanks for the opportunity to have life and the myriad possibilities available to us to become busy serving God through humanity by cheerfully sharing our talents and faith today!

KEY TERMS TO KNOW

- Head of Navigation Site
- Central Place Theory
- Low-Range Goods
- High-Range Goods
- Low-Order Places
- High-Order Places
- World Cities
- Greenbelts
- Ethnic Enclaves
- Central Business District
- Suburbanization
- Zoning
- Gentrification
- Squatter Belts
- Shantytowns

STUDY QUESTIONS

1. Where are urban populations growing most rapidly in the world today? What are some of the challenges these areas face as a result of high rates of urban growth?

_____

_____

_____

_____

_____

_____

_____

_____

2. Compare and contrast urban landscapes in the core with those in the semi-periphery and periphery of the world-economy. What characteristics distinguish urban landscapes in each region?

_____

_____

_____

_____

_____

_____

_____

_____

FURTHER READING

Mark Abrahamson, *Global Cities* (Oxford: Oxford University Press, 2004).

Robert Bruegmann, *Sprawl: A Compact History* (Chicago: University of Chicago Press, 2006).

Stanley Brunn, Maureen Hays-Mitchell, and Donald Zeigler, eds., *Cities of the World: World Regional Urban Development*, 4th ed. (New York: Rowman & Littlefield, 2008).

Joel Garreau, *Edge City: Life on the New Frontier* (New York: Anchor, 1992).

Alan Gilbert, *The Mega-City in Latin America* (New York: United Nations University Press, 1996).

Susan Hanson and Genevieve Giuliano, eds., *The Geography of Urban Transportation*, 3rd ed. (New York: Guilford Press, 2004).

R. J. Johnston, *City and Society: An Outline for Urban Geography* (New York: Routledge, 2007).

Yeong-Hyun Kim and John Rennie Short, *Cities and Economies* (New York: Routledge, 2008).

Paul Knox and Steven Pinch, *Urban Social Geography: An Introduction*, 6th ed. (New York: Prentice-Hall, 2009).

Joel Kotkin, *The City: A Global History* (New York: Modern Library, 2006).

James Howard Kunstler, *The Geography of Nowhere: The Rise and Decline of America's Man-Made Landscape* (Washington: Free Press, 1994).

Robert Neuwirth, *Shadow Cities: A Billion Squatters, a New Urban World* (New York: Routledge, 2006).

Lewis Mumford, *The City in History: Its Origins, Its Transformations, and Its Prospects* (New York: Mariner Books, 1968).

David Smith, *Third World Cities in Global Perspective: The Political Economy of Uneven Urbanization* (Boulder: Westview Press, 1996).

Glossary

adiabatic lapse rate—The loss of energy in the atmosphere as a function of elevation.

AIDS—Acquired immune deficiency syndrome. A deadly disease due to viral infection.

attenuated—An extended or "long" bordered state. An example is Chile.

atmospheric flows—Directed wind or ocean currents.

autocracy—A government where an individual has total power.

Barbadian Slave Code—The legal basis in English law, which ensured perpetual (permanent) slavery until abolished in 1833 throughout the British Empire in large measure due to the work of Christian activists.

bellicosity—The act of being war-like or threateningly hostile.

capital—Any city exercising political authority and hegemony or control over the surrounding areas within a state.

capitalism—An economic system whereby the means of production or ownership of wealth is controlled by private individuals.

caste system—A system of hereditary social status in India and associated with Hinduism.

centrifugal—Cultural forces that act to pull people apart.

centripetal—Cultural forces acting to pull people together.

counter movement—A movement of people usually in a direction opposite of an earlier movement due to related circumstances.

cultural diffusion—The spreading of a way of life generally considered to be in any direction from a cultural hearth.

cultural hearth—The origin of a particular aspect of culture such as a cultural complex (graduation ceremony), ritual (marriage) or tradition (saying prayers at the dinner table).

culture—How humans live, work, worship and act. The transmission of culture from one generation to another is education. The development of culture, its diffusion and the display of rituals and complexes are often survival mechanisms developed to meet the challenges of the physical environment.

curse of South America—Term used to describe the difficulties of establishing networks due to the challenges of physical geography and landforms.

deciduous—Refers to forests where trees generally lose their leaves in fall.

democracy—A system of government where sovereignty rests ultimately with the people.

developing economy—The creation of wealth generally by harvesting resources such as timber, coal or farming.

diaspora—The historical term used to describe the dispersal of the Jewish people from their homeland by the Babylonians.

drawn borders—Artificially constructed lines drawn on maps typically reflective of the western imperial powers after the age of exploration and reflects their attempts to organize and administratively control territory.

dredge—A verb that describes an attempt to channel or deepen a waterway to aid navigation and transport.

epidemic—A disease spreading or diffusing within a region.

escarpments—High-walled canyons often the result of tectonic activity.

failed state—A former nation-state unable to control a portion of its own territory.

feudalism—A political system whereby loyalty is rewarded by the dispensing of land for a fee or an oath of loyalty.

forward capital—A capital city located in an area to encourage movement of people into the area for the purpose of solidifying control.

gateway city—Cities located near rivers allowing access to the oceans. Particularly important during the age of sail.

GNP—Gross national product. The total value of goods and services within a state.

holocaust—A policy used to exterminate a particular people group.

hydroelectric power—The use of flowing water to create electric power.

hydrography—The study of surface waters on the surface of the Earth.

industry—The production of goods or services within an area.

insurgency—A rebellious attempt to gain power over a formally recognized authority.

kudzu—A naturalized species of East Asian legume that is a vine.

leeward—The side of a topographic feature such as a hill or mountain opposite of the direction of prevailing winds or currents where air tends to draw moisture from or dry as a result of a rain shadow effect.

leaching—The phenomenon attributed to heavy rains drawing soil components deeper into the Earth. Particularly important in tropical wet climates where heavy rainfall and slash and burn agricultural techniques can create conditions catastrophic for plant growth.

nationalization—The act of causing ownership to be public property.

natural borders—Areas of the Earth's surface that tend to isolate or act as barriers to the exchange of culture and movement. Usually associated with the border of a state.

networks—A group of interconnecting transportation or communications centers, for example, a radio antenna and a radio receiver in your car. That exchange of information would be an example in communications. Parking your car and getting on a train would be a transportation network.

orographic effect—The tendency for energy to be released at higher elevations where the result is often precipitation such as snow or rain on the side of a mountain facing the oncoming front or current.

pandemic—A disease that spreads from one region to another.

periphery—The parts of the world with less developed economies and less technology than the more industrial or core regions of the world.

permafrost—Soils frozen for indeterminate amounts of time in the arctic and sub-arctic climates (see introduction).

plaza—A public square prominently placed in an urban center.

population pyramid—A schematic diagram used to demonstrate the age of a population by using the total numbers of population on an x-axis while demonstrating the numbers of male and females which are placed in an ascending pattern on the y-axis usually in five year increments.

prairie—Generally shorter grasslands denoting increasing aridity or dryness. Typical of a semi-arid climate such as the southern plains of North America where few if any trees exist.

region—An area of similarity from the standpoint of physical geography or in terms of culture.

shantytown—A generally impoverished area denoted by temporary or expedient structures outside of the cities in most peripheral nations.

slavocracy—A view held in the early to mid 1800's that held to the belief that the slave states of the south would continue to grow in influence into the Caribbean and Middle America with resulting power to slave owners.

smelting—An industrial process whereby metal is derived from ore.

specie—Coinage used as a medium of exchange or money.

tectonic activity—The energy resulting in changes to the Earth's surface as a result of tectonic or plate dynamics.

windward—The side of a hill or mountain facing the oncoming prevailing wind or current and generally moister as a result of adiabatic lapse rates resulting in precipitation.

Political Map of the World, August 2013

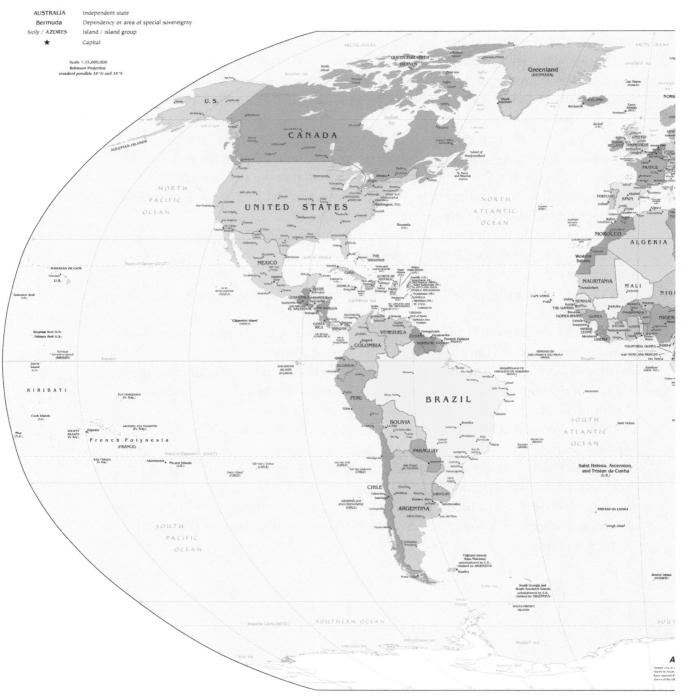

Map Source: *The World Factbook*

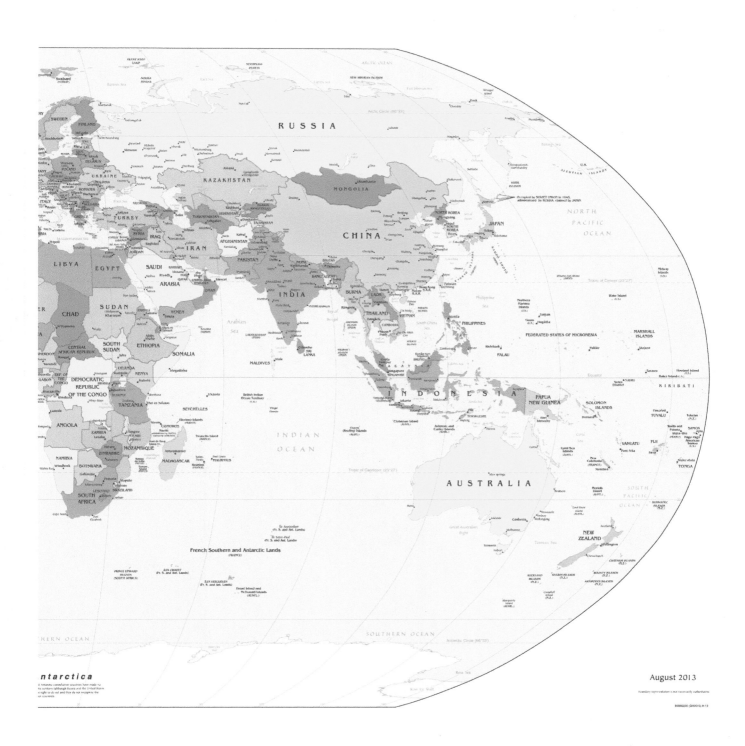

RUSSIA

SWEDEN
FINLAND

KAZAKHSTAN

MONGOLIA

UKRAINE

TURKEY

CHINA

IRAN
AFGHANISTAN

NORTH
KOREA

JAPAN

ITALY

IRAQ
JORDAN

PAKISTAN

NORTH
PACIFIC
OCEAN

LIBYA

EGYPT

SAUDI
ARABIA

INDIA

BURMA
LAOS

YEMEN

OMAN

THAILAND
CAMBODIA

PHILIPPINES

SUDAN

CHAD

ETHIOPIA

SRI
LANKA

MALDIVES

FEDERATED STATES OF MICRONESIA

MARSHALL
ISLANDS

PALAU

CENTRAL
AFRICAN REPUBLIC

SOUTH
SUDAN

SOMALIA

UGANDA
KENYA

DEMOCRATIC
REPUBLIC
OF THE CONGO

British Indian
Ocean Territory

INDONESIA

PAPUA
NEW GUINEA

KIRIBATI

ANGOLA

TANZANIA

SEYCHELLES

SOLOMON
ISLANDS

TUVALU

ZAMBIA

INDIAN
OCEAN

VANUATU

FIJI

NAMIBIA

ZIMBABWE

MOZAMBIQUE

TONGA

BOTSWANA

MADAGASCAR

AUSTRALIA

SOUTH
AFRICA

LESOTHO
SWAZILAND

SOUTH
PACIFIC
OCEAN

French Southern and Antarctic Lands
(FRANCE)

NEW
ZEALAND

SOUTHERN OCEAN

SOUTHERN OCEAN

August 2013